AF606307

SURPLUS - 2
LIBRARY OF CONGRESS
DUPLICATE

Principles of Pediatrics

Series on Nursing

Other titles in this series:

Fundamentals of Social and Preventive Medicine by B. A. Smithurst
Principles and Practice of Nursing by M. D. Emerton

Principles of Pediatrics

G. M. Maxwell
Professor of Pediatrics, University of Adelaide

University of Queensland Press

Typeset by Academy Press Pty. Ltd., Brisbane
Printed and bound in Hong Kong

Distributed in the United Kingdom, Europe, the Middle East, Africa, and the Caribbean by Prentice-Hall International, International Book Distributors Ltd., 66 Wood Lane End, Hemel Hempstead, Herts., England

National Library of Australia
Cataloguing-in-publication data

Maxwell, George Morrison.
Principles of pediatrics.

Index.
Bibliography.
ISBN 0 7022 1412 4.
ISBN 0 7022 1413 2 Paperback.

1. Pediatrics. I. Title.

618.92

Contents

Illustrations

Tables

1 Normal growth and development

In general, *growth* may be defined as an increase in physical size of a part, or the whole, of the child's body. *Development* generally refers to the orderly acquisition of skills and complex functions related to muscular usage, dexterity, and the application of intellectual ability in the child's social context.

It is important to know about growth and development. Firstly, there is much *normal* variation which can be misinterpreted as disease. Secondly, disturbances in growth and development may be early indications of disease in the child.

FACTORS INFLUENCING GROWTH

The main factors are *genetic* and *environmental*. Clearly the genes of the parents will to some extent influence the progeny both in the ultimate size reached and the rate at which this size is attained. Genetic constitution explains the common observation that an individual child tends to resemble the parents in size, and that this resemblance extends to children of the same parents. Since the chromosomes are the agents of genetic transmission (see p. 113), the chromosomal disorders will be associated with growth disturbance. Thus, in mongolism (Down's syndrome), a disorder of the autosome, growth retardation is common; the same holds in disorders of the sex chromosomes, e.g., Turner's syndrome.

Environmental Influences

The major ones are related to the supply of food, and to diseases in the child. On a world scale, it is likely that inadequate nutrition is the major cause of impaired growth. In many affluent societies, however, disease in the child is more important. These disorders may be of single system, e.g., heart or kidney disease, which, however, affect the growth of the body as a whole. Other disease may impair the body's ability to absorb or use food, causing secondary malnutrition and growth failure. Severe generalized infections, especially of the newborn child, may cause growth failure.

GENERAL PATTERNS OF PHYSICAL GROWTH

Growth before birth. This is the stage at which human growth is greatest, both absolutely and in velocity. The major organ systems are present by the second month of gestation, and the remainder of the pregnancy is devoted to their growth and elaboration. This is the stage at which growth impairment by genetic influences is greatest. Diseases affecting the fetus come from the unaffected mother, and are mainly of viral type, although syphilis occasionally occurs. Prenatal malnutrition may result from maternal starvation or ill health, although the former is of less moment than might be imagined. The integrity of placental function is paramount, and disorders of this organ probably explain much growth impairment in neonates.

In practical terms, the fetus has some likelihood of surviving after the 28th week of pregnancy. Growth characteristics and assessments after this stage are then of greatest clinical import.

Growth after birth. Apart from the transient neonatal weight loss, growth in height and weight is very rapid in the first year of life, slowing down in the preschool and school periods, and accelerating again at the time of puberty. This pattern is shown in figure 1.

Head circumference also increases rapidly during the first year, but thereafter at a relatively slow rate until the age of 10-12 years, when adult measurements are reached. Chest circumference measurements have a similar pattern, with, however, a period of increase which continues to the end of adolescence.

Body proportions also undergo considerable change during the total period of growth. In simple terms, at birth the head and trunk are large, and the legs are short. After puberty, the legs are longer than the trunk. The general pattern of proportions at various ages is seen in figure 2.

Growth varies with the sex of the child. Thus, at birth and in early childhood, boys are longer and heavier than girls. This disparity decreases until, in the early school-age years, girls are on the average heavier than boys. Puberty begins earlier in girls than boys, so that they are the heavier and taller between the ages of 10 and 14 years. The situation reverses after puberty.

ASSESSMENT OF PHYSICAL GROWTH

It is essential to remember that although growth is orderly, it is also variable. Failure to appreciate the concept of normal variability can lead to difficulties—mainly in suspecting disease where none is present. Thus average figures for height and weight for any given age are useless, because they cannot encompass the concept of normal variability. The sources of comparison which are used are *percentile tables* (see figure 3) because these allow us to take in to account the

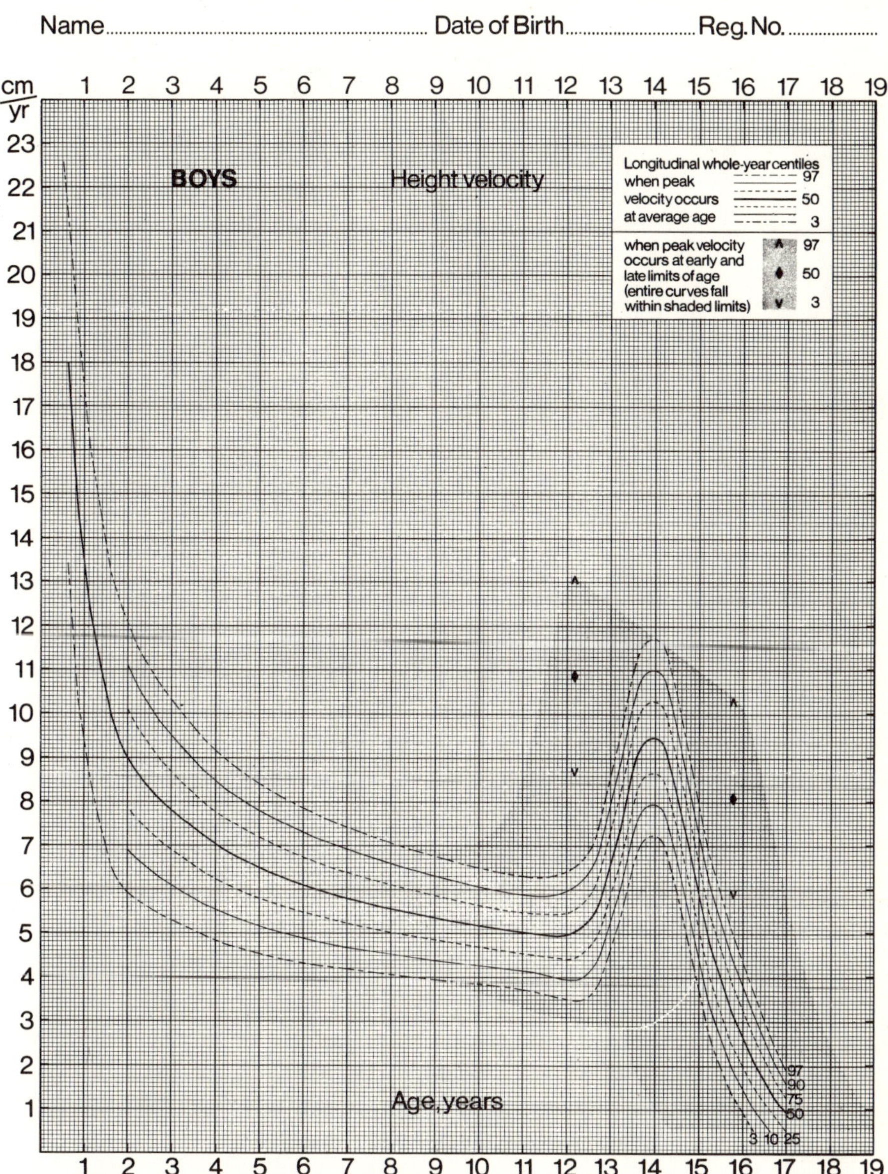

Fig. 1. Height velocity curve for boys. Reproduced with permission from Tanner, J. M. and Whitehouse, R. H., Archives of Disease in Childhood 51 (1976): 170 –79. Chart printed by Creaseys. Ltd., Castle Mead, Hertford, England.

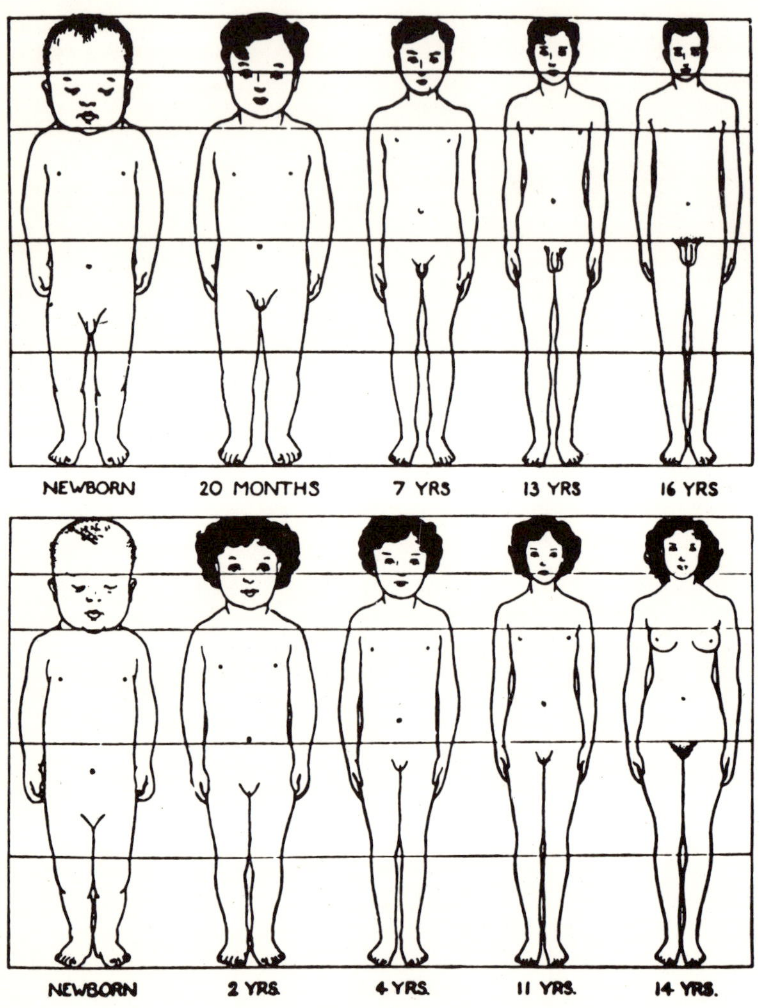

Fig. 2. Body proportions from birth to adolescence.

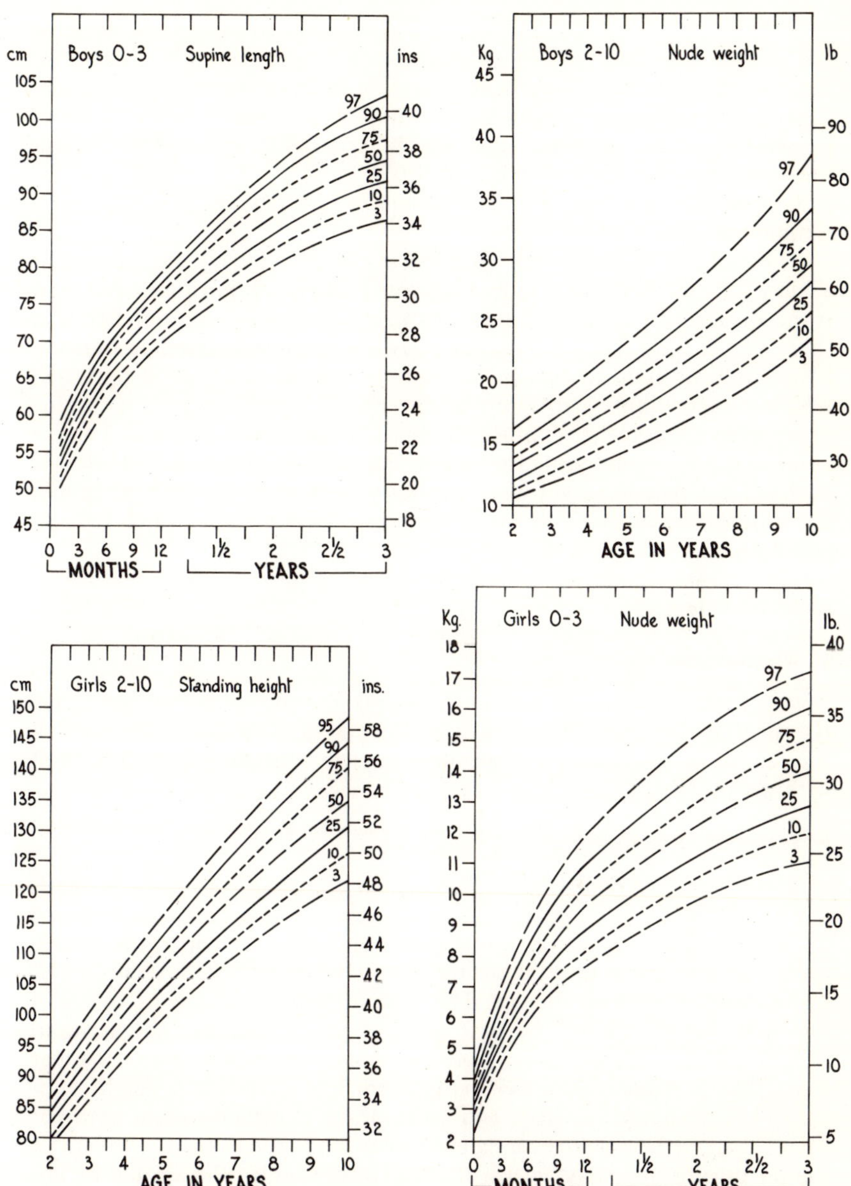

Fig. 3. Typical percentile charts, as used by Adelaide Children's Hospital: *a*, Supine length of boys 0–3; *b*, Nude weight of boys 2–10; *c*, Standing height of girls 2–10; *d*, Nude weight of girls 0–3.

variability in growth achievement. These tables are designed to show the percentage distribution of groups of heights, weights, or other measurements which have been found in a large normal population. Common experience would tell us that in any such group, a small number would be tall and a similar number small. The majority of people would be near the group mean. Small children then would be in the 3rd percentile, and very tall children in the 97th percentile for that particular age group.

Clinically, it is found that children at the extremes of the percentile scale (3rd and 97th) are somewhat more likely to be those who have some disease process. However, it must be emphasized that being in these percentile ranges is also perfectly compatible with being normal. Most children tend to run in the same percentile range for height *and* weight. Accordingly, "differential percentiles" may suggest some disorder even though the separate ratings are themselves normal. Thus, a child in the 97th percentile for height and the 25th percentile for weight perhaps has recent weight loss. Similarly, a child in the 97th percentile for weight and in the 25th for height, may have obesity which reflects some disease.

PRACTICALITIES

1. Prematurity

Assessment of maturity can be made by a suitable percentile table. Recall that it is essential to have a reasonably accurate assessment of the length of pregnancy to use these tables. This matter is also dealt with on p. 37.

2. Infancy, childhood, and adolescence

a. Height and weight. Standard percentile charts (as shown in figure 3) are available for the age groups to 18 years. These are usually based upon British or U.S. surveys. Interpolation within the percentile figures given for the first 3 months of life is somewhat difficult. Accordingly, some rough rules are in order. The normal infant will lose up to 5% of the birth weight during the first week of life. Thereafter the minimal weight gain is 125g per week and the maximum weight gain 250g per week. The average is 200g per week. If one knows the birth weight, subtracts the perinatal net loss, and adds on the expected weight gain per week, then, *within limits* an estimate can be arrived at for the baby's weight during the early weeks of life. These rough rules should be applied only to infants during the first 3 months of life. They are quite unreliable thereafter. Again, useful values for scanning populations are that the infant will double his birthweight during 5-6 months and treble it between 10 and 12 months. There is a good deal of variation in this and the observations should always be checked against percentile tables. These rough rules do not apply to premature infants for whom specific percentile tables should be used.

b. Head circumference. Suitable charts are available for head circumference. Two separate sets are normally used to distinguish the rates of head growth in premature and full term babies (fig. 4). Head circumference measurements tend to reach completion at about the age of 3 years, so such standards are only of value until this time. Again, the general principle is that representation in the low and very high percentiles may argue the presence of disease. Thus the child who has suffered brain damage at birth will tend to appear in the 3rd or lower percentiles for head circumference. Such an observation has useful prognostic value in so far as it implies that cerebral function will probably not ever be normal. On the other hand, children with hydrocephalus or subdural hematoma, or other disease states which tend to increase head circumference, may be found in the 97th percentile of the tables. A useful check of the head circumference is comparison with the measurement for chest circumference at the nipple level, and the crown-rump length. All 3 of these measurements commonly are the same until the age of about 9 months or so. If the child is very fat, the chest circumference may be rather unreliable as a mode of comparison, and in such a case, the crown-rump measurement is to be preferred.

The measurement of head circumference is of greatest moment in the first year. Again, in the absence of percentile tables, useful approximations are that the head circumference increases 1.2 cm a month in the first 4 months, and half of that (0.6 cm) in the next 8 months. Thus, if the newborn head is 35.5 cm in circumference at birth, it is 40.5 cm at 4 months and 47 cm at 1 year. Again these are approximations only.

c. Skeletal maturation. This is the assessment of bone age by x-ray of an appropriate area—commonly both wrists. The radiologist uses tables (some similar to the percentile type) to assess the age from the skeleton. Normally the bone age and the actual age differ by only a few months.

DENTITION

The age at which teeth appear is very variable, and the evaluation of dentition is not regarded as a pediatric routine. A rough guide to the order and age of appearance is shown in table 1.

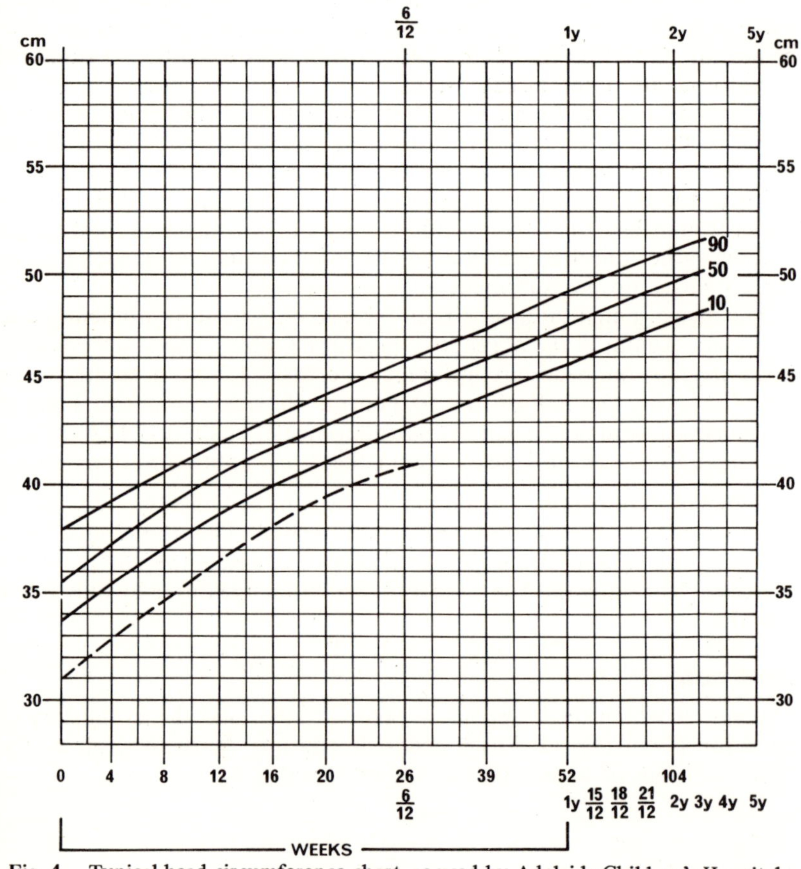

Fig. 4. Typical head circumference chart, as used by Adelaide Children's Hospital.

Table 1. Order and age of appearance of teeth

First Teeth	Age
1. Lower central incisors	5–10 months
2. Upper central and lateral incisors	7–12 months
3. Lower lateral incisors, upper front molars	12–15 months
4. Upper and lower canines	17–24 months
5. Upper and lower molars	24–30 months
Second Teeth	**Age**
1. First molars	5–7 years
2. Central incisors	6½–8 years
3. Lateral incisors	7–9½ years
4. First bicuspids	9–11 years
5. Second bicuspids	10–12 years
6. Canines	10–12 years
7. Cuspids	11–14 years
8. Second molars	11–14 years
9. Third molars	16–20+ years

MOTOR AND MENTAL DEVELOPMENT

The first year. These two are so closely allied at this time of life that they must be considered together. Testing of one (e.g., motor) usually implies some assessment of the other.

Until the second month of life, apparent emotional response is difficult to interpret. Crying is the response to many stimuli, such as hunger, cold, heat, intense light. These are essentially vegetative, and play a part in the infant's survival. The neonate has a less marked response to pain, and does not shed tears. He should not, however, be regarded as a mere bundle of reflexes, although these are clinically of some importance.

By 1 month, the infant can deliberately focus his eyes, and will watch a person. His cry shows some differentiation and will readily indicate hunger or discomfort. At 2 months, the eyes following moving objects, hearing is definitely present, and the infant smiles. Thereafter the infant's abilities progress rapidly. He will reach (and miss!) by 12 weeks, grasp with both hands by 6 months, at which time he can sit with support. At 7 months, the infant can roll over, and manual coordination allows passage of toys from hand to hand, and to the mouth. The infant now discovers the force of gravity—that toys fall from a height. A normal association is to force an onlooker to pick the toy up! At 10 months, he will stand if held, creeps, or hitches (moves on his buttocks) and most use a word meaningfully. He knows names that he has heard repeatedly.

There is little variation in the onset of these abilities in the early stages. Most infants smile between 6 and 8 weeks. By 9 months, however, there is much individual difference, so that one infant may take a step or two, another may just be attempting to crawl. Both are normal. The situation is summarized in figure 5.

The year-old child. Now a distinct personality, the yearling is locomotory, so that he can explore his environment—this is principally manual exploration, with perfection of fine finger movements. He will practise these to perfection, e.g., by putting a ball in and out of a box. Improved dexterity assists in self-feeding, although a spoon is inexpertly handled. Now he has an adult feeding pattern of 3 main meals a day. The emergence of a social conscience is revealed by his sensitivity to approval and otherwise. He may be shy of strangers, showing perhaps an early idea of the differentiation of society. Words and their meaning begin to have stronger association, although advance in vocabulary is relatively slow.

The toddler (2-3 years). The past months have been spent in practising and coordinating movements. Walking is nigh perfect and running usual. Falls are common, partly because of mechanical disadvantages (high centre of gravity), and lack of anticipation of irregularities and obstacles in his path. These difficulties iron themselves out with practice, and by the third birthday he goes up and down steps, and may tricycle with great ease.

By this time too, he is preferentially "handed"—right or left. He will proffer the appropriate limbs when being dressed, and can undress himself (pulling off shoes, socks, etc.) to some extent. He can hold and drink from a cup, and feed himself with some dexterity. This coordination is reflected in other directions—he can use a peg-board or "put the doll to bed".

Speech is fairly skilfully used by the third birthday—he can use short phrases (e.g., "I want milk") and will repeat a 6-syllable sentence. He knows his name and sex, and has a sense of personality. Now begins the self-analysis which will continue throughout his life. His memory begins to function and the toddler will recognize and enumerate familiar objects in a picture. Memory is still short-lived, however, and confusion over instructions is common. The toddler has no real conscience, and cannot be expected to retain any good intentions for more than a short time.

Socially the toddler is not advanced; he is more interested in things than in other children; having no sense of property, and being self-centred, he comes into more or less strife with his playmates. Crying is still his main mode of defence, although when thwarted, temper tantrums (screaming, kicking, and rolling on the floor, breath holding)

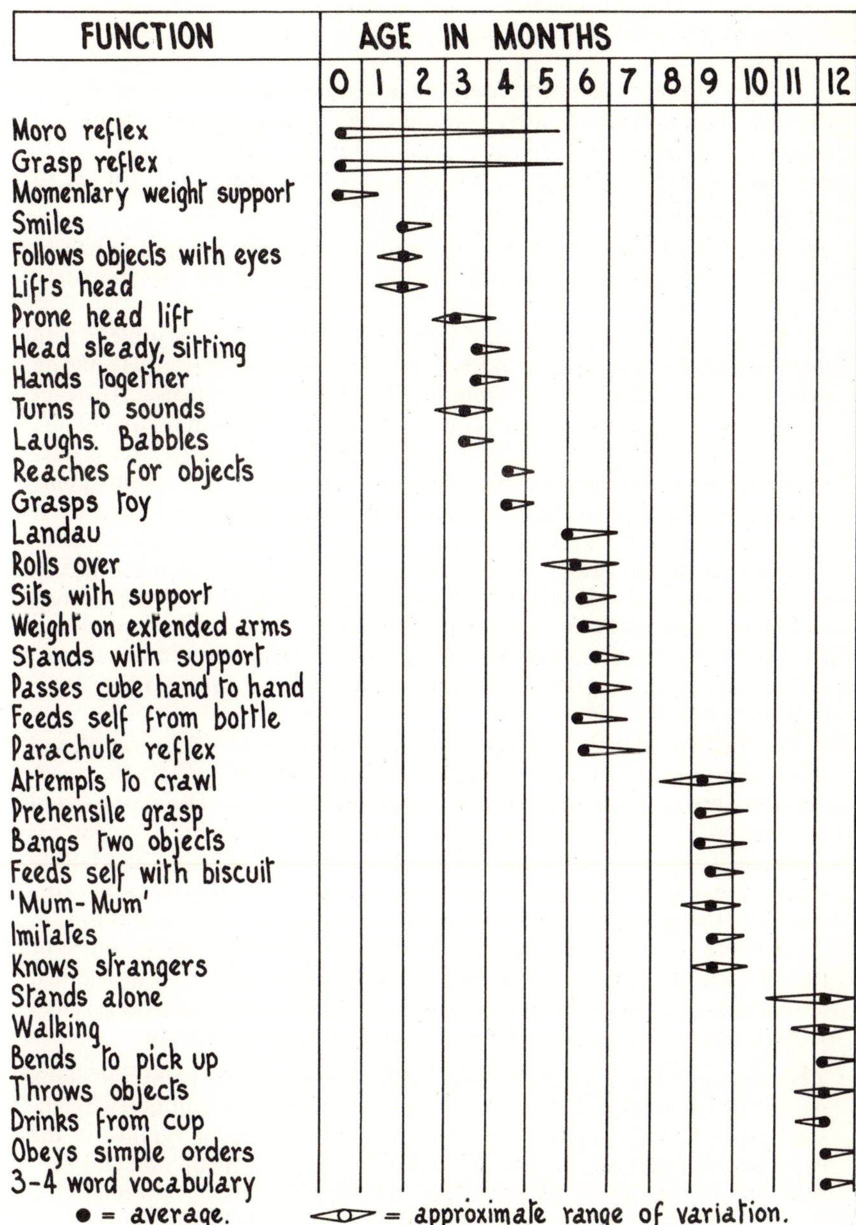

Fig. 5. Chart showing what infants are able to do at various ages.

are perfectly normal. The toddler often fears loud noises, strangers, and falling. Most other fears are inculcated into him by other children and his parents.

At some stage, the toddler will have acquired toilet training during the day. This is usually fairly complete by 2½ years, although diurnal dryness may be incomplete at 3 years. Many children are completely dry day and night by the third birthday, but "accidents" at night are so common as to be normal for a year after that.

The 6-year-old. This is the average age for school entry and indicates that the child can care for himself, and get along with his peers to some extent.

Manual dexterity now approaches adult levels and complete self-feeding and dressing are old skills. New skills have appeared. He has an extensive vocabulary, and combines complex sentences. Abstract thought is revealed in his language, as is a sense of time indicated by the use of the past, present, and future tenses. He lives, however, essentially in the present, and will not be tempted to work to any distant goal.

Socially the 6-year-old is mature, tantrums are unusual, and he is beginning to recognize that crying doesn't solve many problems. His protests are verbal rather than physical, and he can control his impulses in the absence of authority—but not for too long. Conscience is now well developed, and guilt can be an incubus. By this time he has special friends, and is practised in the gambits of flattery, bargaining, threat, and alliance in relation both to his parents and his coevals. He is equally drawn to either sex.

The insight of this age group is still incomplete. Thus radio and television are real to him, as may be stories. Insight rapidly increases and may be quite remarkable by the seventh birthday. The six-year-old has many fears—and will transmit them willingly to his younger associates. These commonly are of the dark, of solitude, fire, and bodily injury. He is a prey to insecurity at school, but familiarity rapidly exorcises his fears; over-compensation, as boasting, is not uncommon.

At some time during this sixth year, he will learn to read—more or less. The effort of identifying word patterns, however, militates against stimulation of ideas or imagination. This he still gets from visual stimuli—picture books, television—and from being read to.

The pre-adolescent (10-12 years). By this age, the child has long perfected his motor abilities, speech is complex and vocabulary extensive (circa 12,500 words). This vocabulary parallels his facility in the expression of experience. The narrative is a frequent form, and will contain all the elements of language. Reading is fluent, although the favourite literary form may be the comic strip. Ideational capacity is well formed and insight maturing. Ideas are best expressed verbally, fluency in writing is still incomplete—blurred perhaps by preoccupation with details such as spelling, punctuation, paragraphing and so on. The concept of number, which was primitive at entrance to school, is now well formed and the common procedures of arithmetic are understood and applied.

Socially there is now a deep rift between the sexes because of differences in pursuits, or the important necessity to conform. Group or gang activities—often physically rough—are typical, and good manners (in the parental sense) are at as much discount as tidiness.

The adolescent. Adolescence is very variable in its time of onset. Menstruation defines it in the female. In the male, the near-adult physique and well-defined secondary sexual characteristics are the definitive marks.

In either sex, difficulties of adaptation beset him. Thus being treated as a child at one time, and being expected to behave as an adult at another time will cause some inner confusion. Socially the adolescent more or less asserts his independence of parental control, but conforms strictly to the standards of his own age group—with whom he spends most of his time. At some time, although not necessarily parallel with the overt signs of maturity, strong heterosexual interests occur; coincidental is an interest in his appearance.

At all ages, it is important to realize the wide degree of normal variation. No book can give an appreciation of this. Simple study of normal children is essential to any understanding of this concept. Emotional development is chiefly dependent upon the pattern of the family; thus, for an individual child, any attempt to understand his emotional life must be based on a knowledge of the total family background, since each child has his personal relationship to his siblings and his parents.

INTELLECTUAL GROWTH

This has been partially considered in the previous section. It is, however, important to realize that there is a distinction between formal intelligence, or the ability to pass certain academic tests, and the contentional intelligence which reveals itself as common sense, shrewdness, and ease in social intercourse. Naturally the two are associated, as is memory, but a good memory does not spell a higher intelligence. The formal tests of intelligence give an indication only of the child's potential, and not of his performance. High performance is a synthesis of formal and contentional intelligence, application and memory. Equally, no child's formal intelligence can be more than roughly assessed by an educational survey. Formal learning patterns will vary within societies, and the same yard-stick must not be applied indiscriminately.

Assessment of mental development

In the first year of life, as has been noted, this is dependent upon observing that the child has acquired the appropriate motor skills, and that his head is growing satisfactorily. The ability to communicate, by speech or gesture, is an important measure of mental development, and so too is the ability to learn. The latter can be tested in many ways, usually by teaching a simple game such as pat-a-cake.

In the second year of life, speech extends, and games and occupations become more elaborate; a discussion with the mother and watching the child at play are good ways of seeing if the child is like his peers in achievement. A word of warning though—a sick, frightened, or lonely child will not perform to his best ability, and much care should be taken to see he is happy and comfortable before any test is applied.

Various questionnaires are available for assessing development. One is the Denver Developmental Screening Test (DDST) which standardizes the achievements likely to be present in various age groups. Such a test can readily be given by nurses. However, it is emphasized that this is a *screening* test, and not a final assessment of the child's ability. A list of achievements for a 3-4-year-old according to the DDST is shown in figure 6.

INTELLIGENCE

This may be imperfectly defined as the basic capacity to benefit from education. It includes the ability to use verbal syllogisms well, to abstract and classify and to see analogies. Accordingly, problem-solving ability is a feature of intelligence. It should be noted that a good intelligence is not a passport to a good education nor to a happy life. Both require emotional and social abilities which are not necessarily found in those with high intelligence.

Intelligence testing

All intelligence tests are comparative, that is they do not give us an answer in completely measurable terms, but only in terms of the behaviour of an individual child as against many thousands of others of approximately the same age. All intelligence tests reflect the culture of those who construct them. Therefore it is not reasonable to apply tests designed for one culture in another. A simple analogy would be that Neolithic hunting men would fare badly in modern English I.Q. studies—but a highly intelligent Australian might fail to survive in a Neolithic culture. Most intelligence tests have a high verbal content, therefore they cannot be applied to a mute child, or in children where a language barrier exists. However, when properly applied, intelligence tests can be reasonable predictions of educational performance—

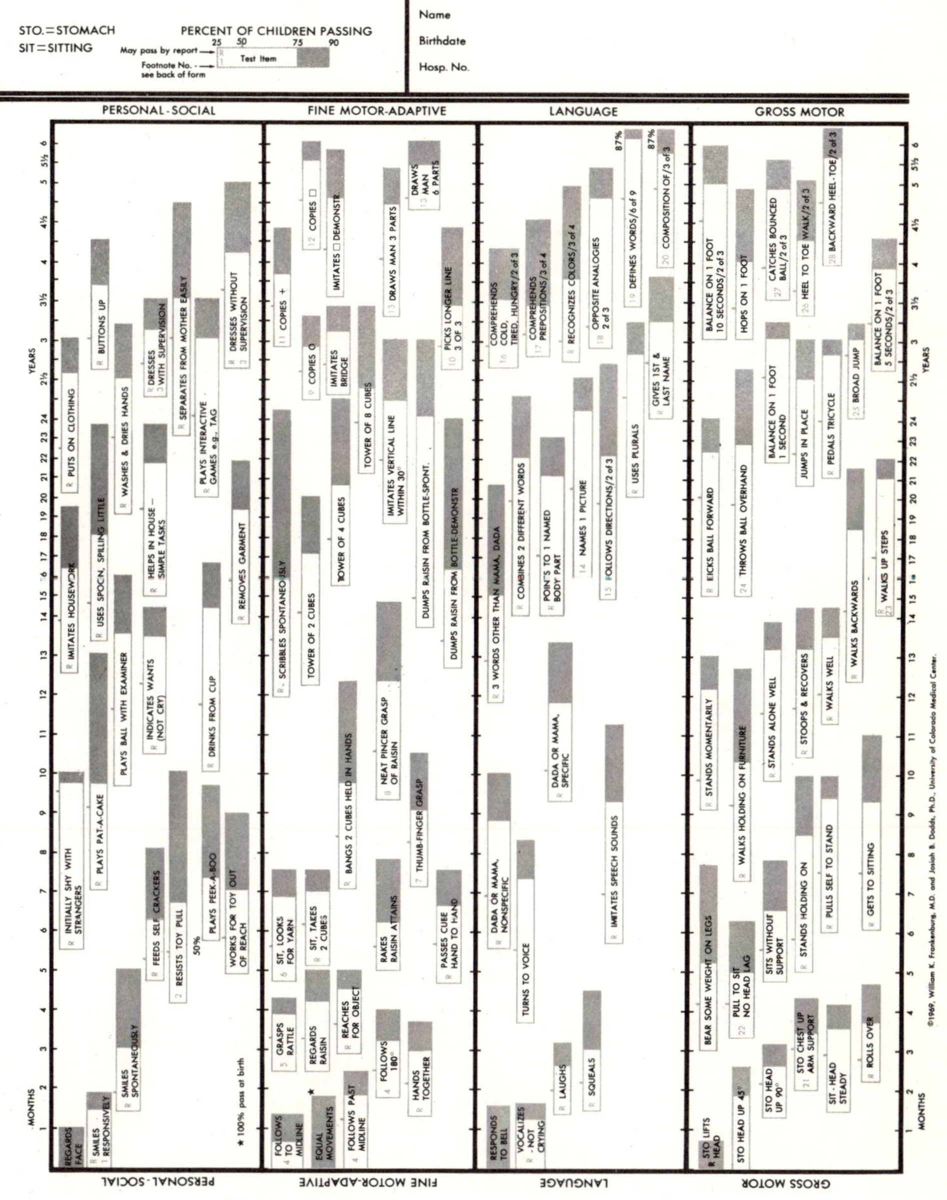

Fig. 6. Denver Developmental Screening Test.

1. Try to get child to smile by smiling, talking or waving to him. Do not touch him.
2. When child is playing with toy, pull it away from him. Pass if he resists.
3. Child does not have to be able to tie shoes or button in the back.
4. Move yarn slowly in an arc from one side to the other, about 6" above child's face. Pass if eyes follow 90° to midline. (Past midline; 180°)
5. Pass if child grasps rattle when it is touched to the backs or tips of fingers.
6. Pass if child continues to look where yarn disappeared or tries to see where it went. Yarn should be dropped quickly from sight from tester's hand without arm movement.
7. Pass if child picks up raisin with any part of thumb and a finger.
8. Pass if child picks up raisin with the ends of thumb and index finger using an over hand approach.

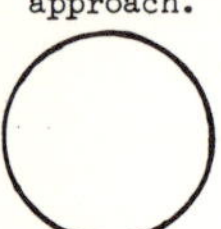

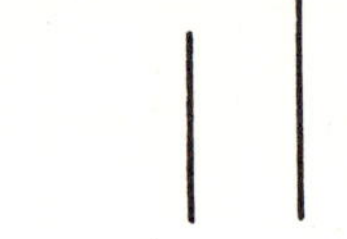

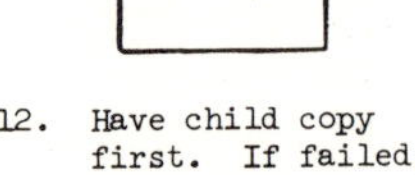

9. Pass any enclosed form. Fail continuous round motions.

10. Which line is longer? (Not bigger.) Turn paper upside down and repeat. (3/3 or 5/6)

11. Pass any crossing lines.

12. Have child copy first. If failed, demonstrate

When giving items 9, 11 and 12, do not name the forms. Do not demonstrate 9 and 11.

13. When scoring, each pair (2 arms, 2 legs, etc.) counts as one part.
14. Point to picture and have child name it. (No credit is given for sounds only.)

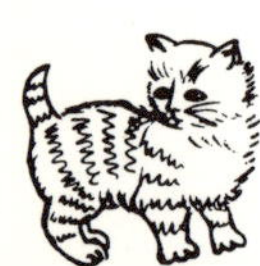

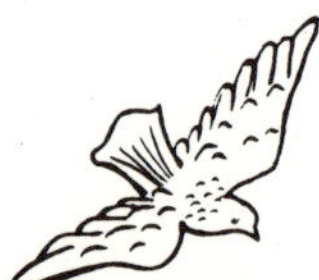

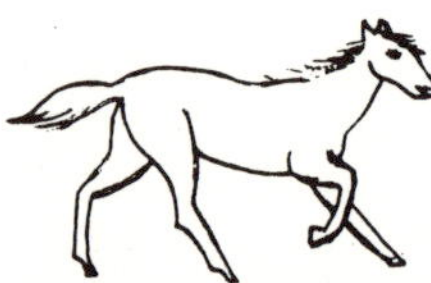

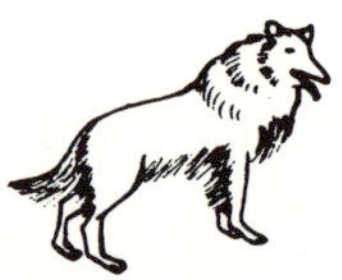

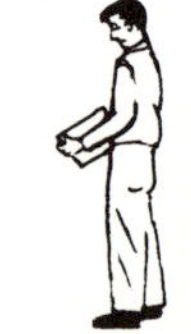

15. Tell child to: Give block to Mommie; put block on table; put block on floor. Pass 2 of 3. (Do not help child by pointing, moving head or eyes.)
16. Ask child: What do you do when you are cold? ..hungry? ..tired? Pass 2 of 3.
17. Tell child to: Put block <u>on</u> table; <u>under</u> table; <u>in front</u> of chair, <u>behind</u> chair. Pass 3 of 4. (Do not help child by pointing, moving head or eyes.)
18. Ask child: If fire is hot, ice is ?; Mother is a woman, Dad is a ?; a horse is big, a mouse is ?. Pass 2 of 3.
19. Ask child: What is a ball? ..lake? ..desk? ..house? ..banana? ..curtain? ..ceiling? ..hedge? ..pavement? Pass if defined in terms of use, shape, what it is made of or general category (such as banana is fruit, not just yellow). Pass 6 of 9.
20. Ask child: What is a spoon made of? ..a shoe made of? ..a door made of? (No other objects may be substituted.) Pass 3 of 3.
21. When placed on stomach, child lifts chest off table with support of forearms and/or hands.
22. When child is on back, grasp his hands and pull him to sitting. Pass if head does not hang back.
23. Child may use wall or rail only, not person. May not crawl.
24. Child must throw ball overhand 3 feet to within arm's reach of tester.
25. Child must perform standing broad jump over width of test sheet. (8-1/2 inches)
26. Tell child to walk forward, heel within 1 inch of toe. Tester may demonstrate. Child must walk 4 consecutive steps, 2 out of 3 trials.
27. Bounce ball to child who should stand 3 feet away from tester. Child must catch ball with hands, not arms, 2 out of 3 trials.
28. Tell child to walk backward, toe within 1 inch of heel. Tester may demonstrate. Child must walk 4 consecutive steps, 2 out of 3 trials.

<u>DATE AND BEHAVIORAL OBSERVATIONS</u> (how child feels at time of test, relation to tester, attention span, verbal behavior, self-confidence, etc,):

mainly in the direction of response to secondary and tertiary education. Again, it must be emphasized that such tests are given only by skilled persons in circumstances which allow the child to perform to his utmost. A typical modern test is the Stanford-Binet scale or the Wechsler intelligence scale for children (WISC). These, and other methods, give a result which is called the Intelligence Quotient (I.Q.). Essentially the test gives a score which approximates to a mental age. When this is divided by the child's actual age and multiplied by 100, the I.Q. is the result. If done repeatedly, and in good circumstances, the I.Q. has value in prognosticating performance—especially if it is low. In terms of subnormality, the WHO classifies I.Q. 0-19 as severe, I.Q. 20-49 as moderate, and I.Q. 50-69 as mild. Except in the lowest levels, there is no absolute relationship between I.Q. and the ability to attain simple skills and social abilities e.g., dressing oneself, toilet training.

For children under the age of 2 years, the infant Cattell test and the Gesell behavioural tests are used. The latter can be used to give a score which is called the Development Quotient (D.Q.). It should be realized that such studies can only be regarded as approximations, and in general terms, the younger the patient, the less reliable the result. Such tests must be applied by experienced clinical psychologists, and usually on more than one occasion. Both D.Q. and I.Q. are only part of the examination of the child's ability, the pediatrician's responsibility is to incorporate them with all of the other evidence, and to synthesize this into a judgment.

SOCIAL DEVELOPMENT

Man becomes a social animal when he recognizes his responsibilities to, and his place in, a group of other humans. His responsibilities to the group will be a balance between what the individual is willing to give the group (as opposed to the family), and what the group demands of him. His place in the group recognizes the balance between what the *group* believes the individual is worth to the group, and what the individual believes *he* is worth (in his own terms) to the group. Now, read all that again, because the social development of the child is determined by what is stated. Eventually the child has to fit in with other people in a way which satisfies them, and which satisfies him too. This is a very complex matter, the more so since the rules are largely unwritten, and change often, and without much warning. Social development is the process of learning the rules, interpreting their change, and winning the chess game between yourself and several other intelligent, and possibly hostile, humans, or, to put it more simply, to bridge the gap between helpless infancy and successful adulthood.

In most societies, social education, and hence development, begins in the family. At first the relationship is entirely between the infant and the mother; the infant learns that crying in a certain way produces food, he begins to recognize when his mother is pleased with him, is stimulated to find pleasure in this himself, and so the cycle of response to another person begins. This is the earliest form of social response and the model for all which eventuates. Into the infant's life now comes another person—the father, who becomes recognizably different. He may not supply food, his voice is different, he is less regular in his attendance, he smells differently, and he has hair on his face. Not only this, but eventually a father is treated differently, and he treats his child differently. But fathers bring pleasure in their own way, and are accepted by the child. Not so strangers—they are quite unrecognizable, and the objects of fear—and the response is a frightened cry, due to an innate sense of caution. Soon the social circle widens, and siblings come into it. The child soon recognizes them as rivals for affection and other favours. To obtain affection (which gives him pleasure) he has several options. The most primitive, and therefore found in young children, is demand—fortified by crying. But this does not always work, and he learns through his siblings (or if a singleton, learns by experience), that ingratiation can work just as well. Ingratiation, simply defined, is the dog who carries the walking stick and wags his tail when he wants a walk—noisy barking doesn't always work!

But now the child can crawl or walk—and explore. He meets the problems of "don't do that—it's bad", and he learns the first painful lesson of conformity, and it is a lesson which is often repeated. Then he meets the tabu—"don't do that" ... "why not?" ... "because I say so", or, "it isn't done in our family". The tabu is a social concept which is often illogical, often archaic, and frequently used by parents because the same tabu was given to them. The initial response to a tabu is defiance; this may be followed by punishment. In most instances the tabu is then obeyed, but its essential illogicality is recognized, and defiance may appear at a later time.

By the age of 2 years, the child communicates well and in most circumstances meets children outside his own family. This poses a new set of problems. Are they equals? Are they superiors? Do I treat them as I do my parents?, and so on, and he has to solve these problems, not only for his own satisfaction, but to meet the approval of his own parents. The child finds too that the group is different from the sum of the individuals within it—that to pee in the centre of the group evokes jeers, whereas to retreat into the bushes with another child is entirely acceptable—or at least it may be during that session of kindergarten. And so to school. Here the children are all of his own age—undiluted by older or younger and without the precious relationship which is called a brother or sister. The class is dominated by a figure of supervision—the teacher—who can punish and praise or define deficiences to the whole group. Now the child has to learn that he has lost his freedom, no longer can he wander about freely, talk when he likes, or go to the toilet immediately he feels the need. To do any of these things will interfere with what is called "education". If he is lucky he has learned the word at home, associates it with some pleasure and the likelihood of being "grown-up", and bends to the situation. Eventually he may find pleasure in his group, assesses its power, and gains satisfaction from its secrets and its growing ability to manipulate the petty events at school. Here he will consolidate—if he has it—his own quality of leadership—the ability to manipulate people and events for good or ill. At least he will see leaders, and assess the techniques which they use—appeal to "tabu" and prejudice, the influencing of subdivisions of the group, threats and intimidation, and excommunication (sending to "Coventry"). Some of this he will report at home—to his surprise he finds that his mother and father may differ on what is good and bad in what he tells them. If he is a boy he finds he is supposed to react differently from his sister—as if he hadn't learned that lesson long ago. On Sunday he goes to another school—Sunday School. Here is a different set of values, and not very measurable either. You can't see them, or hear much about them. You must take them on trust, and soon you learn that these values don't equate with what your parents do, or what goes on at week-day school, so you wonder about it, and realize that there are Sunday values and Monday values, and that Sunday values are principally the old tabus of an earlier time. In all the thinking about these things, the child begins to develop his own ideas—and to modify them after discussion with his friends. But these are now the ideas of a different generation from his parents, and his own ideas about himself and his group begin to determine his ambitions. Because the ideas are different, the ambitions may be different. And now begins another confrontation—and a prolonged one—the confrontation with parents. This is no new thing, the child has been doing it for some years now, but he has a healthy respect for his father and mother, and does not lightly gainsay them. But he continues to try his power and finds a gambit or two which are effective. He gains prowess in argument; his differences with his parents are complicated by the satisfaction with his peers. He is in fact preparing to leave home, but he must shadow-box a few years more—sufficient time to acquire the skills which he now knows are necessary for him. Some of these skills are beyond him. He has to learn the truth of this, and learn to make the truth acceptable to himself. The process is called rationalization and is usually painful. He becomes pubertal, fantasizes his sexual needs, and then, tentatively, takes steps to realize them. And another set of tabus rears up, and are less able to be borne in view of the strength of his sexual drive. He hears nothing of how his mother and father dealt with this problem—

presumably they were different—at least this is how it seems in view of their unwarranted suspicion! His values and their values seem poles apart—they will not see that they are sounding boards for him, and he cannot see that age and exhaustion are impairing their abilities to tolerate him. If he conforms to most of the parental ideas—especially those of educational success—then flying the coop is easy; if he doesn't, then it is wounding to child and parents—and the wounds take a long time to heal.

This is the biography of everyman. Social development will be impaired in infancy if the baby has no mother or is separated from her for a long time. Similarly, although less importantly, the father contributes to the child's social development. After infancy, the child must be recruited into the force which the group (society) has agreed is most valuable to it. For most children this means school. Successful conformity and a modest degree of academic success are reasonable measures of the child's ability to achieve successful social development. Adolescence is a difficult time for parents and child; rebellion is normal and rational. If separation from the parents is achieved with at least continuing communication, then a reasonable degree of adult social development has been achieved.

Measurement of social development

This is largely a subjective measurement by the examiner and related to the common standards of the society at the time of assessment. Thus, in young children, unwarranted fear of strangers, solitariness, and agressive unfriendly behaviour *may* be considered abnormal. So too is stealing, although young children have little or no sense of property. In the school-age years, solitariness, failure to cooperate with teachers, thieving, cruelty, and the premature seeking of sexual experience are also looked upon with disfavour. At a later stage, drunkenness, drug addiction, theft, cruelty, arson, and perversions have the same connotation—at least in society's mind. At another time, in another generation, all of these may have been regarded with equanimity, although it is usually forgotten that modern behaviour would, in another context, have seemed violently antisocial. The values and beliefs of the parents should always be assessed when social development is being considered. Parents are strong mentors and, although they may appear to wish to inculcate a different mode of behaviour, it is likely that their own true code will be reflected in their children.

2 The newborn

PHYSIOLOGY

The unborn baby is supported by the placenta, so that his lungs are without function; his central circulation (see figure 7) is of the *fetal* type, i.e., the oxygenated placental blood traverses the right atrium and enters the left atrium through the foramen ovale and hence to the left ventricle, aorta, and body. The blood which enters the right ventricle and the first part of the pulmonary artery is shunted off to the aorta by way of the ductus arteriosus. The direction of blood flow in the fetal circulation is determined by the resistance to it. Thus flow is directed *away* from areas of high resistance such as the unexpanded lungs, and this is useful and economical before birth. As soon as the first cry is taken, the lungs expand, and their vessel resistance falls greatly. The blood which previously was completely shunted to the aorta now traverses the lungs, to be saturated with oxygen. Simultaneously, the pressure falls in the right ventricle and atrium, so that the pressure level in the left atrium is able to close the flap valve of the foramen ovale. The ductus arteriosus does not immediately close, but the direction of the shunt through it is reversed since the pressure in the aorta is now higher than that in the pulmonary artery. This is known as the *transitional* circulation (fig. 8). Once the ductus arteriosus has closed—and this may take up to 6 weeks—the adult type circulation is present.

INITIATION OF RESPIRATION

Nervous impulses, sent out from the respiratory centre in the brain stem, are intended to stimulate the muscles of breathing. The impulses occur before birth, but are weak until the moment of birth when the baby's face and body receive sensory stimuli; these are sent to the brain, and enhance the output from the respiratory centre. The first effective breath is the *first gasp*, followed by deeper gasps which culminate in regular breathing. At this stage the alveoli are fully expanded and receive an adequate blood supply, so that oxygen can be supplied to the tissues, carbon dioxide be removed from them, and acid base balance be maintained.

Abnormalities of respiration are most likely to occur in prematures especially when the mother receives drugs depressant to the baby's

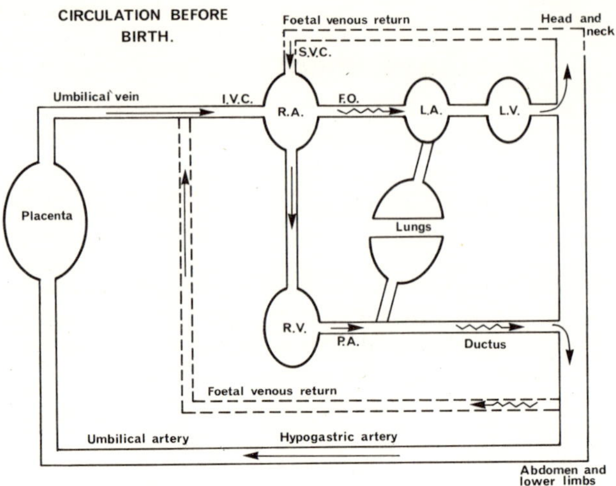

Fig. 7. Circulation before birth. R.A. = right atrium. L.A. = left atrium. L.V. = left ventricle. R.V. = right ventricle. P.A. = pulmonary artery. I.V.C. = inferior vena cava. F.O. = foramen ovale.

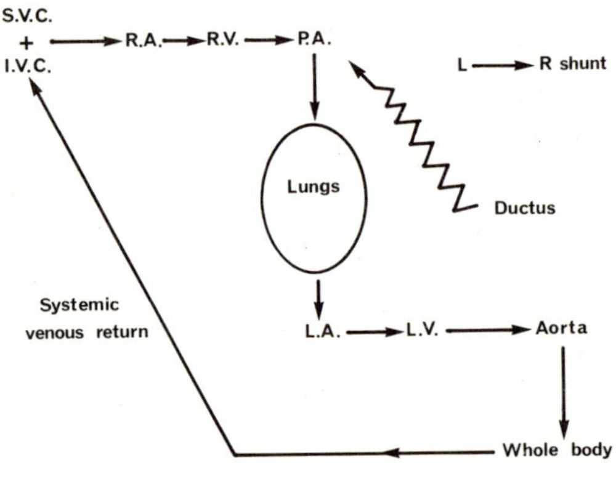

Fig. 8. Transitional circulation. R. A. = right atrium. L.A. = left atrium. L.V. = left ventricle. R.V. = right ventricle. P.A. = pulmonary artery. I.V.C. = inferior vena cava. F. O. = foramen ovale.

respiratory centre, or when the health of the unborn babe has been affected by maternal disorder (e.g., hypertension), or when the placental blood supply has been reduced, as in antepartum hemorrhage. In either case, the infant may never initiate the first gasps or if it does so, does not establish regular breathing, but remains at the gasping stage; when this happens, the resistance in the lungs does not fall, the circulation remains of the fetal type (fig. 7) and neither ventilation of the lungs nor blood flow through them (perfusion) is normal. The venous blood cannot then be arterialized—attain more oxygen partial pressure (pO_2) values, or act as a buffer or transport mechanism for maintenance of normal acid/base values. Continuance of this state of *asphyxia* leads to a reduction in blood volume and cardiac output, which further increases the difficulty of taking oxygen to the tissues.

ENERGY SOURCES IN THE BABY

These are mainly carbohydrate and fat. Glycogen (a carbohydrate) is stored in the baby's liver mainly in the last weeks of pregnancy; the amount is greater when labour begins, but is rapidly used up during birth, and cannot be restored until food is given. Fat is similarly stored and exists as a special type known as brown fat; this can be made quickly available by the baby's catecholamines (adrenaline, noradrenaline). Fat and carbohydrate stores are greatest in normal term babies. They are significantly reduced in premature infants, and to a lesser extent when pregnancy is prolonged.

These energy sources are used not only for the maintenance of vital functions, but also to provide heat. Accordingly, energy loss will occur if the infant is not protected from cold.

PHYSICAL CHARACTERISTICS OF THE NORMAL FULL TERM INFANT (as seen at 2-3 hours of age).

1. Proportions. Average weight 3.2kg, height 50 cm, head circumference 35 cm, crown-rump 35 cm, and chest circumference (nipple line) 35 cm.

The last 3 measurements normally coincide within 0.5 cm. Marked variance of any one may suggest disease.

2. Skin. Variably covered by cream-coloured, waxy material—vernix caseosa, which with the fingernails and cord, may be stained yellow after prolonged pregnancy, or in placental dysfunction. Babies are red at birth, rosy after a few hours. Pallor means blood loss, jaundice means disease, unless it appears after 24 hours. Cyanosis of the hands and feet is usual when the infant is exposed to temperature change, which can also cause a general bluish mottling of the skin—cutis marmorata, or less frequently the harlequin colour change, in which one half of the body (the top) is pale and the other (the lower dependant part) suffused, the response shifting with changes in the longitudinal position of the infant.

Edema (swelling) of the presenting part is normal—the *caput succedaneum*—and is usually associated with some purpuric spots on the face. Abnormal presentations, e.g., face, brow, breech, may be associated with considerable swelling and purpura. *Milia* are small whiteheads best seen on the nose and cheeks. They are due to maternal hormones, are of no consequence and disappear after a week or two. *Capillary hemangiomata* (stork marks) are reddish, flat, irregular marks seen mostly on the upper eyelids, along the posterior hairline, and on the face. They are normal and usually disappear within a few months. In babies of Oriental, Negro, or Aboriginal descent are found Mongolian blue spots. They are diffuse, flat, purplish areas on the lower back and buttocks. They are normal but should be distinguished from bruising.

3. *Respiratory system.* All babies are obliged to breathe through the nostrils, and respiratory distress may indicate that these are blocked (choanal atresia). The respiration rate is 30-45/minute (slower in sleep). Minor irregularity of breathing may occur, but rib or sternal retraction is abnormal, except when the baby cries very lustily.

4. *Cardiovascular system.* The heart rate is 100-110, regular, and best checked by palpation of the upper limb pulses (radial, brachial), or by auscultation of the heart. The blood pressure (flush method) averages 80-90 mm Hg at birth, may fall to 70-75 mm in the first 12 hours, then returns to birth levels. The pressure in the legs measures 10-15 mm Hg. higher than in the arms. Soft systolic heart murmurs occur in about 15% of babies; most are transient and due to a temporarily open ductus arteriosus.

5. *Alimentary system.* All infants, even prematures, can swallow their own saliva. A baby who is bubbling or obviously salivating has a tracheoesophageal fistula until proven otherwise. Small white cysts (Epstein's pearls) are often seen on the hard palate and gums. They are of no consequence. The baby's belly is usually protuberant, if it looks flat and empty then a diaphragmatic hernia may be present. Separation of the rectus abdominis muscles in their upper parts is common and normal. The umbilical cord dries rapidly, but should always be checked for slip of the ligature, and for any bulge or cupping which may suggest a contained piece of gut. The position, muscular tone, and patency of the anal sphincter should be carefully checked. An abnormal anal position in the male is often associated with a rectourethral or rectovesical fecal fistula; in the female the opening may be rectovaginal.

6. The genitals. The female has well-formed labia; a prominent, but not large, clitoris; and a perforated hymen. Undue clitoral enlargement may suggest adrenal overaction, or pseudohermaphroditism.

In the male, there is a well-developed scrotum with testes therein; the penis is well formed, but the foreskin is not designed to be pulled back at this age. If the testes cannot be found, they have likely retracted into the inguinal canals. Simple manipulation or a warm bath will usually reveal them. Hypospadias is the situation where the urethra opens on to the ventral (under) surface of the penis; it is even more common than epispadias, where the opening is on to the dorsal (upper) surface.

THE NERVOUS SYSTEM

The full term baby moves a lot, and in a fairly coordinate way. Failure to move either the whole body, or a part of it (poverty of movement), is a useful clue to brain damage or neurological defect. The muscles have good tone, except during deep sleep, and this tone increases during crying, handling, or after stimulation by noise, cold, pain, or bright light. Flaccidity (hypotonia) of all or part of the body is often a sign of some disease.

REFLEXES

These are present from birth in the full term infant.

The sucking reflex. Put the baby's own finger in its mouth—it will suck. Persistent absence of this response in a full term baby may be a sign of impaired cerebral function.

The grasp reflex. Put your finger in the baby's palm—his fingers should close strongly—enough even to allow you to support him. This sign is present even in quite premature infants. Absence suggests nervous system damage.

The Moro (embrace) reflex. This is most readily elicited by supporting the head and trunk at 45° to the bed and then allowing the head to fall backwards (extend). The full response is extension of the trunk and limbs, with abduction of the latter and later flexion and adduction of the arms and flexion of the legs. This is a long description of embracing. The baby also cries in most cases. The sign is often brought out when the baby hears a loud noise, or when he is laid on a flat surface. Persistent total absence of the Moro reflex raises the suspicion of general neurological disorder. Asymmetry of the reflex, i.e., failure of an arm or leg to move, may make you suspect a limb fracture, nerve plexus damage, hemiplegia, or paraplegia.

The Moro reflex disappears when the infant is 4-6 months old; *persistence* after that time may reflect some nervous system disorder.

The weight bearing reflex. The infant is held upright and firmly planted on his feet. The flexed knees straighten (extend) and the body is clearly supported. In some babies apparent stepping will follow. This reflex is interpreted in the same way as the Moro.

The tonic neck reflex. This is most readily brought out in the premature. The infant is laid on his back and his head slowly turned to one side. This results in extension (straightening) of the limbs on the side to which the jaw points. The limbs on the other side flex. The reflex is very incomplete in most full term infants and disappears within 7-14 days of birth; its persistence or very ready production may suggest cerebral damage.

The tendon reflexes. The ankle, knee, and plantar jerks are difficult to get in the newborn, and their absence should not be overinterpreted. The plantar reflex (scratch the outer sole of the foot) is extensor (by adult standards) and usually accompanied by drawing away the limb, and straightening and fanning of the toes.

The superficial reflexes. These are not easy to obtain in the newborn. The most reliable is the anocutaneous reflex, when the sphincter ani can be seen to contract when the adjacent skin is scratched. Its presence excludes anal paralysis. In males the cremasteric reflex (retraction of the descended testes) is easily obtained by scratching the skin of the upper thigh.

Special sense abilities (seeing and hearing). These are present in the newborn, who will respond to bright lights, large moving objects and loud noises. The pupils contract when exposed to light but the response is not as well sustained as in the older child.

The other sensory functions (touch, pain, etc.) are present, but the responses to the usual tests are more sluggish than in the older child.

It should be noted that all of these reflexes may be impaired or absent if the infant has been given cerebral depressant drugs, such as phenobarbitone, chloral hydrate, or diazepam.

CARE OF THE NEWBORN

Immediate care in the delivery room. The mouth and nose should be sucked out as soon as possible; the infant should be held below the level of the mother's belly for 30 seconds to give it as much placental blood as possible. The cord is clamped and cut *at least* 15 cm from the umbilicus and the baby put on the resuscitation table. A quick estimate is made of its general condition, especially breathing, colour, heart rate, reflex activity, and muscle tone. This is conveniently summarized as the Apgar rating (table 2) and is conventionally measured at 1 and 4 minutes after delivery.

Table 2. Apgar rating

Factor	Score		
	0	1	2
Respiratory effort	None	Irregular and slow	Normal or crying
Colour	Completely pale, cyanosed	Body pink, extremities cyanosed	Pink
Muscle tone	Completely flaccid	Minor flexion of arms and legs	Active movements
Heart rate/minute	<30 or absent	<100	>100

The immediate problem is the establishment of respiration. In most instances this will occur spontaneously, or the first gasp will follow pharyngeal suction. In some babies gasping continues without true breathing. These infants, suffering from minor asphyxia, are cyanosed but have good muscle tone and a rapid heart. They should have bag-and-mask insufflation of oxygen through a pharyngeal airway. If normal breathing does not begin within 2-3 minutes, it is usual to carry out tracheal intubation. The more serious stage of asphyxia is characterized by pallor, limpness, and flaccidity and a slow heart rate. These infants, in the low Apgar ratings, should be sucked out at once, and have an endotracheal tube passed; the trachea is sucked out, and oxygen (40-100%) at a pressure of 30 cm of water (or less) is supplied by intermittent positive pressure breathing (IPPB). In most instances this will relieve the asphyxia and the infant will breathe normally. If, however, pallor and flaccidity continue after 4-5 minutes of IPPB, then a solution of sodium bicarbonate (8.4%) 10 ml bicarbonate in 5 ml 20% dextrose should be given into the umbilical vein.

If the infant is found to have no heartbeat at birth, or if the heartbeat disappears, then external cardiac massage may also be necessary.

After satisfactory breathing has begun the baby should be examined carefully for the more obvious congenital disorders, such as defects of the anterior abdominal wall (exomphalos) or inclusion of abdominal contents in the cord (omphalocele), midline masses over the spine, and ambiguous genitals. None of these require immediate treatment other than protection from infection. The infant is then transferred to a humidicrib with an oxygen supply; temperature is maintained at 36-37°, and he is taken to the nursery. Special care should be given to infants who weigh < 2 kg, who are < 35/52 gestation, who have required considerable resuscitation, or who have some obvious abnormality or illness.

Immediate care of the newborn

The general principles which apply to all babies irrespective of birth weight are:

1. To maintain or reestablish respiration
2. To maintain body temperature
3. To inspect for life-threatening disorders
4. To establish feeding
5. To prevent infection.

Respiration. The procedure after delivery has already been outlined but may require to be used in the nursery. Therefore, bag-and-mask, an oxygen supply, and facilities for intubation should always be available. As most respiratory problems occur in the first 24 hours of life it is good practice to admit all babies to an observation unit during this period. Prematures, and those with neurological or cardiac disorders, should be put in an intensive-care area. Observation and intensive-care units should have more staff and special monitoring apparatus to facilitate checking and treatment.

Maintenance of body temperature. This is very important as variation about the central temperature (37°) causes the baby's oxygen consumption to increase. This makes his body economy less efficient. Extreme loss of heat will kill an infant, and may occur even in tropical climates.

The diagnosis of heat loss (*hypothermia*). The baby may feel cold to the touch, but the only reliable method is to use a low-reading (to 30°C) thermometer. Axillary (skin) temperatures fall sooner than rectal (core) temperatures. The latter is, however, the best method of controlling any rewarming process.

Prevention of hypothermia. The baby should be covered during all procedures. When this is not practicable (as in extensive resuscitation) a source of radiant heat should be used to maintain body temperature. Rapid falls in body temperature may occur during transfer from the delivery room to the nursery, so the infant should be dabbed dry, wrapped in sterile towels, and placed in a preheated crib. For transfer over greater distances, in ambulance or aeroplane, swaddling in aluminium/polyurethane sheeting is useful, but must be combined with the use of a preheated crib.

Most full term infants, who are lightly clothed, will hold their temperature in a crib maintained between 25° and 30°C. However, abilities vary, and the baby's temperature should be checked regularly during the first 24 hours. Premature infants require the improved microclimate of a heated crib, preferably one whose heat output is controlled by feedback from a thermometer (thermistor) on the baby's skin. A baby who becomes cold in spite of apparent adequate heating may have hypoglycemia, septicemia or serious heart disease; these possibilities should be kept in mind.

As the infant has a limited ability to control his temperature, he may become too hot (hyperthermia), especially if heavily insulated, or when being rewarmed. Too high a temperature disturbs the body economy as much as the reverse—watch out then for overheating.

If hypothermia has occurred, the general rule is : the lower the temperature the slower the rewarming, and the greater the chance of hypoglycemia.

Some life-threatening situations. Consideration should be given to the following conditions, which are amenable to treatment if diagnosed early. In many instances the nurse will be the first to suspect their presence. Only a short description will be given, as the disorders are discussed in full elsewhere.

Diaphragmatic hernia. In this condition the abdominal viscera enter the chest due to a diaphragmatic defect. The baby's belly is unnaturally flat and empty looking. As air enters the gut, the lungs become embarrassed and severe dyspnea begins; if treatment is delayed, signs of intestinal obstruction also set in. The emergency care of these infants is to maintain the airway by endotracheal intubation until the infant is on the operating table. Facilities for positive pressure breathing (bag and mask) must be ready, especially when transfer outside the nursery is contemplated.

Choanal atresia. This is where there is failure of canalization in both nostrils. The infant is unwilling to breathe through his mouth, so he tends to suffocate, becoming restless, cyanosed, and develops rib retraction. All of these symptoms are relieved if the mouth is opened, and this is the best method when suspecting the diagnosis, which is confirmed by failure to pass a tube into the pharynx from the nostril. The immediate treatment is to insert an oropharyngeal airway until the nasal blockage can be relieved surgically.

Tracheoesophageal fistula. In this the esophagus may end blindly. If the infant is fed, the esophagus fills up and fluid spills over into the trachea. In extreme cases the baby drowns; more commonly severe coughing and dyspnea occurs, and pulmonary infection invariably follows. The condition is not always easy to recognize. The esophagus is, however, open if a plastic tube can be passed into the stomach, and it is recommended that this simple test be carried out on all infants before they are fed. Otherwise the fistula may be suspected by undue salivation or bubbling by the baby. Since the infant cannot swallow its own secretions this results in a wet pillow. The events subsequent to feeding have already been described.

If tracheoesophageal fistula is suspected, then it is imperative that nothing be given by mouth; the crib must be so labelled, and all staff warned. The further treatment is discussed elsewhere (p. 192).

Pierre Robin syndrome. In this condition, the jaw is greatly underdeveloped (hypomandibulosis) and cleft palate is usually present. The infant's tongue falls back so as to close off the throat and cause breathlessness, rib retraction, and blueness. All of this is most liable to occur with the first feeds. The emergency treatment is to hold the baby face down and with his neck quite straight. Most infants are relieved by doing this, but if respiratory distress goes on, then endotracheal intubation may be necessary.

Bleeding in the newborn. This may be external, as from a slipped ligature, or internal, as in a ruptured viscus. Whatever the cause, the principal sign is marked pallor, usually associated with dyspnea and a rapid thready pulse. The mucous membranes (e.g., inside the lips) are bleached and the blood pressure is low. Such a situation must be treated by urgent transfusion. If the nurse observes pallor in an infant, she should check the cord, adjust the ligature if necessary, and report her findings immediately.

Avoidance of infection

The infant has been living in the sterile womb, so he has not had any infective stimulus to his own immunological defences. Only IgG (immunoglobulin G) has been transferred to him across the placenta. Accordingly he is more liable to infection in general and the risk is greater if he is premature, has abrasions or injuries, fails to breathe normally, or gets respiratory distress syndrome.

Colonization by bacteria (including pathogens) is inevitable, and is well tolerated unless the dose of bacteria is very large, skin abrasions are present, or catheters have been inserted in the blood vessels. Babies infect each other very easily. The principles then are clear—nurseries must not be overcrowded, and barrier nursing should be practised. This means that each infant is regarded as a self-contained unit with his own crib, clothing, utensils, and thermometer, and that the attending nurse wears one gown for each infant's care. She washes her hands thoroughly between infants. Soiled clothing or dressings are placed in plastic bags and disposed of immediately. Infants must be inspected regularly for infection of the eyes, cord, skin, and nails; if any is found, the child should be isolated.

All apparatus used in the resuscitation or care of babies must be carefully sterilized after use, and regularly tested for the presence of dangerous organisms; special care and frequent surveys are needed with things in frequent use, e.g., water supply, suction apparatus, oxygen supply, bags and masks, and baby scales.

Specifics

Care of the cord. The cord is checked to be certain that it has no gut in it, then it is doubly ligatured, shortened to 3-4 cm, and cut cleanly across. An antibiotic spray (e.g., polybactrim) should then be applied. The stump is kept dry, allowed to mummify, and inspected daily. Any discharge, bad smell, or reddening of the umbilical area is evidence of infection. The cord is swabbed, the baby isolated, and the stump cleaned and sprayed with antibiotic.

Care of the skin. A conventional bath is unnecessary for the newborn. Swabbing of the skin with sterile saline is sufficient, followed by *dabbing* with a sterile towel. Weak (<1%) solutions of hexachlorophene are of value, and are dabbed on, but *must* be *thoroughly* rinsed off with sterile water. Hexachlorophene solutions must not touch the eyes, mouth, or any abraded areas of skin.

Clothing. This should be simple and easily sterilized. All clothing should be changed daily, or more often if dirtied. Unsterilized clothing *must not* be issued for use in a nursery.

Prophylactic antibiotics. These are to be avoided as a routine. They may be prescribed occasionally if the membranes have been ruptured for several days before birth, when the mother has a definite infection, or when the baby has had intravascular catheters in place for more than 48 hours.

Gamma globulin replacement. This is normally used only in premature infants in whom a specific deficiency has been demonstrated.

FEEDING THE BABY

The full term infant will require 110 cal/kg*, 150 ml water/kg, and 2-3 g/kg of protein—all per 24 hours. These are average values—more may be required for satiety in some babies. If breast milk, or modified cow's milk mixture, containing 20 cal/30ml is given in sufficient quantity to cover the fluid requirements, then the baby usually gets enough to eat. (See Appendix 1.)

The infant should have been inspected for local problems likely to cause difficulties, e.g., harelip, cleft palate, or Pierre Robin syndrome, and tracheoesophageal fistula must have been excluded. There is little point in expecting normal feeding in an infant who is very breathless from disease, or who cannot be aroused because of the effect of drugs,

*All units in this book, except the unit of energy, are metric. There has been some widespread reluctance to use the term "joule" in place of "calorie". For this reason the existing established nomenclature has been retained. It is expected that the joule will eventually replace the calorie. 1 cal = 4.19J.

or cerebral damage. Accordingly, in these babies food and fluid are supplied through a nasogastric tube.

Feeding babies

Breast feeding. This is the natural method of feeding and has the advantage of sterility, correct temperature, and close regulation of supply to demand. Importantly, a mother who is able to breast feed may be more confident about the baby and achieves a great deal of psychological satisfaction.

Successful breast feeding is usually a tribute to convincing propaganda. The subject should be discussed at the antenatal visits and the advantages of breast feeding outlined. Most mothers have a sense of achievement with the pregnancy and this feeling can be used to encourage the woman towards breast feeding, especially if she is reassured that her figure will not suffer—as it will not. The breasts should be inspected for severe nipple retraction. If this is present, the wearing of glass breast-shields within the bra will help to make them prominent. If at this stage the mother is opposed to breast feeding, the matter should not be pressed; she may feel differently when the baby is born.

It is important for nurses to realize their value as opinion makers for mothers. If the nurse is not herself convinced of the virtues of breast feeding, she will communicate her own doubts to the mother—with failure as the expected result. Differences of opinion about breast feeding should be the subject of rational discussion with the senior nursing staff and with the pediatrician. If the nurse can communicate to the mother her own belief that breast feeding will work, then the battle is half won. Hospital routines are less easy to achieve where breast feeding is widely used and this may be reflected in the need for larger numbers of aides, especially where a central nursery replaces the "rooming in" technique.

Most healthy full term babies can be put to the breast within 12 hours, or as soon as the mother is willing. If complications of pregnancy or labour have occurred, suckling need not begin until the breasts have begun to fill. Delayed suckling does not, however, mean delayed feeding, so that glucose or formula feeds may be given earlier. The mother should have comfort and privacy, and, if she has been given any drugs, she should be reassured that these will not come out in the milk and harm the baby. In most cases, placing the infant's cheek on the breast will cause him to rotate his head and find the nipple; this is called the rooting reflex. Otherwise the mother should gently introduce the nipple into the baby's mouth, while pulling down the chin if the baby is sleepy. At first, only small quantities of milk are available. After the breasts fill—a situation recognizable to the mother by a feeling of tension and heat in the breasts, and to the nurse by the ready extrusion of milk—the milk supply is reasonably assured. It is maintained, however, by regular emptying of the breasts by the baby's feeding from each side for 5-10 minutes. In general, longer periods of suckling tend to cause cracked nipples. The puerperium is a period of maternal tension, and an air of confidence should be generated in the mother by telling her that her milk supply is adequate and that the baby will start to gain weight only after the third day of life.

Timing of feeds. This should be "on demand"—which means what it says. Such a routine is least disconcerting to hospital routine if the mother has her baby in her room. Mothers, especially of first babies, should be told that at first the baby's calls for food may be quite irregular, e.g. 6 a.m., 7.30 a.m., 11.30 a.m., 3 p.m., 5 p.m., and so on. Settling into a 3- or 4- hour interval between feeds occurs when the infant is a few weeks old. Where a central nursery militates against rooming in, sufficient staff should be available to take the baby to the mother for feeding. Often enough this is possible only every 3 hours but this need not discourage the mother from on demand feeding at home.

Care of the breasts. After the early months of pregnancy, the mother should be taught how to express the breasts—the sign of success is the exudation of a little colostrum. In the puerperium, the breasts should be supported by a well-fitting nursing bra. Simple hygiene with soap and water is sufficient and no effort should be made to harden the nipples by local applications.

Difficulties with breast feeding

Problems in the mother. These are few, apart from infectious diseases readily given to the baby. Chronic disease, e.g., of the heart, should not be regarded as an immediate contraindication to breast feeding; this may less fatiguing for the mother than the preparation of bottles.

The most common local problem is severe nipple retraction which may prevent the baby from fixing. Small and nonerectile nipples are compatible with success although they may crack more readily. Cracking is treated by taking the baby off the affected breast for 24 hours while continuing to express the milk by hand. Engorgement of the breast is another common problem. In this the breasts become very full and painful, especially in the axillary tail, the superficial veins dilate, and the periareolar area swells, sometimes to a degree which makes it too big for the baby's mouth, and blocks his nostrils when he does attach. Engorgement is treated by expressing the milk, decreasing the interval between feeds, providing extra support to the breasts, and administering a single large dose of estrogen (say, stilbestrol 5-10 mg).

Lobular engorgement, in which a quadrant of the breasts is similarly affected, should be treated by manual expression. Early treatment of engorgement is important in the prevention of breast abscess.

The excretion of drugs in breast milk. This is seldom a problem, although radioactive and antithyroid drugs may pass in sufficient quantity theoretically to affect the infant. If new drugs are given to nursing mothers, the possibility of milk transmission should be considered.

Bottle feeding of babies. Cow's milk has more protein and less carbohydrate (lactose) than human milk. Accordingly it is usually diluted to humanize it. Dilution reduces the caloric value, and this is restored by adding sugar. Dilution also lowers the higher calcium content of cow's milk but reduces the already low levels of iron. Accordingly, most manufacturers will add iron to their preparation. Although it is true to say that many full term infants have been successfully fed on whole cow's milk, the principle of dilution is accepted and usually demanded by mothers. The basis of the feed may be whole, dried, or evaporated milk. In general this is reconstituted to give a mixture containing 20 cal/30 ml and to contain not less than 1% protein. Many proprietary formulae have added iron, vitamin D and vitamin C. Most countries require that the analysis of the milk be printed on the container. Once a decision has been made as to the product to be used, it is given in quantities sufficient to supply 110 cal/kg and 150 ml/kg fluid daily.

Bottles and nipples vary widely in size and shape but little in effectiveness. The principal criterion should be ease of cleaning and durability for sterilization. The technique of bottle feeding is well known; the infant should be warm and comfortable, and the mother relaxed. She should be taught to test the temperature of the milk by shaking a little on the arm (*not* by sucking the bottle!). This test also ensures that the hole in the nipple is big enough—a regular drip is desirable, no drip is a sign that the hole size should be increased by a red-hot darning needle. Thus assured, the feeding begins. Free access of air into the bottle is necessary as it empties, otherwise the infant cannot suck. Burping the baby during and after a feed is conventional. Most infants finish the bottle in 15-30 minutes. Feeding on demand is usual for bottle fed infants.

Difficulties due to problems in the baby. The causes here may be summarized as (1) anatomical, (2) functional (failure of swallowing mechanism), and (3) those due to coincident disease.

Local causes such as cleft palate are obvious; prematurity and damage to the nervous system are the commonest cause of failure to suck and swallow, and usually exist from birth. If a baby has indeed fed for a day or two and then stops, this may be a symptom of coincident disease, especially infection. *This symptom must always be reported to the pediatrician.* Severe breathlessness, due to lung or heart disease, causes the baby to feed poorly if at all, but the feeding difficulty is only a part of the more serious basic disorder.

A more indefinable situation is that of the "lazy" baby, i.e., one who begins to suckle but does not persist, so that he takes a long time to take in enough food. This condition is most common in low birth weight babies who are being transferred from nasogastric tube feeding to the bottle. Otherwise, the diagnosis should be accepted only after assurance that underlying disease, e.g., minor nervous system disease, is absent and that there are no inborn errors of metabolism.

Treatment. The principle is to maintain fluid and calorie intake by modification of the technique or route of feeding. Thus in the baby with a cleft palate a longer, larger nipple is usually sufficient. Occasionally a nipple equipped with a flange which closes the palatal gap is required. If *prematurity*, *brain damage*, or *breathlessness* are the difficulties, then the infant should be fed by nasogastric tube. It is essential to record carefully the infant's intake of fluid in this situation; any deficit must be reported, so that intravenous fluid may be given if necessary.

In the case of the "lazy" baby, the principal treatment is patience, hence infants may require to be fed more frequently than usual in order to maintain an adequate intake. Mostly the condition is transient, and more disruptive to hospital routine than dangerous to the baby.

Is feeding successful? Contentment and weight gain are the criteria of successful feeding. The former reflects the ability to go for several hours without hunger crying. It is of lesser importance early in life, when the demands for food may occur at close intervals, but after the age of 2 weeks most infants will go for 3-4 hours. If they do not, the quantity of food being offered may be insufficient. Normal weight gain is the criterion most often used in hospital. This means a return towards the birth weight level within 5-6 days for full term babies, and within 10 days for the majority of low birth weight babies. Delay in so doing may of course reflect a disease process, e.g., respiratory distress. If no such cause is present, then the feeding is at fault. After regaining the birth weight, most infants will gain between 100 and 200 g each week. The lower value will apply to smaller infants, or to those who are breast fed.

Why is the baby discontented? Breast feeding is more likely to fail in the first week after discharge from hospital, especially if the nursing mother is thrown straight into the usual domestic turmoil. The symptoms are those of discontent in the baby and a decreasing interval between feeds. The situation is often complicated by the mother's feeling that she is inadequate. The usual treatment is to follow the breast feed by a supplementary bottle feed. This may be sufficient to hold the situation until breast milk production improves. If it does not return in a day or two, then complete bottle feeding is usually to be advised. The mother is then given estrogens to suppress her lactation, and breasts are checked to anticipate the formation of breast abscess.

In the bottle fed baby it should be easy enough to find out how much the infant is taking. If this seems adequate in volume, then the likely cause is too dilute a formula—usually a reversal of the water:milk ratios which have been advised. If the infant is taking enough volume, then some concurrent disorder, e.g., infection, may be present. Prolonged feeding time may be associated with some mechanical problem in the bottle, e.g., too small a hole in the nipple and failure of displacement air to enter. The signs here are vigorous sucking, and frustration crying during the feed. The remedies are usually obvious if the feeding process is watched.

Other problems. A degree of regurgitation, if not actual vomiting, is common in infants. There is no sign of disease, and the infant continues to gain weight. This situation, which is called posseting, may frighten the mother so that she begins to believe that the milk (breast or bottle) is not agreeing with the baby. Simple explanation, weighing the baby, and telling the mother of the normal weight gain form the best treatment.

Similarly, mothers should be made aware of the great variation of bowel habit in normal babies—especially in the breast fed. It is entirely acceptable for a breast fed infant to defecate infrequently (by the mother's standards), e.g., every 2-3 days. Equally, bottle fed babies may have a small, soft bowel action after each feed. In either case the stool is normal. Reassurance and education will again stop unnecessary worry and equally unnecessary changes in the diet.

Overfeeding. This is not a disorder which occurs in the breast fed. In the bottle fed, it is present when the infant drinks a lot and gains excessively. When this happens, enquire into the preparation of the feeds. Often it is found that the infant is receiving far too many calories. This may be due to misinterpretation of the instructions for preparing the bottle, e.g., using heaped instead of level measures. In other cases it is due to misplaced maternal enthusiasm so that her baby will register the most weight gain in the clinic. Overnutrition in infancy may well be the origin of intractable later obesity, so that errors and enthusiasm should be corrected as early as possible.

DYSMATURITY

This describes a group of babies who are born after a short pregnancy, or whose functional state at birth does not correspond with the length of gestation. The commonest type is the *premature* baby, born before the 37th week of pregnancy but of a good size considering the short pregnancy. If the infant is in the low percentile for the duration of pregnancy, then he is described as *small-for-dates*. Such a calculation is made from a table of fetal growth (fig. 9); conventionally babies in the 10th or lower percentiles of weight are considered small-for-dates. *Postmaturity* is not very common, and refers to the baby born at least a week after normal term (42 weeks), and who is found to be of normal length but of subnormal weight for the gestational interval. Postmature and small-for-dates babies are liable to show signs of intrauterine malnutrition.

All dysmature babies are liable to have exaggerated forms of the difficulties found in the full term. Additionally, they are much more prone to asphyxia, apneic attacks, respiratory distress syndrome, hypoglycemia and bleeding disorders. In the long term, they are more liable to have cerebral palsy, intellectual defect, and learning and behaviour disorders.

The causes of dysmaturity. In most cases these remain obscure. The delivery of a preterm infant (simple premature) may be associated with obstetric disaster. Otherwise poor social circumstances, the youthfulness of mothers, and maternal disease such as preeclampsia are the more common factors. The small-for-dates baby has similar associations, although twinning and fetal disease such as chromosome disorder (e.g., Down's syndrome) or viral infections (e.g., rubella) are somewhat more common.

Little is known of the cause of postmaturity.

Clinical features in dysmaturity

1. Simple prematurity. The primary international standard for this is a birth weight of 2.5 kg or less, and the other measurements are concordant, thus head circumference is 33 cm or less, and crown-rump length 32 cm or less. Other external features present at birth are: the skin is usually a deep waxy pink, with vernix covering the trunk, and lanugo (fine hair) on the back. In the heavier premature, breast tissue is definitely present, with a flat areola. As the degree of prematurity increases, breast tissue is less prominent or absent. The hair on the head is fine and woolly in contrast to the silkiness of full term hair. In the male, the testes are found in the inguinal canals, and the scrotum lacks rugae (wrinkles). In the female, the labia are widely separated and the clitoris is prominent. In either sex the ear cartilage is soft, and, if the

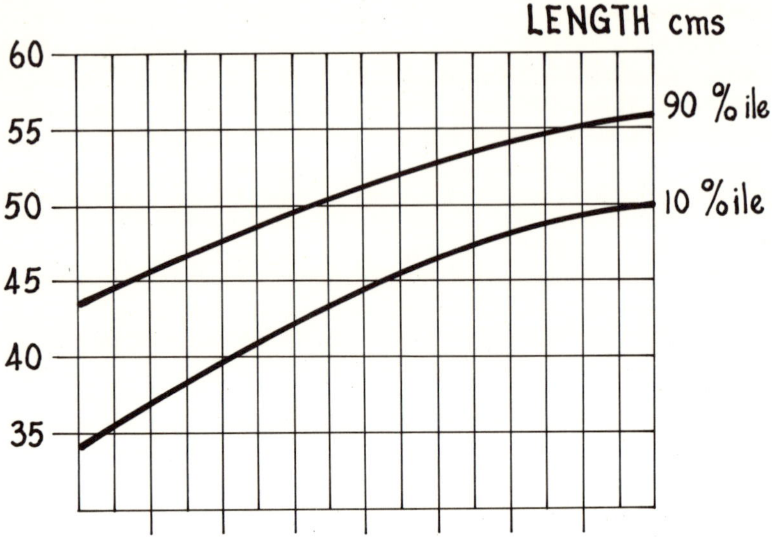

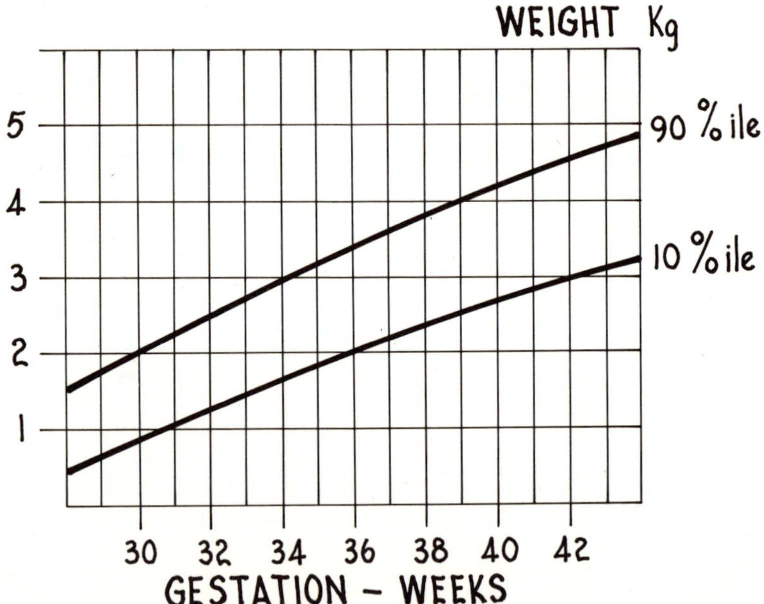

Fig. 9. Fetal growth: *a*, Height for gestational age; *b*, Weight for gestational age.

ear is bent, the return to the normal form is slow. The more shapeless is the ear, the greater the degree of prematurity. The feet show only a single transverse crease.

The simple premature, like all dysmature babies, lacks subcutaneous fat. The resulting thinness of the abdominal wall makes normal gut movements visible. The liver and spleen are able to be felt, exactly as in the full term baby. The chest is conoid in shape, and the respiratory rate (40 per minute) a little greater than in the more mature infant. A little rib retraction is always present, but constant rib or xiphisternal retraction means disease. The cardiovascular system is in all respects similar to that of the full term infant.

The central nervous system is functionally immature. Thus the baby often cannot suck or swallow, and spontaneous movements occur seldom and lack complexity. The limbs tend to be flaccid, and most prematures lie in an extended position. The grasp and Moro reflexes are present in all but the extremely premature, and the tonic neck reflex is easily obtained. The crossed extension test is of value. This is carried out by scratching the foot of an extended leg; the opposite leg should, in the complete response, show flexion followed by extension, with adduction of the foot and toe fanning. If gestation is 30 weeks or less, only flexion is shown, and to 36 weeks, flexion is followed by delayed extension. Only in the full term does adduction appear. The "scarf" sign is elicited by pulling the hand across the body around the opposite shoulder and around the neck. Prematures of less than 36 weeks' gestation can get the elbow past the midline; in more mature infants, the elbow cannot reach the midline. The weight-bearing response is feeble and "tip-toe" in most prematures, and automatic walking absent.

The situation is summarized in table 3.

2. The small-for-dates baby. This diagnosis is tenable only if the clinical state of the infant is discordant with the reported length of pregnancy. Thus, many babies will have the features of simple prematurity as noted above. However, some of the external appearances are different because of malnutrition. Characteristically, the small-for-dates baby has a gaunt, thin face, with obvious bony prominences and a large-looking skull. The skin is dry, often meconium stained, and may show wrinkling, cracking, and a degree of skin shedding (exfoliation) on the hands and feet. There is little subcutaneous fat. In babies who are of short gestation the length and weight percentiles are low, but similar. In term, and postmature, infants, the length percentile is greater than that for weight.

3. Postmaturity. This is the term applied to infants who have a gestation period at least a week longer than normal. In general the infant has a normal length percentile but a lower weight percentile. He shows

Table 3. Estimation of maturity

Factor	32–34 weeks	36 or less weeks	36–38 weeks	39 or more weeks
Skin colour	Waxy red	Waxy red	Deep pink	Bright pink
Lanugo	Face and body	Body only	Less obvious	Scanty
Hair scalp	Fine, fuzzy	Fine, fuzzy	Silky	Coarse and silky
Breast nodule development	Absent	2–3 mm	4–5 mm	7 mm +
Sole creases	Usually absent	Single anterior crease	2–3 creases	Whole foot creased
Male genitals	Testes unpalpable; small, smooth scrotum	Testes unpalpable; small, smooth scrotum	Testes often descended; some scrotal rugae	Testes descended; scrotum fully rugose
Female genitals	Prominent labia minora; labia majora flat	Prominent labia minora; labia majora flat	Labia majora more prominent than minora; few rugae	Prominent labia majora with well-marked rugae
Ears	No cartilage	Still pliable	Cartilage present	Ear quite stiff
Subcutaneous fat	Inobvious	Present	Clearly present	Obvious
Posture	Flexed legs, abducted hips	← Flexed arms and legs →		
Tonus	Hyptonic	Hyptonic	Some tonus	Hypertonic on crying
Scarf sign	Elbow past midline	← Elbow does not reach midline →		
Heel to ear	Usual	Difficult	Impossible	
Reflexes				
Suck	Weak, poorly sustained	Strong – synchronized with swallowing		
Grasp	Weak	Moderate	Strong and well-sustained	
Moro		Complete and reproducible		
Tonic neck		Complete and reproducible		
Crossed extension	Flexion only	Flexion with delayed extension	Flexion followed by rapid extension	Flexion, adductions, and extension
Weight-bearing	Absent	Feeble and tip-toe only	Full weight-bearing	Full weight-bearing and steps heel to toe

similar features to the small-for-dates baby, e.g., meconium stained, exfoliating skin which may show redundant folds, and yellowing of the cord and finger-nails.

Care of dysmature babies

The principles are those already described for full term infants, including attention to resuscitation, avoidance of chilling and infection and frequent detailed physical examination. The dysmature infant is best handled in a special unit equipped with facilities for monitoring and intensive care. After transfer from the delivery room the infant is placed in an incubator and his temperature is maintained at 35.5°-36.5°C, with frequent checking of the temperature by a low-reading thermometer. The infant must be assessed frequently, paying special attention to keeping the airway clear and to anticipating the possibility of respiratory distress (tachypnea, rib and sternal retraction, and expiratory grunt). In very small babies (<1,000 g) apneic attacks are so common that they should be placed on an apnea alarm for several days. Dysmature babies, especially the small-for-dates group, are liable to become hypoglycemic. This should be sought before symptoms appear, usually by Dextrostix examination of heel stab blood. This test should be carried out soon after birth and repeated every 4 hours until the baby has been fed for 12 hours or more. Low Dextrostix readings should be checked biochemically. If the infant has required resuscitation, or develops respiratory distress or prolonged apneic attacks, then arterial pH, pCO_2 and pO_2 should be monitored. This is best done by placing a catheter into the umbilical artery. Otherwise pH and pCO_2 (but not pO_2) can be measured on heel stab blood.

Feeding of the low birth weight baby. Calorie containing fluids should be given early in order to prevent hypoglycemia. In the abnormal premature (e.g., with respiratory distress) this is usually intravenous 5-10% glucose solutions. In the normal premature, feeds of 10% glucose are given by mouth or stomach tube, usually within 4-8 hours of birth. The heavier premature may well be able to suck and swallow. His abilities should be checked by trying him on a sterile dummy. The smaller baby will require to be fed by polythene gavage tube. This is introduced through the nose into the stomach. Its position is checked by the gentle injection of air while auscultating the stomach. The bubbling noise of air in the stomach is characteristic. Although early feeding of dysmature infants is an approved practice, the infants' tolerance of volumes is limited, so do not try to feed too much too quickly. A suitable starting volume of 10% glucose solution is 1.5 ml/kg; if the residual gastric content is small (<2 ml) this may be repeated every hour for 4 hours. Except in the smallest prematures (<1,000 g) the initial volume may then be doubled, and feeds given every 2 hours, with a target of 10-12 ml every 2-3 hours within 24-48 hours, *provided* that the gastric residual remains low (<2 ml) and there is no evidence of aspiration. At this stage a change to expressed breast milk or a suitable formula containing 20-25 cal/28 ml may be made. Low birth weight infants will ultimately require fluid to a level of 150 ml/kg and calories to a level of 110-125/kg; if these levels are attained within 10-14 days you should rest content.

Other dietary supplements. Premature infants require iron and vitamins. Normally these are begun within the first 2-3 weeks of age. An intake (from all sources) of 400 I.U. vitamin D and 1,500 I.U. vitamin A is sufficient. Ascorbic acid (50 mg/day) and iron (6 mg element daily) are also given after the first 2 weeks of life.

Prevention of infection. This is largely a matter of good hygienic practice, with the avoidance of overcrowding. More specifically, intravenous and intra arterial catheters should not be used routinely, and should be removed as soon as possible. The use of injected gamma globulin does not obviously influence morbidity from infection.

Some other problems of the dysmature

The major difficulties are hypoglycemia (low blood glucose), sometimes associated with hypocalcemia (low calcium levels), apneic spells, respiratory distress syndrome, and hypothermia. These are fully dealt with in the appropriate sections of this chapter (pp. 61, 57, 72 respectively). The brain of the dysmature baby is more sensitive to bilirubin levels, so exchange transfusion is done earlier, and on more liberal indications than in big babies. Anemia is common in dysmatures, even when iron has been given. Thus a top-up transfusion may be necessary by the fourth or fifth week of age if the hemoglobin falls to 8 g% or less.

Drug therapy. All drugs should be given with caution in the dysmature baby. Dosage should err on the low side, as their detoxifying mechanisms are incomplete. Thus the dose of digoxin should be reduced, and potentially toxic drugs, e.g., streptomycin, vitamin K analogues, novobiocin, and sulphonamides should be used only on the clearest of indications of benefit to the infant.

The progress of dysmaturity

The immediate mortality is closely related to the birth weight. Thus 75% of infants weighing 1,000 g or less will die, and a substantial number of the survivors will have permanent problems, mainly involving the nervous system. The major causes of death are congenital malformations, respiratory distress syndrome, and apneic spells; with good care, the mortality rate is 30% in the weight groups 1,500-2,000 g, the causes of death being the same as for smaller babies. The mortality rate decreases as the birth weight reaches normal range, and then rises again in postmature babies, even if their weight is normal.

Long-term Prognosis of the Dysmature Baby

There is a correlation between birth weight and the attainment of normal physical and mental attributes—the smaller the baby, the slower in reaching normality. Respiratory difficulties (e.g., apneic spells) or hypoglycemia, increase the incidence of intellectual defect and probably also of subsequent behaviour disorder.

DISEASES AFFECTING THE NEWBORN

Generally speaking, the newborn is liable to most of the diseases of childhood, so that reference to the appropriate chapters of this book is in order. It is necessary, however, to discuss certain disorders which are of high importance in this age group.

Injuries

These are most common when obstructed labour occurs, either because of abnormal presentation of the baby, or narrowing of the birth passages.

Injuries to the skin and subcutaneous tissue

The most minor type is edema of the presenting part. In vertex deliveries this is recognizable as scalp swelling or the caput succedaneum. In frank breech delivery, edema and bruising may affect the buttocks and perineum. In footling presentation, the feet are similarly affected. Most newborn babies have a few purpuric spots in the skin, whatever the presentation.

Cephalhematoma is a fluctuant blood-containing mass, usually over the parietal bone, outlined by the periosteal attachments of the skull. Accordingly, even if present on both sides, the swelling does not overlie the suture line. In most babies no ill-effects occur, although a few may show evidence of blood loss. The mass organizes and calcifies, becoming hard and radiopaque. Treatment is usually unnecessary.

Diffuse *subgaleal hemorrhage* is less common and causes a boggy swelling over the whole head. It is not localized as is the caput succedaneum, nor absent over the sagittal suture, as is a cephalhematoma. In addition to the general scalp swelling, the infant often shows signs of blood loss, e.g., pallor, low blood pressure, and low hemoglobin. High bilirubin levels may follow the break down of the shed blood.

Treatment. Blood loss is made up by transfusion and exchange transfusion may be needed if the bilirubin levels go up. The scalp should *not* be incised or aspirated, as infection readily follows.

Eye injuries

The commonest of these is *subconjunctival* hemorrhage which occurs when the head sticks during delivery. *Retinal* hemorrhage can be seen only by ophthalmoscopy, and has a similar cause. Neither condition needs treatment.

Injuries of the bones

These usually occur in obstructed labour when traction or forceps are used to aid delivery. The clavicle, humerus, and femur are most commonly broken, so that the limb does not move spontaneously or on eliciting the Moro. Local swelling and deformity occur and bony crepitation may be present unless the fragments are kept wide apart by epiphyseal separation.

Treatment. Only those fractures with much deformity are treated, usually by traction sufficient to restore normal alignment.

Skull fractures are usually linear, asymptomatic, and recognized by x-ray. Depressed (pond) skull fractures are quite rare. Treatment is rarely necessary unless the brain is threatened by raised intracranial pressure.

Injuries to the nerves

Pressure by forceps (or by the mother's sacral promontory) is the common cause of *facial palsy*. The affected side of the face does not move when the baby cries, nor does the eye close. These recover rapidly without any treatment. *Persistent* facial palsy may be due to agenesis (failure of formation) of the nerve nucleus within the brain stem.

Injuries to the brachial plexus

Erb's palsy follows damage to the 5th and 6th cervical roots. The arm does not move, is adducted, extended at the elbow, and the hand is pronated. It is sometimes complicated by paralysis of the diaphragm on the same side.

In lesions of the 8th cervical and 1st thoracic roots, *Klumpke's paralysis* results. In this the wrist flexors and small hand muscles are paralyzed. *Horner's syndrome* (drooping of the eyelid and a small pupil on the same side) coexists if the sympathetic fibres are also damaged. Rarely Erb's and Klumpke's paralyses are present together, when the arm is quite motionless.

Paralysis of the *radial* nerve is unusual, and characterized by an active arm but a "drop" wrist.

Treatment of these injuries is conservative. In Erb's paralysis, the supinated hand is fixed beside the head (pin the hand by the head!). In Klumpke's and radial nerve paralysis, the hand and forearm are supported by a cock-up splint.

Injuries of the abdominal viscera

These may follow direct injury, or occur after severe anoxia. The commoner injuries are rupture of the liver or spleen, and hemorrhage into the adrenal. In each the infant becomes pale and shocked, the belly is distended, and a mass can be felt. Blood can be sucked from the abdominal cavity. The treatment is to transfuse the baby, open the abdomen, and stop the bleeding. If the spleen is severely damaged, it is removed.

Intracranial hemorrhage

This is a serious problem, particularly associated with prematurity, anoxia, or as the final complication of respiratory distress syndrome. Most commonly the bleeding occurs into the ventricles and brain substance, but may spread to the membranes around the brain.

Clinical features. If the bleeding occurs before delivery, the baby may have all the features of asphyxia—a low Apgar, and difficult or impossible resuscitation. Breathing, if it is established, begins to fail, so that apneic episodes occur. Evidence of damage to the brain is shown by the baby's failure to move spontaneously (or on stimulation by the Moro reflex) and muscular flaccidity; pallor and low blood pressure evidence the blood loss. Then the baby may seem restless, cries in an anxious fashion, and develops twitching of the arms and legs. The eyes look glassy, and soon the baby stops responding even to irritating stimuli. A bulging fontanelle is common. The spinal fluid contains fresh blood.

Problems in diagnosis

Many of the features described above can occur in hypoglycemia—which also complicates dysmaturity. However, the blood sugar is always low (by Dextrostix) in hypoglycemia, and the symptoms are promptly relieved by intravenous glucose. Meningitis has similar features, but usually comes on later, the cerebrospinal fluid contains pus, and the blood culture is positive.

Treatment. The only thing to do is to make up blood loss by transfusion. This is not a specific treatment, and death is very common.

Subdural hematoma

This condition usually complicates a labour which has been prolonged and in which forceps have been used.

Clinical features. The infant is often normal at birth, but, within a short time, becomes fretful, refuses to feed, and vomits. Convulsions are usual, and a hemiplegia may be noted. The fontanelle is tense. A definite diagnosis is made by putting a needle in the subdural space and sucking out blood or serum.

Differential diagnosis. This is mainly neonatal meningitis, which may have an identical clinical picture, but is characterized by pus in the C.S.F. Hypoglycemia and hypocalcemia cause confusion where convulsions occur, but the patient's fontanelle does not bulge, and the proper biochemical findings are present.

Treatment. Severe anemia is treated by blood transfusion; the subdural tapping is continued, and if dry taps are obtained after a week or so, cure has usually been obtained. If blood or serum persist after this, then the hematoma and membrane are removed surgically.

Neonatal cold injury

Heat loss can occur in any infant, but is most common in prematures. Accordingly, cold injury is always a hazard even in the tropics. The condition may occur in home or hospital, usually in the colder winter months.

Clinical features. The infant refuses to feed, and is apathetic. He does not cry. His face is pink and healthy looking, but he feels cold to the touch. His temperature (taken with a low-reading thermometer) is much below normal. The respiration and heart rates are slow. The skin, especially of the cheeks and buttocks becomes hard, inelastic, and feels waxy; this is called sclerema. Sudden bleeding from the lungs may cause death. The hemoglobin values are very high, but the blood glucose values are low.

Differential diagnosis. This is mainly from disease processes causing hypothermia, especially septicemia, severe congenital heart disease, and dehydrating conditions. None of these children have the rosy, healthy appearance of true neonatal cold injury and each has the features of the underlying disease.

Treatment. The infant should be gradually warmed by putting him in a heated crib. The temperature should carefully be monitored, so as to aim at a return to normal within 24-36 hours. Intravenous fluid (0.18% saline in 5% glucose) is given, and a close watch should be kept for temperature overshoot or for hyperglycemia from the infusion. If pulmonary hemorrhage occurs nothing can be done.

Complications. As some of these children become cretins, they should be carefully followed up.

INFECTIONS OF THE NEWBORN

These are most liable to occur in dysmature infants or in overcrowded nurseries. A division into minor and major infections is somewhat academic, as a minor infection in one infant may spread to become a major one in another. Routine preventive measures, early diagnosis, and prompt isolation are always indicated however petty an infection may seem.

Minor infections of skin, mucous membranes, and subcutaneous tissues

Minor skin infections are common in infants, and cultures usually reveal a staphylococcus, less commonly *Escherichia coli*, or Pseudomonas.

Clinical features. The usual disorder is the skin *pustule*. These are separated, reddened spots, which develop a septic head. The infant is otherwise well. *Bullous impetigo* is the condition in which there are widespread flaccid blisters of pus on the skin, and *Ritter's disease* is a spreading infection which causes the upper skin layer to fall off. Major abscess formations (boils, carbuncles) are rare except as *neonatal breast abscess*. In this the engorged breast becomes infected, with redness, swelling, and the formation of a fluctuant abscess. The baby is fevered, refuses feeds and is clearly unwell.

Paronychia (infection of the nail bed) is also relatively common, and is often found where excess skin overlies an underdeveloped nail. Redness and swelling occur at the nail edge, and pus forms. A *whitlow* (pulp space infection) is an occasional complication.

Umbilical sepsis is recognized by redness and swelling at and around the navel together with an unpleasant odour. The umbilical stump is usually sodden, and if it is taken off, a purulent granuloma is seen. Simple umbilical sepsis does not make the infant unwell; if the baby seems ill then the infection may have spread to the liver by way of the falciform ligament.

Conjunctivitis is nowadays uncommon and seldom due to the gonococcus; the usual organism is the staphylococcus or *E.coli*. The first trouble is a purulent eye discharge, often making the eyelids stick together. Redness and swelling of the upper lid occurs, and conjunctival redness is invariable. A similar picture is seen in the chemical conjunctivitis after silver nitrate eye drops.

General treatment of superficial infections. The lesions should be swabbed to identify the responsible organism. The baby is then washed with weak antiseptic (e.g., hexachlorophene) solution, and rinsed with sterile water. Neomycin/bacitracin ointment should be applied to the infected areas. If the baby is fevered or obviously unwell, antibiotic injections are given, usually as one of the semi-synthetic penicillins.

Gonococcal conjunctivitis carries a risk of corneal scarring so it should be treated by the frequent instillation of penicillin eyedrops and by penicillin injections.

Moniliasis (thrush)

This spreads from the maternal passage, from dirty bottles, or occurs in the infant given broad-spectrum antibiotics. Pale grey patches develop in the mouth, which, if scraped, show a raw bleeding area. A sore bottom is common, the skin around the anus being red and slightly swollen. The organism is readily identified by smear or culture. Generalized moniliasis (indistinguishable from other septicemias) may occur in prematures, or in those older infants with dysgammaglobulinemia.

Treatment. Nystatin solution 100,000 units is put in the mouth every 6 hours for a week.

MAJOR INFECTIONS OF THE NEWBORN

Septicemia

This is a disease which is hard to diagnose but needs early treatment.

Background. It is most likely to occur in low birth weight infants, when the membranes have been ruptured for some time before delivery, or where umbilical catheters have been put into the infant. Overcrowded nurseries, contaminated resuscitation equipment, or other communal apparatus may contribute. Congenital abnormalities of the urinary tract or central nervous system may have a bearing in individuals. Sometimes septicemia follows simple condition such as an infected navel.

The usual bacterial cause is one of the following: staphylococcus, *E.coli*, Pseudomonas, or Proteus.

Clinical features. Of these, the minor manifestations are the more important. The principal early complaint is a slight deviation from normal. The infant is reported to be "not so well", or "looks different". Such a statement should always warn of the possibility of septicemia. Lethargy, sleepiness, and poor feeding are complaints which may emerge on further enquiry. Irregular respiration and apneic spells are also suspicious findings.

Common general findings. The temperature may be increased or subnormal. The latter is perhaps more common in the severer forms of the disease. Loss of weight and dehydration occur.

Major manifestations. Each body system may have its own signs, as shown below, but multisystem involvement is common in the later stages.

The respiratory system. Apnea, or dyspnea with rapid respirations and rib retraction are usual. Cyanosis is nonspecific, but may direct attention to the respiratory system.

The cardiovascular system. A fast heart rate, irregular heart, low blood pressure, and subnormal temperature are all common. Peripheral cyanosis and skin mottling are found in the later stage of the disease.

The central nervous system. Apneic spells, twitching, or obvious fits are found in those who have meningitis as part of septicemia. A bulging fontanelle is a reliable sign in this situation.

Alimentary system manifestations. Vomiting, diarrhea, and abdominal distention are all found, and in advanced disease there is jaundice and enlargement of the liver and spleen.

Other signs. Skin infections are common, and osteomyelitis with abscess may occur. Sclerema of the skin occurs in those who are cold for a long time. Table 4 outlines some aspects of differential diagnosis.

Hematological abnormalities. These are almost always found in the advanced stage of the disease. Pallor, anemia, purpura, bruising, and oozing from injection sites are associated with low platelet levels, and difficulties of the various clotting factors.

Table 4. Septicemia

Manifestations	Differential Diagnosis
Shock, hypothermia, skin mottling, cyanosis	Congenital heart disease, especially left heart hypoplasia
Vomiting, abdominal distention	Intestinal obstruction, especially volvulus. Necrotizing enterocolitis
Jaundice, hepatosplenomegaly	The viremias (rubella, herpes, cytomegalovirus). Erythroblastosis and post-R.D.S. syndrome.
Apnea, twitching, fits	Intracranial hemorrhage. C.N.S. abnormalities. Hypoglycemia.
Dyspnea, rib retraction, and chest signs	Atelectasis. R. D. S.
Purpura, bruising, and hemorrhagic signs	Reaction to thiazide diuretics, viral infections, hemorrhagic disease of the newborn.

Laboratory. The best supporting evidence is a positive blood culture, and cultures from other sites—C.S.F., urine, and umbilicus,—are also valuable clues as to the exact organism responsible. Urine samples are best obtained by bladder puncture. The white blood count is of little value because of the great variations found in normal babies. A normal W.B.C. is entirely compatible with septicemia. Hypoglycemia, acidosis, and hyponatremia are common in the advanced disease.

General treatment. The infant should be kept in an incubator, and given intensive nursing attention. An intravenous infusion should be set up, an apnea monitor fitted, and arrangements made frequently to check blood pH, glucose, electrolytes, and the blood coagulation factors.

Supportive treatment. The fluid requirement is given intravenously as 1/5-1/3 N saline with glucose, according to the estimate of fluid and electrolyte loss. Blood is given to maintain the hemoglobin level at 12-13 g%. If coagulation abnormality is present then Factors I, II, V, and VIII (PPSB) should be added to the infusion.

Specific. The choice of drug will depend upon the resistance pattern of the likely local pathogens. Until the blood culture results are known a useful initial schedule is kanamycin and ampicillin. Methicillin is used if a staphylococcus is suspected or cultured. Pseudomonas infections are an indication for colistimethate sodium. An alternative regime is gentamycin and carbenicillin. The latter is given I.V. at 6-hourly intervals.

Prognosis. This is not good, since death occurs in 50% of all sufferers, irrespective of the bacterial cause. Death is less likely if diagnosis and treatment are prompt.

Osteomyelitis

This condition is commonly preceded by a skin infection, and is usually due to the staphylococcus. The long bones and the maxilla are most commonly affected. Multiple sites of infection may be present.

Clinical features. In most babies the condition is silent, the first sign being the superficial swelling of a ruptured periosteal abscess. Lack of movement or crying when handled are useful signs if the limbs are affected.

A few infants, especially the prematures, are obviously ill with the usual nonspecific observations, viz., refusal to feed, irritability, pallor, and sometimes fever. In these, a careful search should be made for local swelling and tenderness. Extensive early destruction is common in neonatal osteitis, so that obvious deformity and extensive x-ray changes of destruction are seen. Leucocytosis and anemia are common evidence of a severe infection.

Osteomyelitis of the *superior maxilla* causes facial swelling and bulging forward of the eye, as well as the general features described. In all cases of neonatal osteomyelitis careful watch should be kept for metastatic infections such as staphylococcal pneumonia, meningitis, or brain abscess.

Treatment. Blood culture and local aspiration should be done in order to establish the identity and resistance pattern of the organism. Thereafter begin vigorous antibiotic therapy, usually with the semisynthetic penicillins. Transfusion is often necessary for the anemia. Aspiration of abscess may be preferable to open surgery, but the decision must be arrived at on sound orthopedic grounds. The extensive bone destruction implies prolonged, skilful orthopedic follow-up.

Acute renal infection

Pyelonephritis is usually superimposed upon anatomical abnormality and is a common sign of a neonatal septicemia.

Clinical features. The infant is unwell, with refusal to feed, irritability, vomiting, and frequently diarrhea. Dehydration, with shock and hypothermia, may be the mode of presentation. An abdominal mass—an enlarged kidney—may be present. Leucocytosis is usual, and anemia common. The urine contains pus cells, red cells, and casts. The former predominate. Urine and blood culture in most instances reveal *E.coli.* Lumbar puncture should be done in these infants to exclude a coexistent meningitis.

Differential diagnosis. This is from the other causes of severe infection in the newborn—septicemia, meningitis, and gastroenteritis. It should be recalled that the urine passed during any dehydrating episode may contain many polymorphs, not necessarily those due to a true urinary infection. The difficulty in obtaining sterile urine samples is notorious in infancy, so that suprapubic bladder tap is the best method of obtaining cultures.

Treatment. Intravenous infusion of saline is necessary where vomiting is marked and dehydration incipient or present. Antibiotics are begun after appropriate bacteriological survey. Ampicillin or streptomycin are generally used until the sensitivity of the organism is known. The urinary tract should be thoroughly x-rayed after the acute illness has been relieved as surgery may be needed to help any obstructive process.

Gastroenteritis

This condition, due to viral or atypical *E.coli* infection, is happily nowadays rare. It occurs in epidemics, usually in overcrowded nurseries or where formula preparation is unhygienic.

Clinical features. The infant rapidly becomes gravely ill with refusal to feed, vomiting, diarrhea, and dehydration. The stools may be passed explosively. At first mucoid and greenish, they rapidly become to resemble concentrated urine, for which they may be mistaken. There is a gross weight loss with evidence of dehydration—loss of skin elasticity, sunken abdomen, greyish pallor, fast heart, and a low temperature and blood pressure.

The serum electrolytes may be normal or show hypo- or hypernatremia, dependent upon the relative degree of salt and water loss. Hypernatremia is perhaps more common in neonates. Acidosis is not uncommon in neonatal gastroenteritis.

Once an epidemic is established, it is soon found that anorexia and failure to gain weight precede the above symptoms; in some instances the infant is found dead in bed.

Differential diagnosis. This primarily concerns the first case in an epidemic. Neonatal septicemia, meningitis, and pyelonephritis are the conditions which are most likely to cause confusion, since each may be associated with diarrhea. Lumbar puncture, blood culture, and the individual nature of the illness are usually sufficient to gain a proper diagnosis. When several children are smitten simultaneously with a dehydrating illness, consideration should be given to accidental salt poisoning. In this condition, the formula has been made up with salt instead of sugar. The clinical features closely resemble those of infantile diarrhea, but convulsions are usually a prominent feature. There is a gross increase in the blood sodium and chloride values, and the formula tastes salty. Enquiry reveals the error and the propinquity of the salt and sugar dredgers in the formula room is diagnostic.

Neonatal necrotizing enterocolitis

This condition principally affects premature babies, especially those who have been difficult to resuscitate, or who have had respiratory distress. Although the exact cause is not known, interference with the gut blood supply is probably important and umbilical arterial catheterization sometimes has been done beforehand.

Clinical features. The onset is in the first week of life. The main features are vomiting, low temperature, apneic episodes, refusal to feed, distention of the belly, and bleeding from the gut. Evidence of a gut perforation may be present, and dehydration with shock may be early and severe.

X-rays. The abdominal x-rays commonly show pneumatosis intestinalis, i.e., air bubbles and planes of gas outside the gut lumen, but not within the peritoneum. The latter may occur later, as may evidence of gas in the portal venous tree.

Differential diagnosis. This is principally from septicemia of the newborn and from the coagulation disorders giving gastrointestinal bleeding. The x-ray signs described are the best guide to a positive diagnosis.

Treatment. Rehydration is carried out, and antibiotics are given before the belly is opened. At this time resection and anastomosis may be possible, or resection with ileostomy or colostomy in more severe instances.

Viral infections

The 3 viruses which can cause severe illness in the newborn are rubella virus, cytomegalovirus (salivary gland virus), and herpes virus. The first 2 organisms may cause congenital abnormalities in the baby. Premature babies are more prone to have active infection.

General features. The clinical features are often remarkably similar, whatever the virus. Thus, soon after birth the baby refuses to feed, and becomes irritable and drowsy, but seldom fevered. A bleeding tendency is common, with purpura, bruising and sometimes hemorrhage from the gut. Severe early jaundice occurs, usually due to hemolysis. The liver and spleen are greatly enlarged.

There are certain specific features.

In *herpes virus infection*, the mother may have had herpes. The infant's skin will often (50%) show herpetic spots at one stage or another. The features noted above are present, and early death is common. The survivors may reveal spasticity, mental retardation, and chorioretinitis (inflammation of the retina and adjacent area of the eye).

In *cytomegalovirus infection* the only specific finding is of viral inclusion bodies in the urine. As in herpes virus infections, cerebral palsy, chorioretinitis, and intracerebral calcification may afflict the few survivors.

Rubella viral infections. These infants frequently also have congenital cardiac lesions, commonly patent ductus arteriosus. Cataracts or microphthalmia (small eye) may also coexist as well as the general features already described. The survivors of the infection often suffer cerebral palsy, chorioretinitis, microcephaly, deafness and intellectual impairment. In a few, sclerotic decalcified areas occur in the tibia and femur, and are useful x-ray signs of the disease.

Laboratory investigations. Red cell breakdown is common, so the hemoglobin goes down, and the bilirubin rises. The hemolysis causes abnormal red cell shapes and forms to be seen, and the platelets decrease in number. Liver function tests (enzymes, SGOT, SGPT) are abnormal. The cerebrospinal fluid contains excess lymphocytes. By special techniques, the virus can be grown, but this is difficult, especially in rubella infections.

Differential diagnosis. The main problem is to distinguish viral infection from a bacterial septicemia, since the latter can be treated with antibiotics. In general, a viral infection has a less explosive onset, but in all cases a blood culture must be done. A rather rare condition, which resembles the viral disorders, is *toxoplasmosis*. This is acquired from the mother, so that she should be checked for toxoplasmosis by the Sabin test. Special tests done in the baby are for complement fixation against toxoplasma, but as these become positive only after some weeks, they are not very helpful in the acute situation. Congenital *syphilis*, although not common now, can give a similar picture to that of the viremias, so that the mother's and baby's syphilis serology should be tested.

Treatment. No specific treatment exists, so supportive measures, such as blood transfusion or infusion of coagulating substances, or intravenous infusions for the relief of dehydration, are used. The rubella baby will need appropriate care for any heart or eye disorder.

Prognosis. This is not good, especially for the sufferers from herpes virus infection; of those who recover from the initial severe illness, few are normal. A close watch is kept upon the head circumference since failure of adequate skull growth usually argues ultimate intellectual retardation. The hepatosplenomegaly may take many months to disappear, but liver function is ultimately normal. Widespread intracerebral calcification may develop and is frequently associated with spasticity and retardation. Deafness is particularly common after rubella infections. All neonatal viral infections can lead to permanent growth stunting.

Other forms of the rubella syndrome. In many babies the acute illness just described does not occur, and the infant comes in with failure-to-thrive, or may present with congenital heart disease or cataracts. Later in life, the infant may be found to be very deaf, and investigation then proves the diagnosis.

Congenital syphilis

This is nowadays an unusual disease; it occurs often enough, however, to warrant description. In almost every case, the mother's pregnancy has been unsupervised. The responsible organism is of course the *treponema pallidum*, which is distributed generally in the baby's body.

Clinical features. Rarely the disease causes stillbirth. Characteristically, however, the infant seems reasonably well, but within a few days of birth develops a blocked nose (the snuffles) often with a bloody mucoid discharge from the nostrils. After a week or two a skin rash appears, consisting of reddish-coloured, oval areas, distinctly separated and most commonly found around the mouth or anus. The palms and soles of the feet, if involved, soon shed their skin. Scarring of the rash at the mucocutaneous junctions (mouth, anus) gives rise to *rhagades*—radiating linear scars. Condylomata (raised, moist plaques) occur near the anus, but are not very common.

In a few infants, hemolysis with anemia and jaundice occur and these children rather resemble those suffering viral infections. Where the condition has been present for some months, the infection of the bones may be severe enough to cause separation of the shaft from the epiphysis. This is painful, so that the baby does not move the limb (pseudoparalysis). At any age, swelling of the lymph glands and enlargement of the liver and spleen may be present.

X-ray examination. This is done to show the inflammation of the cartilaginous part of the bones, and of the periosteum, which becomes separated from the shaft. The cortex of the bone is irregularly destroyed (moth eaten) and a dense shadow may be seen near the epiphysis.

Other findings. The C.S.F. contains an excess of lymphocytes. The serological tests for syphilis are positive in the blood and C.S.F.

Differential diagnosis. Many infants with short-lived snuffles have a simple viral or staphylococcal infection. Snuffling is also not uncommon in Hunter-Hurler syndrome. The skin rash is seldom to be mistaken for other lesions, except perhaps that of drug reaction (e.g., phenobarbitone).

Treatment. A full course (1-2 weeks) of intramuscular penicillin should be given. This treatment may be repeated if the serological tests again become positive.

DISORDERS OF PARTICULAR SYSTEMS IN THE NEWBORN

The respiratory system

Conditions obstructing the upper airway

These are not common, except for choanal atresia and Pierre Robin syndrome which have already been discussed. Among the other varied causes are congenital cysts of the tongue (e.g., lymphangioma), laryngeal webs or stenosis, and congenital thyroid enlargement (goitre).

Clinical features. Breathlessness, rib retraction, and cyanosis, with stridor on crying, occur soon after birth. The exact condition present is usually recognized when the airway is inspected by laryngoscope.

Treatment. The airway is kept open by placing an endotracheal tube and the situation reviewed to see if the obstructing agent can be removed surgically.

Conditions obstructing the lower respiratory tract

Compression of the lower trachea or bronchi is usually due to an abnormal blood vessel, e.g., an aberrant subclavian or innominate artery, or a right-sided aortic arch.

Symptoms. These are often delayed until the baby is 2-3 weeks old. The main complaints are of stridor on breathing in, and wheezing on breathing out. Vomiting is common, as the gullet may be pressed upon. Thus inhalation of feeds may occur, giving rise to respiratory difficulty and lung infection.

The diagnosis can be established with certainty by contrast x-ray examination of the trachea and bronchi, and the exact course of the compressing blood vessel by angiography.

Treatment. The compressing vessel is surgically rerouted.

Conditions causing compression of the lung

Pneumothorax occurs when air is in the pleural space. When air can get in but cannot get out, it is called valvular pneumothorax, and is much more dangerous because not only is the lung rendered useless, but the largest blood vessels are also obstructed. The condition may follow endotracheal intubation, complicate respiratory distress syndrome, or be a mishap of the continuous positive pressure method of giving oxygen. Often enough, however, there is no obvious cause.

Clinical features. These consist in the rapid onset of breathlessness, rib retraction, restlessness, and sometimes cyanosis. More specifically, the side of the chest which contains the pneumothorax may not move well, and the air entry is poor.

If air has also entered the mediastinum, subcutaneous emphysema (air under the skin) occurs. Chest x-rays show air in the pleural space.

Treatment. The pneumothorax is deflated, in emergency, with a needle and syringe, more deliberately by intercostal catheter connected to underwater sealed drainage.

Lung cyst

This is usually derived from a bronchus. It fills with air and compresses the lung. The symptoms are similar to those of pneumothorax; the treatment is to remove the cyst surgically.

Congenital lobar emphysema

In this condition, one of the lung lobes (usually right upper or middle) swells with trapped air which cannot escape, as in valvular pneumothorax. The abnormal lobe presses upon the rest of the lung and causes dyspnea, anxiety, rib retraction and cyanosis. The chest x-ray shows the enlarged lobe, which may require excision if severe trouble is present.

Chylothorax

This is a very rare cause of pressure upon the lung. It is due to rupture of the cisterna chyli at its entry into the superior vena cava. The escaping lymph gives a pleural effusion which causes the usual symptoms of dyspnea, rib retraction, anxiety, and cyanosis. The affected side of the chest does not move, and is dull to percussion. X-rays reveal a pleural effusion, and pleural aspiration, the yellowish fat-containing chyle.

Treatment. Breathlessness is relieved by sucking out some of the effusion; since the latter contains fluid and salt, care must be taken that the baby does not become dehydrated by this treatment. Surgical repair of the ruptured lymphatic is unnecessary, as spontaneous healing takes place.

Diseases of the lung substance

The most important of these is asphyxia, which has already been described, and respiratory distress syndrome (R.D.S.).

Respiratory distress syndrome (hyaline membrane disease; R.D.S.)

This condition is most liable to occur in prematures, in the babies of diabetic mothers, and in infants severely affected before birth by erythroblastosis fetalis. The latter are usually severely edematous (hydropic). The cause of R.D.S. is not fully known, but there is a definite decrease in the surfactant of the lungs. This is a fatty substance which acts to reduce surface tension (as does a detergent), thus aiding lung expansion at the first breath. In R.D.S. the alveoli collapse, and become lined by a proteinaceous material (the hyaline membrane).

Physiological consequences. Since the alveoli do not function, gas exchange cannot take place across them. Thus oxygenation and carbon dioxide clearance are interfered with. Thus arterial O_2 content (pO_2) decreases, pCO_2 increases, and pH decreases. If blood continues to go to the collapsed alveoli without being oxygenated, then arterial O_2 content decreases again. Also the alveolar disease increases the pressure in the lung vessels, which will tend to keep open the ductus arteriosus, and even cause shunting through it from the pulmonary artery to the aorta—a situation reminiscent of that occurring in asphyxia.

Clinical features. Respiratory distress syndrome is least unexpected in premature babies born with a low Apgar rating and difficult to resuscitate. In these babes the respiratory pattern is never quite normal, and within a few hours of birth there is undoubted distress. This is heralded by an increase in the rate of breathing, soon followed by increasingly labored respiration, sufficient to cause rib and sternal recession, flaring of the nostrils and expiratory grunt. The baby looks tired and the colour goes off—she looks less pink and may have definite attacks of cyanosis. The pulse is rapid and of good quality and the baby can still cry strongly if disturbed. At this stage oxygen is often given, and the distress is relieved. The colour may improve, but the rapid breathing and grunting continue. In many babies, however, episodes of pallor anticipate a return of increasing respiratory distress, increasing cyanosis, and unrelieved rib retraction. In spite of this, the chest is fixed in strong inspiration and little air is coming or going from the chest. No stethoscope is needed to show that air entry is poor. Apart from strenuous breathing, the baby is inactive, then flaccid, and soon there is edema of the hands and feet. Sooner or later the infant becomes exhausted, the eyes become glassy, and breathing slows. Cyanosis is now intensified, there is little response even to a painful stimulus, and the heart slows. Twitching and marked flaccidity warns that bleeding into the brain has occurred, or apneic episodes increase in number and duration until breathing cannot be restored.

Other babies are born crying and vigorous, may take a feed and seem well even for a day or two. Then the babe becomes restless, cries, and is seen to be breathing a little rapidly. The respiration rate invariably increases, rib retraction and grunting begin. The whole may accelerate into the situation described, or happily, may continue only for an hour or two after which the breathing slows, the baby sleeps, and all is well.

Diagnosis. R.D.S. is an emergency, first witnessed by the nurses, who must report it forthwith; the first thing which will follow a rapid examination is a chest x-ray. This is because respiratory difficulty is an unspecific finding, and only x-rays can distinguish such treatable conditions as diaphragmatic hernia, pneumothorax, and lobar emphysema. The main point about the x-rays is that these latter possibilities are absent, since early films of R.D.S. may be reported as normal. Progress films show that the lungs are more transparent than normal, then the disorder of the alveoli shows as a diffuse granular pattern within the lungs. This pattern may coalesce and become coarser, and the air-filled bronchi become abnormally obvious (the air bronchogram). The heart is enlarged in most x-rays of babies with R.D.S.

Other tests. Once respiratory distress is established, an umbilical arterial catheter is usually placed, and in the severe form of the disease, the blood pO_2 and pH declines, and the pCO_2 increases—usually in that order. In mildly affected infants, the pH usually falls, but the pO_2 and pCO_2 may show little change.

In the terminal phase, blood glucose falls, and the potassium and lactic acid values rise.

Prognosis. Death is usual in the small (<1,000 gm) baby with early severe disease. In these, exhaustion, ashen cyanosis, apnea and a slow heart herald death, as does evidence of intracranial bleeding; extreme changes in pO_2, pH, pCO_2 and a fall in body temperature are usually also present. The more mildly affected babies respond to oxygen treatment, breathe less rapidly, and quickly reverse their abnormalities of pO_2, pH, and pCO_2. The respiratory difficulty decreases steadily over 48-72 hours and the baby becomes more active and begins to demand food.

Treatment. Nothing specific is known, and the present modes of treatment rely on giving vigorous oxygen treatment, adjusting pH changes with I.V. bicarbonate, and maintaining hydration and blood glucose levels by glucose/saline intravenous infusions. It is usual to aid oxygen therapy by increasing the pressure at which it is given, and if apnea occurs artificial ventilation may be needed. The indications for and details of these ways of treatment are outlined below. A close watch must be kept for decreased body temperature, and complicating disorders of the lungs such as pneumothorax or infection. The baby who is recovering from R.D.S. not uncommonly developes pneumonia, so antibiotic treatment is acceptable.

Aspiration syndrome

This consists in collapse of the alveoli by inhaled material. Thus, in fetal distress, anoxia stimulates deeper breathing movements while the baby is still in the uterus. This may cause the inhalation of the meconium which is passed as a result of fetal distress. In these babies, unwillingness to breathe, or respiratory distress, is seen at birth. During resuscitation, meconium is seen in the larynx, or wells up through the endotracheal tube. The condition also occurs after birth, particularly in premature babies whose esophageal sphincter more readily allows regurgitation of feeds, or in infants with tracheoesophageal fistula.

Clinical features. Unless the aspirated material is seen at the time of resuscitation, there are no specific features. The baby is breathless at birth, or as soon as the inhalation occurs. Dyspnea progresses to rib retraction, and often cyanosis, and the whole symptomatology may become indistinguishable from R.D.S.

X-rays. These show a coarse granular pattern of lobular collapse of the lung. In gross inhalation, whole lobes may collapse.

Treatment. Laryngoscopy may be done and if material can be seen welling up from the trachea it should be gently aspirated. The treatment is otherwise that for R.D.S. with full antibiotic treatment.

Pneumonia in the newborn

This may complicate aspiration, cause R.D.S., occur as part of a septicemia, or arise of itself. Sometimes it follows prolonged rupture of the amniotic membranes. The inflammation tends to affect small, diffuse areas of the lung—it is bronchopneumonic. Several organisms can cause pneumonia, and of these the most dangerous are staphylococcus and *Pneumocystis carinii* (a parasite) as well as *E.coli* and fungal species.

Clinical features. The infant is commonly normal for a day or two, then develops rapid, difficult respiration, usually with some rib retraction. Refusal to feed is common and the temperature is raised except in the prematures. Cyanosis occurs, but much less often than in R.D.S. A significant finding is that the baby breathes out deeply and effectively—a contrast to the air trapping of R.D.S. Anemia and a high white count are common. In advanced illness, the biochemical findings are those of any severe insult to the lungs—low pO_2 and pH and increased pCO_2.

X-rays. These show obvious patchy, definite consolidation.

Treatment. Broad spectrum antibiotics (e.g., ampicillin) are given until blood or throat culture shows a specific organism and sensitivity. The accelerated breathing promotes water and salt loss, so an intravenous glucose/saline infusion is necessary.

Other respiratory disorders

Some of these are complications of the treatment of sick prematures. Thus, *bronchopulmonary dysplasia* occurs in infants who have required aided respiration for some days. *Wilson-Mikity syndrome* occurs in prematures who are several weeks old. Prolonged exposure to high levels of inspired oxygen may also cause troubles.

The symptoms are of mild to moderate respiratory distress, with minor degrees of cyanosis, but without cough. The exact diagnosis is made largely on the x-ray signs found in the lungs.

Functional disorders of the respiratory system

This affects the low birth weight dysmature infant and is due to failure of the respiratory centre to stimulate the muscles of breathing. The condition presents as:

Apneic attacks

Clinical features. The infant usually has well-marked, periodic breathing which resembles the Cheyne-Stokes pattern of waxing and waning respiration. The apneic gap in breathing prolongs until slight skin mottling is seen, and then is followed by increased efforts to breathe, often sufficient to cause rib retraction. Eventually the spells last long enough to cause cyanosis, sometimes with some trembling of the limbs, and then increase in frequency until the baby cannot breathe by himself. In the early stages, the breathing can be restored by flicking the feet, or moving the child. In the later stages, even painful stimuli are ineffective.

The time of onset of apneic attacks is quite variable, and in very small prematures may exist from the time of resuscitation. In others they begin after a few hours of satisfactory breathing. If apneic spells begin 3-14 days after birth, they may be secondary to septicemia, intracranial hemorrhage, hypothermia, R.D.S., and various metabolic disorders such as hypoglycemia.

Treatment. This is not easy, since there is no specific method of stimulating breathing. The infant should be admitted to an intensive care unit, equipped with some means of signalling that breathing has stopped (an apnea monitor). When breathing stops, the nurse flicks the heels, or moves the child, to restart it. If this stimulates breathing enough to relieve cyanosis, then stay on the alert. If not, then oxygenation should be helped by bag and mask usually with an air/oxygen mixture. If this is insufficient, and arterial blood samples show a fall in pO_2 and pH, and rise in pCO_2, then mechanical ventilation should be started. Essential ancillary treatments are maintenance of hydration by intravenous infusion, the relief of hypoglycemia by I.V. glucose, and the correction of low pH values with bicarbonate.

Prognosis. This is always guarded, especially if the infant's weight is very low. In this circumstance even a few prolonged apneic spells may cause death. Neurological damage may occur in the survivors more or less in proportion to the severity, frequency, and total duration of the disorder.

Heart and circulatory disorders in the newborn

The most serious of these are due to congenital heart disease, which causes an appreciable mortality in this age group.

Cardiac murmurs

These are common in the newborn, occur in up to 20% of normals, but usually disappear by the end of the first week. Most of these are due to the presence of a patent ductus arteriosus—which is not unexpected in view of the pattern of the transitional circulation. In most children the ductus closes unless it is compensating restricted blood flow to the lungs, as in transposition of the great vessels.

Some specific disorders

Only those which often cause trouble in the newborn will be considered. The other disorders are related in another section of this book (p. 260).

Transposition of the great vessels

In this condition, the left ventricle pumps blood to the lungs, and the right ventricle supplies the body. This is the opposite of normal; obviously the baby has no trouble before birth, since his lungs do not function. After birth, life cannot continue unless there is some method of mixing the right and left heart circulation. This can be done by way of a patent ductus, an atrial septal defect, or a ventricular septal defect. If all 3 communications are present, then baby may be fairly well compensated; if only a ductus is present (with its tendency to close anyway) the baby may be in serious trouble quite early in life.

Clinical features. The infant is usually normal at birth. Within a few days he is breathing rapidly and becomes cyanosed, at first intermittently, and then all the time. The weight chart may show excessive gain—an early sign of congestive cardiac failure. Then frank edema occurs, usually as swelling of the hands, feet, eyes, and face. Cardiac murmurs may never be heard, but if they are reported suggest the presence of one of the compensatory defects mentioned above.

The main point in the diagnosis is to consider the possibility before the heart fails. Accordingly, the most suspicious circumstance is cyanosis. Unlike the blueness of lung disease, the cyanosis of transposition is not relieved by high concentrations of oxygen. Other useful clues are a fast heart rate, and an easily felt heart beat at the chest wall.

X-rays. These show an enlarged heart, and lungs which show very prominent arteries (vascular plethora). The root of the heart also seems narrower than normal. If the baby has developed heart failure, hypoglycemia, low body temperature, and acidosis may also be present.

Treatment. It is essential to improve the exchange of blood between the right and left heart. This is done at cardiac catheterization, when the diagnosis is confirmed by angiography.

By this technique radiopaque dye is injected into the blood vessels to show their abnormal origin from the heart. The treatment which is given is to create an atrial septal defect by placing a special catheter, tipped by an inflatable bag, into the left atrium. The bag is filled with dye as a marker and then pulled back forcibly through the foramen ovale (a normal slit separating right and left atria). This rips the atrial septum and allows better mixing of blood to take place. This is essentially an emergency procedure which will allow the baby to survive until more radical operation can be done. It is called the Rashkind operation.

Hypoplasia of the heart

This means that one of the ventricles is grossly underdeveloped, or absent. If this happens, then the blood vessel to which the ventricle pumps blood will atrophy, and the valve at the entrance to the ventricle undergoes the same fate. Thus in left heart hypoplasia, the mitral valve and first part of the aorta are small and often functionless. In right heart hypoplasia, the tricuspid valve and main pulmonary artery are in a similar condition. These abnormalities may be partly compensated by large ductus arteriosus, or by atrial and ventricular septal defects.

Clinical features. The baby is normal at birth, then shortly begins to seem unwell, refuses to feed, becomes increasingly breathless and blue, and becomes cold. Rising body weight is evidence of congestive failure and death may be sudden.

The other features of right and left heart hypoplasia are very similar. In the latter, the best guide to the diagnosis is that the femoral pulses cannot be felt—reflecting the tiny aorta found in this condition.

Differential diagnosis. This is principally from advanced untreated hypoglycemia in which hypothermia, edema, and breathlessness can all occur. In these babies—almost always small—trouble has existed from birth, and twitching is prominent. The blood sugar is very low, and the symptoms are relieved by intravenous glucose. Another important consideration is confusion with septicemia of the newborn; in this the onset of symptoms may be delayed for a day or two, signs of cardiac failure are not prominent, the heart is not greatly enlarged, and the blood culture is positive.

Congestive cardiac failure in the newborn

Transposition of the great vessels or ventricular hypoplasia are the common causes. In a few babies a true inflammation of the heart muscle (myocarditis) due to the Coxsackie virus, or a very fast heart rate from an abnormal focus of stimulation (supraventricular tachycardia), may be relevant.

Clinical features. Those of heart failure are superimposed on those of the primary disease. A common early sign is an increased respiratory rate, often with some rib retraction. Central cyanosis will occur when the venous and arterial blood can mix, e.g., in transposition. The baby gains weight rapidly (or fails to lose, as is normal in the first day or two), and develops swelling of the hands, feet, eyes, and face. This edema may rapidly become generalized. The venous pressure rises and this may best be appreciated by finding a bulging fontanelle. The liver also enlarges as edema becomes apparent. Listening to the heart may reveal murmurs, but the most constant sign is the gallop sound which tells that a ventricle is in trouble. Hypothermia, hypoglycemia, and acidosis complicate congestive failure when it is very severe.

Treatment. The principles are to give digoxin, maintain hydration, and give diuretics with caution. Diuretics cause loss of water and sodium, and more than modest doses may cause dehydration and low blood pressure which can embarrass the circulation more than congestive failure itself.

BLOOD DISORDERS IN THE NEWBORN

Babies can have any of the hematological disorders outlined in chapter 14. However, blood loss, and blood destruction, can be very dangerous to newborns, so these will be given particular consideration.

Anemia due to acute blood loss

There are many causes of this, some of which, e.g., injuries or a slipped cord ligature, have already been mentioned. Causes which exist before birth include accidental hemorrhage in the mother (placenta previa), bleeding from the fetus into the mother, or, in multiple pregnancy, loss of blood from one twin to another. Babies do not tolerate blood loss, so that a bleed of 30-50 ml which would be insignificant in older children can give rise to serious trouble in the newborn.

Clinical features. In rapid blood loss, the baby is pale, breathless, has rib retraction, a rapid heart, an active busy heart beat, and lowered blood pressure. Cold blue limbs is a common association.

In less acute bleeds, pallor coexists with signs of high cardiac output—some increase in respiration rate, quick heart, and bounding pulses. In all bleeding babies the hemoglobin level is reduced.

Treatment. Rapid blood transfusion is given through the umbilical or scalp veins.

As soon as the blood pressure is restored and the baby looks better, the drip is slowed, and the full transfusion given over the next 24 hours.

Anemias due to blood destruction

These are of very great importance since the main product of destruction (hemolysis) is bilirubin. This bilirubin can attach itself to the brain substance, particularly the basal ganglia, causing neurological disease. At worst the interference causes early death, or survival may be associated with deafness, mental retardation, or cerebral palsy.

Thus, the jaundice of hemolysis is more important than the anemia, and the removal of bilirubin may benefit the baby more than giving a blood transfusion.

Some specific entities

Erythroblastosis fetalis

Formerly this was the commonest of the red cell destroying diseases, but it is now largely preventable. The background and genetics are described in full elsewhere (p. 327) but essentially there is incompatibility between the blood of the mother and that of the infant. Thus a maternal blood subgroup is Rh negative and that of the baby is Rh positive. These are also identified by the genotypes D and d; i.e., a mother who is Rh positive has the genotype d, and the baby genotype D. When the mother becomes pregnant, some of the fetal cells escape into her circulation (this happens in all pregnancies irrespective of blood types). She destroys these cells, which are foreign to her body, by making substances called agglutinins. These take time to manufacture, so in her first pregnancy she is stimulated to make them, but her baby is not affected. In the next pregnancy, she makes agglutinins more rapidly, and in sufficient quantity to pass through the placenta and enter the baby. The result is that the baby's red cells are destroyed by these invading maternal agglutinins.

Clinical features. These are quite variable, running the gamut from the stillborn baby to one who has no obvious trouble at birth. The major signs and symptoms are due to the destruction of blood, and the production of excess bilirubin. Stillborn babies are often markedly edematous (hydropic) because the long-continued anemia while in the womb has caused the baby's heart to fail. In most instances, however, the baby looks normal at birth—perhaps yellow vernix may be the only warning sign. If blood destruction is severe, the baby becomes intensely jaundiced within a few hours of birth, pallor is usual and purpuric spots, or even frank bruising, not unusual. The spleen and liver are enlarged, and the baby shows the effect of anemia on the circulation—fast pulse, bounding pulses, and a busy heart when its beat is felt.

In many instances, however, the picture is a less dramatic one, with jaundice appearing only after 12 or more hours, with fewer circulatory signs and only moderate enlargement of the liver and spleen.

Special tests are as follows.

1. *In the mother*
   a. She is Rh positive.
   b. The agglutinins referred to can be tested for in the mother's blood. As a rough rule, the higher the titre (i.e., the greater dilution of the mother's sample at which agglutinins can be found) the more likely is disease in the baby. If several samples from the mother show a rising titre, the baby is again more likely to be affected.
   c. If the amniotic fluid is aspirated from the uterus before birth (amniocentesis) it can be checked for the presence of bilirubin derived from the unborn baby. The higher the reading, the more likely is severe disease in the infant.
2. *In the baby*
   a. The baby is Rh negative.
   b. The mother's agglutinins can be found in a sample of the baby's blood (the Coombs' test is positive).
   c. The baby is anemic—the hemoglobin and red blood count levels have fallen both in cord blood and blood from the baby.
   d. The bilirubin, derived from red cell breakdown (indirect form of bilirubin) is high.
   e. Early red cell forms (nucleated erythroblasts) are found to excess in the blood film. This is evidence only of blood destruction.

Now, why all the noise about this condition? Well, as already noted, babies' brains, especially those of prematures, are very liable to fix the excess of bilirubin and this causes death or permanent disorder. The condition is called kernicterus.

Kernicterus

Clinical features. The baby has been very jaundiced for a day or two. Then he stops moving, refuses to feed, twitches, or even has an obvious convulsion. He is irritable, and develops an unusual high-pitched cry. He tends to lie rigidly at attention—extensor spasm in the name given to this—and it may advance until he is opisthotonic, that is his head, legs, and body are curved backwards like a bow. The Moro reflex disappears, he may become cold and unresponsive and die suddenly with massive bleeding from the lung. All of this is accelerated if he is premature; if he survives, he is likely still not to move or feed well and as time goes on he obviously has developed neurological damage, sometimes mental retardation, and often deafness.

It is to prevent kernicterus that exchange transfusion is the *treatment of erythroblastosis*. The principle here is to remove the Rh negative cells from the baby, and replace them with Rh positive cells; these cannot be broken down by the maternal agglutinins—which soon disappear anyway—so that the excess bilirubin of blood destruction cannot come about. Shortly, this involves removing the baby's blood and replacing it with ABO compatible Rh(D) negative donor blood.

The indications for exchange transfusion in erythroblastosis fetalis are:

1. Prematurity, with Coombs' test positive
2. Clinically affected within a few hours of birth whatever birth weight.
3. Cord blood hemoglobin 15 g or less
4. Cord blood bilirubin 2.5 mg or more
5. Postnatal bilirubin of 18-20 mg% (usually indication for repeat exchange transfusion).

The technique of exchange transfusion

This is described in detail elsewhere. Essentially it consists in removing small quantities of the baby's blood, intermittently or continuously, and replacing this with donor blood until at least twice the baby's blood volume (blood volume in ml = baby's weight in kg x 100) has been exchanged. The procedure may require repetition if the baby's bilirubin values rise again to levels which might cause kernicterus.

It should be noted that exchange transfusion may be required in ANY condition which causes blood destruction, and rise in the indirect bilirubin values—not just in Rh incompatibility.

Erythroblastosis. Due to ABO and other incompatibilities (e.g., Kell subgroup) and generally gives a clinical picture similar to that described for mild or moderate Rh incompatibility. The indications for exchange transfusion are similar, the donor blood given to the baby being compatible with it, except in that factor which is sensitive to the mother's agglutinins.

Hemolysis due to red cell enzyme deficiency

There are many such deficiences (described in full on p. 320), but the commonest is of glucose-6-phosphate dehydrogenase (G6PD). When this is present, the red cell is readily broken down, especially when the baby has been given certain drugs (e.g., sulphonamides, some types of vitamin K) or if he is exposed to broad-bean products (favism). The latter is unusual in the nursery, so drugs are the usual cause.

Plethora of the newborn

This implies an increase in blood volume, hemoglobin level, hematocrit and blood viscosity. It is not a common disorder, usually being found in twin pregnancy, the recipient being plethoric and the donor anemic.

Clinical features. The infant has a slightly purple skin colour. This may darken on crying to simulate cyanosis; other features are usually absent, although coincident respiratory distress syndrome may occur. In an occasional instance, lethargy and convulsions may occur after a day or two. Congestive cardiac failure is a dubious association.

Diagnosis. This depends upon finding a hemoglobin level of >25 g% with a hematocrit of 60%, in a baby who has not suffered fluid loss. It is important to exclude other causes of lethargy and convulsions (e.g., septicemia, hypoglycemia) before accepting that plethora is causal.

Treatment. This is seldom necessary, as the hemoglobin levels fall spontaneously within 3-7 days. If cardiac embarrassment is felt to be due to the plethora, then a slow exchange transfusion may be of value.

Jaundice in the newborn

This has a multitude of causes, most of them discussed in full elsewhere (p. 227). In newborns, hemolysis is the main cause of jaundice. It is physiological for hemoglobin values to fall by 4-6 g% in the first 10 days of life as part of the change of hemoglobin from fetal to adult type.

As the liver is functionally immature at this age, it may not be able to deal with the breakdown products of this red cell destruction, so that a minor degree of hyperbilirubinemia is common, the main part of the bile being the indirect (unconjugated) form. This is the usual cause of the so-called physiological jaundice. The condition is of no clinical moment except in occasional dysmature infants where high bilirubin levels (e.g., 18+ mg%) may indicate exchange transfusion or phototherapy.

Otherwise, the hemolytic disorders already mentioned (erythroblastosis, red cell enzyme deficiencies) make up the major cause of neonatal jaundice, followed by red cell destruction by septicemia or viremia (e.g., congenital rubella). Neonatal hepatitis is a rare disease which causes the liver cells to swell, thus blocking the flow of bile, while the cells proper do not function adequately; both aspects cause jaundice. The jaundice of congenital obstruction of the bile ducts is seldom suspected until after the first week of life. Some aspects of differential diagnosis are shown in table 5 but reference should also be made to the appropriate pages elsewhere (pp. 227-32).

METABOLIC DISORDERS OF THE NEWBORN

These are of major importance in the dysmature infant. The commoner lesions are hypoglycemia, hypothermia, and edema of the newborn.

Table 5. Differential diagnosis of neonatal jaundice

Condition	Association	Time of Appearance	Special Investigations
Hemolytic (increased bilirubin production)			
Erythroblastosis	Rh; ABO incompatability	At or shortly after birth	Indirect bilirubin, high (2.5) Coomb's test positive, low hemoglobin
Extravascular hemolysis	Large enclosed hemorrhage, e.g., subgaleal	1–2 days after birth	Low hemoglobin, high indirect bilirubin
Red cell enzyme deficiency	G–6–PD[9] pyruvate kinase, etc.	1–2 days after birth Drugs: sulphas, Vit. K., Novobiocin, naphthalene	Enzyme deficient in RBCs
Abnormal shape	Familial spherocytosis	1–5 days after birth	Spherocytes visible on film RBC value increased
Impaired liver function			
Physiological jaundice	Deficient glucuronyl transferase	1–2 days after birth Normal fall in hemoglobin accompanies	Indirect bilirubin high especially in prematures
Crigler-Najjar disease	Deficient glucosurosyl transferase	Birth or soon after Kernicterus is common	Indirect bilirubin high NO anemia
Septicemia	Sick infant; jaundice later	Not at birth; 2–7 days usually	Direct/indirect hyperbilirubinemia
Viremia	Rubella: cytomegalovirus, herpes virus – maternal infection; Small-for-dates babies	A few hours to a few days after birth	Direct/indirect hyperbilirubinemia, Associated cardiac, eye defects, virus isolation
Neonatal hepatitis	Maternal infection	1–2 days after birth	Direct/indirect hyperbilirubinemia S.G.P.T.: S.G.O.T. + early
Obstructed biliary system			
Congenital biliary atresia Choledochal cyst		1–2 days after birth	Direct hyperbilirubinemia early S.G.P.T.: S.G.O.T. + late Fecal bilirubin reduced

Hypoglycemia

This may occur in any group of infants. It is, however, more likely in the simple premature, a small-for-dates baby, and in the infant of the diabetic mother; neglected, the disease can cause death, or extensive brain damage.

Glucose values in the newborn are normally lower than in the older child or adult. This difference, however, persists for only a few days, and is presumably related to the low levels of liver glycogen found at birth. Various surveys have been made of the blood glucose values (glucose oxidase method) existing in apparently normal babies. Values as low as 20 mg% have been reported in apparently normal babies. Whether these are in turn associated with total normality (e.g., educability) at a later date is not yet known. For practical purposes, a true blood glucose (glucose oxidase or equivalent method) of$<$40 mg% should be thought of as worthy or treatment, *irrespective of the infant's clinical condition*.

Case finding. This may be based upon biochemical survey, or by waiting for the emergence of suspicious clinical features. Ideally (and this is not impossible), all infants should have a biochemical survey. In any case, infants at high risk—the dysmature infants—must have such tests done.

Methods. These must be based upon the glucose oxidase method. Other tehniques which also measure other carbohydrates (e.g., copper reduction) are useless in that they give spuriously high glucose values. A useful preliminary test can be made by the use of glucose-oxidase impregnated sticks of papers (e.g., Dextrostix). These methods bear a good relation to values obtained by more sophisticated methods at the normal or high range (50 mg%+).

The correlation below these values is imperfect. Accordingly, values read as lower than 50 mg% must be checked by another method, or a decision made that such a reading (Dextrostix$<$50 mg%) is an indication for treatment.

Clinical features of hypoglycemia. In many instances, the early features represent only a minor deviation from normal, and may be missed where nursing or pediatric staff have large numbers of infants to care for.

Common early signs are tremulousness or twitching, which occur spontaneously, unlike the lesser degrees of tremulousness occurring when small babies are stimulated. Exaggeration of the normal periodic pattern of breathing, with apneic spells, and cyanotic attacks, is also common. The latter may appear without any previous symptoms. Difficulty in feeding or refusal to feed is a common although unspecific symptom; frank convulsions are a late sign, as is skin mottling and the appearance of circulatory signs such as tachycardia, gallop rhythm, and low blood pressure. A few infants with these signs will show clinical and radiological evidence of enlarged heart. All of these may be superimposed upon the ordinary appearance of the small-for-dates baby, or the baby of the diabetic mother; the latter is often heavy for the gestation period, has a swollen plethoric face (Cushingoid) and shows peripheral edema. Symptoms of hypoglycemia may also occur in respiratory distress syndrome, erythroblastosis fetalis, severe congenital heart disease, hypothermia, and septicemia of the newborn.

Hypocalcemia is a frequent concomitant of hypoglycemia, irrespective of the underlying disease.

Differential diagnosis. This is principally from septicemia of the newborn, intracranial hemorrhage, and the various unrelated metabolic disorders. The cardinal supporting evidence is the glucose values, and usually the onset of symptoms in the first 24 hours of life. The rapid response of the infant to glucose is also, to some extent, diagnostic. It is usually wiser to carry out blood culture on infants with apparent symptomatic hypoglycemia. Of the metabolic disorders, hypocalcemia (without hypoglycemia) is of later onset (3-7 days), and has the appropriate finding of low serum calcium and high serum phosphate. Hypomagnesemia may complicate exchange transfusion with citrated blood—the citrate binds the Mg^+—or occur as a primary metabolic disorder. Both magnesium and calcium values are low, but the phosphate values are normal. The symptoms of phenylketonuria, maple syrup urine disease, galactosemia, and other metabolic diseases are usually delayed for 2-3 days and have appropriate biochemical findings.

Treatment of hypoglycemia:

1. Prophylactic. There is evidence that the early feeding of infants with 10% glucose solution (say within 4-8 hours of birth) will reduce the incidence of hypoglycemia. This practice is in general to be commended, provided that *small* volumes are given, and that skilled nursing help is available, especially for the low birth weight infant. (see this chapter, p. 000).

2. Active treatment. This consists in the intravenous administration of glucose solution, commonly by way of the umbilical or scalp veins; if the infant has symptoms an initial injection of 50% glucose (1-2 ml/kg) is followed by a maintenance infusion of 10% glucose until the monitored blood glucose values have been stable for 24 hours; in asymptomatic hypoglycemia, as discovered by biochemical survey, 10%

glucose is given intravenously until glucose values have been normal for 24 hours.

If calcium values cannot readily be measured as a routine, or if the results are delayed, calcium gluconate 10% (1 ml/kg) should be added to the infusion of glucose. If these treatments do not promptly relieve the infant's condition, consideration must be given to other serious conditions in which hypoglycemia is only part of a more serious whole.

Prognosis. Most infants suffering isolated hypoglycemia will not die if adequately treated. Damage to the nervous system or intellect is always a possibility, and prolonged follow-up is necessary before a firm opinion can be given concerning this aspect.

Hypothermia (see also "Neonatal cold injury", p. 46)

The dysmature infant tends to lose heat more than the normal infant. This is especially liable to occur during resuscitation, transfer from the labour room to the nursery, or transfer between hospitals. Hypothermia is also an important secondary sign in neonatal septicemia, congenital heart disease, and severe central system disease. Hypothermia is present if the infant's temperature is 35°C or less. Temperatures must of course be recorded with a low-reading thermometer. Peripheral cyanosis and mottling (cutis marmorata) are common accompanying signs, and hypoglycemia and acid/base disturbances may coexist.

Prevention. Labour rooms and resuscitation areas should be adequately heated. Small infants should *always* be nursed in an incubator for the first 36 hours, and then temperatures should frequently be monitored. Small babies should not be transferred from home to hospital except in an incubator. In an emergency warm clothes and a layer of aluminium foil are acceptable.

Treatment. Glucose and pH values should be measured. The infant is placed in an incubator which is set to allow the infant's temperature to increase. Constant monitoring is of course necessary. In mild hypothermia 33.5°-35°C, the return to 36°C should occupy 2-4 hours. In more severe disorders, the rise to the same level will require 12-24 hours.

Simple edema of the newborn

This is almost always found in small babies. The swelling can be seen in the face, legs, genitals, and pubic areas. The skin is shiny, feels puffy, and pits on pressure over the brow, shins, and backs of the hands. In most instances, the edema disappears within 48-72 hours of birth, with a concomitant fall in weight. Edema of a similar sort, but of greater degree, may be seen in the infant of the diabetic mother. Simple edema must be distinguished from the edema of hydrops fetalis, congestive cardiac failure, cold injury, and over hydration due to excessive intravenous or gastric tube treatments. The edema of *idiopathic hypoproteinemia* persists for weeks or months, and has appropriate biochemical findings. Local edema (of the hands and feet) occurs in the Bonnevie-Ulrich-Turner syndrome and in the rare Milroy's disease. In these, a lymphatic etiology is likely.

Other metabolic disorders of importance in the newborn are galactosemia, phenylketonuria, and maple-syrup urine disease. Many such diseases are sought by mass screening studies of blood or urine, and an important responsibility of those caring for newborns is the collection and delivery of such samples. The conditions are considered in detail in chapter 5.

DISORDERS OF THE ALIMENTARY SYSTEM IN THE NEWBORN

These are covered in full elsewhere (chapter 10). Particular attention should be given to the section on tracheoesophageal fistula (chapter 10), neonatal intestinal obstruction (chapter 10), and anorectal anomalies (chapter 10).

Appendix 1: Basic requirements, first 6 months

Fluid 150 ml/kg body weight
Calories 110-120 ml/kg body weight

Formula used

1. *Whole-milk based*

Milk	450 ml
Water	150 ml
Sugar	30 g

2. *Evaporated milk*
   Add 90 ml to 150 ml water, add 15 g sugar per 240 ml formula.
3. *Dried milk*
   Reconstitute with water, 1 part dried milk by volume to 8 of water, add 15 g sugar to 240 ml of formula.

Feeds

Newborn	6-10 feeds daily
1 month	5-7 feeds daily
6 months	4-5 feeds daily

General

Introduce whole milk at 5-6 months.
Introduce mixed feeding at 3-4 months.
Begin with cereal, banana, commercially available baby foods. Spoon feed.
Weaning from the bottle—at baby's discretion.
Stop sterilizing formula when baby crawling on the floor, i.e., 6-7 months, provided a safe whole-milk supply is available.

Comparison of cow and breast milk (g%)

	Human (%)	*Cow* (%)
Protein	1-1.5	3-4
Carbohydrate	7-7.5	4.5-5
Fat	3.5-4	3.5-5
Calcium	0.1-0.25	0.75
Phosphorus	0.015-0.040	0.090-0.196
Iron	0.0001	0.00004*

(*N.B. low level)

Appendix 2: Feeding of premature infants

Weight	**Age of first feeding (glucose solutions)**	
1,000-1,200 g	4-8 hours	unless evidence of hypoglycemia
1,800-2,000 g	6-8 hours	

Ultimate feeding interval

Small premature 1.0-1.6 kg —2-3 hours
Larger premature to 2.5 kg —3 hourly

Foods available

Breast milk, or evaporated/fresh milk mixtures yielding 20 cal/30 ml

Daily vitamins

A 1,500 U
C 50 mg
D 400 I.U. (from all sources)

Amount offered

The fluid requirement will ultimately be up to 150 ml/kg/day; sterile 10% glucose is normally given in the first 24 hours of feeding. Thereafter, the mixture should contain at least 20 cal/30 ml. In the small premature, the first day's feeds should be about 1/6-1/4 of the calculated total 24-hour intake. This is increased daily to reach the full need in 4-5 days. In bigger prematures, this level may be reached in 2-3 days. An intake of at least 120 cal/kg should be reached within 2 weeks of birth.

Appendix 3: Intensive care and aided respiration in newborns

Intensive care of newborns implies more frequent and more sophisticated observations which can be used either to anticipate disease or to treat established disorders more effectively. In modern units, machines are used to measure temperature, heart rate, respiration rate, and blood pressure. This allows nurses to be sure of these observations, and frees them to devote more time to direct nursing care.

METHODS

Measurements of temperature. This is usually done by a thermistor taped to the skin. Its output is taken to an amplifier and then to the display cabinet. Core or deep body temperatures are measured rectally in the same way. A thermistor is sensitive enough for testing to be done by blowing on it. This cools it, and the temperature drop is shown. Misleading readings may occur if the thermistor is placed on the skin near a source of radiant heat.

Pulse rate. This is measured by the electrocardiogram (ECG) usually through 2 chest electrodes. These must make good contact with the skin through a saline conductor in order to give reliable signals. Drying out of the electrode contact pad is a frequent cause of failure.

Respiration rate. This is measurable by a variety of devices. The most common one utilizes the chest electrodes used for ECGs and measures the difference in electrical impedance caused by chest movement. This is displayed at a central console, which usually is equipped with a visual or audible alarm which trips if respiration stops. The *apnea mattress* is an alarm which can signal only that breathing has stopped. It cannot measure respiration rate.

Blood pressure. This is measured from a catheter placed in the umbilical artery and put in communication with a strain gauge; the signal from the latter is amplified and can be calibrated by using a sphygmomanometer.

All such signals can be displayed on an oscilloscope (essentially a T.V. screen). Usually only 2 signals, e.g., heart rate, pressure, can be shown at one time, but the others can be switched in as necessary. Meters or digital readout are also used to display results.

A very great amount of information can be obtained, but much of it is of little interest. The nurse is taught to be able to recognize and report certain important patterns, or to use such patterns to initiate a course of action. Thus, if the respiratory rate and heart rate are both noted to be falling, preparation is made to resuscitate by bag-and-mask oxygen, and pediatric help is summoned, or the apnea alarm goes off and the nurse stimulates the baby's breathing by flicking the heels.

Much intensive care is carried out on babies who are in humidicribs, with arterial and venous catheters in place, and with CPAP or even respirators in use. None of this gear must deter the nursing staff from frequent direct inspection of the baby. Attention to pressure areas and regular shifting of the baby's position as well as routine changing of nappies, etc., are even more essential in babies who are in intensive care. Infection is a constant fear in these babies, partly from any disease present (e.g., R.D.S.) and partly from the intravascular catheters and resuscitating apparatus which may be in use. As far as possible, all such items should be disposable once-only-use type. The permanent equipment should be sterilized regularly and efficiently. Bacteriological surveys should be done often, of both attending staff and permanent equipment.

Again, it should be quite clear that the use of intensive care units demands a large number of nurses for each patient by day and by night. Their time is to be conserved by quick methods of getting information. The conserved time is used to improve the care of the patient. Weaning babies from intensive care, e.g., aided respiration, may be quite tedious and should always be carried out in a situation where the more sophisticated technique can early be restored.

An important aspect of nursing care in the intensive care unit is the collection and delivery of biochemistry samples. The most frequent test which is made is of pO_2, pCO_2, and pH. This is done on a single sample; sealing, identifying, and storing the sample must be done meticulously. A running total of the blood loss due to tests must be kept and the pediatrician reminded when some arbitrary blood loss level has been reached.

Intravenous fluid is often given in the intensive care unit. Because of the small volumes needed, a drip is inaccurate. A motor-driven syringe is used, as it can be accurately preset to deliver small volumes at constant pressure. The latter is essential if intraarterial infusions are given, since ordinary drip sets would stop. Constant infusion apparatus should use as many disposable items as possible. Preliminary calibration of the volume delivery against the machine settings must always be carried out. In prolonged infusions, a special filter, designed to trap bacteria and other particles, may be put in the circuit.

MAINTAINING NORMAL BLOOD OXYGEN LEVELS

This may be needed if the baby has a lung disorder which prevents adequate oxygenation. Where the baby can still breathe strongly, devices which change the normal pressure difference between the lung and the outside air can be used to increase blood O_2 levels. If the device increases this transpulmonary pressure, essentially by pushing air into the baby, it is called the continuous positive airways pressure (CPAP) method. If it depends upon decreasing the external pressure on the chest, then it is a continuous negative pressure (CNP) device. Each device can be used only if the baby is able to breathe. They are not true artificial ventilators, but add to the efficiency of the baby's own breathing.

CPAP devices. There are several of these. Essentially air/oxygen mixtures are supplied to the baby's airway at a pressure higher than that of his chest wall. The differences lie in where the pressure is applied, Thus, it may be applied to the face and mouth by a mask, to the nose by an airway supplying each nostril, to the whole airway by sealing the head in a box, or directly to the lungs through an endotracheal tube. Whatever the point of entry, a major difficulty is to maintain a seal which will prevent leaks, but not cause direct pressure damage to the baby's tissues. Similarly, a safety valve must be put in so that the baby's lungs are not injured by the increased pressure difference across them. An advantage of CPAP is that the baby can be got at for ordinary care such as changing nappies, giving injections, and controlling I.V. therapy. This is because only a small part of his body (head, face) is sealed off.

CNP devices. These do not require a close seal around the airway, but require one around the body. This can be achieved by putting the whole body in a box, or enclosing only the chest. Suction is then applied to the thorax. Leaks must be avoided, not only to keep the apparatus working, but also to avoid a continuous air current which will drain the baby's body of heat. Safety valves are again necessary, since too much negative pressure (suction) will affect the amount of blood pumped by the heart. The advantage of CNP is that damage to the lungs is infrequent, the disadvantages lie in the difficulty in keeping the system sealed, and in getting at the baby to care for it.

AIDED RESPIRATION

1. Why?

Artificial (aided) ventilation is used to assist babies to breathe when they do not breathe of their own accord. This usually happens in prematures, when the respiratory centre in the brain fails to stimulate the respiratory apparatus, or when this apparatus fails to respond to normal stimuli. Now the lungs are used to help maintain normal acid/base (pH) balance in the body, to excrete the carbon dioxide (CO_2) so that blood CO_2 values (pCO_2) are kept within reasonable limits, and most importantly, to oxygenate the blood to a normal degree (pO_2). When breathing is interfered with, then these functions are compromised, often in the order noted. Thus pH decreases, pCO_2 rises, and pO_2 decreases. This combination is called asphyxia. The point of aided respiration is to return these functions to as near normal as possible without upsetting the baby. When blood gas analysis shows pO_2 to be less than 30 mm O_2 (in 100% O_2 atmosphere), a pCO_2 greater than 90 mm Hg, or when pH cannot be corrected by alkali to 7.2, then assisted ventilation is indicated.

2. How?

Normal breathing depends upon a muscular effort to draw air into the lung (inspiration). Breathing out (expiration) is a process which does not require much muscular effort, since the stored energy (elasticity) of the lungs is sufficient to release air from them. Therefore in most instances it is necessary only to inflate the lungs, and to rely upon elastic recoil for their emptying. This is called positive pressure respiration. If the elasticity of the lungs is compromised, then the air must also be sucked out (negative pressure respiration) but this is seldom necessary. The situation is further complicated by the fact that air must be delivered to the alveoli of the lungs since they are the functional units. The trachea and bronchi are transmission channels only, they cannot take part on oxygenating blood. These transmitting tubes make up what is called the dead space of the lungs. This dead space will be increased if connecting tubes are attached to an endotracheal tube, and if precautions are not taken, ventilation of the dead space only will occur. Obviously this does the baby no good. This situation is illustrated by considering the lungs as a half-inflated balloon. If we attach a short tube (small dead space) to the balloon, then injecting a small volume of air will cause a visible change in the size of the balloon. If we attach a long tube (large dead space) then no inflation will be seen, or in the clinical situation, we have ventilated only the non functional part of the lung. Obviously enough too, if we inflate the balloon with too much air, or air under too great a pressure, then it may burst. The same risks are implicit in ventilating babies. So then, we must supply air (or an air/oxygen mixture) at sufficient, but not excessive, pressure and volume through a system which has a small dead space, at an adequate rate each minute.

DEVICES

The simplest form of aided respiration is the *bag-and-mask*. This is capable only of positive pressure respiration, and although it has a blow-off valve which reduces the possibility of excessive inflation pressures, the volume of air delivered is unpredictable. Clearly too, it is unsuitable for prolonged use, and has a high dead space.

A simple, machine-driven bellows with a valve system which allows it to suck in a dose of air and then inject it into the baby is the basis of volume-preset ventilators. Both volume and consequently pressure are regulated by cut-off valves.

Another common type of ventilator depends upon pressure from a cylinder for its operation. This injects air (or air/oxygen) at a given pressure, which in turn determines the volume of air delivered.

All ventilators must have an apparatus for humidifying the gas mixtures put into the lungs. It must also be possible to analyze the exact percentage of oxygen being given to the patient.

Positive end expiratory pressure (PEEP) ventilation is also commonly used. This is analogous to the grunt which occurs in babies with RDS when they breathe out end-tidal air. PEEP can be readily added to volume or pressure regulated ventilators. It is a device which is placed on the expiratory side of the ventilator and slows down the flow of air coming out of the lungs. The resultant increase in pressure tends to keep open alveoli which would otherwise collapse at zero pressure. This causes an effective increase in functioning lung volume, so that the blood circulating around the alveoli can then better take up oxygen.

CONTROL OF AIDED RESPIRATION

In the normal baby, pH, pCO_2, and pO_2 and other information is constantly monitored and appraised by the respiratory centre. This feedback of information tells the respiratory centre what to do, e.g., to increase the speed or depth of respiration, or, in certain circumstances, to decrease them. Such information from the baby cannot be fed to a respirator, however, so that it is necessary, as far as possible, to collect the same information (by sampling) and to use it to control the functions of the respirator. Those items which *must* be monitored are pH, pCO_2 and PO_2 (of arterial blood), as well as heart rate and blood pressure. Generally this means that an umbilical arterial catheter is placed, and arrangements are made for appropriate samples to be analyzed.

Aided respiration must not be carried out for any length of time unless such facilities are available.

PRACTICALITIES

An endotracheal tube is passed (to cut the dead space) and carefully anchored in position. Passage through the nose is to be preferred. The respirator should have been pretested, and a source of humidified air and air/oxygen mixtures should be available. The composition of air/

oxygen mixture should be able to be checked by oxygen analyzer. Care should be taken to keep the infant warm. A ventilating bag should be used to maintain breathing until the respirator is connected and should remain nearby for emergency use. The rate, volume and blow-off pressure (PEEP) will normally be set by the physician, but all figures are a first approximation only. After the first cycles, the baby's chest is inspected to see if expansion is equal (since the endotracheal tube may have blocked off a bronchus if passed too far) and also to determine if *overexpansion* of the baby's lungs is occurring. This is evidenced not only oversplaying of the lower rib cages, but also by an undue delay in the expiratory phase. The blood gases are monitored as soon as a steady cycle has been decided upon, and a chest x-ray should be taken, principally to check that the tube has not caused any lung collapse. Clinical evidence of a good response to ventilation lies primarily in the reversal of cyanosis, fall in the pulse rate, and maintenance of normal blood pressure. Blood gas analysis will help confirm this happy result—pH should rise (to about 7.3), pCO_2 should decrease (to about 50 mm), and pO_2 should increase (to about 80—90 mm Hg). Such improvement may not, however, be maintained, or the respirator itself may overcompensate, especially in excreting CO_2, so regular monitoring continues to be necessary. Table 6 shows *approximately* the response required in relation to the blood gas findings.

Table 6. Ventilator therapy

Measurement	Response
$p0_2$ too low	Check airway Check ventilator Increase ventilatory exchange Ventilate with extra O_2 in air/O_2 mixture X-ray chest
$p0_2$ too high (100 mm+)	Discontinue or reduce O_2 in air supplied
pCO_2 too high ($>$50 mm)	Check ventilator Check dead space Increase PEEP
pCO_2 too low ($<$35 mm)	Decrease ventilatory exchange Decrease PEEP

PROBLEMS OF VENTILATION

The risk of infection is ever present, so prophylactic antibiotics may be used. The tube should be swabbed daily to identify the inevitable pathogens. Drying out of the respiratory tract is partly preventable by using humidified gas mixtures but, additionally, small volumes of saline should be injected into the endotracheal tube and general hydration must be maintained by intravenous infusion.

If oxygen is given in high concentrations for any length of time, then 2 disorders may occur. The most important (because lethal) is that the respiratory epithelium of the small air passages is so damaged as to become functionless. The other is retrolental fibroplasia (see p. 382) in which eventual blindness occurs. Therefore, oxygen should be given in the lowest concentrations, consistent with keeping the baby pink, and for the shortest possible time. In no case should the arterial pO_2 be allowed to get above 100 mm Hg.

FAILURE OF VENTILATOR THERAPY

The evidence for this is that the baby becomes blue, the pulse rises then falls, as does the blood pressure. The hands, feet, and head are cold and this is evidence of falling cardiac output. Blood samples show a rise in pCO_2 and fall in pH and pO_2. The cause may be blockage of the airway, a faulty ventilator, or failure of alveolar function. What is done is to disconnect the ventilator, ensure that the endotracheal tube is open and ventilate the baby manually. If the baby improves then the problem is in the ventilator, and manual breathing should be continued until the fault is traced. If no improvement occurs then the number of functioning alveoli has dropped to a critical level, perhaps because of the presence of inflammation, edema, or bleeding. Sometimes it is possible to confirm alveolar difficulties by an x-ray, and if they are to blame then artificial ventilation can be discontinued with a clear conscience. The other value of an x-ray is of course to make sure that no pneumothorax is present, as this is a treatable cause of alveolar failure.

3 Puberty and adolescence

These two are usually considered together, but in a sense, however, they are separate. Puberty is the attainment of specific, usually incomplete, secondary sexual characteristics, and often with an accompanying growth spurt. Adolescence is puberty with the problems of growing up intellectually, and follows puberty. The problems of puberty and adolescence are psychic rather than somatic.

PUBERTY

In both sexes there is very considerable variation in the onset of puberty, which is easier to define in the female since the time of menstrual onset is usually accurately recorded. Menstruation begins at a mean age of 12.5 years and this implies a range between 10 and 15 years. Accordingly, in any peer group there will be children with or without menstruation. This physiological variance must be appreciated since early or late appearance of menstruation, or any other secondary sexual characteristic, may be considered pathological by the parent. It is also important to appreciate that a girl may regularly menstruate yet physically be a child. There is considerable lack of correlation between secondary sexual characteristics and what might be called sense and sensibility.

The signs of puberty

Females

The onset of menstruation is preceded by a whitish, usually somewhat cyclic, vaginal discharge. This stiffens on the underclothing, and precedes menstruation by as much as 18 months to 2 years. Breast development begins up to 1 year before menstruation, and may initially be unilateral. The latter is normal but may be a cause of parental worry. An increase in transverse pelvic diameter is an early pubertal change. Straight sparse pubic hair occurs before menstruation, axillary hair occurs at a variable time after menstruation. When the latter is well established (1 year +), the breast grows towards the adult type, with definite nipple development and areolar pigmentation. The facial contours (nose, lips) change from the plumpness of childhood towards the more angular features of the adolescent. A strong growth spurt occurs at any stage or throughout all of the described stages of puberty.

Males

The landmark here is less readily detectable, but the amount of peer variation is probably similar to that of the female. The earlier changes are an increase in the size of testes and penis, transient breast swelling, and growth of pubic, axillary, and facial hair. Breaking of the voice accompanies the last. Nocturnal emission is common as soon as axillary hair has developed. A growth spurt usually accompanies pubic hair and precedes facial hair. In most boys, external signs of puberty are visible as early as 10-11 years and usually are present to some degree by 14-15.

ADOLESCENCE

This is essentially a period of psychic development superimposed upon the physical changes of puberty. In general, the adolescent female is 1-2 years ahead of the male. This difference should always be borne in mind. Since adolescence is the time of preparation for a normal and natural independence, it is a period of considerable stress, principally to parents, to a lesser extent to the child. The end point of adolescence is maturity, in the adult sense of intellectual and philosophical integrity. Usually this implies a rejection of parental controls, and a period of exploration of social and personal values. Ultimately the child's philosophy, and these values, tend to resemble those of the parents, but the period of exploration is often painful for both parties. As in adults, there are some sexual overtones to adolescent social activities, and the ambivalent attitude of adults to these sexual overtones may cause considerable problems.

The preadolescent child is, in the ordinary way, family oriented. Thus to some extent he still sees his parents as larger than life, and within fine limits he accepts their standards, their ideas of amusement, and their levels of discipline. In the adolescent, this acceptance is increasingly difficult to maintain, and the orientation and value scale tend more and more to be those of the peer group. This is expressed by the lessening of intimate discussion with the family group, and a corresponding increased association with the peer group. This sometimes results in apparent withdrawal of the adolescent from the family circle, something which may be most wounding to some parents. Normally, however, the phase is transient since, as adolescence advances, a return to the family is usual, although it is not on the same terms as those of the child. This change is normal and natural, but may have to be explained to the parents. The reorientation to the peer group explains to some extent the cult heroes of the teenager, the clothing fads, and so on.

Adolescence is a time of turmoil. The problems faced are considerable, and feelings of inadequacy are normal. These are recognized by the adolescent but are hard to admit. The compensations are loud-mouthed talk, bravado, but seldom overt boasting. Boys are louder voiced than girls, who are more shrill. The end results for the parents are similar. The feelings of inadequacy probably also contribute to the need for conformity with the peer group in clothing (bizarre sometimes). Thus the adolescent in a sense assumes a protective coloration. The rapid changes of adolescent mood and behaviour are more or less stressing to parents who themselves may feel inadequate. A simple explanation that the above behaviour is normal may be a considerable comfort to them. Parents, as well as the adolescents, must reevaluate their attitudes on many subjects. This is because the adolescent is now able to argue logically, and is unaffected by threats which are effective in younger children. The pioneering function of the eldest child often makes his role particularly difficult. He battles with his parents for the adoption of values and attitudes which makes easier the path of the younger children.

The ambivalent attitudes and needs of the adolescent must be appreciated. On the one hand he is striving for independence, on the other hand he appreciates, and needs, a firm parental hand in major decisions. In general, the parents must make up their own minds about what is important to them, and stick to their attitudes. Too often the battles are fought about fringe issues. Exhaustion over these leaves little time or effort for discussion of the problems about which the adolescent really needs guidance. Amid his problems, the child is impatient and aggressive. Generally the parents will have to be patient and firm. This is particularly difficult for those who are receiving adolescent defiance, but who see the same person meekly accept the value judgments of the peer group. Most parents however have considerable insight into adolescent attitudes. No parent should be expected to be a saint but most will be comforted by the recurrent universality of the problem. Commonly enough, when a third party (the physician) analyzes the differences of opinion, these are found to be of detail rather than in principle. The exception is the delinquent child—a separate problem. It is useful and comforting to point out to both parties that they are really not far apart in attitude. In cases of doubt, it is better to stretch the truth rather than the reverse. The adolescent is as capable of remorse as of aggression. His guilt feeling may be quite deep—in his family relationships and otherwise. The medical attendant then may be required to exorcise guilt feelings in the adolescent as well as in his parents. The adolescent usually has a considerable sense of honour—well expressed in the gang syndrome. The same sense of honour may cripple his judgment in the decision as to what he will do with his life. Thus, a child of a father who is, let us say, a physician, may feel almost compelled to continue the family tradition, even if his intellectual abilities and interests lie in another direction. Good parents perhaps will ensure that the child chooses a career which he wishes and which is compatible with his intellectual powers and interests. The physician may occasionally find this conflict of interest in the family, perhaps because of neurotic disorder in the child. He should carefully review the situation and point out the salient aspects to child and parents. He should not himself make the final decisions. This is the right of the child and his parents.

THE SEXUAL SITUATION

The sexual drive must be recognized as part of adolescence, but it should be kept in perspective. Not all adolescent difficulties are directly due to frustrated sexual desires. The sexuality is however sometimes fairly obvious (though not necessarily to the adolescent) and may trouble the parents. In general, the accepted ideas of society are the best standards to which the adolescent should be asked to adhere. The least which society can offer the adolescent is the simplest explanation of the facts of life. The medical man should be prepared to offer simple literature and explanation on the physiology of sex, and the difference between the sexes. For girls he will include the physiology of menstruation, and for boys the explanation of the background of nocturnal emission. These should be dealt with in a matter-of-fact way by the parents, school, or physician at the prepubertal period. The physiological aspects of sex are usually easy to deal with; the social aspects present much more difficulty, and clearly will vary with the standards of society in general, and the family in particular. A degree (minor?) of promiscuity in the older adolescent is a part of our civilization, as is obvious from the level of prenuptial conception. However, the medical profession is obliged to stick to conventional standards, and no person, whatever his individual views, should encourage promiscuity.

It is sometimes thought that boys are sexually aggressive, and that girls are sexually passive. Adolescent opinion may argue on occasion that it is necessary for a girl to accept passionate petting, or even intercourse, as a necessary part of social activity; some may even ask the physician if this is so. Of course it is not, in spite of the blatant sexuality of many aspects of society.

Masturbation is near universal in the male adolescent, and common in females, and a cause of guilt feelings, so that reassurance may be required. Mutual masturbation is not uncommon in male peer groups but is transitory. The importance lies in the fear of masturbation per se, and the fear—latent or overt—of being labelled a queer. Strong, non-sexual, emotional attachments to persons of the same sex are common in adolescents. They are transient and seldom result in formal and permanent homosexual behaviour. The patient may require to be reassured about this.

If the parents seek advice about the conduct of the adolescent, there is still a great deal to be said for keeping him out of "dangerous" situations. Thus teenage parties should always be chaperoned, and a girl should frankly be told what the standards of the family and society are about heavy petting or intercourse.

The need of the teenage for quite savage physical effort is often underestimated, accordingly the parents will find that they will have to deliberately plan for this. The need for socializing with the opposite sex is also fundamental, and sensible parents will provide reasonable opportunities for this.

SPECIFIC PHYSICAL PROBLEMS

Variation in onset of puberty and in the adolescence growth spurt has already been referred to, and while pediatricians may thoroughly appreciate the variation which is compatible with normality, this is frequently not apparent, either to the adolescent or to his parents. Accordingly, with the general need to conform which is a large part of the adolescent's outlook, the patient or his parents may become perturbed because he is physically different from his peers. This may express itself as anxiety, or through symptoms which are tangential to the real problem—the difference between himself and his peer group. Thus, a grade 7 boy who has had an early onset of the adolescent growth spurt, and is already 1.7 m high, may be embarrassed by his stature and the difficulty which he has playing school games with his shorter colleagues. Equally, the immature adolescent who is in high school may contrast himself unfavourably with his tall, heavily bearded, contemporaries. The difference in genital development may also be obvious, and may cause refusal to take part in sports because of the need to undress.

Girls have fewer difficulties, which tend to be concentrated at the early and late stages of puberty. Thus, the well-developed, menstruating child of 10 is obviously different from many of her peer group. This may trouble her. Characteristic is an effort to conceal the secondary sexual characteristics, usually reflected in a hunched-up attitude. Equally, the immature girl who is in high school may contrast herself unfavourably with her more well-endowed sisters. An explanation of the variability of the onset of pubertal characteristics is usually all that is necessary.

Adolescence is a relatively healthy period of life. There are however some problems which tend to occur in it. Most of them pose little danger to health, but in view of the psychic disturbance of adolescence, assume a greater importance than at other stages of life. Perhaps the commonest condition is *acne*. This skin condition accompanies adolescence, to a greater or lesser degree, and may be looked upon as normal. The sensitivity of the adolescent is however disturbed by what can be, in severe cases, an unsightly condition. The principal point in the treatment of acne is indeed for the physician to take the condition seriously and not to laugh it off as something out of which the child will grow. Details of treatment are discussed elsewhere. The pediatrician's principal role is to supervise treatment, reassure the child, and remind him that permanent scarring from acne is unusual.

Nutritional disturbances often come to a head at adolescence, thus obesity may present for treatment although frequently the tendency has been present for some years. If it is due to a faulty diet, the increased adolescent appetite exaggerates the weight gain. Because of the sensitivity of the adolescent, the obesity is complained of more readily than in other age groups. Frank undernutrition is rare in the adolescent, although faulty dietary habits are not unusual. Adolescence is the time at which fad diets occur—usually in an effort to reduce, sometimes in relation to the cult of the adolescent hero. The effects of popular heroes upon adolescent dress are not unknown; the effects of the same upon adolescent diet also occur. In extreme cases the adolescent may develop anorexia nervosa, which is a severe, and sometimes fatal, condition of refusal to eat, symptomatic of a relatively severe mental disturbance (see elsewhere).

Other conditions also occur in the adolescent. In males, *gynecomastia* is a unilateral or bilateral breast enlargement. This is a common situation and requires no treatment except reassurance. Another specifically male condition is *slipped femoral epiphysis*, usually presenting with a limp and pain in the hip joint. In this condition it is important to recall that pain may be referred to the knee. Any limp in an adolescent demands a reasonable examination and usually an x-ray of the appropriate hip.

In girls, a transient enlargement of the *thyroid*, without true thyroid disease, is quite common. It is of little clinical importance. A degree of anemia is not very unusual in girls of this age and responds readily to iron. True menstrual disorders are unusual in the adolescent girl. It should be recalled that irregularity of the menses is normal and that a degree of menorrhagia may occur during a few cycles in the first year of menstruation. Dysmenorrhea may occur also. This is often superimposed upon a medieval family background in relation to menstruation. Thus it is important to make sure that the menstruating girl is not treated as an invalid and is urged to carry out normal activities during her period. Severe recurrent dysmenorrhea should always warrant an investigation into the whole situation to see if there is a psychological overlay. This should be excluded before any surgical treatments are undertaken.

In both sexes, in the adolescent, we have the emergence of disease processes which are unknown or unusual in a younger age group. This includes disseminated lupus, bacterial endocarditis, and cavitating tuberculosis. It is commonplace that diabetes may be more troublesome at adolescence and require more frequent visits and closer control. In this connection, the need of the adolescent for a larger diet should always be kept in mind.

School problems such as "school phobia" again become more common in adolescence. School phobia is not usually consciously planned, and physical symptoms such as abdominal pain or headache are usual. Psychic symptoms alone, e.g., anxiety, may be the presenting feature. It is not very uncommon for the child to blame the school or his teacher for his nervous condition. School phobia implies that a thorough investigation of the environment should be undertaken, a search made for possible precipitating factors, e.g., worry about difference from peer group, irrational fears of disease, and so on. It is rather rarely caused by the nature of the schoolwork, unless the child's ability to cope has been seriously overrated.

EMOTIONAL PROBLEMS

The adult, for mental health, requires to have a feeling of a definite and personally important role in life. The achievement of this feeling is the adolescent's principal preoccupation. The process is called identity formation, or the achievement of a sense of self. In this, the adolescent relates to and takes on the characteristics of valued people and ideas in his environment. He finally achieves more or less independence from these sources while incorporating some of their traits into his own personality. This process takes time, and although ultimate success is usual, the adolescent may have many false starts. The sense of failure associated with these false starts gives rise to emotional problems. The parents are still important people to the adolescent and the loss of one of the parents by death, or the fragmentation of the family situation, e.g., by divorce, may greatly interfere with the adolescent's search for identity. Disillusionment with the family or the parents is common, but in most cases is transitory. If the parents' conduct has, however, been particularly obnoxious in the eyes of the adolescent, it may give rise to permanent disintegration of the relationship and a setback in the search for identity. Intrusiveness on the part of the parents with the adolescent is pretty common and in some cases may delay the success of the process of self-identification. This intrusiveness is perhaps more common in mothers than in fathers, and takes the form of a persistent questioning and sometimes deprecation of the adolescent's motives. Indeed, some adolescents have a hard job to achieve any reasonable privacy at all. However, most children succeed in dealing with their search for identity. The achievement time of an integrated personality is, like any other biological function, a variable one. Indeed, some adults never achieve this state, and function perfectly well socially and economically. This does not, however, absolve us from efforts to help the family and the adolescent. Hopefully we will practise preventive pediatrics when we are aware of the occurrence of death, or family dissolution. If the adolescent presents with emotional problems—which may take many forms—the importance of the search for identity to the adolescent should be appreciated. A not uncommon complaint is apathy and withdrawal from the family. Both are usually parental complaints but may represent, in the adolescent, a stage at which he is temporarily unable to deal with his search for identity, and has decided to opt out for a while. This may present itself as refusal to continue at school, or to carry out a parent's cherished plan. At an extreme it is characterized by the beatnik philosophy. Such a situation requires careful consideration by the pediatrician who should not blindly support parental attitudes, but should carefully explore the whole family situation, especially by personal conversation with the adolescent. Often enough the problem is a fait accompli, and the best the physician can do is to reassure the parents that they are not failures and to point out that a school dropout may still turn into a successful (and conservative) adult. Adolescents may have transient feelings of depression but these should not be overdiagnosed. Organic depressions occur in the older (17-19-year-old) patient, and are commonly associated with gross, frequently expressed feelings of inadequacy. The situation demands early, expert, psychiatric help in this age group.

PREMATURE PUBERTY

The wide variation in the onset of natural puberty has already been noted. In general however, the onset of menstruation or breast changes (usually with clitoral and pubic hair development) before the age of 8 in the female is worthy of investigation. Similarly, in boys the unusually early (<8 years) appearance of pubic and axillary hair, penile and testicular enlargement, and other features of puberty, are generally out with the reasonable limits of normality.

The true precocious puberty is always isosexual (i.e., female changes occur in females) and the progression of external changes of puberty is as in the normal individual. Height, weight, and bone age are also accelerated, but the mental and dental ages are normal.

Clinical features. These are clearly those of accelerated puberty. In true precocious puberty, there is also evidence of gonadal enlargement and the production of sperm or ova. Gonadal enlargement is readily appreciable in the male, but less convincing in the female. In the latter, evidence of cyclic change in the vaginal epithelium, together with estimation of the urinary hormonal output, is useful ancillary evidence of ovulation.

Differential diagnosis. The secondary type is a rare complication of central nervous system disease such as tumour, postencephalitic states, or untreated hydrocephalus, or it may occasionally complicate the McCune-Albright syndrome of polyostotic fibrous dysplasia with skin pigmentation and bone changes.

In most instances of true precocious puberty, investigation is unrewarding. The patient has puberty, with appropriate hormonal changes, at an inappropriate age and that is all.

Treatment. In simple precocious puberty, explanation, reassurance, and careful prophylaxis of disturbance of the family is all that is necessary.

In the other conditions mentioned, the treatment is that of the primary disease.

PRECOCIOUS PSEUDOPUBERTY

This condition may be isosexual or heterosexual (e.g., male type puberty in a female). The condition is differentiated from the primary type in that gonadal enlargement is not present, and sperm and ova production does not occur. The condition is generally due to a process which produces testosterone or estrogen at an early age.

Differential diagnosis. In either sex, the condition is most commonly due to congenital adrenal hyperplasia (described in full elsewhere). The next most common cause is the injudicious prescription of androgens or estrogens, a fact usually available from the history.

In female isosexual precocity, ovarian tumours (granuloma cell, theca cell, or teratoma) may be causal. In the male variety, testicular tumours (interstitial cell, teratoma). Most of these tumours are felt on routine examination. Their removal is the mode of treatment.

4 Nutrition and its disorders

Good nutrition depends upon a diet which is adequate in calories, protein, fat, carbohydrate, and which contains enough of the essential vitamins and minerals to supply bodily requirements and replace any losses. In general, the younger the child is when he is exposed to malnutrition, the more likely is it that he will have permanent ill-effects.

DIET

Caloric requirement. This is highest for premature infants, and falls steadily until adulthood is reached. Table 7 summarizes the situation. The values given are average and not necessarily those which guarantee satiety in every individual.

Table 7. Caloric requirements

Age	Calories/kg/ideal weight
Prematures	120–130
Newborns	110–120
6 months	100
7 years	80
10 years	70
Adolescence	60

Protein requirement. Infants require 2.5 g/kg/body weight/day for good growth. Older children need 2.0 g/kg/body weight/day until adolescence when the need falls to 1.0 g/kg/body weight/day.

Fat. Normally the diet in the first months of life contains 40% of the calories as fat. This is because fat is calorically dense, containing 9 cal/g as against 4.5 cal/g for carbohydrate or protein. Fat also makes food more palatable, and acts as a carrier for certain vitamins. The percentage of fat in the diet falls with age to about 30% in preadolescents, and about 25% thereafter. The essential fatty acids are linoleic acid, arachidonic acid, and linolinic acid, and are necessary in infancy.

Carbohydrates. These make a significant contribution of calories to the average diet, e.g., 50% in the newborn. In poor people, up to 90% of the calories may be taken as carbohydrate. The usual source in infancy is lactose and sucrose—the disaccharides. Thereafter starch (a polysaccharide) is the usual source.

Vitamins, trace elements, and minerals. The daily need for these is shown in table 8. Again it should be noted that these are average values, subject to revision in individual patients or climatic situations.

Table 8. Average daily requirement of vitamins and minerals

Vitamins (daily need)	Infant	Child	Adolescent
Vitamin A (I.U.)	1,500	2,500	4,500
Niacin (mg)	5	10	15
Riboflavin (mg)	0.4	1.0	1.5
Thiamine (mg)	0.4	1.0	1.5
Pyridoxine / Vitamin B_6 (mg)	0.4	1.0	2.0
Vitamin B_{12} (mcg)	1.0	2.5	5.0
Folic acid (mg)	0.05	0.1	0.4
Ascorbic acid (mg)	50	50	50
Vitamin D (I.U.)	400	400	400
Vitamin E (I.U.)	5	10	20
Minerals (daily need)			
Calcium (g)	0.4	0.8	1.0
Phosphorus (g)	0.4	0.8	1.0
Magnesium (mg)	60	250	400
Iron (mg)	6–10	10	20
Iodine (mcg)	40	60	100

DISORDERS OF NUTRITION

These are usually detected by finding variations from a normal growth pattern. Specific deficiencies of vitamins or minerals may give a particular disease pattern. Most malnourished children in the affluent countries have some disease of the major systems. Thus, malabsorption, as in mucoviscidosis or coeliac disease, will cause malnutrition through loss of calories. In chronic renal and heart disease, caloric absorption may be normal, but caloric disposal insufficient, so that impaired growth occurs. The same takes place in the chromosomal disorders and in severe central nervous system disease. The features of the underlying disease however are the major ones, and the impaired growth percentile values the main means of confirming the nutritional deficit.

Undernutrition (malnutrition, marasmus)

This occurs when the diet contains insufficient calories. Protein is usually also lacking. Whole populations may be affected in countries where poverty is rife, or famine occurs. Growth slows down and then ceases when caloric deprivation is marked. The mortality is high usually because of gastroenteritis and chest infections. These disorders may veil the malnutrition unless the child population is adequately weighed and measured. If this is done, large numbers are found to be in the 3rd percentile or less (figure 10). Head circumference values are also decreased.

Clinical features. In the most advanced cases, the child is a living skeleton, with potbelly and wasted buttocks, limbs, and face. There is apathy, irritability, and retardation of motor achievement in infants. The hair is fine and silky, grows slowly, and may be of an abnormal colour. The child usually also has diarrhea and a loose cough. Many die because of dehydration.

In other circumstances, the child may still have a layer of subcutaneous fat, and even seem chubby. Potbelly is usual, however, as is wasting of the buttocks. The child looks younger than its true age, and measurements place it in the very low percentiles. Again, gastroenteritis, chest infections, and chronic E.N.T. problems often coincide. If weight records are available, it is usual to find that the slowing of growth has occurred after the first 6 months of life, and fails at the time of weaning (figure 10).

Kwashiorkor

This is a variant of malnutrition, when protein lack and, usually, low caloric intake coincide. The growth patterns are as described above, but changes in hair and skin colour are more advanced. Thus, black hair becomes reddish in colour. As the plasma proteins fall, edema sets in, evidenced by swelling of the face and body and pleural and peritoneal effusions. Coincident diarrhea is a common cause of death.

TREATMENT OF MALNUTRITION

Associated gastroenteritis, chest infection, and infestation with worms should be treated. Temporary lactose intolerance is common, and may require the use of low lactose milk. Otherwise the child is given a full and free diet. Rapid weight gain then occurs, but restoration to completely normal percentile levels is unusual. However, apathy disappears and motor functions progress rapidly. These are the best early signs of a response to treatment.

Malnutrition (usually of the moderate type) is found also in affluent

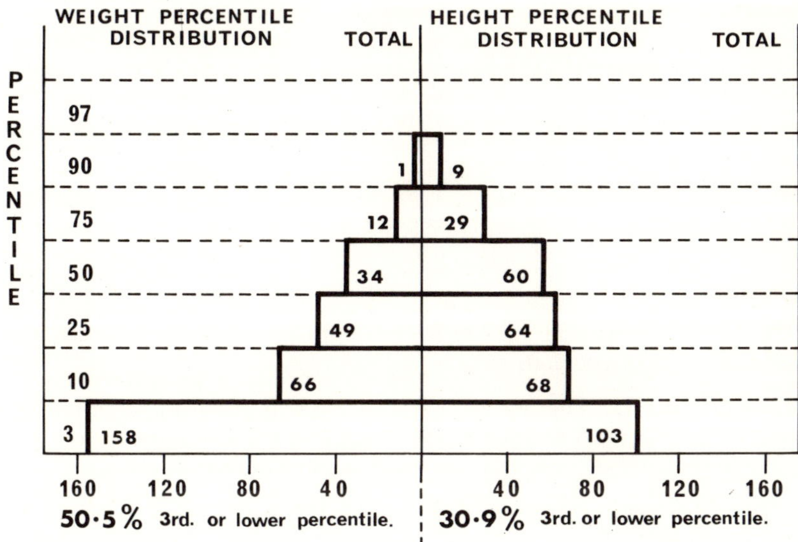

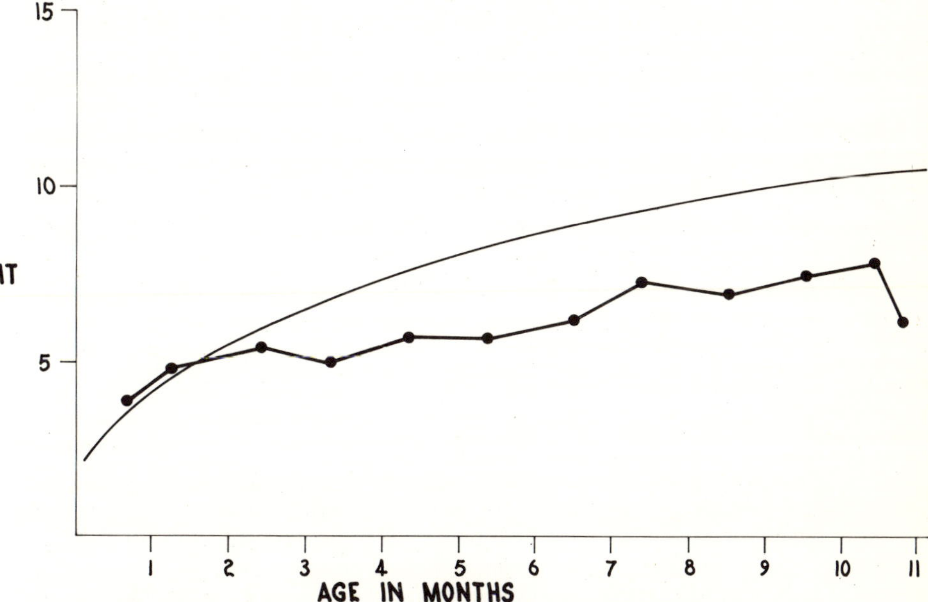

Fig. 10. *a*, Nutritional status: distribution of percentiles in a malnourished population; *b*, Deviation from mean weight values in malnutrition.

societies, usually among poor people, but is also part of the picture of child neglect or abuse. The clinical features are as already described, although the severity of the accompanying diarrhea or chest infection is very much less. The treatment is similar, except that care and education of the parents is also required. Where malnutrition is secondary to some system disorder (e.g., malabsorption) the treatment of the nutritional defect is that of the primary disease.

OVERNUTRITION

Obesity

This is the condition in which the body contains an unacceptable amount of subcutaneous fat.

Clinical features. The main reason for seeking medical attention is a cosmetic one. Thus complaints of being too fat are more common in girls than in boys, and tend to occur around puberty.

Clinical features. The history often reveals that the child has been tall and heavy for her age since early life, has a good appetite and is in good general health. Sudden gain in weight at the age of 8-10 years, or coincident with the onset of menstruation, brings the child to medical attention. The height is found to be within a normal height percentile but the weight is off the percentile scale for the child's age. The excess fat shows mainly on the thighs, buttocks, lower abdomen, and chest. The face and arms are less affected. This distribution is found in both sexes. Where weight gain has been rapid, skin splitting with thin purple scars (striae) is common on the thighs and abdomen. Physical examination is otherwise normal, although a minor degree of hypertension may be found.

Differential diagnosis. This is mainly from syndromal obesity, i.e., diseases of which obesity forms only one part. These are characterized usually by shortness of stature, as well as obesity, and often have other features which are characteristic.

Treatment of simple obesity. The main point is to control the intake of calories. The diet should be surveyed and high calorie items—mainly fat—controlled or excluded. Young children should not be prescribed diets which are insufficient for growth. The diet must be constructed to allow satiety—a feeling of fullness after a meal is important to children. This can be done by the imaginative use of vegetables which are high in bulk, but low in calories. Reasonable goals are set both for parents and patient. The first step then is to ensure that the child does not *gain* weight and this can be done by modest dietary control. As the child sees that he can achieve this step, then more rigorous dietary control will allow actual weight loss. Crash diets are unsuitable for children, since they are unable to maintain the asceticism which such rigorous diets entail. The child should also be encouraged to take adequate and increasing amounts of exercise. Simple ploys to deal with jeering school fellows should also be taught, so that self-pity does not precipitate a compensatory orgy.

The obesity which begins at puberty is treated on similar lines. Particular care is needed to make sure that children in this age group do not embark upon impossible diets. Appetite-controlling drugs are often sought by such patients, but contribute little to the success of any regime.

Syndromal obesity

These are rare conditions. In most cases primary complaints are not of obesity but of some other feature of the underlying condition. All children who suffer from syndromal obesity are short in stature; the only exception to this is the Cushing's syndrome in which height may be normal or accelerated for age. Intellectual retardation is also a common feature of syndromal obesity. Perhaps the commonest is the Lawrence-Moon-Biedl syndrome which is characterized by polydactyly, mental retardation, retinitis pigmentosa, and small stature. The condition is most likely to come to the notice because of the deformities of the hands and feet and the slow progress of the child during the first 2 years of life. Obesity is seldom a marked feature until the third or fourth year. Characteristic retinal changes are present from birth. This condition is due to some unknown lesion of the hypothalamus and there is no primary treatment for it. Orthopedic care is necessary for the deformities and the obesity can, within limits, be controlled by dietary prescription.

Prader-Willi syndrome

This condition is characterized by the association of hypotonia, mental retardation, failure of descent of testicles, dwarfing, and obesity. It is familial but affects only boys. The hypotonia is usually the first complaint and the child may be thought to have cerebral palsy, especially as evidence of intellectual retardation is usually quite early in this syndrome. The testicles do not descend and low percentiles for height are obvious from the early months of life. Frank obesity is rare before the age of 5 or 6 years. No treatment is indicated for these patients.

Tumours affecting the hypothalamus

In these patients, the primary complaints are of raised intracranial pressure, often with visual disturbances. Obesity is more likely to occur after treatment by surgery or x-ray therapy. The stature is short and, though obese, these children are actually in a normal weight percentile for their age group. Treatment is of course that of the primary condition.

Cushing's syndrome

This is rare and is dealt with in the section concerning the diseases of adrenal cortex (p. 361).

Obesity associated with inactivity

This is a not very uncommon situation found in the child who has been rendered bed fast for some reason or another. Thus patients with rheumatic fever, whose activity has been unreasonably reduced, will become obese after months in bed. In the same way, patients undergoing extensive orthopedic treatment are frequently rendered inactive, so that their caloric intake far exceeds their energy production. Obesity results. Care should be taken in such cases adequately to regulate the diet. Appetite is often increased because of the sheer boredom of the situation. Accordingly, appropriate educational and occupational therapy is indicated.

In the same way, patients who are crippled by the results of severe poliomyelitis or who suffer from cerebral palsy are, to a large extent, inactive. Pressures often exist within the family to feed them up. This should be sternly resisted as excess weight in the presence of muscular deficit merely renders the latter a more formidable problem for the patient. Excessive weight gain is often found in the late stages of muscular dystrophy, when the patient is bedfast. Here again, much of the overeating is due to boredom, and appropriate measures should be taken for this, as well as in the prescription of a diet suitable to the activity level.

DISORDERS OF VITAMIN REQUIREMENT

Vitamin A deficiency

This is rare except in severe malabsorption, or in countries where advanced protein-calorie malnutrition occurs. The main features are subjective complaints of night blindness (nyctalopia), followed by painful dry eyes (xerophthalmia), and corneal ulceration which may cause blindness. The treatment is to give 5,000 units daily of vitamin A until cure is achieved and to prevent further trouble by giving 1,000-4,000 units daily, according to age.

Vitamin A excess (hypervitaminosis A)

This gives the symptons of raised intracranial pressure—vomiting, irritability, drowsiness, papilledema and visual disturbances. It is usually due to overenthusiasm in giving mixed vitamin preparations. The treatment is to remove vitamin A from the diet.

Avitaminosis B_1 (beriberi, thiamine deficiency)

Clinical features. The disorder usually occurs in infancy, with loss of appetite and restlessness, followed by the onset of edema of the face and limbs and the signs of congestive cardiac failure. Sudden death is not unusual. Protein-calorie malnutrition is commonly also present.

In older children, the symptons of peripheral neuritis may predominate. These include weakness, difficulty in walking, drooping eyelids (ptosis), and wristdrop.

Treatment. Thiamine 50 mg is given daily.

Riboflavin deficiency

This may cause itching, pain, and excessive tearing of the eyes. The skin (mainly at the corners of the mouth) is also affected, becoming pale, moist, and eventually crusted (cheilosis).

Treatment. Riboflavin 1 mg daily is given.

Pellagra (nicotinic acid deficiency)

This may occur in malnutrition. The main feature is of a rash occurring in the exposed areas. This is red, desquamates and then darkens. Inflammation of the mouth and tongue also occurs.

Treatment. Nicotinic acid is given, and the diet upgraded.

Pyridoxine deficiency

This occurs in infancy, when deficient diets are given. The main symptom is of fits (often myoclonic), irritability, and slowness in achieving milestones. These symptoms disappear with pyridoxine 20 mg/day.

Vitamin B_{12} (cyanocobalamine)

This combines with gastric intrinsic factor and the combination is absorbed as an essential in the production of red cells. Deficiency causes juvenile pernicious anemia (see p. 316).

Vitamin C deficiency (scurvy)

This is mainly a disease of bone, with a slight bleeding tendency, all due to imperfect formation of intracellular cementing substances for which ascorbic acid (vitamin C) is essential.

Clinical features. Symptoms are unusual before the 6th month of life, except in prematures. The first complaint is of irritability and crying, mainly when the baby is handled, as in bathing. This is because bleeding occurs under the periosteum (membrane around the bones) and causes pain. This causes poverty of movement, even to the extent that paralysis is suspected. Purpuric spots in the skin are an occasional first symptom. The pain in the limbs makes the baby assume the position of greatest comfort—the frog position (hips and knees flexed, legs externally rotated). Swelling, tenderness, and fever are common. Bluish gum swellings occur if the teeth are coming in.

Diagnosis. This is confirmed by x-ray which shows early loss of bone substance, and a thickened metaphyseal line. As healing sets in, the subperiosteal blood calcifies and gives a misshapen outline to the bone. Dislocation of the epiphysis may occur.

Treatment. A daily dose of 100 mg of vitamin C is given by mouth for several weeks.

Prevention. All infants should be given 50 mg of ascorbic acid daily. Vitamin C is destroyed by heat, so preparations are put directly into the infant's mouth.

Vitamin D deficiency (rickets)

This is a disorder of bone calcification, usually due to insufficient dietary vitamin D, and often found in children who have scanty opportunity to be exposed to sunlight, which forms vitamin D by its action on our skin. Vitamin D is a fat-soluble vitamin, so rickets may be found in children who have fat malabsorption.

Clinical features. These occur after the first 6 months of life, and are most often diagnosed by finding the signs of the disorder—enlargement of the epiphyses of wrists, ankles, and knee joints, or a rounded swelling of the costochondral (rib epiphyseal) junctions giving the so-called rickety-rosary. In small, premature infants the skull bones soften and can be indented like a Ping-Pong ball. This sign is called craniotabes. Inactivity, lateness in walking, and frequent chest infections are common, but nonspecific complaints. In neglected cases, much deformity occurs in the legs. Tetany may occur when treatment has begun, usually because insufficient calcium has been added to the diet.

X-ray changes. The ends of the bones are enlarged, and the epiphyseal area becomes cupped in shape and irregular. Rarely fractures occur through the abnormal area of calcification.

Laboratory. The phosphate levels and alkaline phosphatase values are increased.

Treatment. 1,000-2,000 I.U. vitamin D is given daily as well as extra calcium. The amount required for prophylaxis is 400 I.U. vitamin D daily.

Vitamin D resistant rickets

This is found in chronic renal disease and has the features noted above together with the renal disorder. Partial healing of the rickets can be obtained by giving large doses of vitamin D.

Hypophosphatasia

This is a familial disorder presenting in early life with vomiting, failure to thrive, and eventual rickets. The enzyme alkaline phosphatase is absent, and the x-ray signs are those of severe rickets. It does not, however, respond to vitamin D.

Excess of vitamin D (hypervitaminosis D)

This results from excessive dosage to prevent or treat rickets. As a result, the serum calcium rises and eventually calcium is deposited in the kidney.

Clinical features. Anorexia, irritability, and vomiting occur, eventually with symptoms of renal disease—thirst, polyuria, growth failure, and episodes of dehydration.

Laboratory. Blood calcium and phosphate levels are greatly increased. Albumen is found in the urine, and the signs of renal failure (e.g., raised blood urea) can be present.

Treatment. Vitamin D is totally excluded from the diet, and steroids (cortisone) given to increase the urinary excretion of calcium.

Vitamin E deficiency

This is unusual in children, but may occur in premature babies when a hemolytic state, with anemia, pallor and jaundice, can occur. The treatment is to give vitamin E as α-tocopherol 100 U/daily.

Vitamin K deficiency

This substance is essential in the formation of the clotting substance, prothrombin. In the newborn, such a deficiency causes the bleeding disorder called hemorrhagic disease of the newborn (p. 346). Much less commonly, prothrombin is deficient in the fat malabsorption states. The treatment is to give vitamin K_1 by injection.

MINERAL DEFICIENCY

Acute situations of sodium and potassium deficit are described elsewhere. Calcium deficiency occurs only where the soil is grossly lime deficient, and is rare. The result is osteomalacia, a disease resembling rickets in which the bones are softened by calcium lack. A similar, though much less severe state, may occur in the disorders with fat malabsorption. The treatment is to give extra calcium lactate in the diet.

The trace elements

These are iron, copper, cobalt, zinc, manganese, and iodine. Iron and copper are both needed in blood manufacture, and deficiencies cause anemia (see p. 315). Cobalt, zinc, and manganese deficiency states have yet to be described in humans.

Iodine deficiency

This occurs in mountainous areas with a high rainfall, when iodides are dissolved from the soil. Plant iodide is low, and total iodine intake insufficient. This gives rise to enlargement of the thyroid gland (goitre), sometimes with failure of thyroxine production (cretinism). Both of these are described elsewhere (p. 356).

The condition is prevented by giving iodide in the diet, usually in the supply of table salt. Established goitres are difficult to treat, but extra iodine may be tried.

5 Disease due to inborn errors of metabolism

These conditions are usually due to a biochemical defect, generally an enzyme deficiency, which affects the handling of the main sources of energy formation, including those needed for growth. The substances (substrates) which can be affected by such enzyme deficiencies are the amino acids, derived from the protein in the diet, or from the body itself; carbohydrates, and the fat (lipids) of the diet or which are made in the body.

The disorder can deprive the child of needed energy sources, or the wherewithal to grow, or it may cause symptoms by causing the accumulation of a product in such a way that disease results. In some children, both of these facets appear at the same time.

DISORDERS OF AMINO ACID METABOLISM (THE AMINOACIDOPATHIES)

There are many amino acids which the body uses, and generally each requires a specific enzyme for its proper metabolism. If the enzyme is absent, then, as a general rule, the corresponding amino acid increases its content in the blood (aminoacidemia) and spills over into the urine (aminoaciduria). The perverted biochemical process may also lead to the formation of abnormal products in the body which may then be present to excess in the blood and urine. Contrariwise, substances of which the affected amino acid is a component may be substantially reduced. All of these features may be used to make a specific diagnoses in individual patients. Among the amino acids which can be affected are phenylalanine and tyrosine, the sulphur-containing amino acids (cystathionine, homocystine, cystine, methionine, histidine) and the amino acids concerned in the formation of urea (ornithine, citrulline, argininosuccinic acid). Other disorders exist due to anomalies of the branch chain amino acids, e.g., involving leucine, valine, methylmalonic acid, etc., and others will certainly emerge in the future.

It is proposed in this section only to give an account of the commoner and more important conditions. An outline of the possibilities can be obtained from the tables. However, some general features should be kept in mind.

Clinical features. The majority of the aminoacidopathies affect the central nervous system. Thus convulsions, mental retardation, and motor and sensory abnormalities are usual. In addition, affected infants feed poorly, gain weight slowly, and are often described as fretful and unresponsive.

Specific diagnosis. This generally depends upon finding the affected amino acid or one of its derivatives in excess quantity in the blood, urine, or both. It may be possible to confirm the suspected enzyme absence by testing the leucocytes or other tissues for its presence.

Screening tests. These must be done in the newborn as irreversible damage soon develops. A typical screening test is the Guthrie technique. In this, a drop of the infant's blood is put on blotting paper, and the levels of various amino acids determined by a microbiological method. Thus, for example, newborns with high levels of phenylalanine, who have the disease called phenylketonuria, can be discovered.

Treatment. Logically the answer would be to replace the missing enzyme. This is, however, impossible so what is done is to remove the offending amino acid (or its precursor) from the diet. This is possible in only a few of the aminoacidopathies, either because it is technically impossible to do so, or because the construction of such a diet would cause other severe deficiency diseases.

Examples of aminoacidopathy

Phenylketonuria (Fölling's disease)

This condition is due to absence of a liver enzyme called phenylalanine hydroxylase (the termination-*ase* implies an enzymatic action). Thus the phenylalanine in the diet cannot be converted to the next stage in its metabolism which is tyrosine. So phenylalanine, and other products of the abnormal metabolism (the phenylketones) accumulate in the blood, and spill over into the urine. Equally, tyrosine, and any substances formed from it, exist in low levels in the body.

Clinical features. In the newborn, vomiting and poor appetite may be noted, as well as a peculiar body odour, described as being like that of mice! In older children, the principal finding is slowness in attaining the motor milestones, insufficient head growth, and eventually, clear-cut mental retardation. Epilepsy may also occur. In general these children are well nourished. Because of the failure of tyrosine formation, the next product, melanin, is also lacking. Melanin is the substance which darkens hair and skin, so that Caucasian children with phenylketonuria tend to be blond and fair skinned.

The diagnosis is confirmed by finding high levels of phenylalanine and phenylketones in the blood and urine. Treatment is by giving a special milk formula which is low in phenylalanine, and continuing to give low phenylalanine foodstuffs when the child is weaned. The effect of the diet is controlled by measuring the blood phenylalanine levels. Dietary treatment is generally of value only if the disorder is diagnosed in the first few months of life. In late (>4 years of age) diagnosed children, the special diet is not well accepted.

Homocystinuria

This is really a disorder of methionine metabolism due to the absence of the enzyme which converts it to cystine. Homocystine is, therefore, found in excess amounts in the urine.

Clinical features. The child fails to grow properly, is mentally retarded, and may develop severe knock knee. Seizures and extrapyramidal tract abnormalities occur, as well as eye problems (dislocated lenses, glaucoma). The condition is diagnosed by urine and blood examination, and the treatment is a low methionine diet, with pyridoxine supplements.

DISORDERS OF THE UREA FORMATION CYCLE

The heart of the problem here is that ammonia is formed in many bodily activities. This is toxic, unless it is converted to urea. Urea formation requires an appropriate set of enzymes which handle the amino acids intermediate in the cycle between ammonia and urea. These amino acids are ornithine, citrulline, and argininosuccinic acid. If an enzyme is deficient then excess ammonia is present in the body, as well as the amino acid which cannot be handled.

Clinical features. These are of hyperammonemia (excess ammonia in the blood) and consist in anorexia, vomiting, irritability, and convulsions in the new born. The baby fails to thrive, and develops the features of cerebral palsy with mental retardation.

The diagnosis of the specific enzyme defect depends on finding a high blood ammonia level, and an appropriate increase of the amino acid (or acids) in the blood and urine.

Treatment. The diet should be low in protein, but this does not guarantee a cure.

DISORDERS OF THE BRANCHED CHAIN AMINO ACIDS

"Maple syrup" urine disease

This is the eponym given to the condition in which the metabolism of leucine, isoleucine, and valine is incomplete. So keto acids accumulate in the body and cause disease. As a result, too, the urine smells of maple syrup.

Clinical features. Apart from the smell of the urine, these are predictable: vomiting, failure to feed, poverty of movement, slowed milestones, and, finally, obvious mental defect. Apart from the aminoaciduria, the blood sugar is often low in the first weeks of life.

Treatment. A synthetic diet low in the guilty amino acids is given, and monitored by appropriate estimates in the blood and urine.

The disorders noted above are examples only of the aminoacidopathies. Table 9 should be consulted for a short account of the others.

Table 9. Disorders of amino acid usage

Substance	Enzyme Defect	Results
Tryptophane	? Tryptophane oxidase	Mental retardation skin disorder
Kynurenine	Kynureninase	Convulsions
Proline	Proline oxidase	Convulsions renal disease
Histidine	Histidine NH_3 – Lyase	Retardation
Isovaleric acid	Isovaleric acid dehydrogenase	Retardation spasticity
Alanine	Pyruvate decarboxylase	Retardation Acidosis Dehydration
Glutathionine	Glutamyl transpeptidase	Mild retardation

In each instance, the level of the amino acid is increased in the blood and urine. Abnormal end products may also be found in the urine, e.g., pyruvate and lactate in alanine disorder.

DISORDERS OF CARBOHYDRATE METABOLISM

There are many of these which affect children. Some are expressed only in 1 cell system, as in some hemolytic anemias with absent enzyme systems. In disorders of the gut ferments, e.g., alactasia, the difficulty with carbohydrate absorption is due primarily to a local defect. Some disorders affecting many systems are described below.

Galactosemia

In this familial condition, the baby can absorb lactose in milk after it has been split into glucose and galactose. However, the enzyme system which in turn converts galactose to glucose is absent. Thus the child lacks adequate energy-giving material and the unusable galactose tends to be stored in various organs of the body.

Clinical features. These occur mainly in the newborn as anorexia, vomiting, loss of weight, jaundice, and sometimes dehydration. Since the baby is hypoglycemic, convulsions occur, and brain growth is interfered with. The liver progressively enlarges, and cirrhosis with liver failure may occur. The child develops cataracts.

In a few children, the onset is less acute, with failure to thrive, retarded motor progress, cataracts, and frank mental retardation.

Diagnosis. The urine contains galactose which may be suspected if it is tested by a copper reduction method (e.g., Clinitest tablets). Galactose does *not* give a positive response to urinalysis by a glucose-oxidase method (e.g., Clinistix). The enzyme defect can also be confirmed by examination of the red cells.

Treatment. The baby must be given a lactose (and hence galactose) free diet, with extra glucose to maintain a normal caloric intake. Lactose should be avoided for life. If begun early enough in life, the child can be expected to grow up normally.

Fructosemia

This is a condition in which the carbohydrate fructose cannot be metabolized. Fructose is a product of the splitting of sucrose (cane sugar), and, as in galactosemia, cannot be converted to glucose because of an enzyme lack. The clinical features resemble those of galactosemia—hypoglycemic fits and brain damage, vomiting, failure to thrive, enlargement of the liver by stored fructose, and mental retardation. Fructose is found in the blood and urine. The treatment is permanent withdrawal of sucrose and fructose from the diet. The caloric level is maintained by giving glucose.

DISORDERS OF GLYCOGEN METABOLISM

Glycogen is a large molecule which is made up from glucose subunits. It is found mainly in the liver and muscles, and acts as an energy reserve for the body. Enzymes are necessary both to form glycogen and to facilitate its release as glucose from the storage areas. Disease can occur either because glycogen cannot be formed, or because it cannot be made available to the body after it *is* formed. In many instances, the child will then have problems either in obtaining enough energy sources or because of accumulation of glycogen. There are about 10 conditions which are due to an enzyme defect in the process of glycogen formation or release. These are summarized in table 10. The more common disorders are discussed in full below. The numbers are those of the Cori classification.

Table 10. Glycogen storage diseases

Type and Enzyme Deficiency		Clinical Features
I	Glucose-6-phosphatase	Failure to thrive, fits, brain damage, enlarged liver (see text)
II	α-glucosidase (acid maltase)	Heart failure (see text)
III	Debranching enzyme	Enlarged liver, hypoglycemia, failure to thrive convulsions
IV	Branching enzyme	Enlarged liver, hypoglycemia, failure to thrive convulsions
V	Muscle phosphorylase	Weakness, muscle pain, stiffness, compatible with fairly normal life
VI	Liver phosphorylase	Similar to type I
VII	Phosphoglycomutase	Enlarged liver
VIII	Phosphofructokinase	Similar to type V, muscle weakness
IX	Glycogen synthetase	Convulsions, mental retardation, no storage signs
X	Phosphorylase kinase	Hepatomegaly

Type I: Glycogenosis (Von Gierke's disease)

This is due to the absence of glucose-6-phosphatase so that glycogen cannot be metabolized to glucose. This gives rise to hypoglycemia.

Clinical features. The infant fails to thrive, and has hypoglycemic convulsions or coma. Brain damage from hypoglycemia is common and leads to mental retardation, abnormalities of nervous system functions, and often early death. The liver enlarges early. The biochemical examination shows a low blood sugar level, but high lipid levels, as the body uses fat as an energy source instead of glucose.

Treatment. No specific therapy is available. Extra glucose will relieve acute symptoms such as convulsions.

Type II: Glycogenosis (Pompe's disease)

This is due to a deficiency of the enzyme α-glucosidase, and leads to the accumulation of glycogen, particularly in the heart muscle.

Clinical features. Soon after birth, the baby develops breathlessness, anorexia, cyanosis, edema, and an enlarged heart. These are all due to cardiac failure. The skeletal muscles are flaccid, but the tongue also enlarges because of glycogen accumulation. The heart is greatly enlarged on x-ray. The enzyme deficiency can be found in liver specimens obtained by biopsy. Treatment is unavailing, and early death is the usual outcome.

Each of the glycogenoses is inherited as an autosomal recessive. Accordingly, appropriate genetic counselling is indicated after the discovery of the index child.

DISORDERS OF GLYCOPROTEIN METABOLISM

Glycoproteins are compounds of polypeptides (protein subunits) with various carbohydrates, e.g., glucose, fructose, etc. If the lack of an enzyme interferes with the formation or degradation of glycoproteins, then disease may occur. In practice this is usually when the metabolism of the substances called mucopolysaccharides (glycose-aminoglycans) is involved. These are formed by the combination of polypeptides with glucose units. If the enzyme which breaks them down (β-galactosidase) is absent, then accumulation of the mucopolysaccharide occurs, and abnormal heparin-like substances are excreted in the urine. At least 5 entities of this type have been identified, but only 1 will be described in full.

Hurler-Hunter disease (gargoylism)

This is an abnormality of mucopolysaccharide metabolism which is heritable as an autosomal recessive. Three principal types are separable, the Hurler syndrome, the Hunter syndrome, and the Sanfilippo type. There is considerable overlap of the clinical types. Each however is characterized by excessive mucopolysaccharide excretion in the urine, together with mental retardation and growth impairment.

Hurler's syndrome

These children usually present with hernias, snuffly nose, and respiratory infections. Delay in attaining the motor milestones and retardation of growth is usual. The bizarre (gargoyle) appearance occurs towards the end of the first or second year. In the fully developed form, there are coarse facial features, with a broad, discharging nose, bulging brow, and apparently large head. The hands are broad, and the back often bowed. The liver and spleen are usually enlarged and the corneae may show cloudiness. Cardiac murmurs are common, and congestive failure may occur.

The Hunter type

The clinical features and facial appearance are similar but retardation of growth and hepatomegaly appear later (1-2 years). Diarrhea is common in this condition and the corneae are normal. Cardiac problems are less common and death is usually due to neurological deterioration or respiratory infection.

Behaviour. These children are hard to get on with, being stubborn, destructive, and reckless. Institutional care is often necessary.

The Sanfilippo type

In these children neurological problems predominate. They are often thought to have cerebral palsy, the more so as athetoid limb movements are found. Intellectual retardation is severe and terminal progressive dementia is usual. The facial appearance is less weird than in the other 2 types, and growth may be normal.

Treatment. No specific treatment is known. The major pediatric contribution is genetic counselling (Hunter's syndrome is X-linked, whereas Hurler and Sanfilippo are autosomal recessive), support of the family, and treatment of the respiratory and cardiac problems.

DISORDERS OF FAT METABOLISM

The major lipids in the blood are bound to protein, and are the free (nonesterified) fatty acids (NEFA), the triglycerides, cholesterol and its esters, and 2 phospholipids—the glycerophosphatides and sphingomyelin. When in the protein-bound state, they are called lipoproteins and are transported as such. Cholesterol and its esters are carried in the β-lipoproteins, and the phospholipids as α-lipoproteins. Both synthesis and transport are dependent upon biochemical mechanisms. If these go wrong, then disease can result.

SOME SPECIFIC DISORDERS

Lipoprotein deficiency states

In *α-lipoprotein* deficiency, the disorder is characterized by accumulation of cholesterol in the tonsils, liver, spleen, and lymph glands. Otherwise there are no symptoms.

In *β-lipoprotein* deficiency, there is failure to thrive with fatty diarrhea (steatorrhea). Mental retardation is common, and ataxia and retinal disease may occur. The condition is associated with thorn-like projections on the red cells when these are viewed by the microscope.

Treatment is usually by varying the type of fat given in the diet.

Conditions with excess of lipoprotein

These are the hyperlipoproteinemias, and may affect either the α or β types. In either case, evidence of storage is present, often in the skin as yellowish plaques called xanthoma. If the triglycerides are increased, then hepatosplenomegaly occurs. If the β-lipoproteins (cholesterol) are increased, there is a greater tendency to develop coronary heart disease. While rare in children, these disorders, if discovered, are worthy of treatment by varying the diet.

THE SPHINGOLIPIDOSES

These are characteristic lipid storage disorders of childhood, which give rise to various ophthalmic and neurological disease states, as well as evidence of storage of the lipid in various organs. Each is due to an enzyme deficiency which occurs in converting a substrate called sphingosine to a series of derivatives which are found in the brain and other nervous tissues. These end substances are called gangliosides or cerebrosides. The possible disease states due to variations in this cycle are shown in the figure 11.

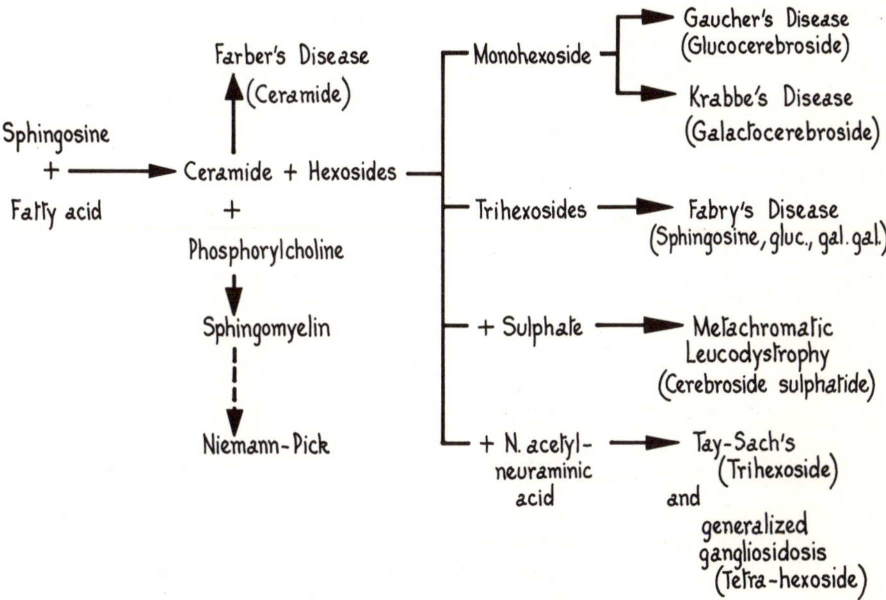

Fig. 11 Origin of the sphingolipidoses.

Some specific disorders

Gaucher's disease

This may occur in an acute infantile form, with failure to thrive, failure of attainment of the motor milestones and progressive, severe nervous system disorder, e.g., bilateral hemiplegia, bulbar paralysis with dysphagia and frequently fatal chest infections. The liver and spleen enlarge.

In the chronic form, which occurs in later childhood, the main problem is hepatosplenomegaly, with anemia due to the consequent Banti's syndrome (q.v.). Some children develop bone pains or fractures in association with the lipid-filled cells which populate the bone marrow. This finding is used at marrow biopsy to confirm the diagnosis of the acute or chronic state.

Tay-Sachs disease (infantile amaurotic family idiocy)

Clinical features. The baby seems normal for a few months. He then ceases to make motor progress. Searching eye movements and other signs of impaired vision develop, and convulsions occur. Ultimately the baby has severe cerebral palsy. Fundoscopy shows the cherry-red spot on the macula. Occasionally hepatosplenomegaly is associated. Nothing can be done for these children. Death usually follows respiratory infection.

The other possibilities are briefly described in table 11.

Table 11. The lipid storage disorders

Eponym	Enzyme Deficiency	Clinical Features
Gaucher's disease	Glucocerebrosidase	Neurological, retardation (see text)
Krabbe's disease	Galactocerebrosidase	Pains in limbs, skin disorder, splenomegaly
Metachromatic leucodystrophy	Aryl sulphatidase	Ataxia, fits, dementia
Niemann-Pick	Sphingomyelinase	Resembles late onset Gaucher's disease
Tay-Sachs disease	Cerebrosidase	See text

SUMMARY

A very large number of the inborn errors of metabolism described above are associated with intellectual retardation. Many cause death early in life, and specific treatment is largely lacking. The problem of early diagnosis relates largely to considering that the problem may exist, or by screening surveys in the newborn. Extension of these screens to the examination of fetal cells obtained in amniocentesis is a further method of timely casefinding for the future.

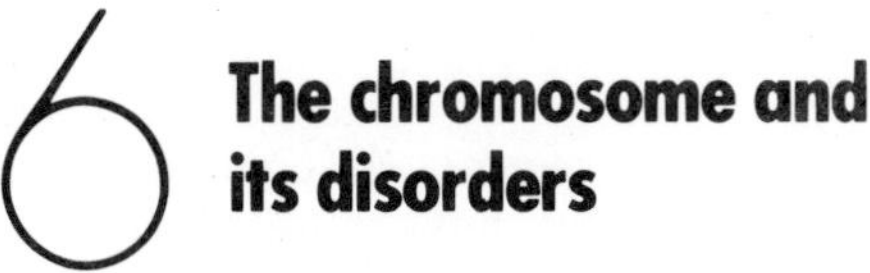

6 The chromosome and its disorders

PRELIMINARY GLOSSARY

Chromosomes: Nuclear chromophilic bodies seen as homologous (identical) pairs in dividing cells. Structurally they are a double helix of D.N.A.

Gene: This is the basic unit of inheritance, occupying a specific site (locus) on the chromosome. Genes structurally are D.N.A. segments, coded to synthesize a specific polypeptide—a protein subunit.

Allele: This is a gene-alternative which may occupy the same site of a similar chromosome. Only 2 alleles can occur in a single individual.

Homozygous: The same allele is present at a gene locus on a pair of similar chromosomes. The genetic instructions given are the same.

Heterozygous: Different alleles are present at a gene locus on a pair of similar chromosomes. The genetic instructions given by each allele are different.

Dominant trait: Generally determined by a heterozygous gene on the autosome.

Recessive trait: Generally determined by a homozygous gene on the autosome.

Sex-linked trait: Determined by a gene on the sex chromosome, invariably the X.

Sex chromosomes: Those determining sex differentiation: female—XX, male—XY.

Autosomes: Other than sex chromosomes.

Karyotype: A conventional description of the chromosomal complement seen at mitotic division.

Phenotype: The outward appearance, or aggregate, of physical characteristics.

Genotype: Genetic constitution.

PHYSIOLOGY

The nuclear chromosomal number of somatic (body) cells is constant for any species. The germ (ova, sperm) cells contain half the number of chromosomes of somatic cells and thus are called haploid. In man, the haploid number is 23, and the somatic cell number is diploid (doubled), i.e., the somatic cell contains 46 chromosomes. The usual diploid complement is of 22 pairs of autosomes, and 2 sex chromosomes. The autosomes consist in 2 identical chromosomes (homologues), 1 of which is maternal and the other of paternal origin. The sex chromosomes in the female are alike and denoted as the X chromosomes. In the male, there is 1 X chromosome and 1 Y chromosome of different shape. Cells may exist with multiples of the haploid number; the general term for these is polyploid cells. Specifically they may be triploid (3 x haploid number) tetraploid (4 x haploid number), etc. Cells which do not contain an exact multiple of the haploid number are called aneuploid, e.g., a cell containing 47 chromosomes is aneuploid.

MORPHOLOGY OF THE CHROMOSOME

Generally the chromosome consists in 2 short arms and 2 long arms attached to a central body—the centromere, the latter being the essential point in identification. The long and short arms attached to the centromere are known as chromatids. Where the centromere is in the middle of the structure, the chromosome is called metacentric; near-terminal centromeres are acrocentrics, those with the intermediate positions are submedian and subterminal chromosomes (see figure 12). These characteristics are used to identify chromosomes grown in tissue culture.

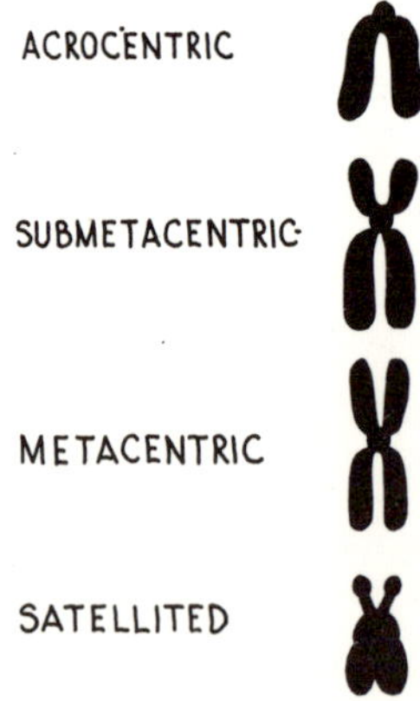

Fig. 12. Chromosal types.

CELL DIVISION

This is constantly occurring both in body (somatic) cells, and in the germ cells. Most chromosome disorders occur because of some change of cell division, so that some knowledge of the process is necessary to understand the causes of disease.

Mitosis

This is the production of body cells identical in chromosomal numbers and genetic material with the parent cell. The chromosomes separate out from the nuclear cytoplasm as rod-like forms which are called chromatids, which in turn divide (except at the centre) at the stage called the metaphase. When division is complete (the anaphase), a completely separate set of chromatids lies at each pole of the cell. Then the cytoplasm divides (telophase) and the pair of daughter cells is now complete. The process is illustrated in figures 13 and 14.

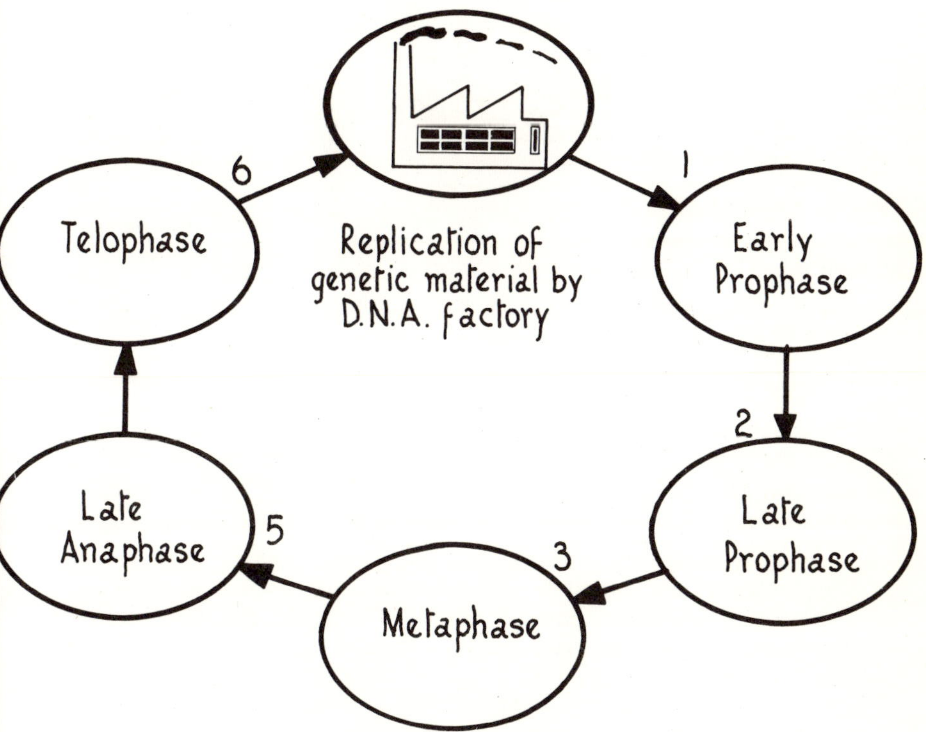

Fig. 13. Events in mitosis.

1. Early Prophase

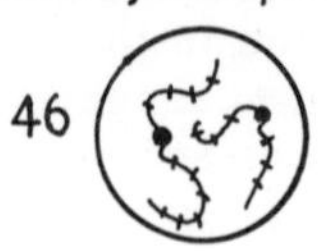

Emergence of thread-like chromosomes. (Not recognisably replicated).

2. Late Prophase

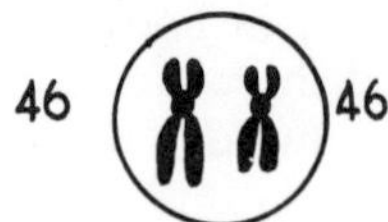

Chromosomes formed of 'lined-up' chromatids, with obvious centromeres (replication now obvious).

3. Metaphase

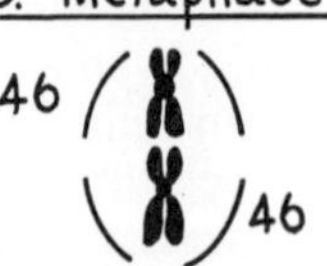

Chromatids in equatori plane of cell. Disintegration of nucle membrane.

4. Early Anaphase

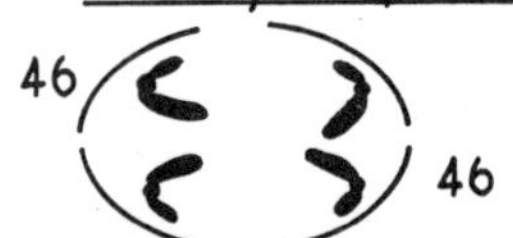

Centromeric division has occurred; complete separation of chromatids.

5. Late Anaphase

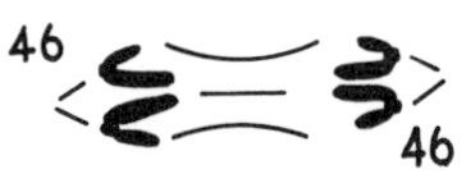

Complete polarization of chromatids.

6 Telophase

46

46

Cytoplasmic cleava occurs.

Fig. 14. Mitotic division: events in the nucleus. Example is of behaviour of 2 paired chromosomes.

Meiosis (reduction division)

This is the process by which the gametes (ova or sperm) are formed, so that the chromosomal number is half of that of the somatic cells, i.e., gametes are haploid. The reduction division is followed by a process of duplication which is similar to that described under mitosis.

The mechanism of meiosis. In the first stage (prophase) the chromosomes are unpaired and threadlike and are called leptotenes. Soon the homologous parts coalesce to form the zygotene (pairs of bivalents). In the later stage (pachytene), the individual chromosomes again reduplicate to form 4 associated chains of genetic material (the tetrad). At this stage, crossing over of genetic material occurs. In a sense the chromosome breaks up and reunites, not with itself, but with its homologue (fig. 15).

1. Early Prophase

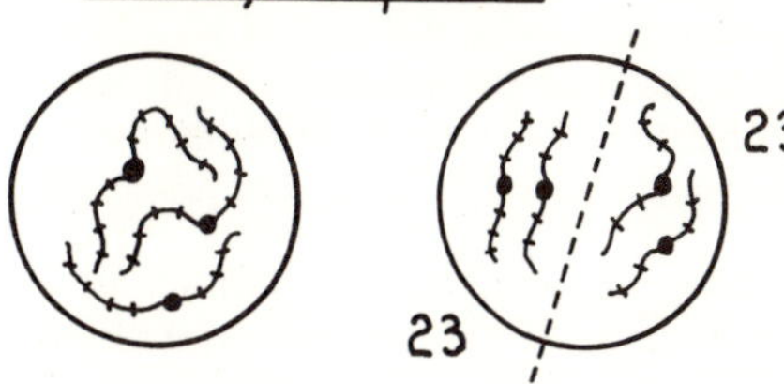

Unpaired threads. The Leptotene.

Paired threads, bivalent The zygotene formation.

2. Late Prophase

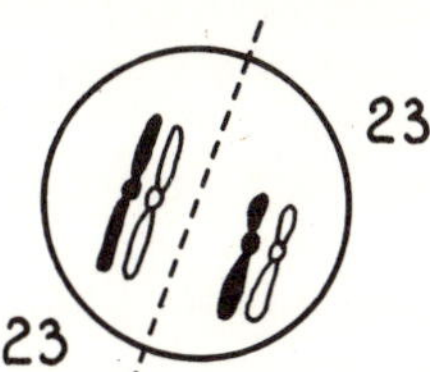

Pachytene formation. Replication has occurred.

3. Late Pachytene

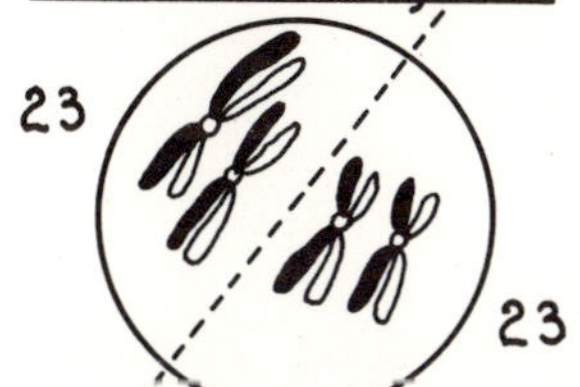

The chromosomes are aligned preparatory to the exchange of genetic material.

4. Diplotene

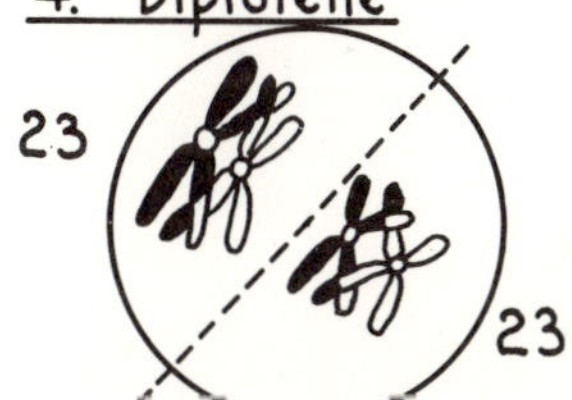

In this phase, diakinesis, (exchange of genetic material occurs (see Fig. 5).

5. First Metaphase

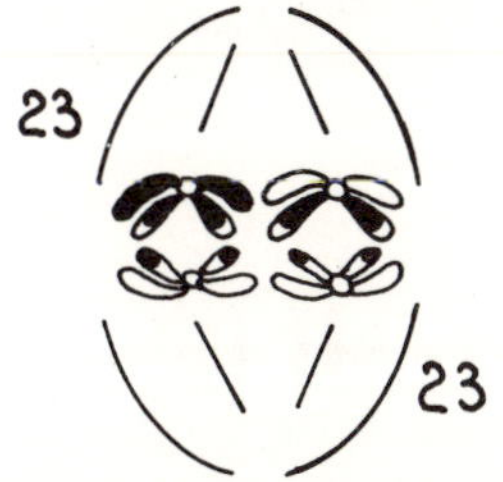

Genetic mixing complete, cell split beginning.

6. Anaphase

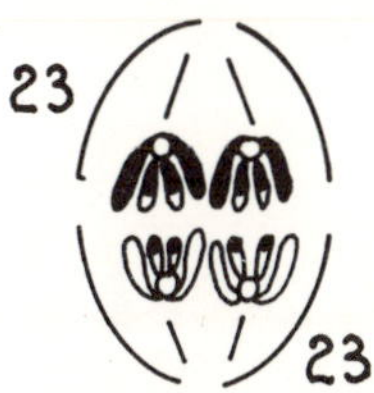

Cell split almost complete.

7. Interphase

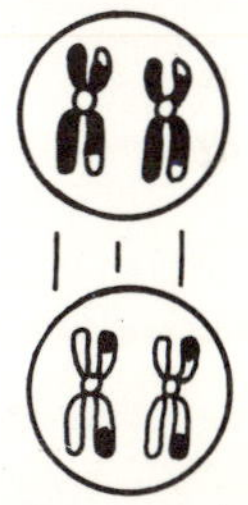

Cell split complete, chromosome number = 23

Fig. 15. Meiosis (reduction division): first meiotic division.

The resultant chromosome need not then be identical with the original parental chromosome (fig. 16). The chromosomal nucleus then goes through the stages (metaphase, anaphase, and telophase) of mitotic division, to give 2 nuclei, each of 23 chromosomes, but with rearrangement of the genetic material by crossover.

In the second meiotic division (fig. 17), the cells which are the products of the first meiotic division split again to give a total of 4 cells, each with 23 chromosomes, and each with a genetically different gametic type. All male haploid (23 chromosomes) cells form spermatozoa; in the female, however, only 1 cell forms the ovum, the other 3—the polar bodies—degenerate.

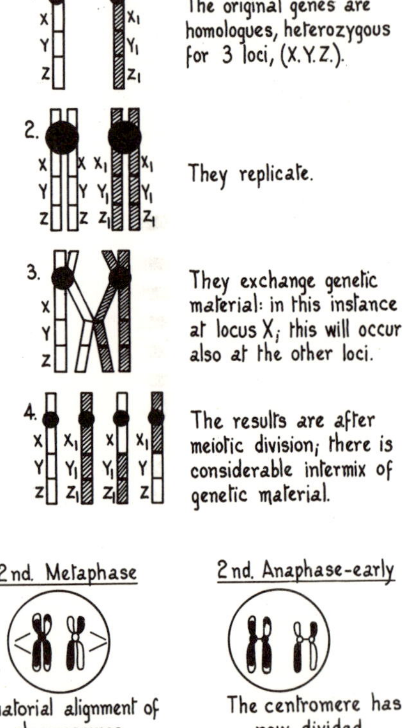

Fig. 16. Details of events during diakinesis to show exchange of genetic material.

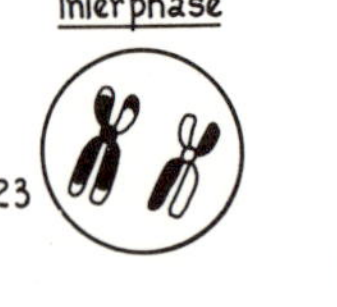

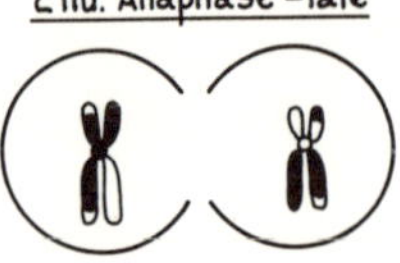

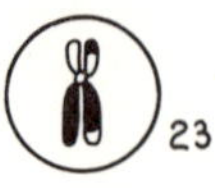

Fig. 17. Meiosis: second meiotic division.

It is clear that in the process of division, the individual sections of the chromosome itself—the genes—may be changed. This may express itself as a mutant single gene, which still controls the same characteristic or process, e.g., an enzymatic process. Mutation here may be associated with a biochemical anomaly or metabolic variant. In any cell, since there are 2 paired chromosomes, the condition where the paired genes are the same is that of *homozygosity*, i.e. the zygote will have the identical gene form. If the genes are quite different (allelomorphs) then 1 may dominate, suppressing the action of the other, which is *recessive*. However, complete dominance or recessivity is not constant. Difference in genes, therefore, is expressed as a difference in specific and (sometimes) a single characteristic. It is compatible with a normal *chromosomal* number and structure.

Fertilization

This is the union of the gametes (haploid cells) to form a zygote. All ova contain the X chromosome, sperm contain either an X or a Y chromosome. The union of an X sperm with an ovum gives a female (XX) zygote; a Y sperm gives a male (XY) zygote. The autosomal number, of course, is the same in either male or female zygotes (see figure 18).

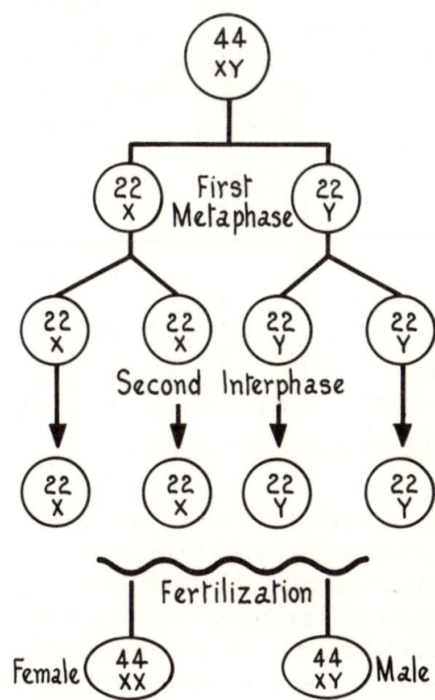

Fig. 18. Gamete formation.

PRODUCTION OF ABNORMAL CHROMOSOMES

1. *Mechanisms which can change genetic content but maintain cell chromosomal number*

a. Inversion. In figure 19 is shown a normal chromosome with identified areas of genetic material (block or crosshatched). In the same figure is shown the situation where genetic material has aligned itself in a different way on the chromosome. Note that the centromeric position is unchanged, and that there is no loss or gain of genetic material, only an inversion of the crosshatched material in relation to the centromere. This is called *paracentric* inversion and may occur in man, apparently without expressing a disease process.

In figure 20, is shown the situation where the centromere also is shifted (pericentric inversion). Again the total content of genetic material is unchanged, and unlike the situation in paracentric inversion, the change in centromeric position may be recognizable when chromosomal analysis is done.

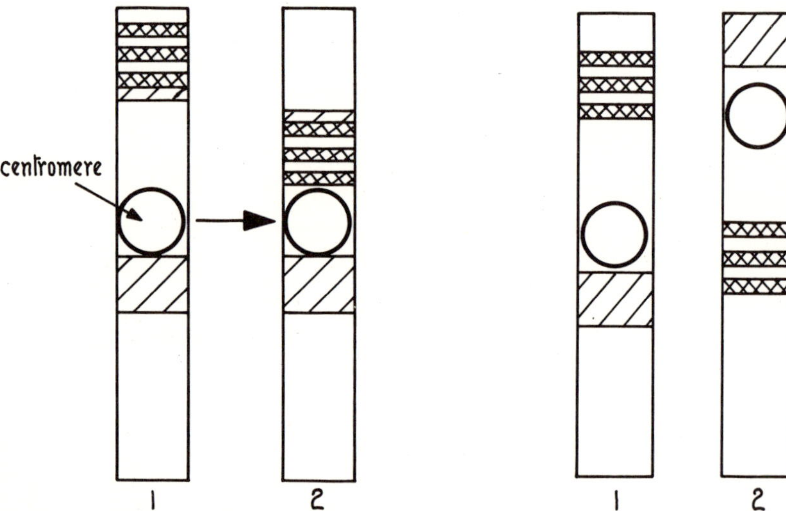

Fig. 19. Paracentric inversion.

Fig. 20. Pericentric inversion.

b. Deletion. This is illustrated in figure 21, where loss of genetic material has occurred. If only a few areas are deleted, the patient may seem normal. Marked loss of genetic material causes severe abnormality. The head-to-tail junction noted in the figure causes the ring chromosome, which may be identified in the karyotype. Its significance is to confirm a loss of genetic material.

c. Translocation. This occurs when a chromosome breaks, and a segment joins to another chromosome, i.e., the genetic material is translocated. If this occurs between 2 paired chromosomes (figure 22), it is called homologous translocation. If to another chromosome, then it is nonhomologous translocation, (figure 23).

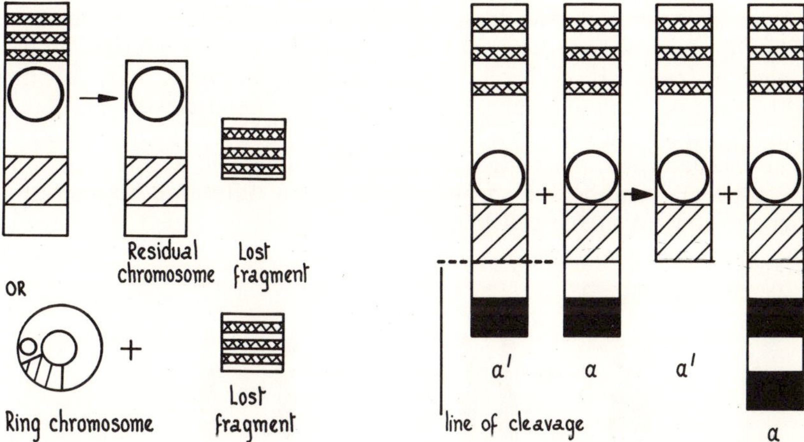

Fig. 21. Deletion of chromosomal material.

Fig. 22. Homologous translocation. The figure shows transfer of extra genetic material to another homologue of a pair of chromosomes.

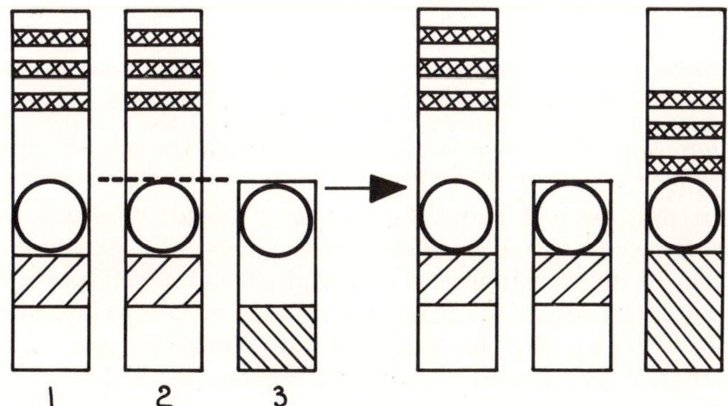

Fig. 23. Nonhomologous translocation. 1 and 2 are homologues, 3 is not.

It should be noted that there is no loss of genetic material in this process, but the chromosome can alter in size and shape. Such translocations without genetic loss are balanced, and do not affect the patient. However, their children may be affected with a chromosomal syndrome.

d. Isochromosome formation. In the anaphase of cell division, a chromosome reduplicates longitudinally by division at the centromere. Thus in general long-arm and short-arm material is present in the daughter cells. If division occurs in the transverse axis of the chromosome, then only long-arm or short-arm material will be present. An abnormal chromosome of this type is called an *isochromosome*. The mechanism is illustrated in figure 24. There will, in this situation, be a normal number of chromosomes, but a difference between the genetic content of the cell lines.

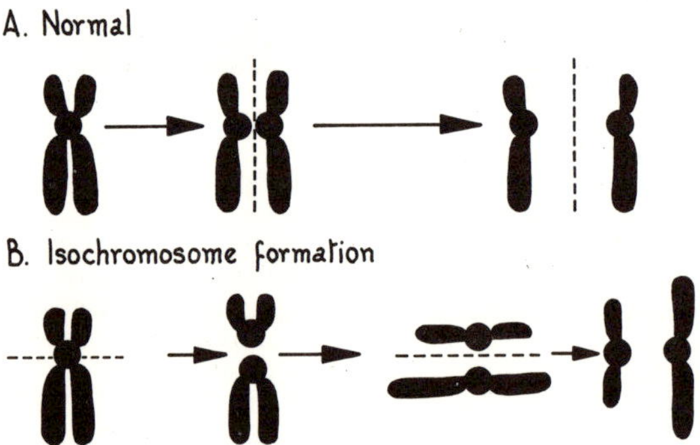

Fig. 24. Events at anaphase. In B, both short and long arms migrate to different cells.

2. *Mechanisms which may change genetic content and increase or decrease cell chromosomal number*

a. Anaphase lag. Anaphase is the stage at which the paired replicated chromosomes migrate to the cell pair. If migration of a chromosome is delayed, it may be lost and the resultant chromosomal cell number would be reduced. The abnormality is theoretically replicable ad infinitum, but in most instances, autosomal chromosomal loss is lethal. Loss of sex chromosome by anaphase lag may be compatible with life, though not with fertility. The condition is illustrated in figure 25. It will be noted that, if the çell line is a gamete, fertilization will supply one of the missing chromosomes in the pair. The resulting zygote will then be monosomic (i.e., lacking one of the chromosomes in any pair).

b. Primary nondisjunction. Disjunction is the process by which the paired, lined up, chromosomes of a single cell at metaphase, separate to migrate to the 2 daughter cells. If the pairs fail to separate, nondisjunction occurs; of the 2 daughter cells, one will have an extra chromosome and the other will lack 1 chromosome. The situation is illustrated in figure 26.

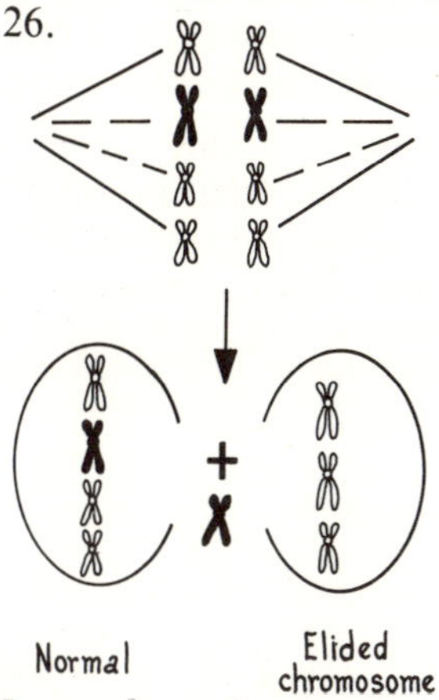

Fig. 25. Loss of a chromosome by anaphase lag.

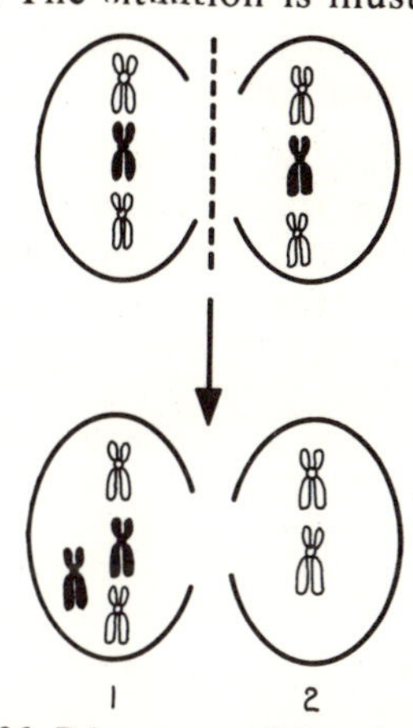

Fig. 26. Primary nondisjunction. Cell in anaphase – movement of "conjoined" homologous chromosomes to daughter cell 1.

If the cell is a gamete (as is common), fertilization with another normal gamete will lead to 2 cell lines. Thus in the zygote derived from the gamete with an extra chromosome (fig. 27), *trisomy* will present, i.e., 2 chromosomes from the original disjunction, plus 1 normal homologue from the other gamete. In this instance, chromosomal number increases, e.g., 24 from the gamete with the extra chromosome, 23 from the normal gamete, total 47; in the other instance, the gamete lacking a

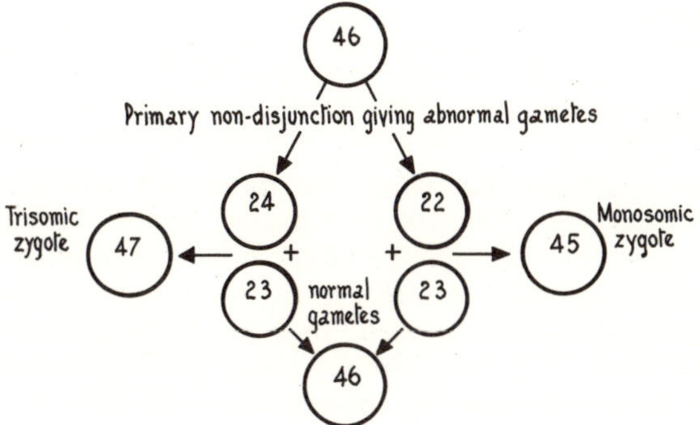

Fig. 27. Origin of trisomy or monosomy.

chromosome joins a normal gamete, which contributes one chromosome of the pair. This is *monosomy*, and total chromosomal number is reduced, e.g., the monosomal gamete has 22 chromosomes, the normal gamete 23, total 45 chromosomes. Abnormal chromosomal number is termed *aneuploidy*. It will be noted that the individual resulting from primary nondisjunction will have only 1 cell line, albeit an abnormal one.

c. *Secondary nondisjunction.* This abnormality follows from the formation of a trisomic gonadal cell following the fertilization of an abnormal gamete. Clearly enough (fig. 28) in the first meiotic division of this cell, 1 trisomic and 1 normal cell will result. Secondary meiotic division gives the same result, with trisomic and normal gametes in equal proportions. Fertilization of these will result in zygotes of which 1 is normal and 1 of which is trisomic.

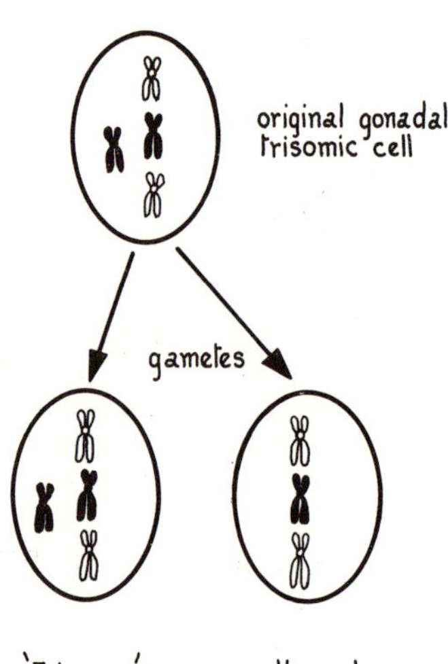

Fig. 28. **Secondary nondisjunction in a trisomic gonadal cell.**

Nondisjunction can also occur at both meiotic divisions of the gonadal cell. The first nondisjunction will lead to cells with 24 and 22 chromosomes as already described (see figures 28 and 29).

The cell ii line (fig. 29) will continue to divide, lacking a chromosome; the cell i line may again undergo nondisjunction at the second meiosis (metaphase). This can lead to the migration of all 4 resultant deviant chromosomes into 1 gamete, or 3 could migrate into 1 gamete, and 1 into the other, or 2 chromosomes could move into each of 2 cells. Fertilization of these gametes by another normal gamete could result in up to 5 chromosomes of the same type occupying a single zygote.

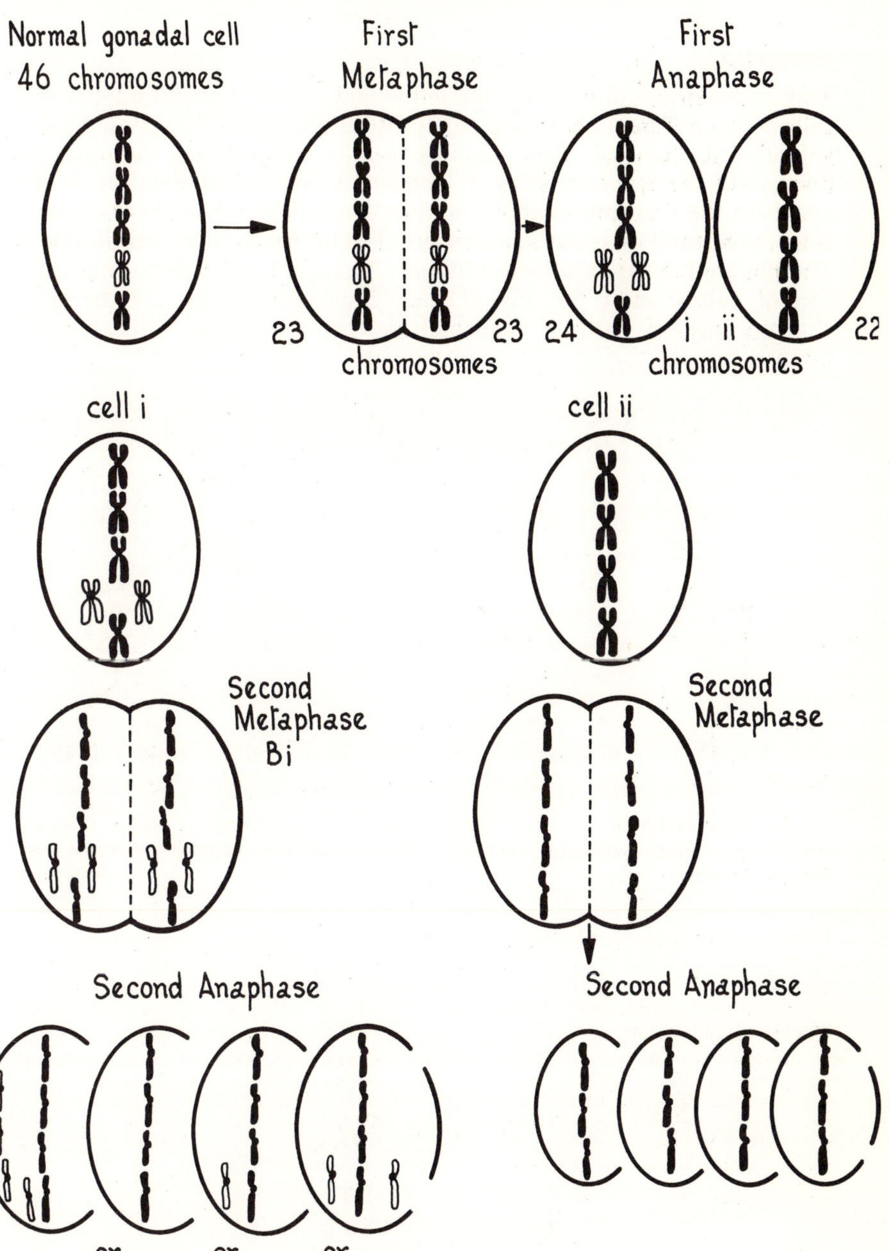

Fig. 29. Nondisjunction at both meiotic phases of the gonadal cell.

Mosaicism

This is the situation in which the individual carries 2 or more types of cells with a different chromosomal constitution. Such cell types are called cell lines (clones). This anomaly usually arises during the mitotic division of the zygote, usually by nondisjunction or anaphase lag. If it occurs in the first mitotic division, then 2 stemlines occur. If at a later stage, abnormal divisions again occur, 3 stemlines may be identifiable. The possibilities are outlined in figures 30 and 31. Such abnormalities can of course exist for any of the 22 autosomes and for the sex chromosomes. Autosomal abnormalities tend to be lethal. Some possible mosaics for the sex chromosomes are shown in table 12.

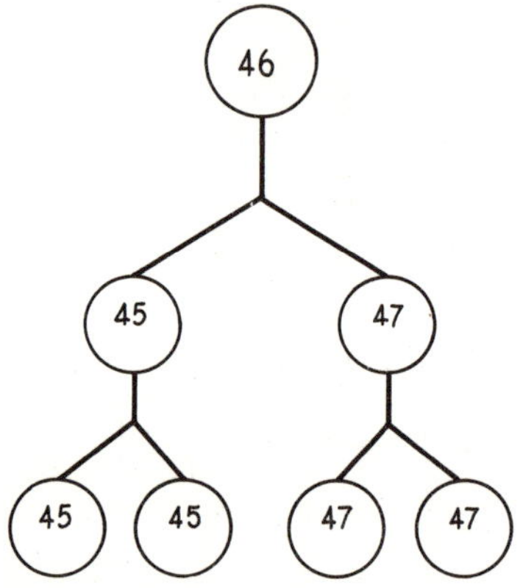

Fig. 30. Nondisjunction at the first mitotic division of the zygote. Two cell lines are formed.

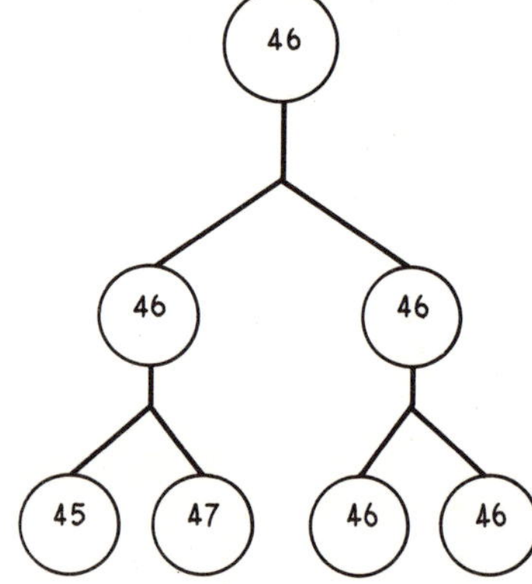

Fig. 31. Nondisjunction after first mitotic division. Three cell lines are formed.

Table 12. Formation of sex chromosome mosaics

Mechanism	Cell Type	Expected Mosaics
Mitotic nondisjunction	XX	XXX/XO
	XY	XYY/XO XXY/XY
	XXY	XXXY/XY XXYY/XX
Anaphase lag	XX	XX/XO
	XY	XY/XO
	XXY	XXY/XX XXY/XY

LABORATORY DIAGNOSIS OF CHROMOSOMAL DISORDERS

This is normally done by culturing the patient's lymphocytes for 72 hours. Cell growth is then arrested at the stage of mitotic metaphase, by treating the culture with phytohemagglutinin. Suitable cells are photographed, and the chromosomes are separately cut from the print. They are then arranged according to the so-called Denver convention, which uses morphological criteria (length and centromeric position) to place the pairs of chromosomes in groups (A-G) and to enumerate those pairs into autosomal chromosomes (1-22). The sex chromosomes (X and Y) are shown separately. The situation is illustrated in figure 32.

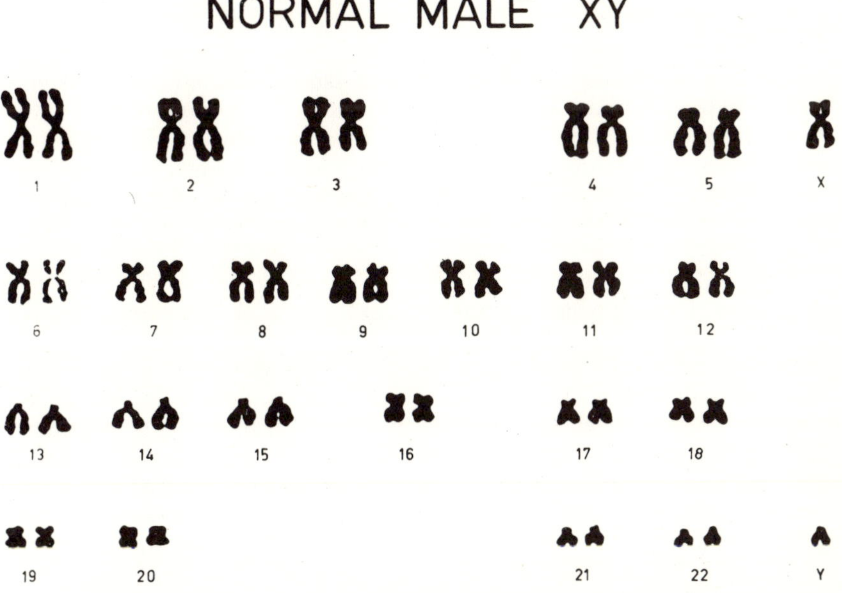

Fig. 32. Example of karotype arranged according to Denver convention.

NUCLEAR SEX

The cell nuclei of many female tissues contains a dark-staining area adjacent to the nuclear membrane which is called a Barr body. It is most readily seen in the cells of the buccal mucosa. The significance of the Barr body is that it implies the presence of a normal female sex chromosome complement (XX). If 1 sex chromosome is missing (XO, as in Turner's syndrome), no Barr body is seen. If the X chromosome complement is increased, e.g., XXX or XXXX, the number of Barr bodies is 2 and 3 respectively, i.e., one less than the number of X chromosomes present.

An accessory lobule (drumstick) is also found in a small percentage of the polymorphs of females, and with an XX complement. These drumsticks are not found in XO complements, and increased X complements (XXX, etc.) are not reflected in drumstick number.

DERMATOGLYPHICS

This is the recording and analysis of finger, hand, toe, and sole prints. These may differ from normal in the chromosomal diseases, and in certain acquired ones such as congenital rubella.

Fingerprints

These are well known to differ between individuals, and also within limits, to have genetically determined patterns. The common basic patterns are loops, arches, and whorls. Loops may open to the radial or ulnar sides. When looking at the palm these are designated radial or ulnar loops. Arches are lines of fairly marked curvature and may be plain or tented. Whorls may be spiral or concentric, or coexist with a loop.

A triradius is the centre of the Δ-shaped point of junction of 3 streams of ridges which are approximately parallel. The same name is used for similar regions in the palm or sole of the foot. A conventionalized palm print is shown in figure 33. From this it will be seen that 4 triradii are placed at the bases of the index, middle, ring, and little fingers. These are conventionalized as triradii a, b, c, and d. Another (axis) triradius is constantly present distal to the wrist (bangle) crease. The height of the triradius is the length from the wrist crease to the axis triradius, and is normally less than 40% of the total palm length. The latter is the distance from the wrist crease to the b triradius at the base of the ring finger. Another way of defining the position of the axis triradius is to measure the angle formed by the axis triradius and the a and d triradii. The normal angle is $< 57°$. The situation is explained in figure 34.

Crease patterns

The normal pattern is shown in figure 33. A fair variation is possible, but a single interphalangeal crease is frequent in chromosomal anomalies. A true complete transverse crease is statistically more common in Down's syndrome, but occurs in 4-5% of normal people.

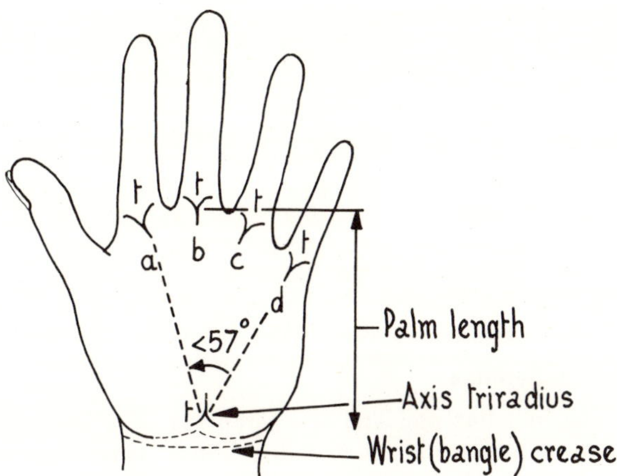

Fig. 33. A conventionalized hand print.

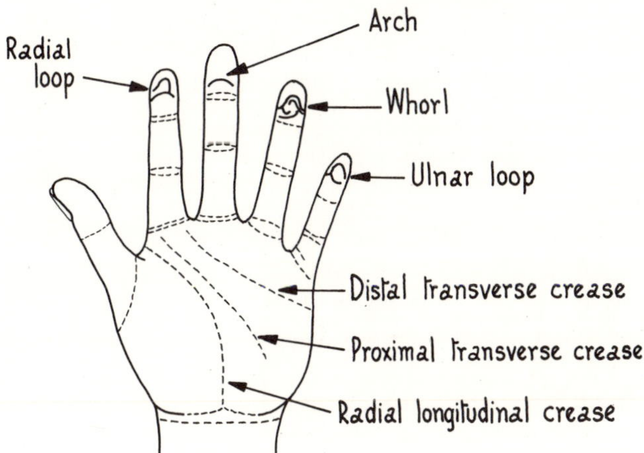

Fig. 34. Triradii of the palm.

Abnormalities in palmar dermatoglyphics

These may be divided into abnormalities of distribution of finger print patterns, and abnormalities of the axis triradial position. A comparison of finger print pattern distribution in normals and Down's syndrome is shown in table 13.

The axis triradius may migrate distally, i.e., towards the palm. This is fairly frequent in chromosomal disorders and, therefore, its height will increase, or the angle forming the a and d axis triradii will exceed 60°.

Table 13. Dermatoglyphics

Left Forefinger Prints		
Pattern	Control	Down's
Whorl	33.4	11.0
Ulnar loop	36.3	82.4
Radial loop	19.4	2.3
Arch	10.9	3.4

Figures are percentage occurrence.

Plantar dermatoglyphics

The sole of the foot has received less attention than the palm, but the principal finding in normals is the distal loop which opens into the space between the hallux and the adjacent toe. The size is variable but the loop formation constant.

In Down's syndrome, a tibial arch (i.e., opening towards the first metatarsal) is very common. A similar arch, opening to the fibular side, may be found in the D_1 trisomy syndrome. The features are shown in figure 35.

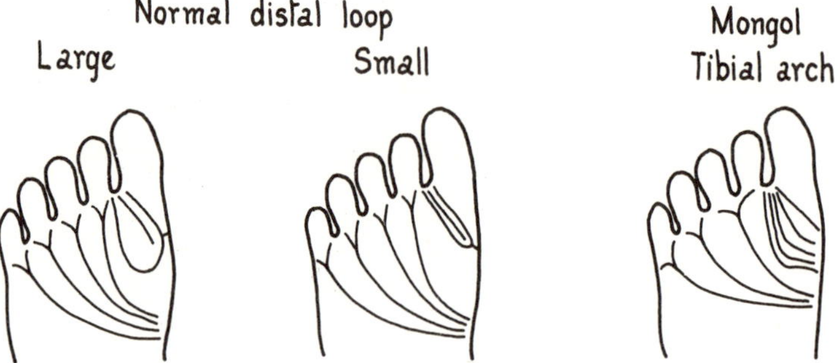

Fig. 35. Normal and abnormal footprints: *a*, Normal distal loop, large; *b*, Normal distal loop, small; *c*, Down's tibial arch.

DISORDERS OF THE SEX CHROMOSOME

Turner's syndrome

This is a form of congenital ovarian deficiency, the fundamental cause is loss of one of the sex chromosomes. Characteristically the patient is monosomic for X and the karyotype is XO, but mosaics, e.g., XX/XO, XO/XX/XXX, isochromosome (XX_1) or partial deletions ($X\bar{x}$), or ring X chromosome formations, have also been described.

Clinical features. The baby is usually of low birth weight and in many there is a symmetrical swelling of the hands and feet due to lymphoedema. This stage is also called the Bonnevie-Ullrich syndrome. Coincident congenital heart disease is frequent, commonly as aortic coarctation, less frequently as septal defects or pulmonic stenosis. In the infant, redundant skin is usual but the classic neck webbing is not yet present. Occasionally the chest may seem to be unduly broad. The baby grows poorly.

The full-blown features are seen in the older child and consist in small stature; cubitus valgus (abnormal carrying angle of the elbows); low hairline; neck webbing; high, arched palate; receding chin; a broad chest with widely spaced nipples; and congenital heart disease. In a few children the above features are present but are not a cause of complaint until delayed puberty is noted. This usually means lack of menses, breast development, and infantile genitalia. Difficulties with education are common and mental retardation may be present.

X-rays. Osteoporosis is common, and I.V.P. may show renal abnormalities.

Laboratory. The buccal smear shows no Barr body and the polymorphs have no drumstick. The patient is chromatin-negative and cytogenetic study usually shows loss of an X chromosome, or any of the possibilities mentioned above.

Treatment. There is no specific treatment. If appropriate, the patient should be reassured that marriage is possible, but the bearing of children impossible. The cardiac defect is treated as necessary. At the appropriate age of puberty (12-14) feminization is induced by estrogen and a progestogen.

Turner's syndrome in the male

Clinical features. The child fails to thrive, is in the low percentiles, and usually has congenital heart disease. Inspection reveals webbing of the neck; bilateral, incomplete eyelid ptosis, giving a suggestive look; and cubitus valgus. The testes are usually undescended and mild mental retardation is frequent. These children do not have the swollen feet of the Bonnevie Ullrich female variant, and the skeletal abnormalities such as the shield chest are less obvious. Sterility is not uncommon.

Polysomy of the X chromosome

In this situation nondisjunction causes a triple X, tetra, or penta-X zygote, i.e., XXX, XXXX, or XXXXX. These children are phenotypically and often functionally normal. The chromosomal abnormality is discovered by chance, usually by buccal smear surveys which show multiple Barr bodies.

Y chromosome and its variations

This chromosome determines masculinity but controls few other factors. Minor chromosomal variations are fairly common, and without clinical significance. Major deletions in the Y chromosome are associated with genital aberrations. The karyotype XYY has been found in some criminal groups, but probably also occurs in normals.

The principal anomaly of clinical importance is Klinefelter's syndrome.

Klinefelter's syndrome

In this the phenotype is masculine. The karyotype is usually XXY or XXXY but XXYY and XXXYY has occurred together with mosaics such as XX/XXY or XY/XXY.

Clinical features. There are few until the age of puberty, although 25% of sufferers show previous evidence of mental retardation. The usual complaint is of smallness of the testes or penis. Such patients tend to be tall and thin, and gynecomastia occurs in those who are of heavier build. Examination reveals minor beard growth, scanty pubic hair of feminine distribution, and a high-pitched voice. Sterility is a common complaint and testicular biopsy shows, at puberty, obliteration of the seminiferous tubules. The buccal smear will show 1 or more Barr body Mental retardation is strongly associated with karyotypes XXXY and mosaic forms.

Treatment. Discretion should be used in explaining the situation and association with femininity avoided. Reassurance as to ability to copulate, but confirmation of infertility is in order. Testosterone will enhance hair growth and sometimes sexual drive. Mental retardation contraindicates active therapy.

DISORDERS OF THE AUTOSOME

The commoner aberrations are Down's syndrome (mongolism) and abnormalities of chromosomes of the E group (trisomy 18) and the D group (trisomy 13-15).

Down's syndrome

Cytogenetics. The commoner type is that called nondisjunction trisomy 21. This is a chance change which is made more likely by advanced maternal age. The mechanism is an incorrect segregation of the chromosomes into the daughter cells at the first or second divisions of the gametes. Thus, 1 cell has a chromosome too many, the other has 1 too few. The resultant zygote, after fertilization, is abnormal, 1 having

3 representatives of the pair. When chromosome 21 is so affected, the syndrome results. The chromosomal number is 47.

Sufferers may rarely appear to have only 46 chromosomes. This is because the extra chromosome is suppressed by *translocation*, which means that the extra chromosome has attached itself to another chromosome, usually to one of the acrocentrics of group D (13, 14, 15), occasionally to another 21 chromosome. This mechanism usually occurs by chance, but also follows when one of the parents has a translocation of 1 of the 21 chromosomes. Such a parent, while having a normal *amount* of gene material, will appear to have only 45 chromosomes. At gametogenesis however, 4 possibilities exist (see figure 36).

If the 21 chromosome is, for example, translocated to number 14, the latter may migrate with the free 21. Fertilization gives a normal infant. The normal 14 may however migrate without any 21 chromosome, so at fertilization there is deletion of 1 21 chromosome, giving an inviable fetus. The 14/21 translocation chromosome may go to a gamete without a 21, which is, however, added after fertilization. This results in an apparently normal child who is a translocation carrier. The possibility is that the 14/21 chromosome is placed in a gamete with the free 21 chromosome, another 21 chromosome is added after fertilization. This zygote gives rise to a sufferer.

Although the translocation state is rare (1-5% of the syndrome), it is of considerable genetic importance, since the translocation carrier state may be found in the parent, and should be sought when translocation is diagnosed in the child. A positive finding implies that 1 in 3 of the *viable* infants will be affected, and that 1/3 will be carriers and 1/3 normal. Appropriate genetic counselling is in order.

Clinical features. The condition may be recognized by the appearance of the child, or suspicion arise because of associated anomalies. At birth, the most important feature is the facial appearance, the most characteristic feature of which is perhaps the small triangular mouth. Epicanthic folds are common but not diagnostic. The eyes usually slant upwards, although this feature may not be clear until a few weeks after birth. The head size is small and flattening of the occiput is sometimes appreciable but becomes more definite after a few months. The ears often look abnormal. Incurving of the little fingers may be noted at birth, and the characteristic dermatoglyphics of the hand and feet (see below) are present. In many instances the baby presents with high intestinal obstruction due to duodenal atresia, and congenital heart disease (often atrioventricularis communis) may also be the first sign.

By early infancy (3-4 months) the characteristic features are usually well established. The face is now typical, with well-marked eye slanting, triangular mouth, snub nose, protruding tongue, and ear anomalies.

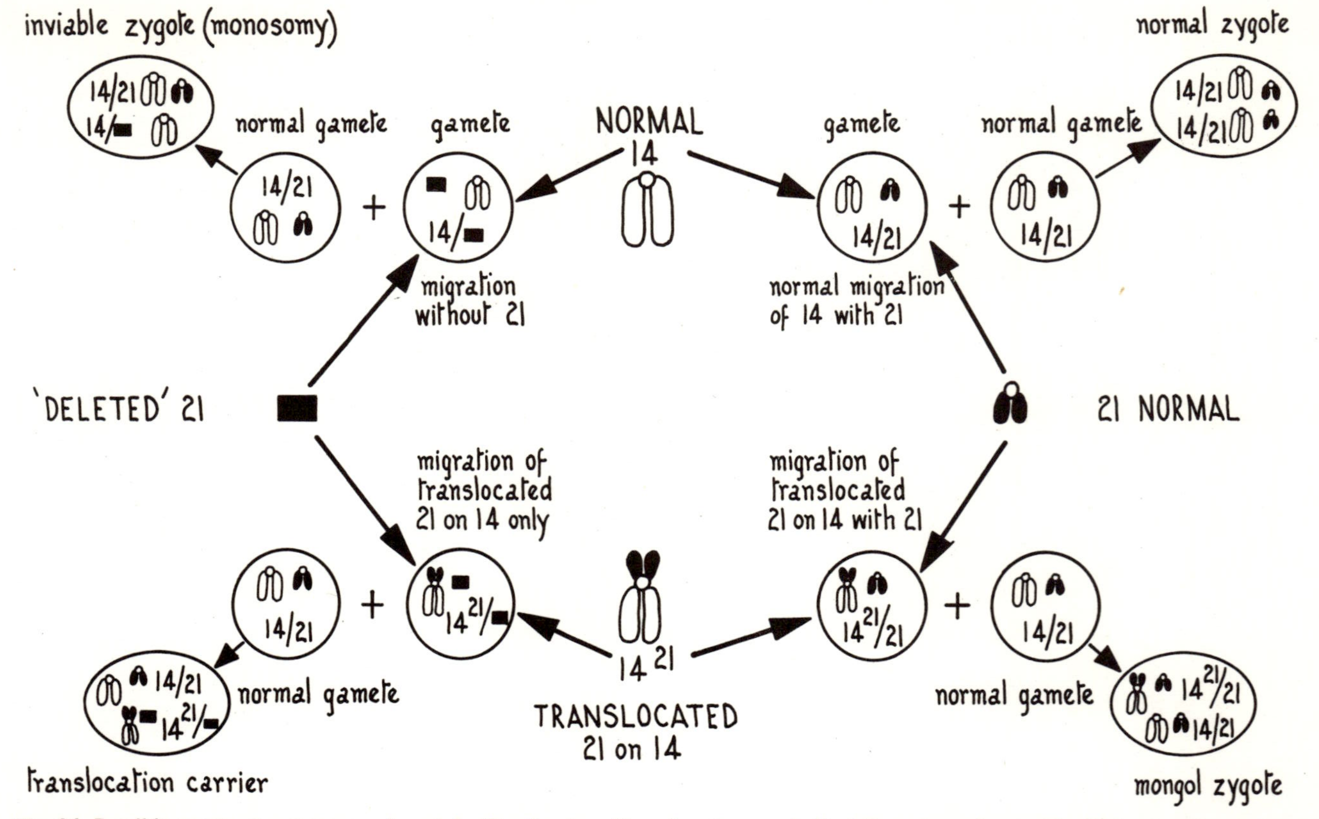

Fig. 36. Possible events at gametogenesis and fertilization in a "translocation carrier" of Down's syndrome. The 21 has translocated on to the 14.

The neck is short and the occiput flattened. The hands and feet are squat with an increased space between the first and second digits. Generalized hypotonia is now well marked. The infant now begins to exhibit delay in the milestones of development. The protruding tongue is often wrinkled by the sixth month. General growth is impaired and all body measurements, including the head, are in the lower percentiles. The infant is undemanding and apathetic and may present a considerable feeding problem.

As the child grows older, the delay in motor development becomes more apparent. Walking is late, and talking may never be achieved. Toilet training is markedly delayed or absent. Muscular hypotonia, however, tends to improve as the child ages. Chronic nasal discharge and frequent respiratory infections are common. Genital development tends to be delayed, as is puberty, although both menstruation and sperm production may ultimately be achieved. In later years, the shortness of stature persists, often with associated obesity. In most instances the child is moderately to severely retarded in intellect. Emotional development is stunted and they are uncomplaining, easy to organize and usually pleasant and affectionate.

X-rays. In infancy, flaring of the hip bones and small acetabular angles may be present. A rudimentary second phalanx in the fifth digit is common.

Dermatoglyphics. A single crease on any digit is suggestive. A transverse palmar crease, although not unknown in normals, has a higher incidence in Mongolism. The representation of digital dermal patterns is different from that of normal children, e.g., whorls of the right thumb in normals average about 38% of the total; in Down's syndrome this will tend to be of the order of 70%.

Treatment. Primarily this lies in the care of the family. If the diagnosis is at all in doubt, another opinion and cytogenetic study is in order. When the diagnosis is certain, there is little point in delaying a thorough explanation. It is well to avoid too much emphasis on the genetic aspects, as this tends to encourage guilt feelings. The parents should be told that the child will never be of normal mentality, but that this does not mean that he will be incapable of acquiring some simple skills. Head size measurement is a useful prognostic measure, the further this deviates from the normal, the more likely is it that severe intellectual retardation will be present. The severely retarded usually require institutionalization, but the child should be retained in the family as long as possible. This gives him a better chance to acquire the simple skills of walking and toilet training which facilitate institutional care. The specific care of the individual patient will vary with the intellectual level and the presence of associated anomalies.

D_1(13-15) trisomy syndrome (Patau's disease)

This condition is seldom compatible with long survival and occurs once in about every 8-9,000 births.

Clinical features. There are multiple congenital abnormalities. The condition is suspected because of the facial anomalies, which are of 2 main types. In one, usually associated with failure of cleavage of the cerebral hemispheres, there is hypertelorism (wide-set eyes), cleft lip, and severe nasal deformities. Ocular anomalies (microphthalmos, buphthalmos) are also common. In the other type, the facial anomaly is less severe, the nose is bulbous, the features coarse, and redundant facial skin folds common. Cleft lip and palate may coexist. Whatever the facial appearance, spade-like hands, with polydactyly and flexion deformities, are usual. Microcephaly is invariable and associated with severe mental defect. In males, genital anomalies are common, and deficiencies of the abdominal muscles, varying from hernias to exomphalos, not uncommon. Most of these children also have severe congenital heart disease and many die in the newborn period.

Dermatoglyphics. Distal axis triradii and horizontal palmar creases are found.

Cytology. Most patients are trisomic in the D group, probably in chromosome 13. Deletions of the B and D groups occur, and mosaicism has been reported.

E trisomy (trisomy 18) (Edwards' syndrome)

Clinical features. The infant is often small and difficult to resuscitate, so that neonatal death is common. The face is small, with micrognathia, hypoplasia of the orbital ridges, and a small narrow head. The ears are low set and deficient in cartilage. The fingers are tightly flexed at the metacarpophalangeal joints, and thus fixed in the palm. The foot is convex, giving a rocker-bottom appearance with a typically short hallux. Eye deformities (microphthalmos, colobomata) occur. The neck may be webbed and a short broad chest, with hypoplastic nipples may occur. The sternum is short, the shoulders hypermobile, and periumbilical herniae occur. Severe congenital heart disease is usual, and serious central nervous system defects, e.g., meningomyelocele, may be associated.

Dermatoglyphics. Simple arches are present on the tips of most fingers. Interphalangeal creases are wanting, and distal displacement of the axis triradius is common.

Cytogenetics. Most (80%) are trisomic at the 18th chromosome; double trisomy and even a normal karyotype has been reported.

Prognosis. 50% of these children die in the first 3 months of life; 90% are dead by 1 year.

Cri-du-chat (Cat-cry) syndrome

This condition is an anomaly of the group B (4-5) chromosomes. Mostly this is a short-arms deletion of the 5th chromosome.

Clinical features. The infant is retarded and microcephalic. He is in the low percentiles for growth. The face is rounded and hypertelorism and slanting eyes are common. The principal feature is the baby's curious cry. This is weak, high pitched, ill maintained, and like the mewing of a kitten. Death is usual in the first year of life.

Cytogenetics. There is deletion, usually incomplete, of the short arms of the 5th chromosome.

Treatment. None is possible.

GENETIC COUNSELLING

This is an area of growing importance to the pediatrician, partly because patterns of inheritance are well established for some disorders, and partly because genetic counselling can be made effective by reliable methods of contraception, or legally available abortion. The increasing sophistication of parents has also increased the demand for genetic counselling.

Minor congenital abnormalities are common, and if treatment is needed, it is easy and effective. Concern arises when the defect is severe or untreatable. In this circumstance, what parents want to know is what is the risk of further disasters to their own future children, and grandchildren. Good genetic counselling is dependent upon an exact diagnosis of the first affected child (the propositus), extensive information concerning his relatives, ascendant, descendant and collateral, and some knowledge of the laws of inheritance.

In relation to the need for exact diagnosis, 2 difficulties arise. First, the condition may be a phenocopy. This is the term applied to a disease process which has an *acquired* basis, but whose clinical features make it look genetically determined. If a phenocopy is misdiagnosed as congenital, then an unnecessary gloomy family outlook may be given. An example would be microcephaly due to rubella being mistaken for an autosomal recessive form of microcephaly.

Secondly, the condition may be one with similar clinical features but with a different genetic background. An example of this is muscular dystrophy which in one form is an autosomal dominant (i.e., affecting either sex) and in another is X linked (i.e., affecting only males). Clearly the genetic prognosis is different in spite of the clinical similarity of the condition.

Known genetic mechanisms

Many of these involve single gene disorders, including the autosomal dominant and recessive forms, and the sex chromosome X linked mode of inheritance. Other familial disease (e.g., pyloric stenosis) may depend on aberrations of several genes.

Dominant trait

The classical situation is that the defect is transmitted vertically through several generations, and one half of any progeny is affected, and males and females are affected indiscriminately (see figure 37).

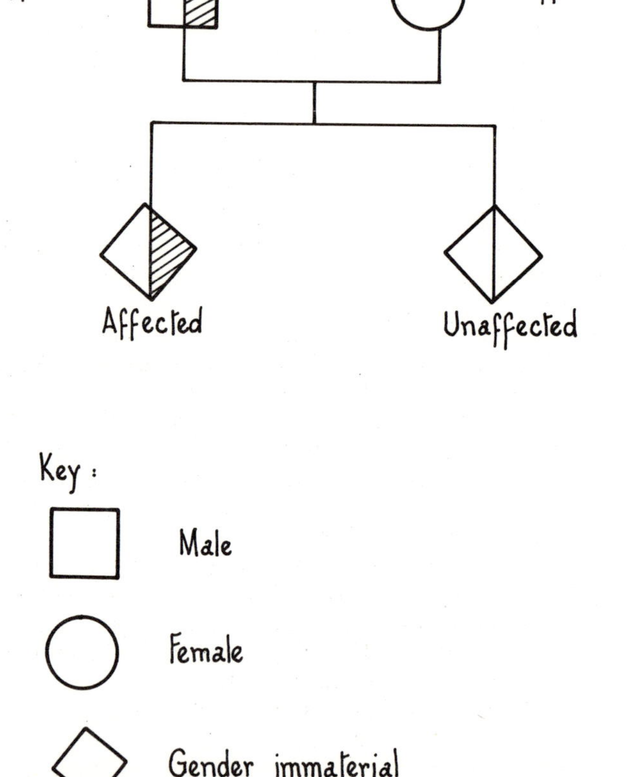

Fig. 37. Autosomal dominant trait. In dominant traits the affected parent is usually heterozygous; in mating with a normal partner, 50% of the offspring are at risk.

If a good family history fails to give evidence of vertical descent, and the disease process is typical of an autosomal dominant (e.g., osteogenesis imperfecta) then it is reasonable to assume that a new mutation (sport) has occurred. In this situation, only the descendents of the affected person will be involved; neither parents themselves, nor the parent's siblings or the siblings of the affected person will necessarily carry the trait, and can be reassured accordingly.

Great care is, however, necessary before diagnosing a new mutation. This is because the true familial disease process may present in a clinically minor way—only part of the disorder is recognizable and, therefore, may be unremarked in the family history. This mild form of the disorder, however, carries the full genetic implication that the parent may produce a child with the full-blown problem.

Many dominant disorders affect the skeleton or the connective tissue and its derivatives, and many are of minor clinical importance. The major disorders may cause death before mating, or have clinical features which militate against it.

Autosomal recessive traits

These make up the majority of the inborn errors of metabolism such as phenylketonuria, mucoviscidosis, and so on. If both parents are heterozygotes for the gene, and are themselves phenotypically (clinically) normal, the children of the union are normal, affected, or carriers (heterozygotes like the parents) in the ratio 1:1:2.

If a heterozygote (carrier) mates with a normal, then only further heterozygotes are generated. If a *sufferer* (homozygote) mates with a normal then carriers are again generated, but if a homozygote (patient) mates with a carrier (heterozygote) then both sufferers and carriers are generated. The situation is summarized in the figure 38.

If the affected gene has a low distribution in the general population, most carriers will mate with normals (situation 2), figure 39, and their children will be clinically normal. This explains the low incidence of any recessive disorder in the cousins (collaterals) of a patient. Knowledge of carriers within the family increases the chances of clinical disease in the children of such a marriage.

The recurrence risk of 1 in 4 is present for each and every child as yet unconceived.

X-linked disorders

These may exist mainly as recessive forms, but the abnormal gene may be transmitted through a *clinically* normal female carrier. In the mother's family there may be affected males, normal males, but carrier females. The latter in turn bear affected males and carrier females.

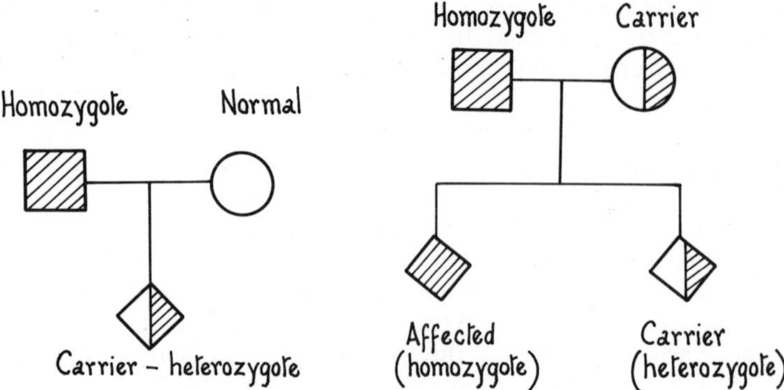

Fig. 38. Autosomal recessive traits: *a*, In this situation the offspring are *clinically* normal carriers; *b*, In this example the unaffected parent is a carrier; 50% of the progeny will be carriers, the others have the disease.

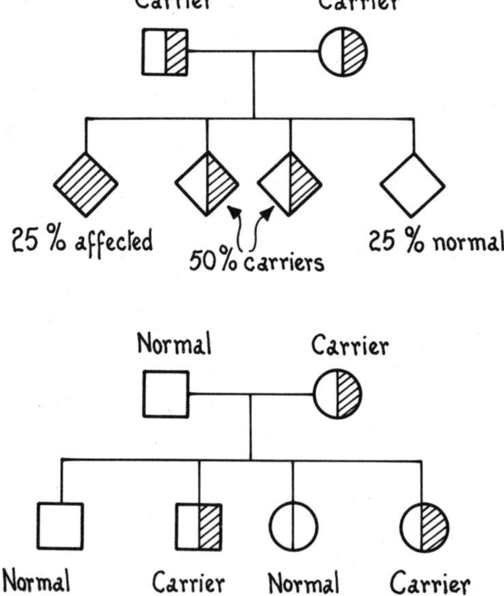

Fig. 39. Recessive traits: *a*, Mating of the heterozygote (carriers). This is the common situation. Diagnosis of the affected offspring implies that the parents are carriers; *b*, This is how undetected carriers are transmitted in a clinically unaffected population.

Transmission is usually in the Mendelian fashion, i.e., in a heterozygous mother, 50% of the male children will be affected and 50% of the females will be carriers. The situation is summarized in figure 40.

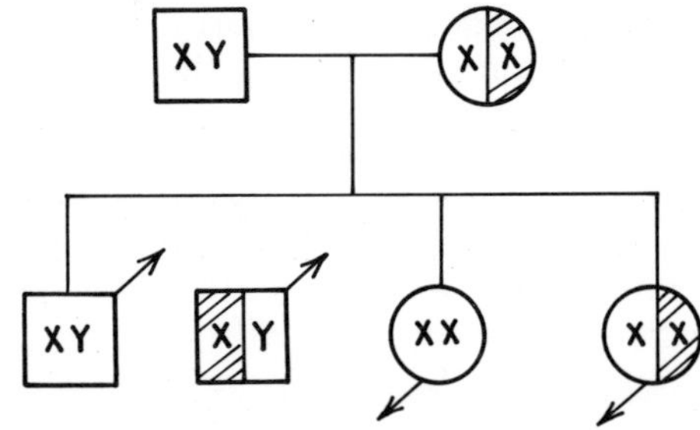

Fig. 40. Sex-linked inheritance: recessive trait.

Note that a female child can only be affected if the father is a sufferer and the mother a carrier. If a male sufferer marries a genetically normal female, then no sufferers result, but the female children are carriers.

The modes of inheritance described above are based upon abnormalities of a single-gene pair, and the explanations can be reasonably simple and direct. There are many other conditions which are multifactorial in origin (i.e., transmitted by several genes) and, therefore, not capable of simple analysis. In this circumstance, genetic counselling is usually based upon the results of experience, together with a knowledge of how widespread the abnormal tendency is within the community.

Table 14 shows some of the rises for various disorders. The higher risk for diabetes is due to the high frequency of the abnormal gene in the community, so that the chances of 2 heterozygotes mating are accordingly increased.

Table 14. Risk recurrence in first degree relatives for various disorders

Lesion	Approximate % Risk Recurrence
Congenital heart disease (all types)	4
Congenital hip dislocation	4
Talipes equinovarus	2
Spina bifida	4
Pyloric stenosis	6
Cleft palate and hare lip	4–5
Diabetes mellitus	20–25

Practical aspects

It is important to recall that the pediatrician can only give the chances and facts concerning the disease. He is not bound to make the decision for the parents. This is their own prerogative. Often enough, however, the decision not to have more children has already been made, on other than genetic grounds, and the parents are seeking some approval of their decision.

In placing the matter in perspective, it should be recalled that 1 in 50 live births suffer from a significant congenital abnormality. In a condition then in which the chance is 1 in 20 or less, the specific family is not taking much more of a risk than the reproductive population as a whole.

7 Immunity and its disorders

Infections and other insults to the body are dealt with by 2 mechanisms, the white cells (mainly the polymorphs), and the immunological system. Normally both work in concert, so that a deficiency in one system may be associated with inefficiency of the other. The disorders of the leucocyte which render the body prone to infection are described elsewhere (p. 337). In this section, the mechanisms of immunity will be discussed.

IMMUNOGLOBULINS

These are proteins which are made by the body. Although the basic structures of the main types are similar, a very great variation in detail is possible. This variability allows the body to respond to an almost infinite number of stimuli. There are 2 broad divisions of reaction, the cellular and the humoral. The cellular immune response is that which, for example, causes rejection of a skin graft from another person, or skin reactions to such substances as streptokinase. The substances concerned in the cellular response are elaborated by lymphocytes of the T (thymus derived) variety, which are in some way dependent upon the thymus.

The *humoral* immune reactions stimulate the production of specific antibodies when challenged by an appropriate antigen (e.g., typhoid vaccination). They depend in the first place upon bone marrow (B type) lymphocytes, for the initiation and maintenance of the response.

Five classes of immunoglobulins (Ig) have been found. The 3 main ones are IgA, IgM, and IgG, each of which plays a definite part in the immune response. IgE is related to allergic reactions; the role of IgD is, as yet, not fully known.

Immunoglobulins are mainly synthesized in response to infection, so that the newborn baby has relatively low levels except for placentally passed IgG. Exposure to various organisms then stimulates the baby to produce the other immune-globulins, although adult levels are not reached until the first birthday. The IgG transferred from the mother also decreases until the baby's own production begins. In general then, it may be said that the baby has a physiological hypogammaglobulinemia in the first 6-8 months of life. It is, however, unusual for a large excess of infection to occur in any except premature babies.

IMMUNOGLOBULIN DEFICIENCY DISEASES

There are many of these. The more important are infantile sex-linked agammaglobulinemia (Bruton's disease), autosomal recessive alymphocytic agammaglobulinemia (Swiss type), and the transient hypogammaglobulinemia of infancy. Each gives rise to a similar picture of repeated severe infections of the skin, upper and lower respiratory tract, and meninges. Viral, fungal, and unusual infections (e.g., with *Pneumocystis carinii*) can also occur.

Bruton's disease

This is a sex-linked recessive, so it occurs in boys.

Clinical features. The baby is normal for a few months, because of transplacental IgG. Then he develops severe recurrent infections (skin, lung, meninges, ears) together with diarrhea and slow growth. If the infant is inoculated with live organisms (e.g., B.C.G., smallpox vaccination) an inappropriate general infection may follow. At first the various infections respond to antibiotics then chronic disease such as otitis or bronchiectasis occurs. A persistent rheumatoid arthritis may follow.

Treatment The child is given vigorous antibiotic therapy and injections of immunoglobulin. The latter are given for life, and in a dose sufficient to maintain normal values.

Autosomal recessive alymphocytic agammaglobulinemia (Swiss type agammaglobulinemia)

This may occur in either sex. Occasionally the infant presents with a fatal response to vaccination against tuberculosis or smallpox. Otherwise, the features are those of severe recurrent infections of the skin, respiratory, and gastrointestinal tract. The responsible organisms may be viruses, fungi, or protozoa. A pertussis-like cough is characteristic. Lymphoid tissue (e.g., tonsils) is absent or rudimentary in these children. Lymphocytes are much reduced and plasma cells absent. Anemia is common. All of the immunoglobulins are markedly deficient, as are both humoral and cellular responses.

Transient hypogammaglobulinemia of infancy

In this, the principle deficiency is in IgG, although IgM and IgA levels may also be depressed. The principal features are of recurrent infections of skin and respiratory tracts. Eventually the immunoglobulin levels return to normal so that the main treatment is to tide the patient over the infections (e.g., by vigorous antibiotic therapy) until this happens.

The other disorders of the immunological mechanisms are rare. Among them are Wiskott-Aldrich syndrome (p. 350) in which eczema and low platelet values are associated with IgA and IgM deficiencies and ataxia-telangiectasia (p. 435) in which IgA deficiency is often found.

An impaired response to infection can occur when T cell production, and hence cellular immune response, is decreased. The clinical features are similar to those already described, e.g., frequent severe infections, often by unusual organisms. The tests of cellular immune response are impaired, but immunoglobulin levels are occasionally normal, or only moderately reduced.

Miscellaneous

Various disabilities of the immunoglobulin system may also occur in patients with Hodgkin's disease, sarcomata, and after the use of cytotoxic drugs. In infants, perhaps the most common cause is a continuing infection with rubella virus.

GENERAL DIFFERENTIAL DIAGNOSIS OF DISORDERS OF THE IMMUNE MECHANISMS

Frequent respiratory infections, failure to thrive, diarrhea and malabsorption are common. This constellation may lead to confusion with mucoviscidosis, especially in the early months, where the sweat test is not as yet diagnostic, and where the physiological hypogammaglobulinemia of infancy is still present. In the common immune disorders, all of the globulins are markedly decreased and the absence of a humoral response is easy to demonstrate. Similarly, the careful evaluation of lymphocyte and plasma cell values is in order in cases of suspected immunological deficiency.

Tests of humoral responses

These must *never* be tested by the use of live vaccines. A useful method is to use DPT vaccine (0.5 ml I.M. each week for 3 doses), and to test for antibodies 2 weeks after the last injection. Pneumococcal or *Hemophilus influenzae* derivatives may also be employed.

Tests of cellular immune responses

These are frequently, although not invariably, associated with low levels of lymphocytes. The skin reaction to various stimuli is also useful. Thus candida antigen (oidomycin) yields a positive response in 80-85% of normal children, and a later challenge may give an even larger harvest of positives. 2-4 dinitrofluorobenzene may be used similarly. If the cellular response is impaired, the skin reactions fail to appear. Other tests include failure of the patients' lymphocytes to go into a mitotic phase when appropriately stimulated.

CONDITIONS CHARACTERIZED BY INCREASE IN THE IMMUNOGLOBULINS

a. A general increase. Such a reaction is characteristic of the child who has had repeated infections and is often found in the child in poor social circumstances.

b. Specific increases. IgG and IgA are often increased in liver cirrhosis and in a variety of collagen diseases. A diffuse hypergammaglobulinemia occurs in disseminated lupus erythematosus. IgG levels may be increased in histiocytosis X, and in children with Down's syndrome.

IMMUNIZATION OF CHIDREN

This is done in order to induce a protective immune state in the child without causing significant disease. One important method is *active* immunization, which can be done by introducing live organisms into the body. The organisms may be attenuated (i.e., capable of inducing immunity but incapable of causing significant disease), e.g., measles vaccine, or they may be similar organisms, i.e., giving cross-immunity, but causing only a minor disorder (as in cowpox vaccination against smallpox). Killed organisms (e.g., typhoid vaccine) are also useful, as are *toxoids*. The latter are toxins which have been treated so that they no longer cause disease—as in diphtheria immunization. Active immunization can be used to prevent tetanus, pertussis, diphtheria, tuberculosis, smallpox, poliomyelitis, mumps, measles, rubella, typhoid, rabies, and certain strains of influenza viral infections.

Passive immunization consists in the injection of an immune serum or gamma globulin into a patient who has been exposed to a specific infection. Passive immunization is inferior to active immunization since it confers only a transient protection. It can, however, be combined with active immunization.

In most societies, the routine immunizations are against diphtheria, pertussis, tetanus, polio, measles, tuberculosis, and rubella. An acceptable schedule is shown in table 15. In areas where smallpox is rare or unknown, smallpox vaccination may be omitted.

In special circumstances, inoculation is possible against cholera, plague, yellow fever, typhus and rabies.

The contraindications to *live* vaccine inoculation are natural immunological deficits, or those following the use of steroids or immunosuppressant drugs. Abnormal sensitivity to the pertussis fraction of DPT may occur and warrants discontinuance of this moiety of the

Table 15. Schedule of immunizations against various diseases

Age	Schedule
2 months	Diphtheria/pertussis/tetanus (DPT)
3 months	DPT
4 months	DPT, oral polio trivalent (OPT)
6 months	DPT
12 months	Measles, BCG if indicated
18 months	DPT, OPT, smallpox
5 years	DPT, OPT
12 years	Mumps, rubella

vaccine. Extensive eczema is regarded as a contraindication to *routine* vaccination against smallpox. Measles vaccine should be given with special care to sufferers from mucoviscidosis, severe cerebral palsy, or severe congenital heart disease.

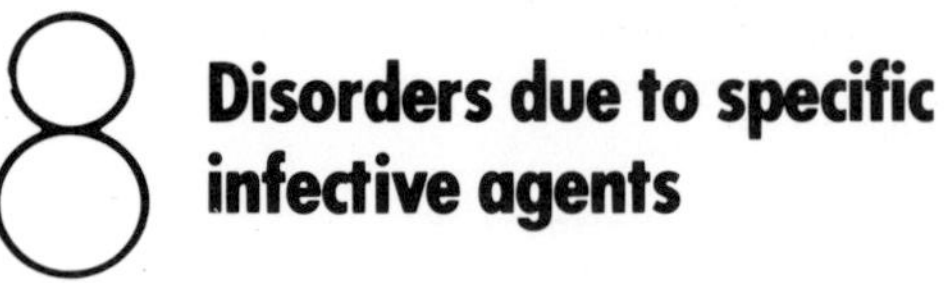

8 Disorders due to specific infective agents

VIRAL INFECTIONS

These are common and important causes of disease in children. Viruses are much smaller than bacteria and biologically much simpler. Thus they have no enzyme system to generate energy and cannot reproduce except within a living cell whose activities can be controlled by the virus. Each virus particle is made up of protein with ribonucleic (RNA) or desoxynucleic acid (DNA). RNA and DNA are never present together in a virus, a property which can be used to distinguish them.

The response of the cell to viral invasion is variable. Often it may be destroyed or damaged, or it is merely colonized by the virus and shows no obvious change. If the patient is immunologically competent, most viruses will sooner or later produce evidence of circulating antibody—a protein produced by the lymphocytes in response to infection, and measurable by special methods. Another substance, which is called interferon, is produced by local tissues (e.g., the nose, gut) and can, in certain circumstances, inhibit viral reproduction in that tissue.

There are few effective antiviral agents, so that control of viral diseases depends upon isolating the patient from other susceptibles (quarantine), increasing his antibody production by a safe method (active immunization or vaccination), injecting antibody prepared in an animal or another human (passive immunization), or controlling the carrier (vector) which transmits the disease to man (e.g., mosquito control in certain types of encephalitis).

SPECIFIC DISORDERS DUE TO MYXOVIRUS

Measles (morbilli)

This disease is endemic in the age group 6 months to 5 years. Epidemics occur in late winter and early spring, but are now much less common because of immunization of susceptibles by attenuated virus preparations.

Clinical features. Frequent early features are irritability, runny nose, cough, conjunctivitis, fever, and photophobia. In young children, vomiting is common; in older children there may be a complaint of sore throat. At this stage, Koplik spots are found on the buccal mucosa. These are pinhead-sized, reddish mauve spots with a pale centre. At this stage, before the true rash appears, the child may appear severely ill, with high fever, delirium, increased cough, otitis media, and bronchitis. Occasionally a prodromal generalized reddish rash appears, which resembles that of scarlet fever. The true measles rash, however, begins on the forehead and around the ears and spreads progressively to the face, trunk, and limbs. The rash, which is not itchy, is at first macular (i.e., the spots are not raised, and are separate one from the other) and then becomes maculopapular (i.e., the lesions are raised but separate). At the height of the rash, the lesions are red, then fade to an orange hue after 3-4 days.

As the rash appears, the child begins to improve, his fever decreases, the cough lessens, and appetite and activity return. The rash fades in the same order as it appears, sometimes with evidence of a little bleeding into it. A true hemorrhagic rash is rare, and a sign of serious disease.

Complications. These occur in the younger child, as otitis media and bronchopneumonia. Encephalitis is rare, usually occurring about 1 week after the appearance of the rash. The clinical features are similar to those of encephalitis from other causes (see p. 469).

Differential diagnosis. Before the rash appears, measles shares with meningitis the symptoms of irritability, anorexia, vomiting, and drowsiness. The rash is mainly to be differentiated from that of rubella (German measles). This is a mild illness, without Koplik's spots, but *with* enlargement of the occipital lymph glands. Anticonvulsants (e.g., phenobarbitone), and antibiotics (e.g., penicillin) also cause morbilliform (measles-like) rashes. However, there is an appropriate history of drug ingestion and absence of Koplik's spots.

Treatment. This is mainly good nursing care and simple sedation. Antibiotics are unnecessary except for severe otitis media or bronchopneumonia. Chest physiotherapy is employed when the cough becomes loose.

Prevention.

Active immunization. This is done with an attenuated live measles virus preparation, given to well children at the age of 1 year. It causes a mild, short-lived illness, sometimes with a transient rash.

Passive immunization. This is done by giving gamma globulin which confers protection for a few weeks. It is mainly used in children with chronic disease (e.g., mucovisdicosis) in whom active immunization might be dangerous, or to cut short an epidemic of measles within an institution for children.

Mumps (epidemic parotitis)

Clinical features. Fever and a complaint of sore face may precede swelling of the salivary glands. One or both parotids may be involved, with the swelling filling in the space between the angle of the mandible and the mastoid. The submandibular glands may also be enlarged. Swollen skin overlies the tender glands, and chewing is difficult and painful. In most instances the symptoms resolve within a week.

Complications. These occur mainly in the older child and adult, the commonest being meningoencephalitis, with fever, headache, vomiting, and sleepiness. The spinal fluid contains an excess of lymphocytes.

Inflammation of the testes (orchitis), of the ovary (oophoritis), or of the pancreas, are very rare complications in children.

Treatment. Analgesics and hot or cold applications to the painful glands are usually the only treatments necessary.

Prevention. Attenuated live virus vaccine is now available and gives good protection.

Influenza

Many strains of the influenza virus can cause disease in children, but the common types are influenza A and B and their mutants.

Clinical features. These vary greatly in severity. Common minor symptoms are fever, anorexia, and cough, with diarrhea in infants. Bronchiolitis is a not uncommon disease state, and in rare instances, the virus may cause a severe respiratory disorder, with severe dyspnea and sometimes cyanosis. A confluent bronchopneumonia is found on x-ray and this may be so severe as to cause death, or severe chronic lung disorder.

Treatment. This is essentially as noted for bronchiolitis (p. 248).

Rubella (German measles)

This disease is a common, mild disease of children, which may, however, give rise to a severe disease in the newborn, or be the cause of congenital defects if occurring in pregnancy. The latter aspects of the disease are considered elsewhere (p. 53).

Clinical features. Mild malaise and fever may precede the rash, but this last is the main feature. The distribution and spread of the rash is as described for measles proper, but it persists for a much shorter time. It is reddish orange in colour, and shows less tendency to coalescence than the macular rash of true measles. The occipital lymph nodes are usually enlarged, but they are seldom tender.

Treatment. No specific treatment is available or necessary.

Prevention. This is recommended because of the possible adverse effect upon the fetus. Accordingly, attenuated virus vaccination is carried out on pubertal girls. In susceptibles exposed to the disease, but unsuitable for active immunization (e.g., pregnant females), passive transient protection may be obtained by the injection of gamma globulins.

Roseola infantum (exanthem subitum)

This is one of the fevers of uncertain origin of childhood, in which the patient has a high, sustained fever without localizing signs other than occasional delirium or a febrile convulsion. The fever falls as the rash appears, and the child recovers. The rash is generalized, and composed of small, separate, pink macules, which may superficially resemble the rash of rubella.

Treatment. None is required except tepid sponging during the febrile stage.

Infective mononucleosis (glandular fever)

Clinical features. The child complains of sore throat and anorexia, and is fevered. Local or generalized enlargement of the lymph glands may be found. A measles-like rash occurs on the trunk in about 25% of patients, and reddish spots are often found on the palate. The throat is usually red and inflamed and occasionally the reaction is so severe as to cause formation of a yellowish membrane. The spleen is frequently enlarged. The diagnosis is usually confirmed by finding atypical lymphocytes in the blood, and by a positive heterophile antibody (Paul-Bunnell) test.

Complications. These are not common but may occur as *hepatitis* with jaundice and abnormal liver function tests, *meningoencephalitis* (aseptic meningitis) or as a blood dyscrasia, with purpura and bleeding states associated with low platelet levels.

Treatment. This is symptomatic with bed rest and simple analgesics for the sore throat.

Infections by the enterovirus group

These viruses cause a large number of diseases. Table 16 summarizes the possibilities. The following describes the disorders not discussed elsewhere.

Table 16. Some diseases due to enterovirus (picornavirus) groups

Group	Disease
Poliomyelitis types 1, 2, 3	Various forms of anterior polio
Coxsackie (A and B)	Aseptic meningitis
	Encephalitis
	Herpangina
	Myocarditis
	Guillain-Barre syndrome (?)
Echo	Diarrhea
	Aseptic meningitis
	Encephalitis

Herpangina

This infection by Coxsackie A virus causes fever, sore mouth and throat, and anorexia. Papules develop on the palate and fauces, rapidly vesiculate and ulcerate, and heal over 1-2 weeks. The condition is very similar to herpetic stomatitis (p. 190) and the treatment is similar—maintain hydration by I.V. fluids if necessary, pain-killing mouth washes, and good oral hygiene.

Hand-foot-mouth disease

In this, fever and anorexia are followed by groups of herpanginal lesions in the mouth and on the hands and feet. Spontaneous cure occurs after a few days.

Fever and rash (Boston exanthem, 6th disease, etc.)

This Echo viral disorder occurs in epidemics, usually in toddlers. The child is fevered, irritable, off his food, and may have diarrhea. He then develops a rash, usually resembling that of rubella, but occasionally with vesicle formation.

Symptomatic treatment is all that is necessary.

Herpes virus infection

This DNA virus group has two types—herpes simplex virus and herpes virus varicellae. The former causes herpetic stomatitis (p. 190) and severe infection of the newborn (p. 53). The latter causes herpes zoster (p. 425) and chicken pox (varicella). The cytomegalovirus (salivary gland virus) is probably also in the same group.

Chickenpox (varicella)

Clinical features. Fever and loss of appetite are common before the frank rash appears. Generally, however, the preliminaries are mild.

Rash. An early (herald) lesion is usually the first thing seen. It is a macule, found on the trunk, and it is itchy. The rash then becomes generalized, beginning on the trunk and spreading to the face, mouth, and scalp. Faint macules rapidly become papules, which become vesicles. The latter become cloudy and then scab. Typically the rash appears in crops, so that lesions at all stages of development are seen. In the mouth, the features are much less stylized than in the skin.

Complications. The skin lesions become infected, so that impetigo with lymphadenitis can occur. Very rarely, encephalitis affecting the cerebellum may occur.

Special problems. Severe or fatal chickenpox may occur in the child who is receiving steroids or cytotoxic agents. In these, the rash may be confluent or hemorrhagic, and hyperpyrexia, dehydration, and shock are common.

Treatment. The nails are cut short to minimize skin injury from scratching. Simple antiseptic baths are given to allay the itch and prevent infection. In the severe disorder, especially in those on steroids or cytotoxics, hyperimmune serum, intravenous fluid and antibiotics may be required.

Cytomegalovirus infection

This occurs in 2 main groups, the newborn and children who are receiving steroids or immunosuppressants.

In the *newborn*, the illness is a severe septicemic-like illness with hemolytic anemia, jaundice, purpura, and bruising (see p. 53). In *children* with impaired immunological competence, the clinical features are fever, malaise, cough, and diarrhea. These symptoms cannot be attributed to any primary disease. The diagnosis is confirmed by finding inclusion bodies (cells containing viral particles) in the urine, or by the isolation of the virus itself.

No specific treatment is available for this disorder. Supportive treatment (e.g., transfusion in the newborn) is all that can be done.

Diseases due to arbovirus

These give rise to encephalitis (e.g., Murray Valley, Japanese B), yellow fever, and dengue. The virus is usually transmitted by mosquito bite.

Encephalitis (Murray Valley)

This occurs in epidemics but only a few of the infected develop significant symptoms. These consist in anorexia, vomiting, and sleepiness which may deepen to coma. Convulsions are common and various neurological difficulties follow. The diagnosis can be confirmed by serological methods. No specific treatment is available. Affected patients are treated as discussed on p. 470.

Dengue.

This occurs mainly in Thailand, Vietnam, and Indonesia. The usual features are headache, fever, and pains in the muscles and joints. In younger children hemorrhagic shock type occurs, in which the child develops purpura and a bleeding tendency, as well as a profound fall in cardiac output and blood pressure. The diagnosis is confirmed by serological methods. The treatment is supportive.

Yellow fever

This occurs in Africa and South America and is characterized by fever, malaise, jaundice, and a bleeding disorder affecting the nose, stomach, and skin. No specific treatment is available but the disease can be prevented by appropriate immunization.

Disorders due to pox viruses

These include smallpox (variola) and vaccinia (cowpox).

Smallpox (variola)

This is a viral disease of wide distribution, endemic and occasionally epidemic in unvaccinated communities. The severity of the disease is variable, probably due to immunological differences. Several clinical varieties occur, these are described below.

Variola major

Clinical features. In this severe form, the rash is preceded by a prodromal period of 5-6 days, during which the patient is fevered, anorexic, obviously ill, with headache, photophobia, backache, and vomiting. The rash begins on the oral mucosa, pharynx, face, arms, and legs (the focal rash), and spreads, with diminishing intensity to the trunk. The initial lesion is a macule which soon becomes a papule. This feels shotty to palpation. Within 24-48 hours the papules are vesicular and these in turn become pustular. About a week after its onset, the rash crusts with scabs which can persist for 3-4 weeks. It is noteworthy that *all of the lesions are at a similar stage of development*, a principal point in the differential diagnosis from chickenpox. In very severe cases, the lesions may cover most of the body (confluent smallpox). Hemorrhagic lesions, although relatively rare, are a grave sign. Pneumonia and dehydration are common complications of severe cases, and secondary infection is usual. The latter contributes to, but is not the primary cause of, death.

Modified smallpox

This may occur in distantly vaccinated patients, or in the babies of vaccinated mothers. The prerash stages are less severe, and the local lesions fewer in number. The virus is, however, just as liable to cause severe disease in the unprotected.

Alastrim

This is a milder form of smallpox, apparently with a longer incubation period (16 days as compared to 12 days for classic variola). The prodromata are mild, and the lesions relatively few and more evanescent than variola major. The mortality rate is low.

Laboratory studies

The virus can be detected by light or electron microscopy in the maculopapular stage, at which time complement fixation tests are also positive. Hemagglutination and antibody studies are positive by the pustular stage. Such studies are of most importance in the minor forms of smallpox, when the differential diagnosis from chickenpox may be difficult.

Differential diagnosis

In the preeruptive stage, this is not easy except in the presence of an epidemic. In the nature of things, conditions such as malaria, dengue, and the commoner (e.g., enteroviral) infections will require consideration. In the eruptive phase, chickenpox is the most difficult problem. In this (varicella), the prodromal illness is mild, and the rash begins as a herald lesion on the trunk which is the area of major involvement. The chickenpox lesions then spread to the face and limbs (centrifugal distribution). The lesions within any area are of *different* types, viz., macules, papules, pustules, coexist.

Treatment

No specific treatment is known. Intravenous therapy is commonly required because of dehydration, and a broad-spectrum antibiotic is of value in containing secondary pyogenic infection. Extensive hemorrhage may demand blood transfusion.

Prophylaxis

Vaccination is advised in endemic areas, or for people (physicians, nurses and their families) heavily exposed. Unprotected contacts should be vaccinated and may benefit, statistically at least, from treatment with the thiosemicarbazones. Isolation of infected patients is a sine qua non, and their excreta, clothing, and dressings should be destroyed or sterilized by heat.

Vaccination against smallpox

This is carried out by introducing a strain of the cowpox virus into the skin. It is usually carried out about the first birthday. At this age, general reaction such as fever, and anorexia are mild and relatively rare. The local lesion goes through the changes described for smallpox, usually leaving a more or less permanent scar. In older children, the primary vaccination may, after the first week, produce a moderate illness with fever, anorexia, headache, and aching muscles.

At any age, vaccinia may become generalized. This is more common in those with immunological disorders, or a skin disease such as infantile eczema. This is a severe complication with multiple lesions and the clinical features of smallpox. Death is common in those with an immunological defect.

Encephalomyelitis may also follow simple vaccination, and is of the allergic type, but with the clinical features of other types of encephalomyelitis. Permanent brain damage or death occasionally occurs.

These complications are the principal arguments against vaccination. Certainly in countries with high health standards the death rate due to vaccination may be higher than that for smallpox itself. In endemic areas, or for those who travel, vaccination is however essential.

Miscellaneous infections

Rabies

This disease is transmitted by bites from dogs, bats, and other animals.

Clinical features. The incubation period is relatively long, commonly 4-8 weeks. The first symptoms are vague sensations of itching and burning near the bite, followed by restlessness, irritability, and feelings of apprehension and ultimately frank terror. At this stage the typical hydrophobia is noted. This consists in remarkable pharyngeal spasm when efforts are made at swallowing. Laryngeal spasm and apnea follow. Then occur meningitic symptoms, headache, vomiting, neck stiffness, and disturbances of consciousness. Coma, fever, and paralysis are terminal events.

Differential diagnosis. This is from tetanus, strychnine poisoning, and meningoencephalitis. In none is there a history of bite, although considerable enquiry may be required to establish attack by a bat.

Prophylaxis. Dogs who bite should be observed for signs of the disease. If there is any doubt that it is rabid, hyperimmune serum should be given the patient, followed by active vaccination. There is no specific treatment for rabies.

Cat-scratch disease

This is of world-wide distribution, but is not very common.

Clinical features. There is always contact with cats and there may be a history of cat scratch. The child becomes vaguely ill, with mild fever, anorexia, and headache. The local lesion at first resembles an insect bite with later redness and swellings. The regional lymph nodes enlarge and this may be the main complaint. Rare complications include local abscess, conjunctivitis, bronchopneumonia and encephalomyelitis.

Differential diagnosis. This is mainly from a simple pyogenic infection, or the skin gland complex following BCG vaccination.

Treatment. No specific treatment is known, and as the prognosis is good, none is necessary.

RICKETTSIAL DISEASES

Rickettsial organisms are intermediate between the viruses and the bacteria, and resemble viruses in that they can only propagate within cells. Unlike viruses, they are susceptible to some antibiotics. The diseases are world wide and include typhus (epidemic and endemic), Rocky Mountain spotted fever, scrub typhus, and Q fever. The first 3 always have a rash as part of the clinical picture. All are transmitted by an insect vector, e.g., lice, fleas, ticks, or mites.

Typhus fever

This is due to *Rickettsia prowazeki.*

Clinical features. Many children have mild illness, with fever, anorexia, irritability, and a rash consisting of rose-coloured, polygonal spots on the trunk. Initially they blanch with pressure, later they darken in colour, and become more permanent. In mild attacks, the rash is transient.

Some children have a more severe illness with fever, rigors, and headache. As the rash appears, delirium, stupor, vomiting, and dehydration occur. Pneumonia and severe meningoencephalitis may occur.

Scrub typhus

This condition occurs in tropical Australia, South-east Asia, India, and some of the Pacific Islands. It is due to *R.orientalis*.

Clinical features. These are similar to those described for typhus. Additionally there is evidence of a mite bite resembling a mosquito bite, but which later ulcerates. The rash is maculopapular, begins on the trunk, and becomes generalized. Enlargement of the superficial lymph glands is usual. Pneumonia and myocarditis are occasional complications.

Rocky Mountain spotted fever

This is due to *R.rickettsii*. It is spread by a mite. The features are fever, anorexia, and a rash. The latter begins in the wrists, ankles, and legs, and spreads to involve the whole body. At first maculopapular, it may become hemorrhagic. Pneumonia, myocarditis, and encephalitis may complicate the course of the disease.

General differential diagnosis of the Rickettsial diseases with a rash

This will depend upon the geographic area. In scrub typhus, malaria needs consideration, especially before the rash appears. In the other conditions, meningoencephalitis (viral and pyogenic) requires exclusion by lumbar puncture. The rash itself may simulate, especially in the early stages, that of typhoid fever or of dengue.

Specific identification

Serologic diagnosis is of value, using antigens prepared from proteus vulgaris strains (The Weil-Felix reaction). Strain OX19 is used in typhus proper, OX2 or OX19 in spotted fever, and OXK in scrub typhus.

Q fever

This is a not uncommon disease in Australia. The clinical features are variable, but include fever, headache, anorexia, and cough. Pneumonia is common, but morbidity and mortality are low. Many instances are diagnosed retrospectively by serologic methods.

General treatment of the Rickettsial diseases

In the severer forms, parenteral fluid therapy is essential. Appropriate treatment should be given for complicating pneumonia or myocarditis. Tetracyclines and chloramphenicol are the more specific antibiotics and should be given in full dosage for 1-2 weeks.

MYCOTIC (FUNGAL) INFECTIONS

Actinomycosis

This parasite causes a chronic granulomatous infection, usually with sinus formation. The commoner form originates from a carious tooth, and causes a progressive enlargement of the jaw or neck glands. The lesion is hard and painless. The overlying skin softens, and sinuses occur. The principal differential diagnosis is from tuberculosis. The sulphur granules of actinomycosis may be seen in exudates, but culture is essential for specific diagnosis. *Thoracic actinomycosis* presents with cough, dyspnea, and empyema. Sinus formation is usual, and the organism is found in the sputum and pleural fluid. In the *abdominal form*, the patient may have had an appendicectomy or may present with what appears to be an appendix abscess—a firm ileocolic swelling. Cutaneous sinus formation occurs and rarely there is intraabdominal dissemination with subphrenic or hepatic abscess.

Treatment. Surgical drainage is employed as necessary. Prolonged courses of penicillin are usually curative, and may be combined with sulphonamides.

Torulosis (cryptococcosis)

This condition occurs in all age groups and has a predilection for invading the lungs and central nervous system. Disseminated infections occasionally occur in the newborn, or in those who have impaired immunological responses.

Clinical features. In the newborn, these may closely resemble the severe viremias or toxoplasma infection. There is hemolytic jaundice, hepatosplenomegaly, failure to feed, twitching, and sometimes development of a cerebral palsy-like state. Hydrocephalus may result but perhaps more common is failure of head growth with evidence of intellectual retardation. Choreoretinitis and intracranial calcification have been described as later manifestations.

In the older child, the C.N.S. symptoms are those of a meningoencephalitis, with anorexia, irritability, vomiting, and sleepiness. The latter may progress to coma. In late cases cranial nerve palsies and papilledema are found. These symptoms develop over a period of a week or two.

The pulmonary disorder has no specific features. There is cough, fever, some dyspnea, and the appearance of scattered bronchopneumonic changes on the x-ray.

Differential diagnosis. In the newborn this is principally from the viral triad (rubella, herpes, cytomegalovirus) and toxoplasmosis. Otherwise it is from meningitis, principally of the tuberculous sort, although half-treated pyogenic meningitis will require occasional consideration.

Diagnosis. This is dependent upon demonstrating the organism in the body fluids.

Treatment. Amphotericin B, intravenously and intrathecally, is the treatment of choice. Side effects are nausea, vomiting, diarrhea, and renal damage.

Histoplasmosis

This is due to the fungus *H. capsulatum.*

Clinical features. These vary greatly: more commonly there are no specific symptoms, the condition being discovered by chest x-ray.

Radiological features of the benign form. In general these are indistinguishable from primary tuberculosis—consisting in a lung process with an associated hilar adenopathy. The latter may be revealed on x-ray, or associated lung collapse may imply its presence. Healing occurs with calcification. Occasionally multiple calcified lesions may be scattered through the lungs.

The severe form is relatively rare. Common features are fever, anorexia, vomiting, diarrhea, and irritability. Older children may complain of headaches and muscular aching. Episodes of cough, with radiological signs of bronchopneumonia are common and meningoencephalitic syndromes also occur. Hepatosplenomegaly is usually present on clinical examination. Ulceration of skin, eye, and gut have been described.

Diagnosis. Ultimately this is dependent upon the demonstration of the fungus. This is most commonly possible in the sputum, bone marrow, and cerebrospinal fluid. The histoplasma skin test is a useful ancillary, with an antigen prepared from the fungus.

Treatment. Amphotericin B may be considered for the severe disseminated disease. The less severe forms have a tendency to heal without specific therapy.

Aspergillosis

This fungal infection assumes importance only in those with severe preexisting pulmonary disease (bronchiectasis, mucoviscidosis), in those with congenital immunologic deficiencies, or those treated extensively with steroids or immunosuppressive agents.

Clinical features. Essentially these are of the underlying disease. In pulmonary disease, there is exacerbation of the preexisting symptoms, and the fungus can be isolated from the sputum. In other conditions (e.g., treated leukemia) pulmonary symptoms begin, and are inexplicable on the basis of the primary disease. X-rays show cavitation and fungus-ball formation. Chronic granulomata of skin and mucous membranes are also found.

Treatment. This is as outlined for histoplasmosis.

PROTOZOAL INFECTIONS

These have their main importance in relation to the common tropical disorders such as malaria and amebiasis, which contribute significantly to morbidity and mortality among the children of the developing countries. Many protozoa are carried by insect vectors.

Malaria

This is due to infection by *Plasmodium vivax*, *Pl. malariae*, or *Pl. falciparum*. The latter gives rise to severe and potentially fatal illness, the former pair to a milder, often recurrent, disease.

Clinical features. These depend largely on the state of the child's immunity. If this is high, as in areas of endemic infection, the sole manifestations may be vague illhealth, splenomegaly, anemia, and evidence of parasitemia. Acute illness is liable to occur in immigrants or in indigenes who suddenly cease prophylactic antimalarials.

In *Pl.vivax* disease, the illness begins about a week after infection, usually with nonspecific symptoms such as change of mood, anorexia, and drowsiness. Fever is usual, and the *Pl.vivax* infestations tend to recur every 48 hours (tertian) or every 72 hours (quartan) in *Pl.malariae* infections. Older children may complain of headache, nausea, and abdominal pain.

In *Pl. falciparum* infections, the fever has no particular pattern, and the child may present with a variety of symptoms. Commonly, these resemble meningitis, viz., anorexia, irritability, and drowsiness progressing to coma, sometimes with convulsions (cerebral malaria). Other symptoms, especially common in the very young, are vomiting, diarrhea, and dehydration.

Pallor of the mucous membranes, functional murmurs, and other signs of anemia are found in all types of malaria. Splenomegaly is usual, especially in *Pl. malariae* and *vivax* infections, and hepatomegaly is found in *Pl. falciparum* disease. The nephrotic syndrome complicates chronic *Pl. malariae* infestations.

Differential diagnosis. This is of greatest moment in *Pl. falciparum* infections, which may simulate meningoencephalitis, or severe gastroenteritis. As these conditions are also common in areas where malaria is endemic, lumbar puncture should always accompany antimalarial therapy.

Laboratory. Anemia is invariable, and the parasite can usually be found in thick blood films.

Treatment. Appropriate supportive therapy—intravenous fluid or blood—is indicated, especially in the young child. Specific drug therapy will depend upon the known resistance patterns of the local parasite, but chloroquine, amodiaquine, and primaquine are commonly used. Chloroquine may be given in an intravenous infusion where vomiting is severe, or very rapid antimalarial activity is desired. Patterns of resistance may demand treatment with combined trimethoprim/sulfalene (a long-acting sulphonamide), and quinine.

Prophylaxis. Chloroquine, amodiaquine, proguanil, and pyrimethamine can all be used. The first two are bitter, and often ill-tolerated by children. The latter two are usually better accepted. The specific drug recommended will vary with the known patterns of resistance. Primaquine is a good suppressant, but liable to give rise to toxic symptoms, especially in those with G-6-P.D. deficiency. Pyrimethamine also has antifolic acid activity.

Amebiasis

This condition is due to the *Entamoeba histolytica.* It is most commonly found in tropical and subtropical areas.

Clinical features. These are principally due to amebic colitis, the principal complaint being of diarrhea, usually intermittent, sometimes with intervening constipation.

A severe form, clinically indistinguishable from gastroenteritis, causes a substantial mortality in children. Among the rarer complications are amebic hepatitis, or amebic liver abscess. These are characterized by fever, loss of weight, and an enlarged and tender liver. Gut perforation with peritonitis may occur in severe colitis.

Differential diagnosis. This is mainly from diarrhea due to salmonellosis or the dysenteries. The coexistence of these latter with amebiasis is not very unusual. Stool examination for the parasite or its cysts is diagnostic in most instances.

Treatment. Intravenous electrolytes and blood are given to relieve dehydration and anemia. Drugs useful in specific treatment are diloxanide furoate, glycobiarsol, and for amebic hepatitis, emetine, chloroquine phosphate, or metronidazole.

Kala-azar (leishmaniasis)

The organism is transmitted by the sandfly, and gives rise to various clinical problems, the most serious being the acute infantile form, in which vomiting, fever, wasting, and agranulocytic syndromes occur. Splenomegaly and lymphadenopathy are common, and death frequent in the untreated case.

In the chronic form, the principal feature is fever and rapid splenic enlargement. The latter may eventually become so large as to cause considerable abdominal protuberance. Secondary infections, e.g., pneumonia, are often found in association with evidence of bone marrow depression.

Diagnosis. This depends upon the demonstration of the parasite in the spleen or bone marrow.

Treatment. Antimony compounds, or petamidine, are given.

Toxoplasmosis

This condition is due to the *Toxoplasma gondii*. The most important clinical variety is the congenital one.

Congenital toxoplasmosis

The infant may be premature, he feeds poorly, develops a severe hemolytic jaundice, with hepatomegaly and splenomegaly and a macular rash which may become hemorrhagic. Head growth is impaired, and chorioretinitis occurs. Intracranial calcification is seen in many cases. The syndrome is clinically difficult to tell from congenital rubella, herpes simplex, or cytomegalovirus infection. The differential diagnosis of these is described in full elsewhere (p. 53).

Acquired toxoplasmosis

This is a rather rare disease which is difficult to confirm. It seems likely that in many instances infestation is not followed by clinical disease. Otherwise, fever, malaise, lymph gland enlargement and a transient maculopapular rash occasionally occur and encephalitis and myocarditis have been reported.

Diagnosis. The organism may be identified in the spinal fluid of the sufferer from congenital type. Toxoplasma antibody levels may also be measured by the Sabin dye test, or less readily, by hemagglutination and fluorescent antibody techniques.

Treatment. A combination of sulphadiazine and pyrimethamine is given for a month, and this therapy would seem likely to eliminate an active infection.

Giardiasis

This is a common pediatric infestation, especially in the younger age group, and more so in those in poor social circumstances.

Clinical features. In many instances there are none, the organisms being discovered on routine stool survey. In a few instances, heavy infestations may apparently be associated with a malabsorptive state. In these, the *Giardia lamblia* may be found in the gut mucosa at biopsy.

Treatment. A short course of Mepacrine is usually curative.

BACTERIAL INFECTIONS

These continue to be common in children, but are now much less dangerous because effective antibiotics are available. Many disease processes due to bacteria are covered in the chapters related to the specific systems. In this section it is proposed to consider the disorders not easily discussed elsewhere.

Tuberculosis

Perspective. In rich countries childhood tuberculosis is now relatively rare, because modern chemotherapy has controlled the infectivity of adults. The major problem today is to find and treat cases of primary tuberculosis, so that tuberculous meningitis can be avoided since this is still a disease whose treatment is unsatisfactory. In the routine care of children, tuberculin testing is important, so that nonreactors may be found, and B.C.G. vaccination done, as well as to find and treat young positive reactors. In western countries, the following entities are rare: abdominal tuberculosis, renal tuberculosis, bone and joint tuberculosis, and miliary tuberculosis. Cavitating lesions (phthisis) can still be found in adolescents. There are 3 varieties of mycobacteria: the human variety, the bovine, and the avian. The first causes most disease, the second causes milk-borne infection, and the third causes only a mild disorder.

The Mantoux reaction. This test is done by the intracutaneous injection of 10 international units of P.P.D. (purified protein derivative). The area is inspected after 48 hours. A positive reaction is an area of induration of at least 10 mm diameter. In interpreting the Mantoux test the phenomenon of anergy should be recalled. Thus a child may have been heavily infected with tubercle bacilli, and have a severe infection before he is allergic enough to produce a positive Mantoux reaction. Atypical mycobacterial infection (see below) also causes a positive Mantoux. Differential Mantoux testing is accordingly indicated in many children, especially those with supposed tuberculous lymphadenitis.

Clinical aspects of tuberculous infection

The primary complex occurs with the first exposure to the infection, and is made up of the reaction to the infection at the point of entry, and the reaction in the lymph gland draining the entry point. The primary complex may occur anywhere, but is most frequently found following invasion of the tonsil, lung, skin, and small intestine. Generally there are no specific symptoms or signs of primary infection, and the danger lies in the possibility of a generalized infection.

Specific types:

Intra-thoracic primary complex

This follows inhalation of *Mycobacterium tuberculosis*. It is made up of the reaction at the area of lodgement (usually in the outer lung), together with the reaction at the hilar gland. The latter can breakdown (caseate) into the bronchus, or into a blood vessel.

Clinical features. There may be none, the condition being sought because the child is a contact of a tuberculous patient, has a positive Mantoux reaction, and has a chest x-ray which reveals the swollen or calcified hilar gland.

In other children, the symptoms are due to blocking of a bronchus, either because of impingement of the swollen gland, or because following perforation of a bronchus, granulation tissue blocks the lumen of the bronchus. In some children with this problem, there is cough, fever and some breathlessness. In others, the collapse is discovered only by chest x-ray.

Tuberculous cervical adenitis

This can be due to mammalian or atypical mycobacteria and occurs when the tonsil and the neck glands make up the primary complex.

Clinical features. The tonsillar infection is asymptomatic, the first complaint being of a painless enlargement of the cervical glands. At first these are movable and separate. Later they mat together, soften, and form a fluctuant, but painless abscess. Eventually the overlying skin will redden, and a sinus form which discharges pus from the caseating glands.

Intraabdominal Tuberculosis

This is due to swallowing a large dose of mycobacteria, often of the bovine type.

Clinical features. Fever, anorexia, fatigue, and loss of weight are common features. There is diarrhea and evidence of malabsorption. If gut ulceration is extensive, colic and bloody diarrhea occur. As in all forms of primary tuberculosis, the caseous gland may rupture to cause tuberculous peritonitis. This latter is usually a chronic process causing painless ascites (peritoneal effusion). Occasionally the process is more acute and causes vomiting, abdominal pain, and tenderness.

Secondary tuberculosis

This is a more severe state than the primary disease, partly because of dissemination, and partly because immune processes now cause more tissue destruction.

Tuberculous bronchopneumonia

This condition usually follows the intrathoracic primary complex. Rarely it may be the presenting problem, if the patient, usually an infant, has inhaled a large dose of tubercle bacilli. In either case, the child shows the usual features of bronchopneumonia, i.e., fever, cough, breathlessness, and often scattered areas of dullness and crepitations. Sometimes the diagnosis is suspected only after chest x-ray.

Tuberculous meningitis

This is the most serious tuberculous disorder of childhood, and usually complicates an untreated primary complex. There are 3 clinical stages: the *irritative* stage, the *meningeal* stage, and the *terminal* stage. By the time the patient has reached the second and third stage, the prognosis for successful treatment is not good. Accordingly, the clinical description which follows will emphasize the earlier stage, which usually occupies about 2 weeks.

Features. The infant or young child becomes irritable, refuses food, and vomits. He may have a fever. In older children a change in temperament is often described, and headache is complained of. Sleepiness is common at all ages. These features are found in any meningitis. The major difference is that in tuberculous meningitis, the whole process is slowed down. Thus, if a contact of a tuberculous patient, or a patient known to have a primary complex, develops anorexia, irritability, vomiting, and sleepiness, diagnostic lumbar puncture is mandatory.

At this stage, neck stiffness, stiffness of the back, and Kernig's sign may be absent. Usually, however, if the history extends over 2 or more weeks, 1 or all of the signs of meningeal irritation are present. As these progress, the patient may develop obvious cranial nerve palsies, his state of consciousness decreases, and paralyses develop, progressing to decerebrate rigidity. Papilledema is usual. Choroideal tubercles may be found at fundoscopy. The terminal stage is associated with ventricular blockage. This is a serious complication which greatly hinders therapy.

Spinal fluid

Pressure. This measurement is of limited value, as the child is usually struggling. If, however, he is quiet, the pressure is elevated.

Cell content. Up to 500 cells per mm^3 may be present, usually as lymphocytes. In the early stage a polymorph leucocytosis is not incompatible with the diagnosis. The protein content is increased, and this gives rise to the characteristic opalescent colour of the spinal fluid, and to the cobweb clot which forms on standing. In occasional cases the sugar level is reduced. This usually is characteristic of the later stages of the disease, so too is depression of the spinal fluid chloride level.

Prognosis. The prognosis for life is usually good with modern treatment, especially if this is begun early. A substantial number may be left with permanent residuals, such as blindness, motor deficits, deafness, and intellectual impairment.

Miliary tuberculosis

This follows blood-borne spread from the primary complex, and is mostly found in association with tuberculous meningitis. The clinical findings are protean, usually taking the form of fever of unknown origin in a child who has been exposed to tuberculosis, or who has an untreated primary complex. General malaise, loss of appetite, and loss of weight are common. If the disease is localized in the lungs there may be appropriate clinical and x-ray signs. The latter show a typical snow storm appearance of infiltrates in the lung fields. Splenic enlargement is common.

Prognosis. This largely depends upon whether the child also has tuberculous meningitis. Where this is not present, antituberculous therapy is usually successful and the lung lesion heals without permanent impairment of function.

Phthisis

This is the term applied to chronic pulmonary disease which produces cavities with surrounding fibrosis. It is a secondary phenomenon of tuberculous infection, dependent upon the presence of allergy to tuberculoprotein, and is rare in children until adolescence has been reached.

Clinical features. None may be present, the condition being discovered by routine chest x-ray; otherwise lack of energy, occasional fever, anorexia, weight loss, and cough are complained of. Hemoptysis occurs if there is cavity formation. Extension of the process, as tuberculous bronchopneumonia, tuberculous urinary infection, or tuberculous laryngitis, may be the first signs.

Radiology. The signs are usually present in the upper lobes of the lung. Initially there is a local infiltration which cavitates with some fibrosis. The process may progress to cause considerable lung destruction.

Laboratory. The only specific finding is the presence of M. *tuberculosis* in the sputum or gastric washings. This may be indicated by appropriate staining or culture.

Treatment of Tuberculosis

The drugs which are commonly used are isoniazid, streptomycin, and para-aminosalicylic acid (P.A.S.). Most patients require treatment, especially the infant. Every effort should be made to establish the pattern of sensitivity of the organism.

Specific situations. The infant or child with a positive Mantoux without other evidence of disease, should be given isoniazid daily for a year. Careful clinical and radiological follow-up should be given.

Intrathoracic primary complex. Unless completely calcified, isoniazid should be given for at least a year.

Granuloma, tuberculous bronchopneumonia, and miliary tuberculosis, should receive isoniazid, P.A.S., and streptomycin. The course of streptomycin should seldom exceed 2 months on a daily basis. In more extended courses of treatment, it should be given on alternate days. P.A.S. and isoniazid are given for at least a year. A similar schedule is used for tuberculous meningitis.

Tuberculous adenitis. If due to mammalian tuberculosis, surgery is preceded and followed by a short course of streptomycin. Isoniazid should be given for at least 1 year; infections due to atypical mycobacteria are commonly insensitive to the usual antituberculous drugs, and surgery is the treatment of choice.

Side effects. Streptomycin interferes with VIIIth nerve function especially if frequent injections (>2 daily) or prolonged (>6 weeks) courses are given. The risk is justifiable, however, in severe tuberculous infections. The drug must always be given with adjuvants (I.N.H., P.A.S.) or resistance rapidly occurs.

P.A.S. This drug is rather poorly accepted by children because of the taste and the gastric irritation. It rarely gives other side effects, although a general reaction, skin rash, hepatosplenomegaly, leucocytosis, and fever occasionally happen.

I.N.H. This is well tolerated. In prolonged therapy pyridoxine should be given.

Other drugs. These include cycloserine, viomycin, and ethionamide. They should not be used unless the organism is totally resistant to the usual drugs, and significantly sensitive to those mentioned.

Infection with atypical mycobacteria

Infection with this organism will cause a positive Mantoux reaction and occasionally give rise to disease. The common types which have been reported are the Battey type, and *M.Kansasii.* Infection of the lungs is very uncommon in children, in whom superficial lymphadenitis is the usual presentation. This is most common in the lymph glands of the neck, but inguinal lymphadenitis has also been reported. The atypical mycobacteria may be isolated from the tissue but more commonly differential Mantoux tests are done. This implies a simultaneous injection of P.P.D. derived from a mammalian strain, and from the other organisms described above. A Mantoux reaction is present for both P.P.D's but that stimulated by the atypical P.P.D. is larger.

Treatment. Atypical mycobacteria are resistant to the ordinarily used antituberculous drugs. In lymphadenitis in children, the treatment of choice is surgical excision.

Scarlet fever (scarlatina)

This condition is infectious, endemic, and occasionally epidemic. Nowadays it is mild and not very common. It is due to streptococcus.

Clinical features. In the average child these are sore throat with a rash, and discomfort and swelling in the neck may point to enlargement of the tonsillar glands. Inspection of the throat reveals red fauces with enlarged edematous tonsils with follicles of pus on their surface. The uvula and tonsillar pillars are also swollen. The breath smells and fever, vomiting, anorexia, and restlessness are usual. Swallowing may be difficult.

The rash appears after a day or two, is bright red and faintly papular, beginning in the skin folds (neck, axillae, groins) and rapidly becoming generalized. It blanches on pressure. The tongue is heavily coated and the papillae are prominent, (white strawberry tongue), later desquamation occurs, leaving the surface generally red, with swollen papillae (red strawberry tongue). The rash begins to fade after a few (3-7) days, and desquamation follows.

Differential diagnosis. Scarlatiniform rashes occur as a reaction to atropine, penicillin, and other drugs. An appropriate history should be sought; the exanthems more commonly confused with mild scarlatina are rubella and exanthem subitum. In the former, the mildness of the sore throat and the enlarged occipital nodes are usually sufficient points of differentiation. In the latter, the throat is usually normal, and the rash preceded by several days of nonspecific fever, which abates as the rash appears.

Complications. These are mostly extensions of the sore throat and include otitis media, sinusitis, peritonsillar abscess, and laryngitis. Septicemia or meningitis and endocarditis are nowadays rare.

Treatment. Supportive therapy, sometimes including I.V. fluids, is given, and intramuscular penicillin administered.

Staphylococcal infections

This organism is found everywhere, and causes both minor and severe illness. Skin infections (boils, paronychia, cellulitis) are in the former category, and pneumonia, meningitis, and osteomyelitis among the latter. The newborn, and patients with impaired immune function, and sufferers from mucoviscidosis are more likely to acquire severe disease. The organism may also be responsible for wound sepsis in surgical or burns units.

The details of the disorders mentioned above are covered in the appropriate sections of this book.

Diphtheria

This condition is due to the *Corynebacterium diphtheriae*, which most commonly invades the pharynx, although infection of open sores or wounds can occur. The infection is spread by droplet and mainly affects toddlers. It has a short incubation period.

Clinical features. These depend largely upon the site of the primary infection, and the mechanical effects of the diphtheritic membrane.

Pharyngeal diphtheria

This causes sore throat, often with much difficulty in swallowing. The membrane is dull grey in colour, and mainly affects the tonsils, but spreads on to the faucial pillars, the uvula, and palate. It cannot easily be removed and attempts to do so cause bleeding.

Laryngeal Diphtheria

This is a severe form which may precede or follow pharyngeal diphtheria. It gives rise to respiratory blockage, clinically indistinguishable from that described under acute laryngotracheobronchitis. Laryngoscopy will reveal the characteristic membrane.

Nasal diphtheria

This is a relatively rare variety, giving rise to a serosanguineous nasal discharge.

Other features

Bad breath is a characteristic sign of diphtheria, as is glandular enlargement in the neck, which may be so marked as to cause bull-necking. Fever is not prominent but general toxemia, pallor, inactivity, anorexia, and tachycardia are usual. Hypotension and coldness of the hands and feet imply that the heart is involved.

Complications

Myocarditis

This occurs in the first 2 weeks after the disease has begun. Common early signs are hypotension, gallop rhythm, and bradycardia which reflects atrioventricular block. Signs of congestive cardiac failure are uncommon.

Polyneuritis

This usually begins in the second or third week of the disease. A usual first sign is of palatal paralysis with regurgitation of fluid through the nose. The eye muscles are affected later with paralysis of accommodation, or even total ophthalmoplegia. Paralysis of the pharynx, larynx, and skeletal muscles are late (5-6 week) occurrences.

Laboratory studies

The corynebacterium may be identified in, and grown from, the membrane.

Differential diagnosis

1. Pharyngeal and tonsillar diphtheria

The diphtheritic membrane may be simulated in acute streptococcal infections, and by the exudate of infectious mononucleosis. In tonsillar infection by Vincent's organisms, ulceration coexists with membrane formation. In all instances of suspected diphtheria a swab is mandatory.

2. Nasal diphtheria

In this, the principal differential diagnosis is from foreign body in the nostril. A careful history and immaculate local inspection will usually exclude/include this possibility.

3. Laryngeal Diphtheria

This is the differential diagnosis of acute laryngotracheo-bronchitis which is discussed elsewhere. It almost always, however, coexists with faucial diphtheria.

Treatment

The *specific* treatment is antitoxin. This should be administered *on reasonable suspicion* that diphtheria exists, and especially if the history suggests that active immunization has been neglected. An average dose would be 30,000-40,000 units given by slow intravenous injection.

Supportive treatment

Severe dysphagia may need intravenous feeding. The treatment of laryngeal obstruction is discussed elsewhere, but essentially consists in per-nasal tracheal intubation, or tracheotomy. Myocarditis may demand digitalization. Penicillin will eliminate the carrier state. The convalescent patient should receive routine immunization against diphtheria.

Pertussis (whooping cough)

This disease is due to *Bordetella pertussis*. It is readily transmitted to any age group but serious disease occurs only in infants.

Clinical features. These are divisible into bronchitic (catarrhal) and spasmodic phases. The bronchitic stage is characterized by the onset of a loose, nocturnal cough. This gradually becomes diurnal also and the spasmodic phase begins. This is characterized by an uncontrollable episode of coughing, followed by a compulsory indrawing of breath which gives rise to the typical whoop. Vomiting of food and mucus follows. The child then seems normal. During the episode, the eyes bulge, the face becomes red, and slight cyanosis may follow. In infants the picture is somewhat different. The cough may sound looser, there is much less evidence of whooping, but vomiting is prominent. Physical signs in the chest are infrequent, and if found, imply that a pulmonary complication (see below) has occurred.

Complications: These may be divided into 2 types: pressure phenomena and pulmonary complications.

Pressure phenomena. This results from the large increase in systemic pressure, capillary pressure, intraabdominal pressure, or airway pressure. This increase in airway pressure may lead to pneumothorax with the appropriate physical signs. Subconjunctival hemorrhage is associated with rupture of the capillaries, and the occasional intracranial hemorrhage is assumed to be associated with a rise in systemic pressure. Prolapse of the rectum is an accompaniment of the straining associated with the coughing spells. Subconjunctival hemorrhage and ulceration of the frenum of the tongue are the commonest complications. The latter exists only of course if the child has teeth.

Pulmonary complications The commonest is bronchopneumonia, and occurs mostly in infancy and early childhood. Persistent collapse of the lung with or without bronchiectasis or pulmonary fibrosis is nowadays rather rare.

Blood examination. This is of value only in the late bronchitic or early spasmodic stage. There is leucocytosis due to lymphocyte proliferation.

Differential diagnosis. This is most important in the younger age group. Two conditions should be born in mind when a diagnosis of pertussis is suspected. One is fibrocystic disease. In this condition the first respiratory episode may closely simulate whooping cough. Simple tracheobronchitis mimics the nocturnal bronchitic stage of pertussis, but there is much less vomiting and distress, and more evidence of a general reaction such as fever. It is important to realize that vomiting may occur in episodes of coughing which are due to tracheobronchitis. In the older age group the catarrhal stage of measles may be confused with the early stage of whooping cough. Patients who have inhaled a foreign body may have a paroxysmal cough, usually without any whoop, although it may be severe enough on occasion to cause vomiting.

Progress. The whooping cough lasts for at least 6 weeks and on occasion may extend its course for as long as 4 months. The return of symptoms with intercurrent infections such as the cold is common.

Prevention. In early infancy, before the age of usual inoculation, young infants who have been exposed may be given hyperimmune gamma globulin. The ordinary immunization course with triple vaccine should begin at 3 months, especially if the disease is endemic. Few children suffer reactions from these injections. If, however, fever and convulsions occur during a course of triple vaccine therapy, they are usually due to the pertussis fraction, and it is usually unwise to persist.

Treatment. The patient is usually isolated for 4 weeks. Normally 2 weeks after the spasmodic stage has begun, he is no longer infective, although he may still be coughing. There is no specific treatment for whooping cough, and in small infants with severe choking spells, hospital treatment is best, since they may require oxygen and gavage feeding. Bronchopneumonia may require antibiotics.

Pseudomonas infections

These are of considerable importance in pediatrics. Such infections are not uncommon in the newborn, as a complication of burns, and following treatment by wide-spectrum antibiotics in such conditions as mucoviscidosis. They also occur in persons given steroids or immunosuppressive drugs, and in those where intravenous catheters are left indwelling for a prolonged period.

Clinical features. There is nothing specific in these, although purpura and necrotic skin lesions are usual in severe septicemias.

Prevention. This is particularly important in the newborn nurseries, where water taps, humidifying apparatus, and cribs may harbour the organism. Otherwise, the judicious use of antibiotics, with frequent swabbing of those on the broad-spectrum variety, should be carried out.

Treatment. Antibiotic therapy will depend largely on the local pattern of resistance; generally, however, kanamycin and chloramphenicol are to be considered, as is the recent penicillin-variant, carbenicillin.

Tetanus

This is due to the *Clostridium tetani*, and can only arise as a result of injury, which is usually a relatively deep puncture wound.

Clinical features. The incubation period is 6-14 days. The generalized form has a subacute onset, with progressive muscle stiffness. This is usually first noticed in the jaws and neck, Trismus or difficulty in mouth opening is an early sign, as is difficulty in swallowing, headache, and pain in the limbs. Occasionally a convulsion is the first complaint, and a few patients have early rigidity of the abdominal muscles, which may cause confusion with an acute abdomen.

In the well-developed disease, the child shows characteristic spasms, with stiffening of the limbs and fist clenching. The head is opisthotonic and the teeth bared (risus sardonicus). Muscular contraction is violent, and the fixation of the respiratory muscles (intercostals, diaphragm, larynx) causes cyanosis and anoxia. Sweating and fear are usual. Hemorrhage into the muscles, or fractures are rather rare complications. In the progressive case, the spasms increase in frequency and severity, with a decreasing threshold of stimulation. Fever is low grade, leucocytosis inconstant and the spinal fluid normal. Death, if it occurs, is due to anoxia or pulmonary complications.

Diagnosis. The principal condition to be considered is strychnine poisoning. The difference in a sense is academic, as the treatment is similar. Absence of a wound, and access to the poison are the principal points. Local stiffness of the jaw, due to mumps or cervical adenitis, is usually obvious enough in the differential diagnosis of trismus.

Prevention. A full course of tetanus toxoid should be given to everyone. A child receiving a wound should be given a booster dose of tetanus toxoid. If not immunized, tetanus antitoxin should be given after a preliminary skin test. Tetanus toxoid should follow a few weeks later.

Treatment. This must be carried out in a specially staffed and equipped hospital. The wound must have suitable surgical care, and the patient kept sedated in a quiet environment. If spasms occur, he should be anesthetized, have an endotracheal tube passed, and then paralyzed and ventilated mechanically. Tetanus antitoxin therapy is also usually given. Assisted respiration is continued for about 7 days, until the spasms cease.

Salmonella Infections

There are many varieties of the salmonella organism, most cause gastroenteritis, the clinical features of which are described elsewhere. *Salmonella typhosa* gives rise to a somewhat more severe clinical syndrome—enteric, or typhoid fever.

Typhoid fever

Clinical features. In the *infant*, symptoms of gastroenteritis are common, occasionally a septicemic picture is seen, with jaundice, splenic enlargement and meningitis. In some, mild fever with refusal to feed are the sole problems, the diagnosis being arrived at by laboratory methods.

In the older child, the early phase is characterized by listlessness, anorexia and fever, and abdominal pain. Diarrhea and constipation occur almost equally. Bronchitis is usual, and pneumonia may follow. Splenomegaly and a rash appear after about 7 days illness. The latter is described as rose red in colour and macular in type, appearing in crops on the abdomen and trunk. Some degree of dehydration is common, as are headache and neck stiffness. Examination of the abdomen will reveal some distention, diffuse tenderness, and splenomegaly. Delirium, confusional states, and coma are much less common in children than in adults.

Complications. The commonest in children is an extension of the bronchitic state to a true pneumonia. Extensive hemorrhage into the gut from the typhoid ulcer is characterized by sudden pallor, hypotension, and tachycardia. Perforation of the gut gives rise to the symptoms of peritonitis—severe abdominal pain, shock, and generalized tenderness. Hepatitis, osteomyelitis and pyelonephritis may each complicate the course of typhoid, perhaps less often than in the adult. Osteomyelitis is more likely in sufferers from sickle-cell anemia.

Laboratory studies. The organism can be grown from the blood early in the disease, and from the gut after the first week or so. Agglutination studies (the Widal reaction) are reliable in the second week.

Differential diagnosis. In the early stage, this is principally from other causes of dubious fevers such as dengue, viral pneumonia, and malaria. The gastrointestinal symptoms may mimic appendicitis, or occasionally intussusception. Meningeal symptoms are not very uncommon in typhoid, and diagnostic lumbar puncture should not be neglected.

Treatment. Chloramphenicol and ampicillin are the drugs of choice, and both should be given until the pattern of sensitivity is known. Supportive intravenous therapy is usually necessary. Hemorrhage will require transfusion, and gut perforation, laparotomy.

Prevention. The avoidance of contaminated food and water is primary. Prophylactic inoculation with a reliable antigen gives reasonable protection for 2-3 years, after which booster doses are necessary.

The carrier state. This occurs for 6-8 weeks after recovery from the disease process. The organism is excreted in the feces and urine. In most instances spontaneous clearance occurs. In a few persons (rarely children), carriage is more permanent, resistant to antibiotic courses, and sometimes relieved only by cholecystectomy.

Shigella infections

These cause the bacterial diarrheas and are spread by infected food, water, or food handlers. The common varieties are *S.sonnei*, *S.flexneri* and *S.dysenteriae*.

Clinical features. The incubation period is short (2-3 days) and the disease presents as gastroenteritis of variable severity (see p. 204). Specific diagnosis is made by stool culture. The treatment is to relieve dehydration and, occasionally to give appropriate antibiotics.

Cholera

This disease, caused by the *Vibrio cholerae*, is spread by infected water or food.

Clinical features. The main problem is diarrhea with early and severe dehydration, and the other expected clinical features of gastroenteritis (see p. 204).

Treatment. This is as described for severe water and electrolyte depletion, no specific drug therapy is of great value.

Prevention. Cholera vaccine is of considerable value in individual prevention, although good standards of hygiene are the basic methods of protecting communities.

Brucellosis

This disease is due to *Brucella melitensis*, which is transmitted by domestic animals.

Clinical features. These are very varied. In the *acute* form usual symptoms are fever, anorexia, headache, and respiratory infection. Intervals of well being are not uncommon. Alimentary symptoms include constipation and abdominal pain, and occasionally diarrhea. In younger children, lymphadenopathy and hepatosplenomegaly are found. Rare manifestations include meningitis and eye disorders (uveitis, keratitis, and optic neuritis.)

The chronic form is associated with malaise, poor appetite, low-grade fever and minor joint pains.

Diagnosis. In the acute disease, the organism may be cultured from the blood or urine. Specific agglutinins appear after the 10th day of illness.

Treatment. Tetracycline will commonly cure the condition.

Tularemia

This disease of rodents, which occurs in man, is found principally in the northern hemisphere and usually in those having close contact with rabbits and other animals harbouring the disease, or the infected vector (usually a tick or flea).

Clinical features. These vary with the mode of infection; if this has been a bite, a papule which ulcerates and causes an associated lymphadenitis is common. After ingestion of infective material, a severe pharyngotonsillitis (resembling that of diphtheria) is common. If the organism is inhaled, a severe bronchopneumonia results.

Diagnosis. An agglutinin appears after 2 weeks of illness, and a skin test may be positive early in the disease. The organism (*Pasteurella tularensis*) may be recovered from animals inoculated with the patient's blood or secretions.

Treatment. A weeks's course of streptomycin is usually curative.

SPIROCHAETAL INFECTIONS

The most important of these of syphilis, which is much less common nowadays since congenital infections can readily be prevented by treating the mother.

SYPHILIS

Clinical features. Those in the newborn are described elsewhere, briefly the principal manifestations are nasal snuffles with a blood discharge, a discrete maculopapular rash, and, in a few infants, hemolysis with jaundice. After a few months, bone infection may be severe enough to cause epiphyseal dislocation and loss of limb movement (pseudoparalysis).

Later manifestation of congenital syphilis. The most common presentation is keratitis, in which there is lacrimation, eye pain, and photophobia. The cornea is reddened, and may later scar. Choreoretinitis and optic atrophy also are found.

Osseous lesions. These occur in a minority of patients. The usual pathology consists in a periostitis, readily recognizable by x-ray. Sabre-shin (boomerang) tibia is due to thickening of the anterior surface of the bone and is a characteristic deformity. Pain may also be present and, in young children, epiphyseal subluxation occurs. In the same age group, bossing of the skull occurs. A painless arthritis (Clutton's joints) is characterized by effusions in the large joints. The secondary dentition may also show characteristic changes; peg-shaped incisors, sometimes with a notch (Hutchinson's teeth) and malformed cusps of the molars (Moon's deformity) both occur.

Skin and mucous membrane. Condylomata may persist among older children, as do perioral radial skin scars (rhagades). Various rashes (syphilides) also occur. In the early years these tend to be papulopustular, in the later stages they resemble adult tertiary disease, commonly presenting as localized ulcers (gummata), or serpiginous nodular lesions.

The nervous system. Meningovascular syphilis is characterized by progressive intellectual deterioration and involvement of the cranial nerves and pyramidal tracts. Taboparesis with dementia, ataxia, pupillary (Argyll-Robertson) aberrations, and cachexia is nowadays virtually unknown. Paroxysmal hemoglobinuria, a late manifestation, is described elsewhere.

Laboratory. The blood and spinal fluid will show the characteristic V.D.R.L. reaction. In meningovascular syphilis, abnormal C.S.F. pleocytosis and globulin values occur.

Treatment. Penicillin is used; a suitable regime is to use procaine penicillin 200,000 units/kg total, given at 48-hour intervals. Full serological reversal occurs 18-24 months after treatment.

LEPTOSPIROSIS

This disease may be spread from rats (*Leptospira icterohemorrhagiae*, Weil's disease) or from the dog (*L.canicola*).

Clinical features. This usually presents with a septicemic picture—fever, rigors, headache, and vomiting, followed by jaundice and purpura. Oliguria or complete renal shut-down may occur. A meningoencephalitis is another mode of presentation, with anorexia, irritability, vomiting, and drowsiness.

Laboratory. A polymorph leucocytosis is usual. The urine shows albumen and red cells. The spinal fluid initially will contain polymorphs and then lymphocytes. The organism can be cultivated from the blood and urine.

Treatment. Penicillin in large doses should be given and the usual supportive therapy begun.

RAT-BITE FEVER

This is due to infection by the *Spirillum minus*, and as the name implies, inoculation follows rat bite.

Clinical features. After healing of the initial bite, an indurated area forms which then ulcerates. The corresponding glands enlarge, and a reddish macular rash appears on the face and trunk. Improvement and relapse is characteristic of the general symptoms. The organism may be seen in scrapings from the ulcer.

Treatment. Penicillin is recommended.

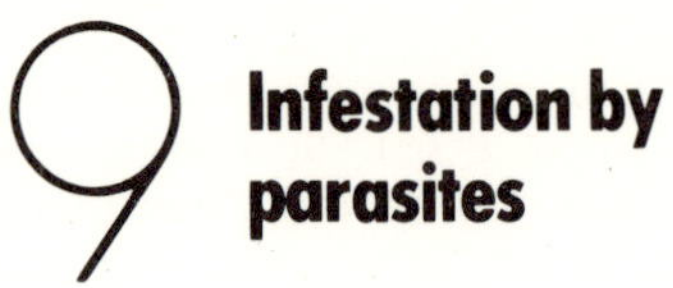

9 Infestation by parasites

These are common in children, especially in tropical areas, or where social circumstances are poor. Perhaps the most widely distributed of them is round worm infestation (nematodiasis). Some common nematodes include the following.

Oxyuriasis (threadworm, pinworm)

This common infestation is caused by the passage of eggs from person to person. These develop in the duodenum and parasitize the cecum and appendix.

Clinical features. In most instances there are none, the thread-like gravid females being observed among the feces. Itchiness of the anus, especially after going to bed, is a usual complaint. In females, a vaginal discharge may occur. In a few instances, an acute appendix is found to be stuffed with threadworms.

Diagnosis. This is made by identifying the eggs, which readily adhere to transparent adhesive tape applied to the perianal area.

Treatment. The whole family or other group, should be treated with piperazine citrate, or by a single dose of pyrvinium pamoate.

Ascariasis

This means infestation with the large roundworm, and usually results from the ingestion of the worm eggs from food, or from contact with fecal-contaminated soil. The eggs hatch in the duodenum, enter the gut wall, and pass, via the lymphatics and veins, to the inferior vena cava and lungs. There they develop in the alveoli, and eventually reenter the gut by migrating to the epiglottic area whence they are swallowed.

Clinical features. Usually there are none, occasionally a mild atypical pneumonia has been reported after heavy pulmonary invasion.

Diagnosis. This is made by identifying the eggs in feces.

Treatment. This is with piperazine citrate, which affects only the worms in the gut. Reinfestation is common, so that repeated courses of treatment may be necessary.

Toxocariasis

This implies infestation with the cat (*Toxocara felis*) or dog (*Toxocara canis*) roundworm. The animal passes the eggs to the soil where embryos form and are ingested by children. These go through the stages of development noted for ascaris, except that the adult type worm cannot survive in the human gut.

Clinical features. In many instances there are none, otherwise visceral larva migrans (*T.canis*) has been reported. This is associated with a reaction to the migrating larvae, and occurs most frequently in the liver or lungs, or occasionally in the eye. Fever, an allergic type pneumonia with eosinophilia, and hepatomegaly occur. There is some evidence that *T.canis* may be a vector for toxoplasma infections.

Diagnosis. The larva must be demonstrated histologically.

Treatment. Thiabendazole appears to be the drug of choice.

Prevention. Cats and dogs should regularly be dewormed with piperazine.

Ancylostomiasis (hookworm infestation)

This is widely distributed in tropical areas. Geographic eponyms exist for sub varieties of the *Ancylostoma*, viz., *americanus*, *ceylonensis*, *braziliense*, etc. The eggs are shed in feces, embryonate in the soil, and reenter the human body through the skin of the lower limbs. Thence they enter the venous system and migrate to the lungs, develop there, and return to the gut as already described for ascaris. The worm is nourished from the gut capillaries.

Clinical features. Usually there are none until heavy infestation has occurred. At this stage, blood loss causes symptoms of anemia, viz., pallid mucous membranes, fatigue, venous thrills, functional murmurs, and gallop rhythms. Occasionally some varieties cause a skin lesion—cutaneous larva migrans.

Diagnosis. The eggs are readily recognizable in the feces.

Treatment. The parasite is treated by giving bephenium hydroxynaphthoate. The anemia will respond to iron.

Prevention. Foot gear should be worn in endemic areas, and hygienic practices instituted.

Strongyloidiasis

This is a threadworm-like parasite which occurs principally in tropical areas. Its life cycle and mode of reentry to the human is essentially as described for hookworm.

Clinical features. These are rather varied; in most instances there are none. In other children, diarrhea and malnutrition have been reported.

Diagnosis. The larvae can be identified in the stool.

Treatment. Thiabendazole is the drug of choice.

Trichinosis

This is due to eating pork infected with *Trichinella* cysts. The larvae hatch in the duodenum and enter various tissues, principally the muscles.

Clinical features. These are liable to occur in the older child. Eating heavily infected pork causes acute gastroenteritis. Invasion of the muscles causes much aching and pain, with stiffness of the skeletal muscles, and dysphagia if the muscles of deglutition are invaded. Fever and periorbital edema occur.

Diagnosis. This is best made by the demonstration of the larvae in a muscle biopsy.

Treatment. None is satisfactory. Thiabendazole may be of some value.

Infestation with cestoda (tapeworm)

The larval stage—the cysticerus—may be carried in beef (*Taenia saginata*) or in pork (*T. solium*). The cysticercus grows into the segmented adult worm in the gut, where it may attain a considerable length. Human ingestion of the eggs (from fecal material) is followed by migration of the larvae to various soft tissues, e.g., the muscles, eyes, brain, etc.

Clinical features. These are few. Commonly the infestation is not noticed until the passage of mature proglottids (segments) occurs. Very rarely there is diarrhea, or intestinal obstruction.

In larval migration, the cysticercus may cause visual troubles, or, rarely, epilepsy if to the brain.

Treatment. Mepacrine, followed by a gentle purge with examination of the stool for the *complete* worm is the routine treatment. Niclosamide (yomesan) or dichlorophen can also be used. With the latter drugs, the stool should be examined after 3 months for gravid segments.

Infestation with the dwarf tapeworm

This is common in children. The worm is *Hymenolepis nana*, whose eggs are passed from child to child by fecal contamination. There are no symptoms. The diagnosis is made by finding the eggs in the stool and the treatment is with mepacrine. Reinfection is frequent, so that repeated courses of treatment are necessary.

Diphylobothriasis

This is infestation with the fish tapeworm, and occurs in fish-eating populations, especially when the fish is not cooked. There are few symptoms, except the passage of proglottids. However, macrocytic anemias have been reported in adults. The eggs can be demonstrated in the patient's feces. The treatment is as already described for other tapeworms.

Hydatid disease

This condition is due to invasion of the body by the larval phase of a small canine tape worm. The eggs are passed in the dog dung, and the larvae develop in any animal (including man) which ingests them. The sheep is readily affected, so that hydatid disease appears in them. Eating the uncooked mutton by dogs or man, carries the cycle on.

Clinical features. These are entirely due to the presence of the cyst. In many instances these can grow to large size without causing much trouble. Hydatid cyst of the liver causes hepatomegaly, or, in rare cases, vague pain in the right hypochondrium. Pulmonary hydatids are usually found at chest x-ray, often when hydatid disease has not been entertained as a diagnosis. In very rare instances, the cyst ruptures into a bronchus, causing severe coughing and dyspnea.

Hydatid cyst of the brain causes focal neurological signs (fits) or signs of raised intracranial pressure (headache, vomiting, papilledema). Visual disturbances may betoken a small cyst in the eye. In any position, rupture of the cyst may be followed by severe, occasionally fatal, anaphylaxis.

Prevention. Dogs should be thoroughly dewormed, and infected mutton adequately cooked.

Treatment. This is surgical, with isolation, aspiration, and excision of the cyst.

Infestation with flukes (trematodes)

There are 2 such groups. The intestinal (*Schistosoma mansoni* and *S. japonicum*), and the vesical (*S.haematobium*). In either instance, the adult forms live in the small veins draining the gut or bladder. The eggs which are laid ulcerate into the gut, or bladder lumen. Entry to the body takes place by bathing in infected water.

Clinical features. In a few instances, the patient notes irritation and pain at the place where the larva penetrates the skin. Although the larva has to traverse the venous and systemic circulations in order to reach its favored site, this stage seldom gives rise to specific symptoms, other than urticarial skin reactions. In the intestinal afflictions, the release of the eggs causes dysentery, fever, and prostration. In the vesical type, hematuria and frequency are usual. With healing, fibrosis occurs and this may cause intestinal obstruction, hepatic cirrhosis, or in the vesical infections, interference with bladder function, and the formation of bladder stones.

Prevention. This is dependent upon destroying the intermediary host, usually a water snail.

Treatment. Antimonial drugs, e.g., Stibophen, are of great value, although repeated intravenous treatments are usually necessary.

Liver flukes

The most important of these is *Fasciola hepatica*, which thrives in sheep. Human infestation is not very common, and symptoms occur because the fluke invades the bile ducts, giving rise to cholecystitis. Biliary cirrhosis is a usual concomitant, and the principal cause of death.

Treatment. This is by giving several courses of emetine hydrochloride.

Lung flukes (paragonimiasis)

This infestation occurs after the ingested cyst has become a larva in the gut; from there it bores its way to the lung where it becomes adult. The eggs are coughed up, and thus spread again.

Clinical features. There is a cough, with bloody sputum. X-rays show a nonspecific infiltrate. Abscesses may form at any point of the larva's track of migration.

Treatment. Bithionol may be of some value in this condition.

Filariasis

This is a small, thread-like worm, the larvae of which (microfilariae) enter the victim as a result of a bite by an insect vector. *Wuchereria bancrofti* is the more widely distributed species. *Brugia malayi* occurs in Southeast Asia and the South Pacific. The microfilariae enter the lymphatics after the insect bite and may develop to the adult form at any stage of its passage in the lymphatic system.

Clinical features. There are repeated attacks of lymphangitis with lymphatic gland swelling. Fever usually accompanies these episodes. Eventually lymphatic blockage occurs with local lymphedema and much tissue distortion—elephantiasis. The adult worms cause painless enlargement, especially on the scalp and near the long bone ends.

Diagnosis. The microfilariae can be demonstrated by films of nocturnal blood.

Treatment. Hetrazine is often used but more modern therapy consists in giving diethylcarbamazine.

10 Diseases of the alimentary tract

PHYSIOLOGY

The principal activities of the alimentary tract are taking in food (ingestion); digestion; absorption of food elements; and, to a minor extent, excretion. Some of these activities can go on at the same time.

Ingestion

In the older infant the food is broken up by chewing, the process being aided by the secretions of the salivary glands (parotid, submandibular, and sublingual) which produce a watery solution containing mucus—a lubricant—and ptyalin (amylase—an enzyme which splits starch). These glands are under control of the autonomic nerves; the sight of food, or the presence of food in the mouth signals the medullary secretory centre which initiates glandular activity. Mastication is followed by swallowing (deglutition) which is quite a complex business, beginning when a bolus of food reaches the pharynx. This has a rich nerve supply, so that the brain knows at all times the exact position of the bolus, so preventing food entering the air passages. Impulses sent from the pharynx to the medulla are handled at the *deglutition* centre, which coordinates the information and initiates the act of swallowing—basically a movement in which the muscle ring around the food contracts, while the area below relaxes. The same actions occur in the esophagus by the same mechanisms. The process of alternate contraction and relaxation (peristalsis) requires closer local control by means of nerves in the muscular part of the esophagus. Deglutition ends when the food enters the stomach.

Gastric function

This is a storing and mixing area which produces acid, mucus, and enzymes. The acid (dilute hydrochloric) is produced in the parietal cells and kills swallowed bacteria. The mucus, apart from its lubricant function, helps protect the stomach wall against its own acid, and also contains the AB blood group antigens, as well as intrinsic factor—an important protein which combines with dietary vitamin B_{12} to allow the latter to be absorbed and used in red cell formation. In infants, the stomach also produces *rennin*, the ferment which curdles milk, and *pepsin*, an enzyme which begins the breakdown of protein. The stomach then has some digestive ability, but a main function is to act as a reservoir which gradually releases food for further processing down stream.

Gastric secretion is partly reflex, following the sight of, or arrival of food in the stomach. The latter stimulus will also cause the secretion from the pylorus of a hormone called *gastrin*; this is carried by the blood to the secretory cells of the stomach. *Enterogastrone*, another hormone secreted by the small intestine, stops gastric secretory activity.

Function of the small gut (duodenum, ileum, jejunum)

This is the body's main digestive and absorptive area. The duodenum produces an alkaline mucus, which together with the alkaline pancreatic juice, neutralizes the acid food transmitted by the stomach. The pancreatic juice also contains proteolytic enzymes (mainly trypsin), fat splitting enzymes (lipase), and amylase, which degrades starch. Bile also enters the duodenum and is used to aid fat digestion and absorption. The jejunum and ileum act mainly to absorb food products, but secrete quantities of protein and fat-splitting enzymes. The small gut also deals with simple carbohydrates, mainly the disaccharides. It does so by secreting an appropriate enzyme (e.g., lactase, for lactose degradation) which reduces the disaccharide to a monosaccharide, suitable for direct absorption. The small gut also absorbs vitamins, calcium, and the trace elements such as zinc, manganese, and copper.

Function of the large bowel

This comprises the area from the cecum to the rectum. The first half (to the splenic fixure of the colon) is an important area for the reabsorption of water and electrolytes such as sodium, chloride, and potassium. The rest of the large bowel acts as a reservoir for feces, but also can reabsorb water and some electrolytes.

DISORDERS OF FACE AND MOUTH

Hare lip and cleft palate

These occur about once in every 600 births, usually together and occasionally occur in association with congenital heart disease or a chromosome disorder.

Anatomical features. These are quite variable. The major difficulties in treatment arise if the upper jaw is also cleft through the gum line (the alveolus). A simple classification is:

A. Prealveolar clefts
(i) Only the lip involved—incomplete
(ii) Lip and nostril involved—complete

B. Alveolar cleft — Lip, maxilla, and palate involved
C. Postalveolar cleft — Only the palate is affected.

In cases A and B, the defect may be in one or both sides. In simple cleft palate, the defect may involve the soft palate alone, or involve both the soft and hard palates. These conditions are readily seen at birth.

Other clinical features. These occur only in the more severe types and consist in difficulty in sucking and swallowing, with regurgitation of milk through the nostrils. If not treated, chewing is difficult because of a subsequent poor dental arch and speech is also indistinct. Infections of the ear are common.

General care. The ugly appearance of the baby distresses parents, so they should be reassured that effective treatment is possible. Warnings about the duration of treatment should be postponed until the parents have accepted the situation.

Babies with difficulty in sucking and swallowing may need to be tube fed for a day or two. Thereafter, they can usually manage to suck if they are sat up, and a long teat is used. The mother should herself look after the baby from the earliest opportunity.

Specific treatment. The principles are to restore the parts of the face and palate to their normal position by plastic surgery. Thus the face grows normally and the ability to masticate, swallow, and speak is conserved. All of this also improves the baby's appearance. Dental assistance is sought from the earliest stage. The lip deformity is closed first, usually in the early months. If the alveolus is split, the dentist begins early to realign the dental arch using special appliances. The cleft palate is closed at a later date, but always before the baby begins to speak. Prolonged follow-up is necessary, especially to ensure that the child talks normally. Accordingly, a speech therapist will see the infant before, and for a considerable time after any surgical procedure.

Microstomia and macrostomia

These terms mean respectively that the mouth is smaller or larger than usual. Microstomia may be associated with mental defect. Macrostomia is often most associated with generalized bone abnormalities.

DISORDERS OF THE TEETH

Minor variations in the shape and number of teeth are common in children. Abnormalities of the dental arch, e.g., buck teeth, crowding of teeth, and irregularity of the tooth line are also frequent. These usually require long continued orthodontic treatment in which the teeth are braced and gradually brought to a normal form.

Enamel hypoplasia

This is a serious disorder of the first teeth; in it the teeth pit and groove easily, and soon decay. It occurs in children with brain disorder, e.g., severe cerebral palsy, and in serious cyanotic heart disease. Yellow staining of the teeth occurs when tetracycline (an antibiotic) has been given early in life.

Dental caries

This is the most common dental disease of childhood, with involvement and destruction of all dental tissue. Lack of oral hygiene and a high carbohydrate intake are contributary; especially to be condemned is the practice of coating the dummy with honey or sugar as a more efficient pacifier.

There is clear evidence that the provision of fluoride in the drinking water, or as tablets, will reduce the incidence of caries. Fluoride will not, however, compensate for poor dental hygiene or faulty dietary habits.

Mandibular hypoplasia (Pierre Robin syndrome)

In this condition, the lower jaw is under developed. Cleft palate is often present, and the tongue is also smaller than normal. Problems occur only in the newborn.

Clinical features. The pharyngeal airway blocks when the tongue falls back, and this gives rise to attacks of breathlessness, rib retraction, and cyanosis. Difficulty in sucking and swallowing are usual. The underslung jaw and "Andy Gump" profile are sufficient to suggest the diagnosis.

Treatment. The airway must be maintained; in the newborn nursery this is commonly done by endotracheal intubation. The baby is tube fed, and nursed and fed in the prone position. Care of the airway is necessary for up to 8 weeks, after that spontaneous improvement is usual. Treatment of any associated cleft palate should be delayed until the baby can maintain his airway without trouble.

DISORDERS OF THE TONGUE

A macroglossia (large tongue) may occur as a single inborn defect, or be a secondary finding in cretinism, Down's syndrome, and other forms of mental retardation. Variations in the surface of the tongue, e.g., fissured or geographic tongue are of no importance. The frenum of the tongue (attachment on the lower front of the tongue) may be short (so called tongue tie) and is often wrongly blamed for delay in speech. However, treatment is very seldom necessary.

DISORDERS OF THE MOUTH

Aphthous stomatitis

This is an inflammation of the mouth caused by the herpes simplex (cold sore) virus which occurs in pre-school-age children.

Clinical features. The child is unwell, fevered, and cannot eat because of the inflamed, painful mouth. In young children, refusal of fluids may lead to dehydration. At first the mouth, lips and pharynx are red and inflamed, then crops of vesicles come out, rapidly lose their tops, and show as small gray ulcers. The submandibular glands enlarge.

Treatment. In young children, intravenous fluid may be needed for a day or two, otherwise pain-relieving mouth washes are given before feeding the child. If pain is severe and continued, sedatives are given.

Recurrent aphthous ulcer

In this condition, a small, painful vesicle develops in the mouth or on the tongue. It ruptures and ulcerates, but remains quite small. Multiple ulcers are usually widely separated. They recur over a period of years. No method of prevention is known. Treatment is with pain killing mouth washes.

Thrush

This is due to the fungus monilia (candida) albicans, which, in the newborn, may originate from the mother's birth passages. Otherwise it tends to follow the use of a broad-spectrum antibiotic.

Clinical features. In many children there are no complaints, the disease being suspected when the mouth is looked at and the grayish white, *longitudinal* strands of exudate are seen. These occur on the inside of the cheek, the gums, and tongue. If rubbed lightly the strands separate to leave a raw, bleeding area. Fever, irritability, and refusal to feed occur if the infection is extensive. If the infant is clearly very ill, breathless, and anoxic, then the infection has spread to the lungs. This dangerous complication occurs only in children with disorders of the immune system, or when prolonged broad-spectrum antibiotic treatment has been given.

Treatment. Antibiotics should be discontinued and an antifungal agent (e.g., nystatin) given by mouth.

Cancrum Oris (noma)

This is a rare, severe infection which causes ulceration and gangrene of the cheek. It occurs only in malnourished, debilitated infants. The treatment is supportive, with intravenous feeding and antibiotics. If tissue destruction is great, plastic surgical repair may be required.

DISORDERS OF THE SALIVARY GLANDS

Mumps (epidemic parotitis)

This is a common viral disease occurring mostly in the winter, the incubation period is about 3 weeks.

Clinical features. Fever and sore throat are occasional preliminaries, but the commonest first complaint is of a sore face in the area of the parotids. These glands swell, filling the area behind the angle of the lower jaw and extending towards the mastoid behind the ear. The overlying skin may be edematous, but there is no redness. The glands are tender to touch and painful on jaw movement so that difficulty occurs with eating. Fever is usual at this stage. Occasionally the submandibular glands are also affected. The orifices of the parotid duct may be red. The swelling goes down in a few days and all symptoms are relieved.

Complications. The commonest is meningoencephalitis, with fever, headache, drowsiness, and vomiting. Rarely are there convulsions. Lymphocytes are found in the spinal fluid. Spontaneous recovery is usual. In adolescents testicular inflammation (orchitis) or ovarian involvement (oophoritis) are rare complications.

Treatment. Soft, easily chewed foods are given, together with warm mouthwashes. External heat or cold to the face is comforting, and analgesics are used. Isolation of patients is usual until the swelling has gone down.

Prevention. Older children may be given a specific mumps vaccine.

Recurrent parotitis

Clinical features. The parotid swells, and is a little tender, but the patient feels well and has no fever. The swelling subsides without treatment, but recurs again within a week or two. The whole cycle is repeated at varying intervals, and between attacks the gland is quite normal. The sialogram (x-ray after injection of radiopaque dye into the parotid duct) shows dilation of the smaller duct divisions.

Treatment. This is symptomatic only, with hot and cold applications to the parotid, and the use of mild analgesics.

DISEASES OF THE ESOPHAGUS

Tracheoesophageal fistula and esophageal atresia

These are common inborn defects, sometimes coexisting with congenital heart disease or pyloric stenosis. The mother often has hydramnios.

Clinical features. These are divisible into 2 groups, those existing before the baby is given his first feed, and those occurring after this. The pre-feed features are the most important, as the outlook is much better if feeding is avoided.

Pre-feed features:

1. On routine passage of a stomach tube at birth, resistance is felt about 10 cm from the lips. If this occurs, forbid feeding and inform the medical officer who will arrange confirmatory x-rays.
2. At, or soon after, birth the infant is noticed to drool from the overflow of unswallowable saliva. The pillow may be wet from this. There are no respiratory symptoms at this stage. Again forbid feeding and report the finding.

Features at first feeding. The baby sucks well, but immediately coughs, chokes, returns the feed, becomes breathless, and may become cyanosed. The whole cycle recurs if he is fed again, because the gullet fills up and the food spills over into the wind pipe. If milk has been given, breathlessness tends to persist, and x-rays of the chest will show scattered areas of consolidation and collapse.

The diagnosis is confirmed at this stage by failure to pass a gastric tube, and injection of air into the tube outlines the blind-ended (atretic) esophagus; contrast media (e.g., lipiodol) should only be injected by the radiologist.

Treatment. This is surgical, the principle being to join the upper and lower segment of the esophagus and to close off any communication with the trachea. A plastic tube is left in place for feeding the baby, or, occasionally, an opening into the stomach (a gastrostomy) is made to do the same thing.

Outlook for the patient. This depends on whether the baby has been fed or not, so all babies should have a tube passed in order to be sure that the gullet is open. If milk is inhaled, this gives rise to a severe pneumonia which aggravates the surgical difficulties. So, give all babies glucose solution as their first feed. This ameliorates the disaster of a missed tracheoesophageal fistula. Babies with this condition should always be checked for congenital heart disease. If postoperative vomiting is persistent, then pyloric stenosis (see below) may be present.

Tracheoesophageal fistula without atresia (H-type fistula)

Clinical features. The features at birth are less dramatic, since the baby can swallow. There is a communication between the esophagus and trachea (see figure 41) so that liquid enters the windpipe causing coughing, breathlessness, and recurrent respiratory complaints, often considered to be pneumonias. The diagnosis is confirmed by special x-rays which show the communication (fistula) between the gullet and wind pipe.

The treatment is surgical, to close the fistula.

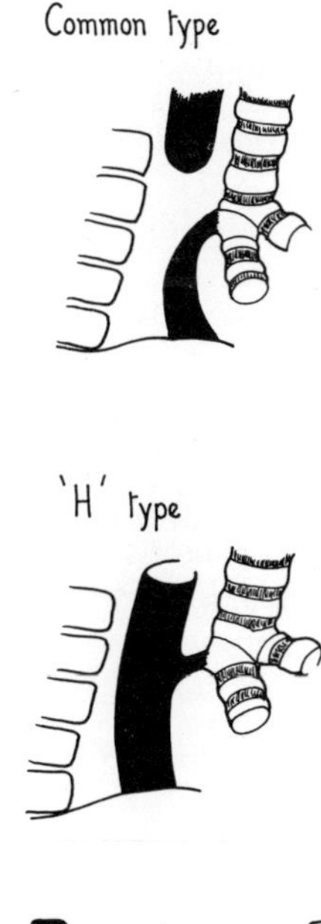

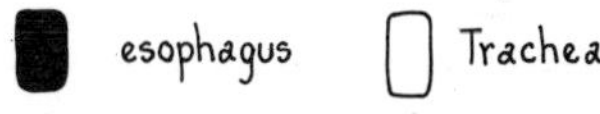

Fig. 41. Diagrammatic lateral view of tracheoesophageal fistula.

Esophagitis

This means inflammation of the gullet, and is due usually to a foreign body, e.g., a feeding tube, in it. It also occurs where the patient has a poor immune response such as agammaglobulinemia, when the cause is usually a fungus.

Clinical features. Swallowing is difficult and painful. Vomiting, often of blood, is common, as are fever and irritability. X-rays show abnormalities (raggedness) of the mucous membrane, especially in fungal infections.

Progress. Perforation of the gullet may occur, with the development of a fatal mediastinitis. If the patient survives the primary infection, narrowing (stenosis) of the gullet is common and causes renewed difficulty in swallowing, followed by vomiting.

Treatment. Remove any foreign bodies, relieve dehydration with a drip, and give vigorous antibiotic and antifungal therapy. The surgeon may decide to pass a tube through the gullet for feeding, or short circuit it with a gastrostomy until healing has occurred.

Esophageal burns

These are usually due to caustic soda or hydrochloric acid. They occur mainly in toddlers.

Clinical features. The material is available to the child, and he rushes in with his lips and mouth burned and painful. He salivates a lot, and cannot drink or swallow. The mucous membrane of the mouth looks swollen and gray.

Treatment. The mouth is so painful that the use of dilute antidotes (e.g., acid for alkali burns) is impossible. The child should be sent to hospital where an anesthetic is given and the mouth, pharynx, and esophagus looked at. Often enough it will be found that only the mouth and pharynx are burned, and not the esophagus. Burns of the esophagus can only be diagnosed confidently by looking (esophagoscopy).

Fluid is supplied by intravenous drip and the surgeon passes a plastic tube through the gullet to keep it open and allow feeding. Steroids are given for 7-10 days to try and prevent scarring. Antibiotics are given to prevent infection.

Follow-up. Scarring and narrowing may occur; dilatation of this stenosis is carried out by the passage of flexible plastic rods (bouginage).

Diaphragmatic hernia

This is an emergency of the newborn, which is due to a hole in the diaphragm allowing the gut to enter the chest. This pressure on the lungs may strangle the baby, or the gut itself may be obstructed.

Clinical features. The baby may be difficult to resuscitate at birth, and the belly looks flat and empty. More often perhaps the infant seems normal for a little while, and then becomes very breathless, with rib retraction and cyanosis. This is because the gut in the chest swells when swallowed air enters it after birth. When the baby is looked at, the abdomen again seems empty, and chest movement, although labored, is ineffective. The heart is difficult to hear and the cardiac impulse (apex beat) may be felt on the wrong side.

X-rays show gas-filled gut in the chest, with shifting of the heart shadow.

In some instances, respiratory difficulty is not so dramatic, and vomiting and failure to pass meconium herald intestinal obstruction.

Treatment. Since the lungs are being pressed upon, an endotracheal tube is passed, and positive pressure breathing begun in order to keep up respiratory function. *This must be continued until the child is on the operating table.* Treatment is surgical, the principle being to remove the gut from the chest and repair the defect in the diaphragm. Since the abdominal cavity is quite small, special plastic procedures may be needed to make it big enough to take the returned gut.

Hiatus hernia

In this condition, the area of the stomach joining the gullet (the cardia) slips above the diaphragm. The esophagus is also short. This means that stomach contents reflux up the gullet, and may ulcerate it.

Clinical features. Vomiting is constant, may be forceful, and often blood stained. Much food is lost, so that the baby is crying with hunger, fails to gain, then loses weight and is constipated. Adding solids to the diet may partly relieve the vomiting. After some time, the inflamed esophagus may scar, aggravating the vomiting and causing obvious difficulty in swallowing (dysphagia). The baby looks hungry, anxious, and may be pale from blood loss. Sometimes stomach contractions (gastric peristalsis) can be seen when the belly is inspected. The diagnosis can be confirmed by special x-rays which show the reflux from the stomach up the esophagus.

Special points. Vomiting is common in the first months of life. The main thing to distinguish from hiatus hernia is posseting, which is a harmless condition in which the baby returns some of its feed but is happy, gains weight, and looks well. Otherwise, pyloric stenosis needs thought. In this, vomiting doesn't occur for a few weeks after birth, is forceful (projectile) is not associated with hematemesis (blood in the vomit) and while showing gastric peristalsis, also has a lump (the pyloric tumour) which can be felt by the doctor.

Treatment. The feeds are thickened with cereal, and the baby is kept—day and night—in an upright position in a special chair. Most babies respond well, but if there is much bleeding or narrowing of the esophagus by scarring, then surgery is undertaken to replace and maintain the stomach in its proper position.

Esophageal varices

These are dilated (varicose) veins at the lower end of the gullet. They bulge when their pressure is increased as in cirrhosis of the liver. Because of this they bleed easily. This is the main symptom—hematemesis—which may be slight or so profuse as to cause serious blood loss and shock. The immediate treatment is sedation and blood transfusion. The other treatment is noted under cirrhosis of the liver. (p. 230).

DISORDERS OF THE STOMACH AND INTESTINE

Stomach (peptic) ulcer

This is not common in children. There are 3 types.

1. Acute peptic ulcer of neonates

Clinical features. The baby seems normal at birth and feeds well. He vomits some blood, and then the ulcer perforates to cause peritonitis and intestinal obstruction, with more vomiting, abdominal distension and constipation. Dehydration, with rapid pulse, low blood pressure, and low urine output follow. Fever may be present. X-rays show gas in the abdominal cavity, and dilated gut from the intestinal obstruction.

Treatment. The baby is given I.V. fluids to combat the shock and dehydration, and surgery carried out to close the perforated ulcer. Antibiotics are given for the peritonitis.

2. Stress stomach ulcer

This can occur at any age. It can follow an extensive burn (Curling's ulcer) severe central nervous system disease (Cushing-Rokitansky ulcer), or some extensive surgical operations, e.g., open heart procedures. Steroids and salicylates (aspirin) are possibly the common causes nowadays, especially if these drugs are given together.

Clinical features. The predisposing condition (e.g., the indication for steroid therapy, burn, etc.) is present. The patient may vomit blood, or the passage of blood into the gut be suspected because the stools are black or contain altered blood (melena). All too often the child has a large hemorrhage but shows only the symptoms of shock—pallor, sweating, breathlessness, with a rapid thready pulse and low blood pressure. Note that abdominal pain or discomfort are *not* present in this type of ulcer, unless perforation and peritonitis have occurred. If the ulcer has been due to steroids, pain is absent even in peritonitis.

Treatment. Blood transfusion, sometimes massive, is essential. If drugs have caused the ulcer, stop them. If bleeding continues, the ulcer may need to be repaired by the surgeon.

3. Chronic peptic ulcer

This is rare, occurring in school-age children.

Clinical features. The main feature is pain in the abdomen, often epigastric, and usually in the same place, but not particularly related to eating. It may occur through the night. Vomiting, sometimes of blood, can happen, but less commonly than in grown-ups. Pallor and anemia are not uncommon and weight loss may be present. The child often looks (and is), anxious and tense. Marked hematemesis is unusual, but melena is well known. Barium x-rays will show the ulcer crater.

Special features. Abdominal discomfort is common in children, and is mostly due to a desire to receive attention. This functional bellyache is very variable, mild, shifts its position a lot, and has no associated vomiting or anemia. The child is also well grown and has a good appetite. These features are usually enough to exclude peptic ulcer.

Treatment. Causes of nervous strain (e.g., school) should be investigated and antacids and antispasmodics given. Dietary measures are less important in children than adults, although items which definitely cause increased discomfort should be limited. Iron is given for anemia. Surgery is very seldom used in children except for extensive bleeding or perforation of the ulcer.

Pyloric stenosis

This is a narrowing of the stomach outlet due to thickening of the muscle. It is inborn and may occur in several family members. It affects both sexes, but mainly boys. The usual age of onset is the first month of life; it occurs earlier in prematures.

Clinical features. The history is important and characteristic. The baby vomits, often forcibly (projectile vomiting) but is hungry and ready to feed again afterwards. The mother then changes the feed, believing the previous one to be unsuitable and the infant is relieved for a short time. Then the vomiting comes back and is more frequent and severe. He is hungry, so he cries with discontent. He stops gaining weight, then loses weight, and becomes constipated. Vomiting, but never of blood, becomes more and more prominent and he may eventually become dehydrated and collapsed. In the usual situation, the baby has lost condition, looks hungry, and whines a lot. He is underweight, and if he is fed, he shortly vomits. At this stage gastric peristalsis may be seen.

These are waves of stomach contractions running from the left side of the belly towards the umbilicus—it looks like golf balls running under the skin. The enlarged muscle can be felt and is called a pyloric tumour.

Special features. Some confusion may occur with hiatus hernia, but this condition causes vomiting, often bloodstained, soon after birth, and while gastric peristalsis may be present, no pyloric tumour is present. Another condition, also occurring at birth, is *duodenal atresia*, but again the age of onset, and absence of a pyloric tumour are of help. Another dangerous condition in which vomiting is a prominent symptom, is the adrenogenital syndrome, in which in females the clitoris is enlarged (masculinization) and both gastric peristalsis and a pyloric tumour are absent.

Treatment. As the baby has lost fluid and salt, an intravenous saline drip is set up before surgery. The curative operation consists in splitting the enlarged muscle down to the mucosal surface of the pylorus (Rammstedt's procedure). The baby is fed glucose-saline within a few hours of operation, beginning with small volumes (e.g., 5 ml) and doubling this every hour for 4 feeds; if there is no vomiting, dilute formula is given to the infant's requirement, and full strength feeds restored after 24-36 hours. Persistent post-operative vomiting may be due to coincident unappreciated hiatus hernia. Medical treatment of pyloric stenosis, e.g., with antispasmodics, is not recommended.

DUODENAL OBSTRUCTIONS

These occur in the newborn, particularly in association with Down's syndrome. The commonest cause is failure of the duodenum to canalize (atresia). Less often a part of the pancreas may encircle and obstruct the duodenum (annular pancreas); a twist and external band (malrotation of the gut) is responsible on even fewer occasions.

Clinical features. The baby develops a high intestinal obstruction within a few hours of birth. Vomiting is early and severe, and dehydration rapidly develops, with rapid heart rate, falling blood pressure, and failure to pass meconium and urine. The baby loses weight dramatically. The upper abdomen (epigastrium) may look swollen, while the rest of the abdomen is sunken with dehydration. The diagnosis can be confirmed by x-rays which show a double bubble of air—the stomach and the distended part of the duodenum preceding the obstruction.

Treatment. The dehydration is relieved by I.V. saline and the duodenum joined to the jejunum, thus bypassing the obstruction. The drip is continued postoperatively and the stomach sucked out regularly. If the aspirate is small, the anastomosis is probably functioning well, and the passage of meconium confirms this. Indeed, small, frequent bowel actions are commonly found in the early postoperative phase.

Outlook. Duodenal atresia is a serious condition, as the anastomosis may not function adequately and intestinal obstruction may recur. The problems of the associated Down's syndrome should also be recalled.

INTESTINAL OBSTRUCTIONS

In the newborn

The commoner causes in this age group are congenital atresias of the jejunum or ileum, meconium ileus, malrotation of the gut, and congenital megacolon (Hirschsprung's disease). Rarely the gut is paralyzed by drugs given to the mother before the baby is born. Hydramnios is often a feature of the mother's pregnancy.

Clinical situation. Whatever the cause, the features are the same. The earliest reliable sign is distention of the abdomen, contractions of the gut can be seen, and constipation is usual, although meconium may previously have been passed. The baby develops copious bile-stained vomiting and loses so much fluid and electrolyte that dehydration is rapid. Thus, there is much weight loss, the baby looks pale and pinched, the skin loses its elasticity, the pulse is rapid and thready, the blood pressure falls, and the scanty urine secretion stops altogether.

Plain x-rays show distended loops of gut with fluid levels inside them. These levels shift as the baby's position is changed. Intestinal obstruction, if neglected, may cause perforation of the gut, with peritonitis and aggravation of the dehydration and shock by the toxins of infection.

These are general statements which are modified by the level of obstruction. Thus, in high (jejunal) obstruction, vomiting is early and severe, abdominal distension less, and often more obvious in the upper abdomen. In congenital megacolon, which is a low obstruction, general distension is an early sign, and vomiting is a later one.

Some specific disorders

Atresias (obliteration of the gut tube) and stenoses (narrowing of the gut) are the commonest causes of obstruction. They can occur anywhere in the small bowel, sometimes in several places. Often the exact type and level of the defect is established only at operation.

Meconium ileus

This is associated with mucoviscidosis, a disease in which the pancreas does not produce the enzyme (trypsin) which can digest protein. The fetal gut contents (meconium) then stay solid and plug the gut. A family history of mucoviscidosis may be present, otherwise the picture is that of any intestinal obstruction. The abdominal x-rays can help in that air bubbles in the solid meconium give a granular look to the gut loop. Sometimes the obstructed gut has perforated before birth. This causes a sterile peritonitis which heals by calcification. Thus, chalky masses can be seen on the x-ray.

Volvulus of the mid-gut

This is due to an abnormality of the mesentery, the structure which supports the gut, and which carries the supplying blood vessels. Thus the gut is not well anchored and the narrow mesentery is liable to twist upon itself. If this happens then a high (duodenojejunal) obstruction occurs, and the blood supply to the mid-gut (mainly ileum) is interrupted. The first condition gives rise to the situation already discussed under duodenal atresia, the second leads to small-gut obstruction. The coincidence of the two is such that the surgeon always looks for the other if he suspects or finds one.

Congenital megacolon (Hirschsprung's disease)

In this the nerve supply to the colon is interrupted. This means that the gut contents cannot be propelled onwards, so that obstruction results. In the newborn, the distension may deflate when a thermometer is placed in the rectum. This is because the lowest part of the colon is most commonly affected. The disease, however, may be severe enough to cause all of the features already described, or mild enough for trouble to be avoided until later childhood.

General treatment of neonatal obstruction

The infant must be resuscitated with intravenous fluid and electrolyte, a stomach tube is placed and any fluid aspirated from it is measured and made up in the calculation of the total fluid and electrolyte need. The baby is given antibiotics if gut rupture and peritonitis are suspected. Surgery is done when hydration, blood pressure and urinary output have been restored. The principles of surgery are (1) to establish continuity of the gut by suitable junctions (anastomosis) or, if this is impossible, to allow the gut contents to discharge externally, e.g., by colostomy; (2) to remove any gut which cannot survive; and (3) to make sure that the whole gut is inspected and passed as normal before the abdomen is closed. The last is important because multiple obstructions are often present. In the postoperative phase, intravenous feeding is maintained, and antibiotics given if infection is suspected. In meconium ileus the treatment for mucoviscidosis is begun.

Intestinal obstruction in the older child

Congenital defects are now a rare cause of obstruction, although occasional problems occur with megacolon, congenital bands, or volvulus. Important causes are intussusception, paralytic ileus with peritoneal infection (usually due to appendicitis) and obstruction due to neglected herniae.

Clinical features. Complaints of colicky abdominal pain are common in this age group, and loss of appetite (anorexia), vomiting, and constipation occur. Abdominal distension and visible peristalsis are features of established obstruction. Dehydration is less liable to occur because the patient resists vomiting better and comes earlier to medical attention. The x-ray signs are those already described.

Special points in diagnosis. The abdominal pain, vomiting, and varying degrees of dehydration may be confused with *medical* conditions having the same symptoms. The main thing to be considered is *gastro-enteritis* where vomiting and pain may precede diarrhea. Another important condition is *diabetic coma*, in which vomiting, abdominal pain, constipation, and gut distention are common, and in which x-rays may also show distended loops of gut. Routine urinalysis for sugar will prevent disastrous laparotomies in these patients.

Somewhat similar symptoms occur in anaphylactoid (Henoch-Schonlein) purpura, but these patients have urticaria, purpuric spots, and bruising—usually on the buttocks and legs.

Treatment. This consists in repairing fluid and electrolyte defects and relieving the obstruction by the surgical principles already outlined.

Intussusception

This occurs when one piece of gut slips into the lumen of another piece. The blood supply of the inner section (the intussusceptum) is cut off, so that obstruction occurs. The most common type is invagination of the small gut into the colon (enterocolic) (see figure 42). Mostly there is no obvious cause, occasionally infiltrations of the bowel wall (e.g., tumour, leukemia) or a Meckel's diverticulum may be the cause.

Clinical features. Most patients are between the ages 4 and 12 months and most are previously healthy boys. The child then develops severe abdominal pain, evidenced by screaming and drawing up the legs. At the same time he turns pale, sweats, may seem to faint, and often vomits. Seemingly exhausted the infant then appears better. Then the whole cycle recurs, vomiting becomes more frequent and profuse, and sooner or later the baby has a loose, bloody bowel movement—sometimes only of bloodstained mucus, sometimes of frank whole

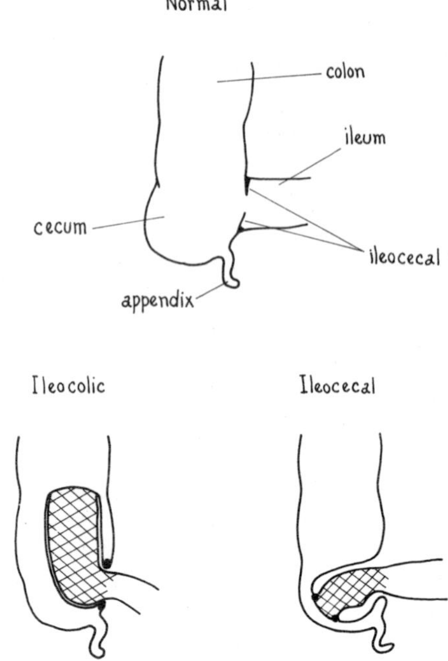

Fig. 42. Types of intussusception. • • ileo colic valve
intussusceptum

blood. This may recur, simulating diarrhea. If nothing is done, obvious intestinal obstruction sets in with profuse vomiting, abdomen distention, gut peristalsis, and dehydration. Shock may be profound because of the addition of blood loss to the fluid and electrolyte deficit.

The intussusception can usually be felt by the surgeon as a sausage-shaped mass which is concave towards the umbilicus and roughly in the line of the colon. The rectum contains bloody mucus and occasionally the tip of the intussuscepted gut.

Early the x-ray (barium enema) will reveal the intussusception. At a later stage the findings are only those of intestinal obstruction.

Special points in diagnosis. The main point of confusion is with gastroenteritis in which pain, abdominal distention, and diarrhea occur. The latter at first contains liquid feces, and blood appears later. No intussusception can be felt, and dehydration occurs earlier.

Sudden acute bleeding, as from a Meckel's diverticulum also causes the pallor and sweating already described but the appearances are permanent rather than episodic as in intussusception.

Treatment. Dehydration should be relieved, and blood transfusion given if necessary. In early cases the intussusception may be reduced by barium enema under x-ray control. Many surgeons, however, will open the abdomen, make sure the gut can survive, reduce the intussusception directly, and reestablish gut continuity if necessary.

INFLAMMATION OF THE INTESTINE

Appendicitis

This is the commonest surgical emergency of childhood, occurring at any age, but mostly between 3 and 10 years. In children, the inflammation is more rapid than in adults so that perforation occurs earlier, causing peritonitis rather than local abscess. The position of the inflamed appendix is variable, e.g., retrocecal, splenic, or pelvic, the latter being harder to diagnose with certainty.

Clinical features. These vary with age; the younger the patient the less specific the complaints.

1. *In the infant* (say to 18 months) the illness is obscure, with irritability, loss of appetite and vomiting. Diarrhea may occur, and dehydration is common and early. Fever is inconstant. The child resents being handled, and lies with the legs bent to relieve his discomfort. Careful examination of the abdomen will reveal tenderness, which is hard to localize. Rigidity of the abdomen is very variable. In some children the first real complaints are those of intestinal obstruction, due to perforation and secondary peritonitis.
2. *In the older child* the complaint is of colicky central abdominal pain which is followed by vomiting. The site of the pain shifts to the right lower abdomen and becomes constant. Fever is low grade, constipation is common, but urinary symptoms (frequency, painful micturition) unusual. The child tries to relieve his belly-ache by curling up and bending his legs. The characteristic sign is tenderness and muscular guarding (rigidity) in the lower right abdomen. Sometimes the child needs sedation before he can be properly examined. Rectal examination must be done, not only to find local tenderness, but to feel for a pelvic abscess. Signs often seen in adults (Rovsing's, psoas) are much less frequently found in children.

Differential diagnosis. The more important are the conditions in which surgery should be avoided, such as tonsillitis with vomiting and abdominal pain. The red, inflamed tonsils are diagnostic. Pneumonia (especially of the right lower lobe) may also cause abdominal pain and vomiting, but the respiratory rate is increased and there are appropriate clinical and x-ray signs. In urinary infections, symptoms such as frequency and the finding of pus in the urine (pyuria) are suggestive of the correct diagnosis.

Complications

Appendix abscess

In addition to the history of appendicitis, a lump may be felt in the right iliac fossa. More often the abscess is felt as a tender mass at rectal examination. Fever and leucocytosis are prominent and intestinal obstruction may develop at any stage of the illness.

Peritonitis

The history of appendicitis progresses to that of intestinal obstruction with vomiting, constipation, and abdominal distension. There is general rigidity of the abdominal muscles, fever, leucocytosis, and dehydration.

Treatment. Fluid deficits are replaced, and laparotomy carried out to remove the source of infection. Broad spectrum antibiotics are given if there is any suspicion of perforation, abscess, or peritonitis.

Gastroenteritis

This is an important pediatric infectious disease, being particularly prevalent where hygiene is poor, and where children are malnourished. The condition is dangerous in those under the age of 6 months, and carries a high death rate if it occurs in the newborn.

Cause. This is, for the most part, a viral invasion, otherwise infection by bacteria, e.g., salmonella, shigella, and pathogenic *E.coli* are responsible.

Clinical features. In most children, the main problem is diarrhea. This varies in severity from the passage of a few loose stools to the constant squirting of apparently clear fluid (which may be taken for urine). Mucus is commonly found in the stools, as is bile—giving them a greenish hue. Bloody diarrhea is more common with bacterial (e.g., *Shigella*) infection, and varies from slight staining to the passage of thick blood. Vomiting is less often found, and may occur only at the beginning of the illness. It is not common in the younger child. Abdominal cramping is a complaint only of older children.

The main danger of gastroenteritis is dehydration—which implies not only loss of fluid, but of sodium, potassium, chloride, and bicarbonate. Sometimes the process is so rapid that the child arrives moribund in the casualty department. More often the history is of diarrhea of increasing severity, together with failure to take food or fluid. A cold or other minor respiratory infection may coexist, and in the young child, there is often the story of drowsiness.

On examining the child the findings are quite variable. Many older children appear to have nothing much amiss. Otherwise the main signs are those of dehydration—loss of skin elasticity, dryness of the mouth, depression of eye balls (and of the fontanelle in the baby), a scaphoid abdomen, and measurable recent weight loss. In the severely affected child there is circulatory collapse with greyish pallor, cold hands and feet, and rapid weak pulse, and a fall in blood pressure. In these coincident acidosis due to loss of bicarbonate, may cause the breathing to be deep and sighing (Kussmaul breathing).

Special tests. The loss of water may give rise to hemoconcentration, i.e., the ratio of red cells to total blood fluid (the hematocrit) increases. Electrolyte (Na:K) values are often normal, even in severe dehydration. This is because the salt and water losses occur in parallel. If relatively more water than salt has been lost, then the serum sodium may rise (hypernatremia), if sodium loss exceeds relative water loss, then serum sodium values fall (hyponatremia). It should be noted that serum sodium values are no guide to the total loss of sodium suffered by the patient. Accumulation of acid hydrogen ions or of hydroxyl (alkaline) ions may also occur, and is diagnosed by measuring the pH of arterialized capillary (or arterial) blood.

Differential diagnosis. Other common causes of diarrhea include antibiotics, which change the range of bacteria normally present in the gut. Otherwise, dietary indiscretion (green apples) or food poisoning, may be responsible. In either case, the history will be helpful. In the young child with bloody diarrhea, think about intussusception, and in the infant with diarrhea, dehydration, and signs of intestinal obstruction, spare a thought for appendicitis. If the child develops repeated loose stools, malabsorption syndromes should be considered. These include celiac disease, intestinal enzyme deficiencies (e.g., alactasia) and occasionally mucoviscidosis.

Treatment:

Mild cases. In the older child (2 years or more) treatment is largely dietary. Ample fluids (containing electrolyte and dextrose) should be prescribed and the mother given a definite target, i.e., the normal daily fluid requirement + 10%. If the child is hungry, biscuits (soda and saltine crackers) may be given. Some ingenuity is occasionally necessary to ensure an adequate fluid intake. Soft drinks, with salt added, are often well taken. Care should be taken not to overprescribe salt in the younger child. As the diarrhea subsides, the child may return to his accustomed foods. A minor degree of fat malabsorption is common in the convalescent period from gastroenteritis, and fat restriction is commonly practised during the first week after the disappearance of diarrhea.

Moderate cases. The patient who, while having severe diarrhea is not dehydrated should be carefully observed. Electrolyte-containing fluids should be pushed by mouth and if necessary given by gavage. Again careful measurement of intake is necessary. Weighing the child will help decide whether the oral intake is adequate or not.

Severe cases. If dehydration of any degree is present in a child of six months or less, intravenous therapy is imperative. The principles are outlined elsewhere. In both mild and severe cases, the child, while not in water or electrolyte imbalance, may continue to have diarrhea. In this situation, 24 hours of maintenance intravenous fluid may be useful as a gut-resting regime to clear up the diarrhea.

As in the mild cases, fat restriction may be helpful in early convalescence. It is, however, not to be used for any length of time, in the bottle-fed infant.

Symptomatic treatment. The use of kaolin or other inert substances, such as pectin or carob flour, is seldom necessary and should never obscure the fundamental treatment of gastroenteritis, which is *salt and water*.

Antibiotics. These have some value in treating the carrier of pathogens and in the septicemia which may coexist. Again, their use must not replace the patient's need for fluid and electrolyte. Diarrhea is a common side effect of antibiotics, such as tetracyclines and chloramphenicol. If it is felt that antibiotics must be used, therapy should be delayed until a definite intestinal pathogen has been isolated, and its antibiotic sensitivity determined. The uselessness of treating a viral gastroenteritis is obvious.

Carrier states, usually of salmonella, shigella, and atypical pathogenic *E.coli* usually clear spontaneously; if they do not, then treatment with the microbiologically indicated antibiotic is in order. Such treatment should not however exceed a few weeks in duration, as there is some evidence that prolonged antibiotic therapy may in fact increase the duration of the carrier state.

In the treatment of the acute or carrier state with antibiotics, the danger of fungal overgrowth should be recalled. This usually occurs in younger children who have already a 'candida' infestation, so concomitant antifungal treatment may be needed.

Finally, remember the basic treatment of infantile gastroenteritis is with salt and water; all other treatments are of marginal importance.

Prognosis. In general this is a function of age, being worst in the newborn. It also depends upon the previous nutritional status of the patient—malnutrition worsens the prognosis. Specifically the outlook is related to the rapidity and skill with which intravenous therapy can be instituted and maintained.

Ulcerative colitis

The cause of this rare condition is not yet known, but an autoimmune or allergic basis has been considered.

Clinical features. The usual complaints are of a slowly increasing diarrhea, occurring especially at night. Blood and mucus are present in the stools. Fever, loss of weight, and anemia are common. In a minority of children the condition is very acute, resembling severe gastroenteritis, with early and severe dehydration. The identity of the disease may be confirmed by special x-rays which reveal dilatation and ulceration of the colon, together with lack of a normal outline. The rectum and lower colon may be inspected directly (proctoscopy) to show a velvety looking, swollen, bleeding mucosa which has shallow ulcers.

Complications. Arthritis and skin rashes (erythema nodosum) occur rarely. Liver function disorder is common, and if the patient survives for a long time, cancer of the colon is frequent.

Treatment. The child with the fulminant disorder is treated as if he had a severe gastroenteritis. Blood transfusion is also necessary. Steroid enemata, sometimes also with steroids by mouth, are also given, but must be covered by a broad-spectrum antibiotic for fear of a disseminated infection. If this has no effect, then short-circuiting the colon by an ileostomy may be needed.

The chronic case. A high calorie, low residue diet is given, anemia is corrected, and the child and family given much moral support. Steroid enemata are tried and if unsuccessful should be followed by a full course of steroids given by mouth. This regime should continue for a long time before any surgical treatment (ileostomy) is considered.

SOME DEFECTS OF STRUCTURE

Meckel's diverticulum

This is the remains of the omphalomesenteric duct which in fetal life connects the ileum to the placental yolk sac through the umbilical cord. The duct shrinks after birth, but occasionally persists as a tube, or blind-ended segment.

Clinical features. The most important is sudden bleeding, which is due to ulceration of acid producing (gastric) mucosa in the diverticulum. The child, previously well, becomes pale, shocked, and passes bloody stools; lesser degrees of bleeding cause only the latter symptom. Very occasionally the ulcer may perforate to cause peritonitis. In infancy when the whole duct persists, feces may appear at the umbilicus, but this type of fistula is very rare.

Treatment. If bleeding has occurred, the patient is transfused. The diverticulum is surgically removed after resuscitation.

Congenital aganglionic megacolon (Hirschsprung's disease)

This is due to a congenital absence of the parasympathetic nerve supply to a portion of the gut, usually the colon. Thus peristalsis is ineffective, and the gut contents accumulate just before the site of the abnormality.

Clinical features. In the *newborn* the commonest pattern is of intestinal obstruction, whose features have already been described, i.e., failure to pass stools, abdominal distention, vomiting, and dehydration. It is not unusual for the obstruction temporarily to subside, sometimes spontaneously, more often following rectal examination.

In the *older child*, the main feature is of obstinate constipation, usually associated with abdominal distention. "Spurious" diarrhea is common. In this the liquid iliac contents ooze past the loaded colon into the normal rectum. Growth failure is the rule, and acute intestinal obstruction may supervene at any time. The abdomen may become very large due to the remarkable collection of feces. Poor general health, loss of appetite and energy, and anemia are very common. Rarely the ureter may also be dilated (hydroureter) and predispose to urinary infection.

Specific diagnosis. This is usually made by x-ray study of the colon, which has been previously cleared by saline enemata. The narrowed segment is outlined by the barium, together with the dilated area above it. A biopsy of the rectum (or lower colon) when suitably prepared for microscopy will often reveal the abnormality of the nerve cell distribution.

Differential diagnosis. In infancy this is from other causes of intestinal obstruction. In the older child, one must exclude simple, severe, constipation, which is sometimes called *psychogenic megacolon*. In this condition, growth and general health is good, and the abdomen is seldom greatly distended although masses of feces can be felt. The perianal area is soiled with feces, which also pack the rectum to the sphincter.

Treatment. If obstruction has occurred, it is relieved by colostomy. Later the abnormal gut is removed, and continuity restored by joining the rectum to the normal colon.

ANOMALIES OF THE ANUS AND RECTUM

There is a large variety of these, so only the more important will be discussed.

Rectal atresia

In this the rectum stops short of the anus, which is usually absent, although the sphincter ani may still be there. Abnormal openings (fistulae) may occur into the vagina, bladder, or in boys, into the posterior urethra. Feces are passed through these fistulae.

Clinical features. Usually the anal abnormality is seen at birth; occasionally the passage of meconium from the vagina or bladder may be the first clue, as may be the onset of intestinal obstruction. The portion of the blind-ended rectum may be estimated by x-raying the upside down infant while marking the anal area with a coin.

Imperforate anus

This is usually associated with rectal atresia; in a few only a thin membrane prevents the passage of meconium. The anus and its sphincter are normal in this instance. The clinical features are essentially as described for rectal atresia.

Prolapse of the rectum

In this the rectum, in part or whole, is extruded through the anus. In some children, usually with simple constipation, only the mucous membrane of the rectum comes out. If the whole rectum protrudes, the association may be with meningomyelocele, a severe abnormality of the bowel and bladder, or malnutrition.

Clinical features. The appearance is characteristic and painless to the patient although distressing to the parents. The rectum usually goes back in by itself.

Treatment. Gently press the rectum with a saline-soaked swab, but soothe the child first—crying prevents reduction. Strap the buttocks together to keep the rectum in, and ensure that constipation is treated.

External hernias

Umbilical hernia

This is a common problem which probably gives few symptoms, although many are ascribed to it. The usual complaint is of a bulge at the belly button when the infant cries or strains. Very large umbilical herniae are unusual, and incarceration (inability to push the mass back) or strangulation, are rare. These hernias are often found in cretinism, mongolism, and Hunter-Hurler syndrome (mucopolysaccharidosis). Examination reveals a lump at the umbilicus which can be pushed back into the abdomen through a defect easily felt by the fingertip.

In older children, an umbilical hernia may appear during the ascites (accumulation of fluid in the peritoneum) of nephrotic syndrome, or cirrhosis. It also occurs in severely malnourished children. The features are as already described, plus those of the underlying disease.

Differential diagnosis. This is entirely from the benign condition of cutis navel in which the skin of the abdomen continues further along the cord than is usual. The tag will apparently 'swell' when baby cries, but no muscle defect can be felt under it.

Treatment. In most cases reassure the parents and do nothing for at least 6 months. The hernia will usually heal spontaneously during this period. Surgical repair in early life is done only for large hernias, and the smaller ones which persist for longer than 12 months. "Bandage and penny" treatments are quite useless; the apparent success is in the coincidence with spontaneous cure.

Inguinal hernia

This is usually of the indirect type, i.e., the gut passes through the structures normally traversed by the testes, or in the female the canal of Nuck.

Clinical features. The usual complaint is of a painless 'lump in the groin'. If incarceration—inability to reduce the content into the peritoneal cavity— occurs, crying and apparent discomfort may be alleged by the parents. Strangulation (which is pressure sufficient not only to prevent reduction, but to cut off the gut circulation) leads to intestinal obstruction.

The hernia is usually visible only when the infant cries or strains. Large hernias show as an obvious bulge and clearly contain gut. In young infants, the enlarged inguinal ring can be felt when a finger is pushed up from the scrotum. This defect can enlarge, giving rise to bigger hernias, which can pass down into the scrotum.

Treatment. Surgery should be carried out forthwith. The principle is to repair the muscular defect at the inguinal ring. Trusses and other external appliances should be avoided.

FOREIGN BODIES IN THE ALIMENTARY TRACT

These are common in children but most are passed without trouble. A foreign body may, however, lodge at any level, especially if it is pointed or longitudinal. Most pass readily into the stomach and there are few symptoms except when the child becomes frightened or the object is missed.

Esophageal foreign bodies

If these stick, there is difficulty in swallowing, choking and retrosternal discomfort. Perforation of the esophagus may lead to mediastinitis.

Gastric foreign bodies

These seldom give rise to trouble except for the rare trichobezoar or hair ball, which complicates the neurosis of trichotillomania (compulsive pulling and eating of the hair). The complaint is of vomiting and loss of weight. The mass is sometimes visible on plain or contrast x-ray.

Intestinal foreign bodies

If smooth and rigid, these usually pass without trouble. Fibrous foreign bodies, e.g., orange pith, may cause intestinal obstruction.

General treatment of foreign bodies

An x-ray should always be done to locate and determine the nature of the swallowed object. All stools should be collected and examined to see if it passes. If a sharp object (safety pin, bobby pin, glass, etc.) stays in the same place for more than 3-4 days, surgical removal should be contemplated. Objects impacted in the esophagus should be removed forthwith.

DISORDERS DUE TO ABNORMALITIES OF FUNCTION

Abnormalities of bowel function are common in children. They run the whole gamut of severity, from minor discomfort to life-threatening disease.

Constipation

This is a common problem of function, which, as already noted, may be a symptom of disease, as in aganglionic megacolon; most often, however, the condition is harmless to the child although it may cause much worry to the parents and, through them, anxiety in the patient.

Definition. Constipation is the passage of hard stools, usually infrequently. If the bowel movements are of normal consistency, then constipation does not exist, whatever the interval between them. So a breast-fed baby who has a soft stool every 2-3 days is NOT constipated, he is normal for his age and diet.

Causes of constipation. In infancy, infrequent firm stools are often due to insufficient fluid in the diet, whether or not he is receiving enough calories. Otherwise, the commonest cause of transient constipation is an acute feverish illness, such as tonsillitis. This may be accompanied by vomiting, and refusal to eat, which results in a hard stool being passed with difficulty. The delicate mucous membrane of the anus may be thus overstretched, causing an acute 'split' which is called a fissure in ano.

Constipation may be a minor complaint in major diseases such as dehydration, intestinal obstruction or metabolic disorders such as cretinism (thyroid deficiency). In these, as in mental retardation and severe cerebral palsy, the constipation is overshadowed by the other features of the disorder.

Simple chronic constipation (acquired megacolon)

This is a common childhood problem. The child is often brought to the physician after the parents have tried domestic remedies for some time. The history may then be found to go back to the early months of life. A febrile episode, with sudden constipation and a history of blood on the stool shortly thereafter is often found. This story implies a fissure in ano which leads to pain and refusal to defecate. A vicious circle is set up of purges, suppositories, enemata, and parental preoccupation with the child's stools.

In many cases the history is only of constantly increasing constipation and parental concern. Often there is encopresis—soiling with spurious diarrhea. Scybala (hard fecal masses) are usually felt in the abdomen, the perianal area is soiled, and the rectum and anus packed with hard feces. It is noteworthy that these children, unlike sufferers from Hirschsprung's disease, have a normal growth pattern. A plain x-ray of the abdomen will reveal remarkable dilatation of the colon by the contained fecal masses. Active or healing anal fissures are commonly visible.

There is little doubt that the parent/child relationship is strained in this situation. Charges of wilful and traumatic 'bowel training' by such parents are probably exaggerated, although the common parental preoccupation with their children's bowel activities may lessen the child's confidence if he is unable to produce. Overuse of laxatives is an unusual cause of constipation in children, and psychological causes are perhaps too frequently adduced as a cause of constipation, although these certainly occur in children who live in an unusual environment, e.g., school, hospital, relatives, remand home, or where the toilet facilities are unknown or unattractive. In a proportion of these children the acute constipation period is followed by a fissure in ano which causes the process to continue. In severe primary psychic problems, e.g., autism, brain damage, anorexia nervosa, the constipation is a minor part of the parental complaints.

Treatment. The parents must first be reassured. If fecal retention is marked, the child should be admitted to hospital and, after suitable explanation, given a saline enema. These should continue until the colon is empty. Suppositories are useless if the rectum is packed. If a fissure is present it should be treated by the frequent (x5 daily) and generous application of a local anesthetic ointment. The toilet facilities available to the child at home and at school should be inspected for privacy and suitability. Normal bowel function is obtained after rectal washout by retraining the child. The parents are told to be encouraging but not obsessive. The child too should be told that his stools are not a matter of life or death, but a normal function which will readily return. A gentle purgative, e.g., Senokot granules, is given for a week or two, in a dose sufficient to give a soft stool. This is especially important where a fissure is present. Care and observation should go on for at least 3 months. The criterion of success is a normal family attitude, and a soft, although not necessarily frequent, stool. In some instances the normal bowel frequency in these children settles down to once every 2-3 days.

MALABSORPTION

This is the term applied when fat, protein, carbohydrate, vitamins and minerals are not properly processed by the gut for use in the body. Several components in the diet may be affected at once, but fat malabsorption is important because this substance contains twice as many calories as protein or carbohydrate. Thus energy sources are more quickly impaired if fat is not taken in.

The causes of malabsorption follow the physiology of absorption in the following ways.

1. The absorbing surface may be too small. This occurs after massive surgical gut removal (e.g., in volvulus of infancy), in intestinal short-circuit, destruction of the mucosal surface by disease process (e.g., celiac disease, ulcerative colitis), or when the mucosa is covered with small parasites (e.g., *Giardia lamblia*). In such instances all dietary components, including the fat soluble vitamins, are poorly dealt with.

2. There is insufficient time for absorption. This must occur in the short gut situation above, but is more common in diseases which cause purging, e.g., gastroenteritis. This shortened 'transit time' is common in other malabsorptive situations, since excess of unabsorbed dietary components may act as gut irritants.

3. Insufficient bile. Bile is not a digestive agent in the sense that it chemically changes food. Its detergent properties are, however, necessary for the proper mechanical handling of fat, and in the fat splitting action of lipase. Blockage of the bile duct, or failure of bile production will then compromise fat absorption.

4. *Absence of enzymes which digest food.* This is the most common cause of malabsorption. Digestive enzymes are supplied by the pancreas and by the small gut itself. Thus, in mucoviscidosis (pancreatic fibrosis) the proteolytic enzyme trypsin is absent, as is pancreatic lipase. Some difficulty will then occur in food handling.

The intestine also produces enzymes which break down the common sugars which enter it. These substances are lactose (enzyme lactase), maltose (isomaltase), sucrose (sucrase). The enzymes may be deficient because they have never been there, or because disease has destroyed the cells which produce the enzymes. Infection such as gastroenteritis, is the common cause of the last situation, and the deficiency may then last only as long as the acute disease.

5. *Interference with gut transport mechanisms.* This is uncommon, occurring more often in conditions causing gut hurry. Thus, glucose and galactose, which are monosaccharides not requiring digestion, may not enter the body normally in mucoviscidosis. Rarely the energy-giving mechanisms for carrying them from the gut to the blood are absent.

It will be recalled that fat is eventually passed from the gut wall into the lymphatics (lacteals) and hence to the blood by way of the cisterna chyli. Diseases such as tumours or leukemia, which infiltrate the lymphatics or lymph glands, will prevent the adequate absorption of fat, causing back-up and loss in the intestinal cavity.

6. *Secretion into the gut cavity.* This is grouped under the malabsorption disease although, strictly speaking, absorption is normal but dietary components are lost into the gut. The commonest causes are ulcerative colitis, and congenital defects of the lymph channels (lymphangiectasis). These cause a leak of protein into the gut, with appropriate calorie loss. The leak may cause diarrhea, in turn impairing the handling of other dietary components.

Tests of absorptive function

Several methods are used; one is to measure the amount of dietary material going in, and the amount coming out in the feces. This is most often done for fat, and is called a balance study, i.e., one can calculate the amount of fat absorbed. The collections are made over at least 3 days (duplicate food and feces), the normal fat absorption is 85-90%. A cruder method is to label fat with iodine. Thus iodized fat is given by mouth. In the process of digestion/absorption the iodine is split off and comes out in the urine. The urinary iodine level, which is easy to measure, is then a rough test of fat absorption.

Another test of gut absorbing power is the xylose tolerance. Xylose is a substance which is not used by the human body, but which is dealt with by the gut as if it were a foodstuff. A dose is given by mouth and the xylose blood levels measured afterwards. If absorption is normal, then the blood xylose levels rise to a definite peak. Another check is to find the percentage of xylose which comes out in the urine in the 6 hours after it is administered.

In demonstrating gut enzyme deficiencies, a common test is to give the food substance by mouth, then measure its own (or its derivatives) level in the blood. Thus, if lactase deficiency is suspected a dose of lactose will fail to raise the level of its derivative (in this case glucose) in the blood. The same would apply in tests for maltose and sucrose malabsorption. Most tests of absorptive power are approximate. They are not used if the child has active gastroenteritis.

In the diseases where food substances are secreted into the gut, then that substance is labelled and injected into the blood. It is then sought in the feces. Thus albumin can be radioactively tagged, injected into the blood, and the stools examined for radioactivity. A positive test implies a protein-losing state.

Many malabsorptive diseases can be investigated by getting a sample of the gut wall. This is done by passing a tube with a cutter on its end. The sample of mucosa can be tested for the presence of an enzyme (e.g., lactase) within it, or the typical changes of these diseases sought for in its microscopic appearance.

General clinical features of malabsorption

The failure to absorb calories means that the child fails to gain weight, and then loses it. The gut contains an excess of the unabsorbed food, or an abnormal product of digestion, and this causes diarrhea. The latter may itself convert malabsorption of a single component to a general failure of absorption. In some instances the diarrhea is severe enough to cause severe salt and water loss, but this is not very common. The stools are usually foul smelling, and, in fat malabsorption, are bulky. The malabsorbed food products are irritating and thus a sore bottom is characteristic. The history is often very helpful; if the disease begins in early infancy one might suspect difficulty with lactose—which is the main sugar found in milk. If the condition is due to wheat (as in celiac disease) the symptoms are delayed until wheat products are given. If the disease is due to inability to handle one single item, the diarrhea will disappear if that food is excluded from the diet.

SOME SPECIFIC DISORDERS

Disaccharide malabsorption

This commonly involves lactose, sucrose, or maltose. The condition dates back to the introduction of these substances into the diet. Thus, in lactose intolerance, the onset is at birth or soon afterwards. The baby develops diarrhea, often with sour smelling stools, and excoriation of the anus. The abdomen may be distended with gas; weight is not gained, and then is lost. The condition improves if the suspected substance is excluded from the diet, and the appropriate tolerance test is positive. It should be noted that abnormal lactose tolerance tests may coexist with good health in some racial groups, e.g., Aborigine, Chinese, Africans. The treatment is to exclude the mishandled foodstuff from the diet and make up the food value from some other source, e.g., substitute glucose for lactose in lactose malabsorption.

Monosaccharide malabsorption

This is rare, and involves mainly glucose or galactose (the latter comes from lactose). The symptoms are similar to those of disaccharide malabsorption, but begin at the first feed. Wasting is early and severe, and dehydration not uncommon. Diarrhea ceases as soon as intravenous feeding is begun. The urine may contain the sugar which cannot be dealt with.

Treatment. Fructose is used to replace the sugar which cannot be used.

The Celiac syndrome

This is caused by an abnormal reaction of the gut to wheat protein (gluten) so it is also called gluten-induced enteropathy. The absorptive gut surface (the villi) waste away, and a general malabsorption ensues.

Clinical features. These usually begin in the second 6 months of life or whenever wheat products are given to the baby. The complaint is of diarrhea, and the first episode may be mistaken for gastroenteritis. Alternation of diarrhea and constipation may follow. In a short time the child loses condition, falls below his expected height and weight, lacks appetite, and becomes fractious. The abdomen may be distended and in most cases, the foul greasy bulky stools are noted by the parents. Rarely may the loss of secondary minerals and vitamins lead to rickets, scurvy, or certain types of anemia.

Diagnosis. It is necessary to exclude mucoviscidosis in which chest complaints are common, and where pancreatic trypsin is absent. In celiac syndrome the stool and duodenal secretions contain trypsin and this test is always done. Fat malabsorption is found by balance study, and general malabsorption by xylose tolerance. The gut biopsy shows wasting of the villi.

Treatment. This is to give a gluten-free diet, usually for life, and certainly for 5-10 years. The symptoms disappear, growth goes towards normal, and the abnormal findings disappear in the gut biopsy. The food pattern is planned by a dietician. The mother must be warned not to give new foods until she is sure that wheat is absent from them.

Mucoviscidosis (pancreatic fibrosis)

This condition is discussed in full elsewhere. The main problems are intestinal obstruction in newborn (meconium ileus), or severe respiratory disease, rather than malabsorption, although the latter is one mode of presentation.

Clinical features. Apart from the respiratory problems, the features resemble those of the celiac syndrome. A notable difference is, however, that diarrhea and growth failure often occur in the first few months of life. The diagnosis is made by failure to find trypsin in the stool or duodenum, and by an excess of sodium and chloride in the sweat (a positive sweat test).

Treatment. The malabsorption can be partly compensated by giving pancreatic extract in large quantities. The child is also given a more readily absorbed form of fat—a mixture of medium and short-chain fatty acids. This food is not very palatable, and must be started early in life if the child is to acquire a taste for it. The treatment otherwise is of the respiratory disorder.

TUMOURS OF THE ALIMENTARY TRACT

These are rare in childhood, the commonest being benign polyps of the lower gut and rectum.

Clinical features. Juvenile polyp is an adenomatous hemangioma (simple blood vessel tumour) which causes bleeding from the rectum. This may be obvious and stain the stools with bright blood, or it may be covert, giving rise to anemia. Occasionally the polyp prolapses through the anus when profuse bleeding may occur. The polyp can be readily seen at proctoscopy.

Treatment. The polyp should be excised.

Multiple polyposis

This is familial and gives rise to symptoms of diarrhea and bleeding at the time of adolescence. The tumours are finger-like masses which are seen in huge numbers on the rectum and colon. Neoplastic change is inevitable, and is the main reason for removal of the affected gut.

Peutz-Jeghers syndrome

This is another familial polypoid condition of the small gut. The skin, lips, and mouth display brownish spots. Symptoms are due to bleeding from the gut, or the onset of intussusception.

Carcinoids

These are tumours of the argentaffin cells. Most commonly they are asymptomatic, being found at appendicectomy.

The *malignant carcinoid syndrome* is caused by the production of vasoactive polypeptides (serotonin, bradykinin) in some of these tumours. Episodic facial flushing, asthma, and diarrhea occur as a result, as may heart failure. Large amounts of 5-hydroxyindoleacetic acid (a serotonin metabolite) are found in the urine.

Treatment. The symptoms may be partly relieved by anti-serotonin drugs, but cure lies in the surgical removal of the tumours.

Lymphosarcoma

This may present with intestinal obstruction, or occasionally with swelling of the abdomen due to a bloody peritoneal effusion. Malabsorption may coexist. In occasional instances the patient may present with a superior vena caval syndrome (swelling of the face and upper body) due to obstruction in the chest. Metastasis to the liver is early and usually obvious at laparotomy, which is the usual mode of diagnosis. Surgical relief of obstruction, and cytotoxic agents are the usual mode of treatment.

DISORDERS OF THE PANCREAS

Physiology

The pancreas is controlled by the sympathetic and parasympathetic nerves, and also responds to the hormone 'secretin' (upper intestinal tract origin), and pancreozymin (from duodenal mucosa). The exocrine products are trypsin and chymotrypsin, which split proteins into polypeptides, and the fat-splitting enzyme, lipase. Amylase, which splits starch to maltose, and small amounts of carboxypeptidase, which splits polypeptides to aminoacids, are also produced. The principal endocrine (secreted into blood) product is insulin.

Tests of pancreatic function

Direct tests, involve duodenal intubation, aspiration of its contents, and estimation of enzyme activity. In practice, only trypsin is measured. The ability to digest the gelatine coat on an x-ray film is a screening test; more quantitative studies are made by diluting the juice and observing its digestive effect upon tubes of gelatine. Such tests are, however, unreliable in the first 3 months of life.

Indirect tests of pancreatic function relate to stool trypsin estimations on photographic plate gelatine. These tests may be vitiated by the presence of trypsin from intestinal bacteria, or by the age of the child, since stool trypsin is normally low or absent after the 3rd or 4th birthday. Other indirect tests are those of fat malabsorption, viz., fat balance, lipiodol absorption. These are described in full elsewhere. The sweat test is characteristically abnormal in mucoviscidosis.

Disease processes

The commonest condition is mucoviscidosis (pancreatic fibrosis) which is described in detail below. Other congenital anomalies include *generalized hypoplasia*, which is rare, and gives rise to a general malabsorptive syndrome. It is principally to be differentiated from mucoviscidosis by the absence of respiratory disorder and a normal sweat test.

Annular pancreas

This is a cause of duodenal obstruction early in life, and is described elsewhere. Ectopic pancreatic tissue, usually located in the duodenum, may be a cause of intussusception. Multiple congenital cysts are asymptomatic, but may be discovered on routine examination. They may complicate cystic disease of other organs, e.g., the kidney.

Acute pancreatitis

This complicates mumps in the older child. It is, however, not very common.

Clinical features. These occur about 5 days after the mumps begin, with severe abdominal pain, nausea, vomiting, fever, and sometimes diarrhea. Investigations may reveal polymorph leucocytosis, hyperglycemia, and raised serum amylase level. Hemorrhagic pancreatitis is similar to the above, but often more severe, and associated with early dehydration. Frequently it is diagnosed only at laparotomy.

Differential diagnosis. This is principally from other abdominal catastrophes, especially intestinal obstruction.

Cystic fibrosis of the pancreas (mucoviscidosis, pancreatic fibrosis)

This disease is transmitted as a recessive. It is an inborn error of metabolism affecting the exocrine glands. Thus, in the respiratory tract, the mucus is abnormally tenacious, predisposing to airway obstruction and infection. The end results include obstructive emphysema, bronchiectasis, and pulmonary fibrosis.

The viscid pancreatic secretions cause obstruction of the duct system, with failure of forward flow, and fibrosis of the gland. The liver is the seat of bile duct obstruction and, in some cases, of biliary cirrhosis. The sweat glands are involved, and the secretions are abnormally high in volume, sodium, and potassium.

Clinical features. The condition may present in the neonate as meconium ileus—one cause of neonatal intestinal obstruction. Otherwise, the majority of patients show evidence of pulmonary or gastrointestinal disease during the first year. Both alimentary and respiratory systems are affected simultaneously. The initial respiratory symptom is a nonproductive cough. In early life this may be paroxysmal and simulate pertussis. Secondary infection is usual and the child may present with a history of several bouts of bronchitis; a considerable degree of bronchospasm is common in these bouts, so that a diagnosis of asthma may sometimes be entertained. In the majority of cases, staphylococcal infection occurs at some time or another, giving rise to a severe pneumonitis with marked toxemia. Empyema, pneumothorax, and the other complications of staphylococcal pneumonia occur. In a few cases, the child, previously well, suddenly develops a fatal pneumonia, with pancreatic fibrosis being demonstrated at autopsy. Other children may first see the E.N.T. specialist suffering from nasal polyps.

The absence or insufficiency of pancreatic trypsin, amylase, and lipase causes a malabsorption syndrome which usually coexists with the respiratory problems. Thus, the child fails to gain or grow properly, and may have bulky, foul-smelling and fat-laden stools. Malnutrition may ultimately be very severe. The malabsorption may be complicated by anemia, usually of the iron deficiency type. Rickets is seldom found and other vitamin deficiences, e.g., vitamin K, are rare. Rectal prolapse is not, however, uncommon.

As the disease progresses, there is increasing evidence that the child is becoming a respiratory cripple. Clubbing and cyanosis appear, the blood count rises, poor chest expansion is aggravated, and evidence of heart enlargement occurs. Cirrhosis, initially expressed as enlargement of the liver, is common, and this may progress to portal obstruction (see below). Respiratory infection usually ends the story, although death in congestive cardiac failure, or from the effects of liver cirrhosis, may occur in older patients. In a few sufferers, the excessive loss of electrolyte in the sweat leads to death during hot weather from low salt syndrome.

Diagnosis. Apart from meconium ileus, the diagnosis is confirmed by demonstration of an abnormally high sweat electrolyte level (sweat test) and by examination of the duodenal contents for trypsin.

The sweat test. This is reliable after the third month of life. Adequate quantities of sweat are collected after stimulation by pilocarpine iontophoresis. Analysis of the sweat shows increase in the chloride, sodium, and potassium levels to above 50mEq/1 for sodium and chloride, and above 10 mEq/1 for potassium. The test is positive in over 90% of patients with the disease.

Measurement of tryptic activity. This is done as already described.

Other laboratory investigations. Tests of intestinal malabsorption, such as the fat balance, xylose tolerance, chylomicra blood counts, and tests of vitamin A and iodized-oil absorption are commonly abnormal. Blood examination often shows hypochromic anemia. Leucocytosis during acute chest infections is usual. Hypoproteinemia is not unusual. In advanced cases, arterial oxygen saturation is reduced and pCO_2 increased. Lung function tests at this time confirm reduced vital capacity, evidence of poor alveolar ventilation, and increased airway resistance.

X-ray changes. Young infants may show no changes in the chest x-ray. Episodes of chest infection, such as bronchopneumonia, cause the x-ray changes usual in this condition. At first these clear but the films begin to show permanent change. Initially these are irregularity of aeration with collapse and emphysema. As the disease progresses, patches of fibrosis appear and segmental collapse and prominent peribronchial shadows are common. The hilar nodes are also enlarged. If staphylococcal pneumonia occurs, the characteristic x-ray signs of this condition are seen. The advanced case shows heart enlargement, usually of the right ventricle, with prominence of the main pulmonary artery.

Differential diagnosis. In the newborn this is from other causes of intestinal obstruction, and is discussed elsewhere. Otherwise, the diagnosis is from other causes of failure to thrive, of malabsorption syndromes, and respiratory infection. Simple deficiency of calories and evidence of other systemic disease (cardiac, renal) occasionally cause difficulty. Of the malabsorption syndromes, gluten-induced enteropathy (celiac disease) perhaps gives rise to most difficulty. In this disease, respiratory symptoms are usually absent, and the poor appetite contrasts with the good food intake of the patient with fibrocystic disease. Again, the glucose and xylose absorption tests, commonly abnormal in celiac disease, are often normal in mucoviscidosis. Finally, in the celiac syndrome, intestinal biopsy has characteristic findings on microscopy.

In relation to the respiratory problems, pertussis may present some difficulty. The absence of prophylactic inoculation, the presence of an epidemic, and lymphocytosis are here useful guides. More difficult is the child who has several attacks of bronchitis or bronchopneumonia. In these children, it is necessary to do the sweat test in order to exclude fibrocystic disease. The patient with congenital heart disease may suffer from failure to thrive and frequent respiratory infections, but only in rare cases are the cardiac signs obscure. Patients who present with asthma early in life should be considered carefully for possible evidence of fibrocystic disease. The chronic respiratory problems which are common in cerebral palsy, Werdnig-Hoffman disease, dysautonomia, and agammaglobulinemia, are usually so obviously superimposed on the primary condition that little difficulty arises.

Treatment. The situation should be thoroughly explained to the parents with emphasis on the need for frequent evaluation of the patient. The pediatrician will require to devote much time to family support, especially in the direction of exorcising guilt feelings. The necessity for preventive treatment should be carefully explained, and an attitude of realistic optimism engendered. It should be emphasized that the disease can only be controlled, not cured.

The treatment of the patient divides itself into 3 aspects: The treatment of chest infections, the prevention of chest infections, and the treatment of intestinal malabsorption. The last is handled by the prescription of a diet which is high in calories and protein, and relatively low in fat. Pancreatin is given in large doses; for an infant this is ½ teaspoonful of pancreatin powder (viokase) with each meal. The dose for older children is increased pro rata. Pancreatin preparations are frequently not well taken, and much ingenuity may be necessary to ensure an adequate intake. The success of the pancreatin therapy may be gauged by the disappearance of symptoms of fat malabsorption and by some increase in weight. Acute respiratory infections require vigorous therapy with antibiotics, steam, oxygen, and bronchodilators. As some of the severe bouts are associated with staphylococcal infection, therapy with the semisynthetic penicillins may be needed. Supportive intravenous therapy is commonly needed, and physiotherapy is useful in convalescence.

The prevention of respiratory infections is important. The child's home should be inspected and appropriate adjustments made in the environment. Postural drainage and breathing exercises should be taught to the parents, and carried out daily. In dry climates, the room should be kept moist. Prophylactic antibiotics are not invariably to be prescribed and the broad-spectrum antibiotics (tetracyclines, chloramphenicol) avoided if possible. Oral semisynthetic penicillins are again of value. Routine aerosol therapy is often helpful, especially in those who have almost continuous low-grade respiratory infections. An aerosol tent may be used in the home.

General care will include inoculation against the usual diseases, especially pertussis, and the modification or prevention of measles in contacts by gamma globulin or measles vaccination. The parents should be warned of the need to give extra salt in hot weather.

If the child becomes a respiratory cripple with diffusion defects and hypoventilation (inefficient breathing) greater attention to the prevention of respiratory infection and breathing exercises is necessary. Oxygen should be used with care. Cardiac failure will require digitalis and diuretics. Bleeding from esophageal varices and rectal prolapse demand appropriate therapy.

Prognosis. If diagnosed and treated early, the general prognosis for five years of life is fair. Much depends upon the number and severity of the chest infections. If there is evidence of diffusion defect and heart involvement, the life expectancy is short. The degree of malabsorption bears little relationship to the general prognosis. If serial lung function tests reveal a deteriorating situation, the outlook is not good.

Pancreatic insufficiency with neutropenia

The cause of this condition is unknown. The child fails to thrive and has malabsorption, without respiratory symptoms, and with a normal sweat test. The other tests of pancreatic function are abnormal.

Pseudocysts of the pancreas

These follow abdominal injury, often vehicular accident. The only symptom is an abdominal mass, roughly midline, which does not move with breathing. In a few instances, the cyst enlarges to a degree which causes a complaint of abdominal enlargement. The diagnosis is confirmed by laparotomy; the treatment is surgical marsupialization.

Tumours of the pancreas

Only the insulinoma (islet cell adenoma) occurs in children. This causes hypoglycemia, the clinical features of which are described elsewhere.

Substitution therapy in pancreatic disorder

This is indicated in defective exocrine secretion, with evidence of malabsorption. The substance used is animal pancreatic extract, which contains trypsin and a variable amount of the other pancreatic enzymes. Many therapies are repugnant to children, and the more concentrated preparations are best tolerated. The earlier in life these can be introduced the better; the same philosophy applies to the use of medium chain triglycerides which may aid caloric intake by the fact that they do not require digestion. Other dietary aids are a high calorie/high protein content with extra fat soluble vitamins (A and D); iron and folic acid are added if necessary.

DISORDERS OF THE LIVER

The liver has a large number of functions. These are especially concerned with the synthesis, storage, and interconversion of fat, carbohydrate, and protein. Additionally it forms and excretes bile, synthesizes urea, and metabolizes drugs and endogenous hormones. However, it is only in advanced disease that these faculties are interfered with. It is obvious from the summary of functions that the liver is well endowed with enzyme systems.

Carbohydrate metabolism

The liver has an important role in maintaining normal blood glucose values. This it does by responding to catecholamines (e.g., adrenaline) and glucagon (produced by the pancreas) which activate liver phosphorylase. This enzyme catalyses the first step in glycogen catabolism which begins the breakdown of glycogen to glucose. The liver can also *synthesize* glycogen through a variety of enzymatic reactions. Glycogen is thus the tactical reserve to supply glucose by the methods mentioned; glycogen formation may occur from glucose, or indirectly from non-sugars such as glycerol and the amino acids. The whole process is called *gluconeogenesis*.

The liver and protein metabolism

As already mentioned, the liver may convert amino acids into a carbohydrate equivalent. Equally it can synthesize them into the plasma proteins, principally albumen, although these and globulins can also be formed.

Urea synthesis

This is an important hepatic activity which ensures that the potentially toxic NH_4^+ (ammonium ion) is converted to urea. The reaction is known as the ornithine (Krebs-Henseleit) cycle. Disturbances in this process, because of enzyme defect, can result in the clinical disorder which is labelled hyperammonemia. The same will occur in extensive damage to the liver.

The liver and fat metabolism

The process of fat absorption is aided by the secretion of bile. The liver itself can synthesize triglycerides, phospholipids, and cholesterol, and can degrade long-chain fatty acids to acetyl CoA, a simple substance which can then be used in the energy-producing citric acid cycle.

Formation and excretion of bile

The bile salts are formed in the metabolism of cholesterol as *cholic and chenodeoxycholic acid*, and are conjugated in the liver with taurine and glycine. These compounds are excreted in the bile, and act as emulsifying agents which assist in fat digestion.

Bilirubin. This is formed principally from hemoglobin breakdown. It is transported to the liver in a protein-bound form (unconjugated). There it is exposed to the hepatic microsomal enzymes, which convert it mainly to bilirubin glucuronide, by conjugation with glucuronic acid. This is carried out under the influence of *glucuronyl transferase* which transfers the required glucuronic acid from uridine phosphoglucuronic acid (UDGPA). Some bilirubin sulphate is also formed. These are the *conjugated* forms of bilirubin which give the direct reacting tests. The conjugates are metabolized by the gut bacteria to form stercobilinogen which is oxydized and excreted in the feces as stercobilin. A moiety of the stercobilinogen is resorbed, converted in the body to urobilinogen, and excreted in the urine as urobilin.

It is clear that excess unconjugated (albumen bound) bilirubin can accumulate in the body if hemoglobin breakdown is excessive. The same will occur if the hepatic microsomal system is relatively inefficient. This is likely to be the case in newborns, especially the premature, and is the probable cause of physiological jaundice in this age group. In Crigler-Najjar disease there is a permanent deficiency of glucuronyl-transferase. It is usual for bilirubin conjugation to be affected in liver cell disease, and also in biliary obstructive states.

Inactivation of hormones and drugs

This too is an important facet of liver physiology. Cortisol, aldosterone, testosterone, and certain thyroid hormones are all converted to inactive forms, mostly to be excreted in the urine. Many drugs are disposed of by oxidation, reduction, conjugation, or methylation—processes which alter the pharmacological properties and tend to enhance excretion, often by increasing their solubility. The naturally occurring glycosides (e.g., digitalis) are so dealt with, as are a large variety of synthetic compounds. So drug dosage must be carefully watched if the liver is damaged.

Storage functions

There is evidence that the liver can store both the water soluble (B_{12}, folic acid) and fat soluble (A,D,E, and K) vitamins. The latter is essential for the synthesis of prothrombin and related coagulation factors. Severe liver disease may compromise both the absorption and the storage of the fat soluble vitamins.

Tests of liver function

There are many of these, some of which do not become abnormal until very extensive liver damage has occurred. Perhaps the most sensitive are estimates of the levels of the amino-transferase enzymes, which test for liver cell damage. The ones usually measured are serum glutamic-oxaloacetic (SGOT) and glutamic-pyruvate (SGPT) transaminases. Elevated transaminase levels can of course occur in other disease, e.g., cardiac infarct, and must be interpreted against the clinical background. Lactic dehydrogenase (LDH) is also elevated in hepatic cellular disease; this exists in several forms (isoenzymes), the one involved in liver tests being the slowest migrating type (LDH_5).

Tests of excretory function

The usual test is to measure bilirubin level, both as conjugated (indirectly reacting) and unconjugated (directly reacting) forms. This will give some indication as to whether the hyperbilirubinemia is due to hemolysis (conjugated +) or to an obstructive process (unconjugated +).

In the posthepatic biliary obstructive conditions, urobilinogen levels are low, as is fecal bile content. Other liver function tests are normal in the early stages of obstruction, but become abnormal as the hepatic cell is involved. Thus, after prolonged biliary obstruction, there may be elevated levels both of conjugated and unconjugated bilirubin, as well as increased enzyme levels (SGOT, SGPT). The other tests of excretory function usually involve testing detoxicating mechanisms, e.g., bromsulphalein excretion, rose bengal excretion. They are relatively insensitive, reflecting only advanced level disease.

Tests of synthetic capacity

In advanced liver disease, there are low levels of plasma protein, principally albumen and prothrombin levels.

Other tests of metabolic activity

Raised levels of blood ammonia, often concomitant with hypoglycemia, occur in acute extensive liver damage.

Nonspecific studies

These do not directly test any aspect of hepatic function and thus they are of rather variable value in the diagnosis or prognosis of liver disease. Typical of these are the thymol turbidity and cephalin-cholesterol flocculation test.

Anatomical studies

These may be carried out on liver biopsy specimens, which may be obtained at laparotomy, or by needle biopsy.

JAUNDICE

From the discussion above, it is clear that jaundice may occur in situations of excessive hemolysis, hepatic enzymatic deficiency, and in obstruction of the intra or extra hepatic bile ducts. In the clinical situation, more than one of these causes may operate.

In the newborn

The differential diagnosis here is wide, but some general points are worthy of recall. Jaundice appearing within a few hours of birth is due to *hemolysis* until proven otherwise. In the nature of things, this is most likely to be due to Rh incompatibility. Jaundice occurring after 24-36 hours, in a full term infant, is usually physiological. This type is not associated with bilirubinuria, and the stools are normal in colour. If these last features are present, infection of the viral (rubella, cytomegalovirus, herpes virus) or septicemic types should be excluded. A prolonged physiological jaundice may suggest cretinism.

The *jaundice of prematurity* may occur within 24-48 hours of birth, especially if the infant has not been fed, and will persist for longer than in the full term infant. Care must be taken to ensure that the premature infant does not have a hemolytic disorder due to red cell enzyme deficiency.

Obstructive jaundice in the newborn may complicate an hemolytic state. If jaundice is delayed until after the first week, an anatomical obstruction such as biliary atresia, or choledochal cyst, may be present.

Hemolytic states, other than Rh or ABO incompatability, can present with jaundice at any age, and are discussed in full elsewhere. In general, however, jaundice in the older child is usually due to infective hepatitis or occasionally to mononucleosis. Jaundice of obscure origin in the older child may be an adverse reaction to drugs, the possibility of toxic reactions, especially to those taking drugs such as chlorpromazine and certain anticonvulsants, e.g., troxidone.

Table 17 shows, in simplified form, the likely changes in biochemical tests in jaundiced patients. These are not as specific as they look and much overlap occurs in individual patients.

Table 17. Biochemical tests in jaundice

Factor	Hemolytic	Hepatocellular	Obstructive
Urine			
Urobilinogen	+	± (early), + (late)	+
Bilirubin	N	+	–
Feces			
Urobilinogen	+	± (early), + (late)	–
Bilirubin	N	–	–
Blood			
Conjugated bilirubin	+	– (early), ± (late)	–
Unconjugated bilirubin	± (late)	+	+
SGOT	N	+	+ (late)
or			
SGPT	N	+	+ (late)
LDH	N	+	+ (late)
Nonspecific	N	+	+ (late)

N = Normal.
\+ = Increased.
– = Decreased.
± = Minor increase.

Some specific entities (see also section on newborns, pp. 68-69)

Physiological jaundice

This occurs in a large percentage of normal newborns, but the exact mechanism is not yet fully explained. Possibilities have included progesterone-like substances (pregnanediols) from breast milk which could inhibit liver enzyme activity, resorption of bilirubin from the gut, persistent patency of the ductus venosus, as well as excessive red cell and chromoprotein breakdown; in general the process is more marked in premature infants.

Clinical features. The infant shows mild jaundice beginning at about 36 hours but is otherwise well. Characteristically the jaundice begins to fade at about the fifth day. The serum bilirubin levels are not excessive (less than 12 mg%) except in some prematures.

Differential diagnosis. This is principally from the hemolytic syndromes of infancy, especially perhaps ABO incompatibility. A prolonged physiological jaundice may lead to a suspicion of cretinism or bile duct atresia.

Treatment. None is usually necessary, but in some babies, exposure to light (phototherapy) will hasten the disappearance of the jaundice. Ex change transfusion may rarely be required in prematures with persistently high levels of bilirubin.

Crigler-Najjar disease

This, happily rare, condition, due to absence of hepatic glucuronyl transferase, is familial, and causes kernicterus.

Clinical features. Jaundice begins at birth or within a day thereafter. The child is not anemic, but has a high indirect bilirubin level, and rapidly develops evidence of kernicterus with lethargy, failure to feed, head retraction, extensor spasms, and convulsions, progressing to opisthotonos. There is poverty of movement and depression of the Moro and grasp reflexes. The child may die at this stage, or survive to be stricken with cerebral palsy with intellectual retardation and deafness.

Differential diagnosis. This is principally from other true hemolytic diseases, giving high levels of indirect bilirubin. Principal among these are the Rh, ABO, and other incompatibilities, which should thoroughly be sought for. Red cell enzyme deficiencies as of glucose-6-phosphatase and pyruvate kinase should be excluded. Neonatal infection, especially with cytomegalovirus, rubella virus, or herpes virus should not be forgotten.

Treatment. Exchange transfusion should be repeated until it is no longer technically possible. Thereafter, little can be done except to institute phototherapy. In this, the child (with his eyes protected) is exposed to daylight-type fluorescent tubes for some hours each day. There is evidence that this converts the bile to a less toxic and more soluble form.

Familial nonhemolytic jaundice (Gilbert's disease, Dubin-Johnson syndrome)

These are rare causes of neonatal jaundice which give an accumulation of direct bilirubin, suggestive of an obstructive process. The main things to exclude are congenital biliary atresia and the conditions giving rise to hemolytic jaundice. Treatment is usually unnecessary.

HEPATIC CIRRHOSIS (FIBROSIS)

This follows damage by infection, biliary obstruction, or poisons. It causes increased portal venous pressure and liver failure.

Clinical features. Anorexia, anemia, and growth failure are common. Portal hypertension causes hematemesis from esophageal varices, abdominal distension from ascites (excess peritoneal fluid), and splenomegaly. Failure of liver function is associated with jaundice, a bleeding tendency, hypoglycemia, and hyperammonemia. Coma is a terminal event. Most liver function tests are impaired, and needle biopsy is confirmatory.

Treatment. Portal hypertension may sometimes be helped by joining the splenic and renal veins. Otherwise only supportive measures are indicated.

TUMOURS OF THE LIVER

Most of these are secondary. The rare primary tumours are the simple hemangioendothelioma or the malignant hepatoma. They occur early in life.

Clinical features. A mass may be found, or the tumour may cause obstructive jaundice or ascites. A vascular hemangioendothelioma causes heart failure. An exact diagnosis is made at laparatomy, and the treatment is surgical.

DISORDERS OF THE BILIARY SYSTEM

Congenital biliary atresia

This is a not uncommon abnormality which results from a persistence of the solid cord stage of the bile ducts. Both the intrahepatic and extrahepatic ducts are involved and the gall bladder is usually tiny or absent.

Clinical features. The infant is normal at birth, but develops persistent jaundice within a day or two. An occasional child is asymptomatic until it is a few weeks old. Suspicion is usually aroused when the jaundice fails to disappear in the second week of life. Thereafter, until death or successful operation, the jaundice is constant although often variable in degree. The meconium is normal, but the stools thereafter are pale and acholic. In the stage of intense jaundice, a thin layer of bile may coat the outer layer of the stool which, however, remains internally clay coloured. The pale stools may be noted before the jaundice. The infant fails to gain weight and soon becomes thin and emaciated, apathetic, and has febrile episodes. The urine is bile-stained from early in life and the liver and spleen enlarge progressively. If unrelieved, biliary cirrhosis rapidly occurs causing prominent abdominal veins and ascites.

Biochemical examination. The serum bilirubin is increased, principally in the conjugated (direct) form; signs of cellular damage are early reflected in abnormally high S.G.O.T. and S.G.P.T. values. The urine contains much bilirubin but no urobilinogen. The nonspecific tests of liver function (flocculation tests) are abnormal. Anemia is common after some months of unrelieved disease. The stool is fatty and malabsorption of fat is present. Defects in prothrombin synthesis cause a bleeding tendency. The blood cholesterol may rise and in occasional patients, especially those who survive many months, there is a reduction in the serum proteins.

Diagnosis This should always be confirmed by laparotomy, preferably before the age of 2 months, before which time cirrhosis may not be permanent. The principal conditions to be considered in the differential are *neonatal hepatitis*—a diagnosis which may be reached in retrospect if the jaundice clears completely, but which is best made by an operative cholangiogram and liver biopsy. Other causes of jaundice are excluded by the tests already described.

Treatment. Exploratory laparotomy, with cholangiogram if feasible, should be done as soon as the diagnosis is suspected. Vitamin K is a normal preoperative precaution. A liver biopsy is usually obtained at the time of laparotomy. If possible, an anastomosis of the remnant of the biliary tract to the gut is carried out. If the situation is inoperable, the principal measure is support of the family. Infections are treated as they arise. No special dietetic measures are indicated.

Prognosis. In the absence of effective surgery, the disease is invariably fatal, although most children survive for at least 6 months, and occasionally into the second year.

Choledochal cyst

This is a dilatation of the common bile duct, usually of unknown etiology, although infection has been suspected in some instances.

Clinical features. The disease begins early and the initial feature is jaundice of the obstructive type usually associated with a mass in the belly, which may progressively enlarge. Fever and failure to thrive is common, and the onset of biliary cirrhosis relatively rapid.

Treatment. This is surgical and consists in drainage of the cyst and anastomosis of the proximal bile duct to the gut, usually the duodenum. Complicating cirrhosis may persist even after relief of the cyst.

Cholelithiasis

This, the presence of stones in the biliary system, is rarely found except in children with chronic bilirubin-producing hemolysis, e.g., congenital spherocytosis.

Clinical features. Nausea and vomiting are common, together with abdominal pain which is ill localized except by the older child who will describe it as being in the right hypochondrium. Fever, abdominal tenderness, and muscle guarding may be present, with jaundice if biliary obstruction occurs.

X-rays. The stones may be seen on the plain x-ray or be revealed by contrast examination after the injection of a dye excreted into the bile.

Treatment. The stones are removed surgically, and the gall bladder too, if it shows chronic inflammation.

Cholecystitis

Clinical features. Inflammation of the gall bladder and biliary ducts causes anorexia, vomiting, fever, abdominal pain and distention of the belly, and often dehydration. Tenderness is found in the right abdomen. It is often difficult to differentiate cholecystitis from appendicitis, so that laparotomy may be the ultimate way of recognizing the disease.

Treatment. Dehydration is relieved, pain-killing drugs given, together with broad-spectrum antibiotics. If diagnosed at operation, the bile ducts are explored for stones, and the gall bladder aspirated.

11 Disorders of the respiratory system

PHYSIOLOGY

The nose and throat transmit filtered, warm, moist air to the lungs. The nose is the end organ of smell, and the larynx that of speech. The bronchi and bronchioles carry the air to the alveolus, the functional unit of the lung, which is surrounded by a network of blood vessels. At the alveolus, oxygen is given up to the blood, and the carbon dioxide taken out of it. The last process is facilitated by an enzyme called carbonic anhydrase. The process of respiration also contributes greatly to body acid/base regulation. Perfusion is the process of supplying blood to the lung and normally parallels ventilation. Perfusion of an unventilated alveolus will lead to the return of unoxygenated (desaturated) blood to the left atrium, and general systemic circulation. This occurs only to a minor extent in normals. If caused by disease, central cyanosis (blueness) results.

Breathing is stimulated by the respiratory centre of the brain which is located in the brain stem near the 4th ventricle. The centre gives out an upper motor neurone which descends in the spinal cord, connects with the lower motor neurone, and drives the diaphragm and intercostal muscles. The primary outputs of the respiratory centre are modified by sensory impulses from the lungs, respiratory muscles, the cerebrum, and the circulation. In relation to the last, the chemoreceptors are peripheral (the carotid and aortic bodies) and central (in the 4th ventricle) and supply information mainly about blood oxygen tension (pO_2) as well as the acid/base status of the body. The carotid and aortic bodies also transmit information about the systemic blood pressure (baroceptor response).

The responses from the lung are mainly concerned with the prevention of overshoot in the direction of inflation or deflation. They are integrated as the Hering-Breuer reflex. The information from the respiratory muscles proper may be concerned with the amount of work done. The respiratory centre is also sensitive to temperature change and to some extent to impulses from the higher entities (the cerebrum). All in all, with the rich variety of information available to it, the respiratory centre is able to evaluate and react to a large variety of circumstances.

The subdivisions of the respiratory tract

The respiratory dead-space includes the nose, pharynx, bronchi, and bronchioles which cannot take part in oxygen/carbon dioxide exchange. These contribute the major amount to the resistance of the airways, vary in volame with the phase of respiration, and provide an evaporative surface from which water loss can occur. The total lung capacity (TLC) is the volume contained in the respiratory passages after the deepest possible inspiration, and includes dead space volume. The expiratory reserve volume (ERV) is the amount which can be forced out after a normal expiratory effort. As the lungs cannot be completely emptied the remaining air in them is called the residual volume. The total volume (TV) is that air which is moved in and out from the end of a normal expiration to the end of a normal inspiration. A forced inspiratory effort after a *normal* inspiration gives the inspiratory reserve volume (IRV). Vital capacity (VC) is the sum of the ERV, TV, and IRV. Functional residual capacity (FRC) is the sum of ERV and RV.

Measurement of the above

This is not usually possible under the age of 5 years. A simple gasometer system, called a spirometer, is used to measure TV, IRV, ERV, and hence VC. The speed of release of the air is also measured as the percentage of the VC which can be breathed out in 1 second; this is labelled FEV_1 and is used as a test of obstruction in the airways. Measurement of FRC means measurement of RV, and entails special methods of gas dilution within the lung or by putting the body in a box with the face communicating to the atmosphere. This is called a plethysmograph.

DISORDERS OF THE UPPER RESPIRATORY TRACT

Disorders of the nose

Choanal atresia has already been dealt with. Congenital disorders of the nose include *deflected septum*, in which the nasal cavities are unequally divided. This is often found without symptoms, but in severe deflection there is nasal blockage. The septum itself may occasionally perforate following tuberculous or syphilitic ulceration, but this is now rare.

Epistaxis (nose bleed)

This is most often due to minor injury to a vascular part of the anterior septum (Little's area), usually by nose picking. The bleeding is usually only from the nostril.

Epistaxis may also reflect general disease, such as rheumatic fever, salmonella infections, and the disorders of blood coagulation. The obvious symptom of external nose bleeding may be associated with hematemesis secondary to the swallowing of blood.

Treatment. Most nose bleeds stop by themselves, external pressure controls most of the others and in only a few instances is packing (with or without adrenalin) necessary.

Foreign bodies in the nostril

These are usually beads, plastic, peas, beans, or peanuts. The child may report what has happened, or, if he doesn't, may complain of a blocked nose. More often, however, the first complaint is of a bloody, smelly discharge from one nostril, which may be associated with swelling of the nose itself. The object can be seen through a speculum, and this is the way of differentiating the problem from nasal diphtheria, which has similar clinical features. Removal of the offending object is curative, but usually requires a general anesthetic.

The common cold (coryza)

This is caused by a large variety of rhinoviruses and can be quite troublesome to babies and young infants, mainly because they find it difficult to breathe through their mouths, and so are unduly affected by a blocked nose.

Clinical features. In little children, sneezing, a watery nasal discharge, and fever are common. Then the nose blocks and irritability and a small amount of respiratory distress follows. Vomiting of thick mucus may occur. Examination confirms redness of the nose and pharynx. The tonsils and ear drums are often also mildly inflamed. The whole may proceed to acute otitis media, or an attack of laryngotracheobronchitis or bronchiolitis.

In older children, the symptoms are too well known to bear repetition, but a running nose and blockage may be followed by sinusitis with purulent discharge.

Diagnostic problems. In the young patients, this is mainly from the invasive stage of measles and other exanthema. In older children, *allergic rhinitis* (hay fever) requires consideration. Hay fever is seasonal, is associated with itchy eyes, a watery nasal discharge, and has no redness of the interior of the nose.

Treatment. Decongestant nasal drops (¼% neosynephrine) and humidifying the room are of value in treating babies.

Nasal polyps

These are stalked excrescences of mucous membrane arising from the maxillary antra. They are rather rare, but may occur in mucoviscidosis. The polyp causes a nasal discharge and blockage of the nostril. Sometimes it may extend into the nasopharynx and block both nostrils. The treatment is surgical removal.

Infection of the paranasal sinuses

This is rare in infants, but is a relatively common, although mild, complication of the common cold in older children.

Acute sinusitis

The nose is blocked and there is mild fever with a purulent nasal discharge.. Mild bronchitis and otitis often coexist. Pressing over the sinuses is painful.

Chronic sinusitis

This is mainly associated with large adenoids. The main problem is a purulent nasal discharge, and nasal block. There is little complaint of pain, but tenderness over the affected sinus (usually the ethmoidal) is common. X-rays reveal opacity in the sinus, but this sign is reliable only in children over the age of 3-4 years.

Treatment. The principle is to drain the sinus, usually by cleaning the nose and putting in vasoconstrictor drops. Acute infections require antibiotics. Chronic sinusitis may require surgical drainage (antral washouts). Enlarged adenoids are removed if they are hindering drainage of the sinuses.

Acute tonsillitis

This is a common disease, and a part of the ill-defined upper respiratory tract infection disorder. The cause is usually a virus, although streptococcal infections are important because they may later cause nephritis or rheumatic fever.

General features. In the first few years of life, there may be few localizing features. Fever, irritability, and loss of appetite are common, vomiting less so, and a febrile convulsion only an occasional mode of onset. The older child complains of sore throat, difficulty in swallowing, and of painful neck glands. He too is usually fevered and off his food, may have ill-localized abdominal pain, but is less likely to have a febrile convulsion.

Local features. In mild cases, the tonsils are red and swollen and the palate and pharynx red and congested. Small follicles of pus are present on the tonsils, and these can be easily wiped off. It is seldom possible to predict the cause (virus, strep.) from the local appearance. The tonsillar glands of the neck enlarge and are tender in all but the mildest form of the disease.

Diagnostic difficulties. Measles may give rise to the features described, so that Koplik's spots (q.v.) should be sought. In septicemia and mononucleosis, the tonsils are covered by a membrane rather than having separate follicles of exudate; the palate and larynx are usually also involved. A diphtheritic membrane is hard to remove and bleeds if you do so. In mononucleosis the membrane separates cleanly. A specific diagnosis is made by throat swab and culture.

Treatment. In mild disorders, no treatment is needed apart from giving plenty of fluids. If a streptococcal infection is suspected, penicillin should be given for at least a week.

Chronic tonsillitis

Clinical features. There is a definite history of frequent attacks of acute tonsillitis. Between these attacks, the child complains of sore throat, often in the morning. There is no fever or other systemic disturbances, although the appetite is often impaired. Difficulty in swallowing is unusual unless the tonsils are very large, but the tonsillar glands are almost always enlarged.

Treatment. Tonsillectomy should be carried out.

Peritonsillar Abscess (quinsy)

Clinical features. This usually follows a streptococcal tonsillitis. There is severe sore throat, fever, inability to open the mouth (trismus), difficulty in speaking, and earache on the affected side. The tonsillar glands are enlarged and tender. The whole throat is seen to be inflamed and swollen especially above the affected tonsil, and the uvula is pushed away from it.

Treatment. Penicillin is given, and the abscess incised unless spontaneous drainage occurs. Tonsillectomy is done later.

Retropharyngeal abscess

This begins in the lymph glands of the pharynx, usually as a result of a local infection, occasionally as a spread from tuberculosis of the spine. It occurs in young children.

Clinical features. The infant is fevered, irritable, and cannot swallow, so saliva trickles from the mouth, and he will not feed. Accordingly, he may become dehydrated. The swelling can press on the airway causing noisy, rapid breathing, sometimes with rib retraction. The bulge of the abscess can be seen and felt in the lower pharynx—usually more on one side than centrally. In cases of doubt, an x-ray of the neck will show the tissue bulge.

Treatment. Antibiotics and intravenous fluids are given, and the baby is intubated if there is pressure on the airway. If the abscess is fluctuant, it is carefully incised after an endotracheal tube has been placed.

Indications for tonsillectomy and adenoidectomy

These operations are often combined but may be done separately.

Adenoids. Common symptoms are persistent mouth breathing, snoring, nasal block, and frequent attacks of otitis media. In the older child, sinusitis and deafness also occur. The adenoidal mass may be felt or seen on an x-ray of the neck. These features are indications for operation.

Tonsillectomy. This is indicated if the child has recurrent tonsillitis (documented by the doctor, not the parents). A minimum of 3 attacks for 2 years is acceptable. In most instances the tonsils are irregular and craggy although not necessarily enlarged. The tonsillar glands are invariably palpable. Very large tonsils are not an indication for surgery, unless difficulty in swallowing and alteration of speech coincide.

It is to be emphasized that tonsillectomy and adenoidectomy should *not* be carried out as treatment for such disorders as asthma, enuresis, or cough, unless the above indications are present.

Disorders of the ear

Congenital variations in shape and position are common. Low-slung ears, especially if abnormally shaped, may be found in babies with autosomal or kidney abnormalities. Accessory ear tissue is occasionally found on the cheeks and is of little significance. The commonest clinical problem is that of bat ears, where the pinnae stick out from the head in a cosmetically unacceptable way.

Disorders of the auditory canal

Cerumen (ear wax) is a normal finding, but may worry parents who see it. If removal is attempted by amateurs, the wax may impact painfully upon the ear drum. Rather rarely, hearing loss occurs with impacted wax. The treatment is simple—syringe out the wax after softening it with oil.

Otitis externa

This is an infection of the skin of the auditory canal. If it is localized, it has the characteristics of a boil, with pain and discomfort made worse by tweaking the ear. The nearby glands enlarge, and the boil can be seen with the otoscope.

In *generalized* otitis externa, there is discomfort, itching, and a purulent discharge rather than pain. Itching is particularly common in swimming pool ear where the skin is macerated by constant moisture.

Treatment. A boil in the meatus is best left to open spontaneously. Analgesics are given to relieve the pain. Diffuse otitis externa is treated by removing the exudate by gentle syringing and then packing the meatus with medicated gauze.

Foreign bodies in the auditory canal

The common ones are beads, peanuts, pieces of plastic or paper, or flies in the case of children with running ears.

The child may be frightened enough to say that he has inserted the object, more often he presents with a painful otitis externa and the object is seen at otoscopy. In those who have a running ear, a fly seldom causes much discomfort, and is usually found at examination after the syringing.

Treatment. If the foreign body is loose, and not of a type which swells with water, then it may be syringed out. Otherwise, it is pulled out by alligator forceps.

Acute otitis media

Generally this spreads from infections of the nasopharynx, so it occurs as part of the URTI syndrome, measles, and the common cold. Poor drainage of the middle ear predisposes to infection, so that otitis is common in adenoidal enlargement.

Clinical features. In the infant, there may be few features to direct attention to the ears. Fever, irritability, anorexia, and vomiting are all common, and a febrile convulsion occasional. Sometimes the first sign is pus running from the ear.

The diagnosis is made by inspecting the ear drum. In the early stage there is blushing of the tympanic membrane with loss of the normal light reflex. The membrane later bulges, is greyish red, and may show a fluid level. Perforation shows as a bead of pus exuding from the drum.

Treatment. If the drum is not yet bulging, then nasal vaso-constricting drops and antibiotics will suffice. Significant bulging of the drum, and a visible fluid level behind it indicates the need for its incision (myringotomy) as well as the medical measures noted above.

Chronic serous otitis media (glue ear)

This is found in children rather than infants, and is due to the accumulation of viscous fluid in the middle ear. The cause is not fully known, but seems to be due to failure of middle ear ventilation through the eustachian tube.

Clinical features. Intermittent mild earache and deafness are the common symptoms, the latter may come to attention because of difficulties at school. Inspection reveals that the drum is greyish or greyish yellow in colour, has a dulled light reflex, and is immobile. It may be retracted or bulging. Hearing tests reveal a conductive loss in the low frequency range.

Treatment. Myringotomy and the placement of a plastic tube in the drum is the usual mode. The tube comes out by itself after a few weeks or months, but may need replacement if the fluid reaccumulates.

Chronic suppurative otitis media

This follows the acute state, and is more common in those who live in unhygienic conditions. Deafness is a common complication and mastoid infection may occasionally develop.

Clinical features. The main complaint is of a running ear, without constitutional symptoms such as fever. The ear drum is always perforated, indeed the tympanum may be entirely destroyed and granulations be visible. Large central or anterior perforations are the safe types, in that complicating mastoiditis is unusual. The superoposterior (atticoantral) perforations are more commonly associated with mastoid infection. However, such descriptive subdivisions are only relatively accurate, and any child may develop complications, whatever the description of the perforation.

Treatment. The risks of reinfection should be reduced by improving the social circumstances. Local treatment is to remove the exudate by gentle syringing or aspiration. Dry mopping is of value when the discharge is reduced. Topical antibiotic therapy is of dubious value and cannot be effective if there is much pus. Ventilation of the middle ear should be ensured—by adenoidectomy if necessary. If the underlying cause can be cleared and the discharge stopped, then the drum may be repaired by a plastic procedure (tympanoplasty).

The treatment of atticoantral disease often requires mastoid surgery to ensure free drainage and to remove a characteristic complicating foreign body, the *cholesteatoma*. This is a cast of the inner ear cavity made up of products of infection and shed epithelium.

Mastoiditis

This is not a common problem nowadays, and is always preceded by middle ear disease, usually of the chronic type with attic perforation and the formation of a cholesteatoma.

Clinical features. The older child complains of earache, headache, and deafness. Fever is usual. The eardrum is inflamed; there is acute tenderness over the mastoid process. The swelling overlying the mastoid process may push the ear forward. In infancy, the symptoms are of fever, vomiting, and restlessness. There is mastoid tenderness and a fluctuant mass may form in the same area. This may be the first localizing sign of the disease if the patient is very young.

X-rays. These show clouding of the mastoid air cells in the older child. They are valueless in infants.

Treatment. Antibiotics (usually a penicillin) should be given in full dosage. This is usually sufficient if ear drainage is free and cholesteatoma absent. Otherwise, simple mastoidectomy is carried out.

Disorders of the larynx and adjacent structures

These are common and important disorders which, in children, cause respiratory obstruction because of the relatively small larynx. Thus, the characteristic symptom is stridor.

Stridor. This is the equivalent of hoarseness in the adult, and has many causes, which are divisible into those directly involving the larynx (intrinsic) and those due to external pressure upon the larynx (extrinsic). Some examples of these are shown in table 18. All are rare with the exception of acute viral laryngotracheobronchitis.

Table 18. Disorders causing stridor in children

	Intrinsic	Extrinsic
Infective	Acute laryngotracheobronchitis	Epiglottitis Retropharyngeal abscess
Tumours and cysts	Papilloma Hemangioma	Cystic hygroma Thyroglossal cyst Hemangioma
Anatomical defect	Laryngomalacia (congenital stridor) Laryngical web	Congenital goitre Vascular ring
Neurological	Hypocalcemia Cranial N. (9 and 10) paralysis Recurrent laryngeal N. paralysis	
Other	Foreign body, injury	Esophageal foreign body Pierre-Robin syndrome

The type of stridor may be a help to the exact diagnosis. Thus, in *supraglottic* (i.e., above the vocal cords) diseases, the stridor is mainly on inspiration and there is also difficulty in swallowing, but the voice is normal. In conditions involving the larynx proper, *glottic* stridor may occur in both phases of breathing and the voice is hoarse, weak, or absent. The stridor of disorders below the larynx (subglottic stridor) is mainly expiratory, although some inspiratory dificulty may occur. Again the voice is normal in obstructions at this level.

SPECIFIC DISORDERS:

Congenital laryngeal stridor (laryngomalacia)

In this, the epiglottis is distorted and the larynx floppy; trouble begins soon after birth, is worst at 3-6 months and then improves, to disappear by the age of 2.

Clinical features. The baby has stridor which is increased by crying. Breathlessness, difficulty in feeding, choking, and vomiting are common associated problems. The voice is normal. The presence of rib and sternal retraction means severe respiratory obstruction. The diagnosis is confirmed by laryngoscopy, when the distorted epiglottis and larynx can be seen.

Treatment. This is needed only if infection increases the laryngeal obstruction. Then the airway is maintained by intubation.

Acute laryngotracheobronchitis (ALTB)

This vital disease occurs mainly in preschool children, is most dangerous to infants, and is the main cause of the so-called croup syndrome. In spite of the name, the tracheal and bronchial components are of minor importance.

Clinical features. The child develops a cold, which is followed by a hoarse cough, noisy inspiration, stridor, and breathlessness. These may rapidly progress to a state of suffocation, with the child restless, anxious, and cyanosed. Other signs of airway obstruction such as rib retraction, and indrawing of the suprasternal and supraclavicular areas are common. Tachycardia is usual, fever may be absent. Eating and drinking become difficult, so that dehydration is common.

Other considerations. The main one is epiglottitis, in which the red, swollen epiglottis is readily seen. Laryngeal diphtheria generally is associated with the pharyngeal type in which the typical whitish membrane is seen in the throat. Enlarged neck glands are also present.

Treatment. The principles are to keep the airway open and maintain hydration. This is best done in hospital. Mildly affected patients respond to gentle sedation and humidified oxygen. Otherwise, intubation, or occasionally tracheotomy is done to relieve the anoxia of obstruction. The main sign of anoxia is *restlessness* in the presence of respiratory distress and tachycardia. If these signs persist after giving a sedative and oxygen, then intubation is considered necessary. Cyanosis is a late (often too late) indication for the relief of airway obstruction. Intravenous fluid is given to maintain hydration. Antibiotics are not used, unless complicating bronchopneumonia has occurred.

Epiglottitis

This is usually due to invasion by *H influenzae.*

Clinical features. These closely resemble those of ALTB, with the addition of difficulty in swallowing,—evidenced by the drooling of saliva. The older child complains of sore throat. The main symptom at any age is respiratory obstruction with *inspiratory* stridor and an *expiratory* grunt. The disease progresses more rapidly than ALTB, so that the results of severe respiratory obstruction—restlessness, tachypnea, rib and tissue retraction, cyanosis, and shock—are more common in epiglottitis.

Diagnosis. This is made by looking down the throat, where the swollen, fiery red tip of the epiglottis is visible; in advanced disease, this can be done by simply depressing the tongue; in lesser inflammation, mirror laryngoscopy is needed.

Treatment. This is exactly that outlined for ALTB, with the addition of ampicillin to eradicate the *H. influenzae* infection.

Acute laryngitis

This is a viral infection which occurs in the older child.

Clinical features. The patient gets a cold, followed by huskiness, cough, and mild respiratory distress. Discomfort on speaking may progress to almost complete loss of voice. The cough is harsh and barking. Fever is not common, but restlessness is usual. Laryngeal obstruction (as described above) may occur in a few patients.

Treatment. The room is steamed and simple analgesics are given. Talking should be forbidden. If respiratory obstruction occurs, it is treated as already described.

Injuries to the larynx

Many of these are due to the inhalation of physical or chemical agents, e.g., steam, acids, irritant gases. In the newborn, swelling of the cords may follow clumsy attempts at intubation. At any age, diagnostic bronchoscopy may be followed by hoarseness and mild dyspnea. The principles of treatment are those outlined for ALTB.

Foreign body in the larynx

A large, impacted foreign body may cause death by strangulation; otherwise there is cough, hoarseness, and respiratory obstruction. There is always a history of opportunity and the sudden onset of symptoms.

Differential diagnosis. This is principally from epiglottitis and acute laryngotracheobronchitis. Each of these usually has its onset at night, the symptoms are variable in their severity, and endoscopy is negative.

Treatment. Endoscopy and removal of the object.

Laryngeal paralysis

Unilateral paralysis is often asymptomatic, as speech may remain normal. Rarely is the condition due to birth injury, occasionally it coexists with congenital heart disease, where the recurrent nerve is nipped between adjacent blood vessels. *Bilateral* paralysis is associated with respiratory obstruction and is found in infants with severe brain damage, most commonly the Arnold-Chiari syndrome.

Summary. Laryngeal conditions are dangerous in infancy, but are readily recognized by the presence of dyspnea, stridor, and voice change. Restlessness and anxiety are signs of anoxia. The prime treatment of all of these is endotracheal intubation for relief of the obstruction and maintenance of fluid and electrolyte balance.

DISORDERS OF THE LOWER RESPIRATORY TRACT

These include disorders of the tracheobronchial tree and of the alveoli. They make up a large proportion of pediatric disease, most are mild viral disorders, a few are life threatening.

Diseases which principally affect the dead space (trachea, bronchi, bronchioles) cause an increase in airway resistance. The smaller the child, the greater is the resistance increase, so younger children are more likely to be disabled. Disorders of the smaller bronchi are usually associated with alveolar disease, which interferes with the diffusion of oxygen into the lung capillaries.

Specific disorders

Acute tracheitis

This occurs mostly in older children as an association of laryngeal and bronchial infections, or the early stages of measles.

Clinical features. There is a harsh, frequent, irritating, unproductive cough, and a scratchy retrosternal sensation. Fever and breathlessness are not common unless bronchitis or pneumonia follow. In most children the disease is short lived and requires little treatment apart from moist air and simple analgesics.

Acute bronchitis

This again is a disorder found in older children. It is constantly found in the early stages of pertussis and measles, but most commonly complicates a simple URTI.

Clinical features. Cough and fever are the principal symptoms. The cough is at first dry, but within a short time the child can produce mucoid or mucopurulent sputum. Breathlessness is not common unless bronchopneumonia has occurred.

Treatment. This consists in providing ample fluids, steaming the room, and the provision of postural drainage and percussion when the cough becomes loose. Antibiotics and cough mixtures are not indicated in simple bronchitis.

Chronic bronchitis

This follows repeated pulmonary infections, or can complicate long standing asthma.

Clinical features. There is a constant, loose cough which is often worse in the morning. Mucopurulent sputum is produced, but fever and other systemic symptoms are unusual. The main sign is the productive cough which can be produced on demand. Episodes of wheezing may occur. These problems may be present for several years without much complaint from the patient or his parents. In a few instances, air exchange is interfered with by lung collapse or fibrosis. At this stage, dyspnea, clubbing, and cyanosis may appear. At any stage, attacks of acute bronchitis can occur and cause fever, dyspnea and aggravation of the cough.

X-rays. In many sufferers the chest x-ray is normal, otherwise prominent thickened bronchial shadows are seen.

Other considerations. Mucoviscidosis with growth failure and a positive sweat test should be excluded, as well as the occasional case of missed foreign body. Bronchiectasis (which may closely resemble chronic bronchitis) is diagnosed by bronchography.

Bronchiectasis

This means dilatation and destruction by infection of the bronchi. It commonly follows collapse of a lung segment either by external pressure upon, or blockage of, a bronchus.

Clinical features. There is a history of frequent chest infections and chronic cough productive of purulent sputum. Hemoptysis (spitting of blood) is found only rarely and in the late stages. The whole situation resembles that of severe chronic bronchitis, and, as in that disease, episodes of wheezing and pneumonia are common. Considerable destruction of lung tissue may cause clubbing and cyanosis, but this is rare. Growth failure is frequent in long standing bronchiectasis.

X-rays. These are quite variable, but generally demonstrate prominent dilated bronchial shadows. Areas of collapse are common, and intercurrent infections may be associated with pneumonia. Specific diagnosis is made by *bronchography*, i.e., x-rays following the injection of contrast medium (iodized oil) into the suspected bronchi.

Differential diagnosis. This is mainly between conditions causing bronchiectasis, such as mucoviscidosis (positive sweat test, early onset), missed foreign body (history, bronchoscopy) and conditions in which resistance to infection is impaired (agammaglobulinemia). Chronic bronchitis may be so similar that only bronchography is diagnostic.

Treatment. This is based upon constant postural drainage and chest percussion, with antibiotics to control acute infections. If the bronchiectasis is localized, e.g., in the left lower lobe, surgical removal may be contemplated.

Mucoviscidosis

This follows the secretion of abnormally viscid mucus. The disease is described in full elsewhere, but since the serious aspects relate to the lung, these will be recapitulated now.

Clinical features. There may be a family history, or the child may have had neonatal intestinal obstruction (meconium ileus). Within a few months of birth, growth slows down, and a cough is heard. At first this may be spasmodic and mimic pertussis. Frequent chest infections occur until the child has lung trouble most of the time. The recurrent chest infections may take the form of bronchiolitis, bronchitis, or bronchopneumonia. The last is commonest. Breathlessness, clubbing, and cyanosis appear sooner or later. Occasionally an attack of staphylococcal pneumonia is the first evidence of the disease. The diagnosis is suspected by the presence of multiple respiratory infections in a child with impaired growth. It is confirmed by finding an excess amount of sodium, potassium, and chloride in the sweat (a positive sweat test).

X-rays. In the early stages, the changes are those of bronchiolitis or bronchopneumonia; collapse and fibrosis soon occur, and are permanent. The signs of bronchiectasis are usually also present.

Treatment. The details of the general care are described elsewhere. The lung disorder is treated by constant postural drainage and physiotherapy, inhalation of moisture to loosen the bronchial secretions, and antibiotics for acute infection. In spite of all treatments, slow deterioration is the rule, and respiratory failure occurs within a few years.

Bronchiolitis

This is a viral disease, affecting mainly the smaller airways, and causing much trouble in infants and young children. It is found at all seasons, but mostly in the winter.

Clinical features. The baby gets a cold, then begins to cough, and becomes breathless. Wheezing and fever may be noted. The appetite fails, and the intake of food and fluid suffers, threatening dehydration. The degree of breathlessness increases, with rib and soft tissue retraction. The baby is restless and looks anxious. All these symptoms may improve a little, especially during the day, to return again in a more severe form. The paramount problem is always breathlessness; observant parents may notice some cyanosis. Sleep is fitful and restless.

Examination shows a pallid, breathless, restless baby with an anxious expression—all tokens of anoxia. In severely affected babies, there is obvious cyanosis. The heart rate is rapid, and some degree of dehydration is almost always present. In spite of the heavy respiratory efforts, the chest is fixed in the inspiratory phase, and air exchange is limited.

X-rays. These show evidence of air-trapping—the diaphragms are low, and the lungs hyperlucent with abnormally prominent bronchial shadows.

Complications. Dehydration is common, due to increased evaporative loss and impaired intake of fluid. The intrathoracic pressure is high, so that a rupture of the lung substance can lead to pneumothorax, air in the mediastinum (pneumomediastinum), which may track into the face and neck, giving rise to subcutaneous emphysema. Lung collapse can follow crust formation in the airways, and pneumonia is a constant threat.

Diagnosis. This is mainly from other chest infections. Acute LTB is excluded by the presence of hoarseness and stridor. X-rays will exclude pneumonia. Salicylism in which aspirin precipitates respiratory distress by causing acidosis should be considered either as a primary problem or as a complication of bronchiolitis. It is excluded by a careful history. Diabetic ketosis, which also causes hyperventilation, is excluded by examination of the blood and urine for sugar. Asthma is distinguished by the presence of high-pitched rhonchi which indicate bronchospasm and the relatively rapid response to I.V. fluid and bronchodilators.

Treatment. The principles are to prevent or relieve dehydration, give humidified oxygen to help anoxia, and to observe the patient for possible complications. In most instances, antibiotics are not indicated. If the infant is clearly exhausted, is making feeble respiratory efforts, has a falling pO_2 and rising pCO_2, then *aided respiration* is indicated. The general methods outlined for the newborn apply in this circumstance.

Asthma

This is defined as episodic attacks of bronchial spasm which increase airway resistance, causing breathlessness and decrease of alveolar ventilation. The condition may be due to an allergic mechanism which releases substances e.g., histamine, which cause the bronchi to contract. It often follows infantile eczema, but in most cases arises spontaneously after the second birthday.

Clinical features. The first attack usually comes on at night, and without apparent cause. The child suddenly becomes breathless, and wheezes audibly. He is fearful. Most of the difficulty is in expiration, so that the chest fixes in the *inspiratory* position. An expiratory grunt, rib recession, and action of the accessory breathing muscles of the neck are extra evidences of the dyspnea. Fever is absent. The attack may stop suddenly with the coughing up of thick, gluey mucus. The wheeze disappears at the same time. Some wheezing is common between acute attacks, especially after exercise. Parents soon notice that infections, change of weather, and temperature can bring the attacks on, but the pattern is very variable. As an attack of asthma is a frightening experience, secondary psychological upsets are not uncommon.

X-rays. In an acute episode, the lungs are seen to be large and hyperlucent, with prominent bronchi and straight ribs. All of this reflects the air trapping present in the condition.

Other investigations. Theoretically the responsible allergens could be eaten (ingested) or inhaled. Asthma due to ingestants is not common, and best confirmed by a careful diet scan designed to show the relationship between asthma and what is eaten. If anything suggestive eventuates, the suspected substance is eliminated from the diet; if this apparently cures the patient, then it is reintroduced as a provocation. Only if this again causes asthma should the item be held responsible and totally eliminated from the diet.

If the asthma is seasonal then a search sould be made for plant allergens (e.g., grasses) as the cause. This may be done by a careful history and also by skin tests to the suspected items. Positive skin tests are not, however, proof that the reacting substances are the true cause of the asthma, but indicate the direction in which provocation tests may go. In many children who have year-round (perennial) asthma, skin tests are positive to many plant allergens and yet desensitization has little effect.

Excess eosinophils are found in the blood and nasal secretions of many asthmatics. This confirms that an allergic state exists, but does not give a guide as to the exact cause or severity of the condition.

Differential diagnosis of the acute attack. This is most difficult in the initial episode, which in the younger child is most likely to be taken for bronchiolitis. The presence of cough and fever favour the latter. Wheezing may be a feature of mucoviscidosis, but a long history, and the presence of growth failure usually support the correct diagnosis. Inhaled foreign body may cause acute distress and wheezing, but can be confirmed by a careful history and appropriate x-ray findings.

The course of asthma. This is very variable. Most asthmatics have relatively few episodes and many are totally cured by puberty. In others, wheezing is never really absent, and chest deformity, with growth failure, occurs. A constant hazard is the development of chronic bronchitis in these children. This is heralded by the onset of a constant, loose cough, with purulent sputum. Permanent pulmonary crippling is unusual, occurring only in those with frequent attacks in which lung collapse or infection has occurred.

Treatment: General measures. The recurrent nature of the disorder, the need for frequent medical care and also the generally good prognosis should be carefully explained to the parents. Parental and child anxiety is best helped by a reasonably optimistic attitude, but with frankness about the need for occasional hospitalization. Undue restrictions on the child and family are to be avoided. Dust is an irritant to all asthmatics, so simple, easily cleaned furniture is advisable. Dogs and cats should not be banished, but shampooed frequently. The vacuum cleaner is the best agent to cut down on household dust, and should be used fully. Breathing exercises and postural drainage should be taught to all asthmatics.

In seasonal asthma, obvious causes such as grasses or pollens should be avoided. If this is impossible, them desensitization may be tried *although it is seldom curative*.

In perennial asthma, there are two problems, to prevent attacks and to treat the established attack of asthma. Prevention may be tried by giving drugs. One is disodium cromoglycate, which is inhaled, and is said to stop the release of histamine and related substances which make the bronchi contract. This technique can only be used in children who are old enough to inhale the substance, viz., more than 4 years old. Below this age, or when the cromoglycate does not work, then small doses of bronchodilator (e.g., orciprenaline, salbutamol, terbutaline) may be needed. All such treatments should be assessed by keeping a daily diary. It should be specially noted that antihistamine drugs are *not* used in asthma, especially in the acute attack. These measures will control many patients except when they acquire a chest infection.

In the severely affected child with short intervals between attacks, bronchodilators may be given by inhalation, but again this treatment is helpful only in the older child. When growth is slowing, much school is missed and hospitalization frequent, then *intermittent* steroid therapy may be considered. This decision should not be taken lightly, and the possible consequences (growth failure, Cushingoid state, etc.) fully considered and explained to the parents. Steroids are given in the smallest possible dose, and on alternate days. Every effort is made to replace steroids by some other mode of treatment, or by increasing specificity by giving them in an inhalable form.

Status asthmaticus

This is when a severe attack of asthma persists for 6-10 hours, and is unaffected by the usual treatments. It is often precipitated by infection, and insufficient fluid intake is a usual association.

Clinical features. There is severe bronchospasm as already described; fear, exhaustion, sweatiness, and some cyanosis are usually also present. The patient is thirsty, but too breathless to drink, and signs of dehydration are common. Air exchange is poor, in spite of severe respiratory efforts. The heart is fast and active, and the blood pressure increased. If unrelieved, respiratory efforts decrease, cyanosis increases and slowing of the heart, restlessness, decrease of arterial pO_2 and increases of pCO_2 may herald terminal exhaustion and death.

Treatment. The patient is placed in humidified oxygen, and an intravenous saline infusion set up. Subcutaneous adrenaline is given when rehydration is established and this may decrease the attack. Xanthines (aminophyllin) may be used with care in the same circumstance: if the spasm persists, then hydrocortisone is given intravenously. A chest x-ray should be done so that infection or lung collapse may be diagnosed and treated. If these measures are unsuccessful, and in the presence of exhaustion, a low pO_2 and high pCO_2, then artificial ventilation may be required. This is, however, a rare event.

When the acute stage is over, vigorous physiotherapy should begin in order to prevent plugging of the bronchi by mucus.

Foreign body in the bronchi

This occurs in younger children who are able to get at whatever is inhaled. Pieces of plastic, nuts, carrot and popcorn are the common offenders.

Clinical features. The child has been well, then while eating or running, he begins to cough, choke, gag, and becomes breathless. Stridor and dyspnea may occur, but all of these may abate after a short time. Cough and breathlessness come back sooner or later, especially at night. An obstructing object soon causes fever, increasing cough and dyspnea. If the obstruction is check-valve, air can get into the affected area of the lung, but cannot get out. The segment inflates, and may move the mediastinum, causing the cardiac apex to shift and sometimes obstructing the return of blood to the heart. In total obstruction, dyspnea is less, although the lung segment collapses, but infection is inevitable. The physical signs of a foreign body are not reliable, and x-rays and bronchoscopy should always be carried out if there is the slightest doubt. The x-ray signs will vary with the type of obstruction, thus lung *hyperinflation* occurs with the check-valve type, and *collapse* with total bronchial obstruction.

Missed Foreign Body

This situation arises usually when the parents underestimate the significance of the acute symptoms and do not seek medical care. Occasionally the physician is too unsuspicious to carry out an x-ray.

Clinical features. There are 3 main modes of presentation: the usual one is a history of repeated respiratory infections, and chronic cough. X-rays, if taken, usually fail to show complete clearance of any consolidation present. The second is bronchiectasis—the child develops a respiratory infection and is found by x-ray to have a localized area of collapse and bronchial crowding; he does not respond well to antibiotics and physiotherapy. Less common is sudden, often repeated, hemoptysis in the older child.

Differential diagnosis. The child is commonly too old for serious thought to be given to mucoviscidosis, although this disease is often considered. Pertussis is perhaps a more common suspicion, as is unresolved pneumonia. A stern search for opportunity to inhale, an x-ray review, and endoscopy should always be carried out in pulmonary disease of undetermined origin. It may be due to a foreign body.

Disorders of the Alveoli

Essentially this means pneumonia, which is most often due to a virus, or to *Mycoplasma pneumoniae*. Bacterial pneumonia (staphylococcus, pneumococcus, *Klebsiella*, *H. influenzae*) are much rarer although often more serious. Protozoal pneumonia (*P. carinii*) may occur in premature or more commonly in children given cytotoxic agents, or in agammaglobulinemia, where body defence mechanisms are lacking.

Viral pneumonia

The commonest organism is the respiratory syncytial virus, and the usual type is bronchopneumonia. The disease is often an extension of bronchiolitis.

Clinical features. Respiratory distress, cough, irritability, and refusal to feed are constant. Fever is less so, or a later feature. The degree of dyspnea is variable, but rib retraction and air trapping are common in young infants. Auscultatory signs (e.g., crepitations) may be intermittent or minor, and the exact diagnosis is often made by x-ray. Dehydration is a common accompaniment.

Treatment. Antibiotics are not indicated. The principles of treatment are those outlined for bronchiolitis, viz., fluid, humidified oxygen and physiotherapy.

Bacterial pneumonia

The most important (and common) type is that due to the staphylococcus. In the younger child, the disease is primary, in the older patient, a complication of osteomyelitis or other staphylococcal infection. The disease occurs in mucoviscidosis or in children who have impaired respiratory ability, as in amyotonia congenita, muscular dystrophy, or severe cerebral palsy.

Staphylococcal pneumonia in infancy

The infant is unwell for a day or two, and then is smitten with cough, fever, and breathlessness. Anorexia and dehydration occur early, and are aggravated by the bacterial toxins to produce a shock-like state with pallor, restlessness, and hypotension. The child looks gravely ill.

Breathlessness increases, and abdominal distension is common. Cyanosis and exhaustion are frequent. Any sudden increase in the degree of dyspnea suggests a complication such as pneumothorax or empyema.

Other features. Impaired movement of one side of the chest may suggest an empyema, and dullness on percussion is confirmatory. Leucocytosis and anemia are invariable, and the blood culture usually positive.

X-rays. At first these show diffuse bronchopneumonic infiltrates in the lungs, which later coalesce. Cavitation soon occurs with the formation of air-filled spaces within the lung substance (pneumatocoeles). Air or fluid in the pleural cavity is diagnostic of pneumothorax or effusion.

Complications. The commonest are *empyema* and *pneumothorax*. The first may be an early part of the illness. If large, the empyema may cause mediastinal shift and dullness to percussion. If small it may be suspected only after x-ray.

Pneumothorax occurs when the disease causes a fistula between a bronchus and the pleural space. A check-valve obstruction may be present, so that air can get into the pleura but not out. If this happens, then the child (even if previously improving) is seized with extraordinary dyspnea and a sense of suffocation. Gross rib retraction, tachycardia, and cyanosis are common, and death may occur rapidly, especially if the venous return is impeded by mediastinal shift. Very rarely there is metastatic infection to the brain or pericardium.

Treatment. The child is given intravenous fluid and blood if need be, and is nursed in humidified oxygen. Antibiotics (methicillin) are given after a blood culture is taken. If an empyema is present, it should be drained. The patient is closely watched in case he develops a pneumothorax. If this is suspected the pleural space is aspirated by needle and syringe until intercostal drainage can be obtained. The antibiotic may need to be varied according to the sensitivity of the staphylococcus, and should be given for at least 2 weeks. Several blood transfusions may be required during this time.

Staphylococcal pneumonia in the older child

The child may have osteomyelitis, and then develops chest pain and dyspnea together with signs of pneumonia. Chest x-rays are confirmatory. The complications and mode of treatment are those noted above.

Aspiration pneumonia

This occurs in infants where some disorder of deglutition is present, such as tracheoesophageal fistula, cerebral (bulbar) palsy, and the amyotonia congenita syndromes.

Clinical features. At or soon after feeding, the child gags, chokes, coughs, and may become blue and breathless. Rib retraction sets in, and fever follows within a short time. Massive inhalation can cause rapid death. Smaller inhalations cause consolidation and collapse in the lung, which is readily confirmed by x-ray.

Treatment. The immediate incident is treated by suction, posturing, and patting. If unrelieved, bronchoscopy should be attempted although it is often unrewarding. A prophylactic antibiotic (e.g., ampicillin) should be given, and the child nursed as if he had bronchiolitis.

Kerosene pneumonia

This is due to the inhalation of kerosene at the time of swallowing it. There is usually a history of coughing in close association with the vomiting of kerosene. Within a short time the child is breathless, fevered, and is coughing, and x-rays show a scattered bronchopneumonia.

Lipoid pneumonia

This is due to the inhalation of various oily materials, principally liquid paraffin. It occurs if oily nose drops are given, or where forcible attempts are made to give unpleasant substances, such as castor oil, olive oil, or cod liver oil.

Clinical features. The child presents with a cough and minor breathlessness. The latter is at first only on exertion, but later is constant. Fever and general upset is not common, and the association with the causes noted above may be hard to confirm. Progressive breathlessness is usual, since the oil causes pulmonary fibrosis, and can never be recovered from the lungs.

X-rays. These may show localized collapse (e.g., the right upper lobe in young infants); more often there are scattered bronchopneumonic changes, which do not regress. Pulmonary fibrosis is found later.

Treatment. No effective cure is known. Complicating infective episodes are treated with antibiotics.

Lobar pneumonia

This is usually due to the pneumococcus, occasionally the staphylococcus is responsible.

Clinical features. The child suddenly develops fever, shivering, cough, and breathlessness. Pleural pain is fairly common and may be referred to the abdomen. In *upper lobe* pneumonia (especially on the right) headache and stiff neck—meningismus—may dominate the clinical picture. Examination reveals a febrile child with tachypnea, active alae nasi, and an expiratory grunt. Chest movement is less on the affected side. There may be dullness, diminished air entry, or a pleural rub. Bronchial breathing occurs, but much less frequently than in adults. In general, the most constant physical signs are diminished chest movement and crepitations. The x-ray evidence is usually more marked than the clinical signs.

Differential diagnosis. Most problems arise where there is pleural pain referred to the abdomen, or where meningeal symptoms are present, as in upper lobe pneumonias. Occasional cases of diabetic coma or salicylism presenting with breathlessness may cause difficulty. The possibility of foreign body should never be forgotten as a cause of pneumonia.

Complications. These are few. A small pleural effusion may occur which is usually sterile and does not require specific treatment.

Treatment. Penicillin given intramuscularly for a week will cure most children. Intravenous fluids are given if necessary, and vigorous physiotherapy is begun when the cough becomes loose.

Pulmonary edema

This implies the presence of fluid in the alveoli and the fine bronchioles. It is almost always secondary to heart disease, but may occasionally follow the inhalation of irritant gases such as sulphur dioxide.

In the newborn, pulmonary edema usually implies the presence of severe congenital heart disease, and is particularly associated with the hypoplastic left heart syndromes. In older children, *fibroelastosis* of the left heart, or left ventricular failure secondary to *myocarditis* or *paroxysmal tachycardias* may be the cause. Rheumatic fever occasionally presents with severe left ventricular failure, giving rise to widespread pulmonary edema—the so-called rheumatic pneumonia. Acute glomerulonephritis with hypertension may also be so complicated.

Clinical features. Those of the primary condition are present and dyspnea and rib retraction are usual. Sometimes the diagnosis is made only on inspection of the x-rays. The bloody, frothy, sputum of adult pulmonary edema is rather unusual in children.

X-ray appearances. These are bilateral, fluffy exudates in the lungs, most marked near the hila, and in the lower lobes.

Treatment. The primary disease requires care, and as this is usually cardiac, digitalization and diuretics are in order. The pulmonary edema of acute glomerulonephritis will often subside without active treatment.

Disorders of the pleura

Pleurisy

This means inflammation of the pleura, and can be due to many organisms. Most commonly it occurs as part of a pneumonia, most often of the pneumococcal or staphylococcal type. In young children, pleurisy gives little in the way of symptoms unless an effusion develops. In older children, there is pain on breathing, a short painful cough, and rapid, shallow breathing. The chest moves poorly on the affected side, and auscultation reveals a pleural rub—a leathery creak present in both phases of respiration. The treatment of pleurisy is that of pneumonia.

Pleural effusion

This may be sterile or purulent (empyema) and usually complicates a pneumonia. Large effusions cause marked dyspnea, small effusions may only be suspected by x-ray. Empyemata additionally cause high fever, rigors, rapid anemia and severe toxemic illness.

Tuberculous pleural effusion

This is a rare primary form of tuberculosis occurring in older children and adolescents. Dyspnea is the main complaint, together with malaise and a feeling of heaviness in the chest.

The signs of pleural effusion vary with its size. Definite effusions may be found on x-ray in the absence of obvious physical signs; usually, however, an effusion of reasonable size gives rise to dullness on percussion, diminished thoracic movement, and suppression of breath sounds. Mediastinal shift, usually expressed as movement of cardiac position, is a feature of large effusions. Aspiration of the pleural fluid is the principal mode of confirmation of diagnosis, and differentiation of its cause. In inflammatory effusions, the fluid has an SG >1015, with some cells (leucocytes or lymphocytes), according to etiology. The fluid should always be examined for bacteria, pyogenic or tuberculous.

Treatment. Unless mediastinal shift is present, only diagnostic aspiration is necessary. In most instances, the effusion will spontaneously absorb. Purulent transformation of the effusion demands underwater sealed drainage by way of a rib space.

Other forms of pleural effusion

Hydrothorax is mostly associated with the nephrotic syndrome, or other conditions causing hypoproteinemia, e.g., advanced cirrhosis of the liver, protein-losing enteropathy. Congestive cardiac failure is also occasionally causal. Hydrothorax fluid is of low (>1015) SG and has a minimal protein and cellular content.

Chylothorax is rare, occurs in newborns, and most often due to traumatic rupture of the thoracic duct. The fluid is milky and contains fat and protein. Aspiration is needed if mediastinal shift is severe. Otherwise, spontaneous recovery may be expected in most instances.

Hemothorax. This is usually traumatic, and due to vehicular accident. Apart from the primary thoracic signs, shock is commonplace. Bloody effusions may be also due to pleural involvement in the neoplastic or collagen diseases.

Pneumothorax. This is the name given to the presence of air in the pleural cavity. It occurs in the newborn, de novo, or as a result of the respiratory distress syndrome.

In older children, severe suppurative lung disease with bronchopleural fistula also causes pneumothorax, often in association with empyema when it is called pyopneumothorax. Severe asthma may also cause pneumothorax, frequently in association with subcutaneous or mediastinal emphysema. The clinical features of pneumothorax, and its treatment, are described elsewhere.

Tumours of the respiratory system

These are rare in childhood, most are secondaries from kidney, adrenal, or bone tumours; of the primary tumours, only hemangioma of the larynx, and simple bronchial adenoma are more than the greatest rarities. The former affects the newborn, is usually subglottic, giving rise to a hoarse cry, and evidence of respiratory obstruction. The latter protrude into the bronchial lumen, and act as a foreign body. They cause cough, recurrent respiratory infection, and occasionally hemoptysis. X-rays will reveal emphysema or collapse, depending upon the degree of obstruction present. The principal differential diagnosis is from foreign body, and endoscopy is always needed. The treatment is entirely surgical.

Tumours of the mediastinum

Many of these are secondary; of the primary tumours, the usual type is teratoma, or its cystic variant, *dermoid* cysts. Duplications of the esophagus and cystic masses derived from the trachea, bronchus, or gastroenteric remnants, all may simulate tumours. True tumours are usually found in the anterior mediastinum, the benign cysts in the posterior mediastinum.

Clinical features. None may be present, the condition being suspected at x-ray for an acute respiratory infection. Otherwise, the symptoms are those of compression. If this is upon the air passages, there is cough and dyspnea; multiple respiratory infections may be associated. If the compression is vascular, the superior vena caval syndrome occurs, with venous dilatation and edema of the face, head, and neck.

X-rays. These will usually reveal the mass. In teratoma, bony elements, or teeth, may be visible.

Treatment. This is by surgical removal.

12 Disorders of the heart and circulation

In children, most of these are due to inborn defects of the heart's structure and many can now be cured by operation. In school-age children, rheumatic fever can cause damage to the valves of the heart. Viral infections of the heart muscle (myocardium) are rare, but can occur at any age; so too can variation in the heart's rate or mode of contraction—these abnormalities are called arrhythmias.

PHYSIOLOGY

The heart is a double pump, the right atrium receives the venous (low oxygen content) blood, and transmits it to the right ventricle, which pumps it into the pulmonary arteries which divide finely until the blood is in contact with the air in the alveoli of the lung. There it is oxygenated and this blood (arterialized, i.e., high O_2 content) returns by the pulmonary veins to the left atrium, then to the left ventricle which pumps the arterialized blood to the body. The right atrium and ventricle are separated by the tricuspid valve, the right ventricle and pulmonary arteries by the pulmonary valve. The left atrium transmits blood to the left ventricle by the mitral valve, and the latter to the body through the aortic valve.

The 2 atria and ventricles are separated by the atrial and ventricular septum respectively. Each ventricle does work divisible into flow work and pressure work. Flow work is done by the ventricle contracting upon the volume of blood entering it through the proximal valve, i.e., the tricuspid for right ventricular flow work and the mitral valve for left ventricular flow work. Pressure work is done against the resistance at the distal valve, i.e., the pulmonary valve for the right ventricle, and the aortic valve for the left ventricle. An increase in flow will increase work, so too will an increase in the resistance at the distal valve. Changes in ventricular work load can often be recognized by x-ray, or by electrocardiogram (E.C.G.). Normally the left ventricle does most work, since systemic resistance is greater than the resistance in the lungs. This in turn produces higher pressures in left atrium and left ventricle as compared to the pressure in the right ventricle.

CONGENITAL HEART DISEASE

There are 3 general divisions of these disorders. The first is the *left-to-right* shunt which is so called because the direction of the leak of blood is from the left atrium, ventricle, or aorta, into the corresponding right atrium, ventricle, or pulmonary artery. The direction is fixed by the fact that the pressures are higher on the left side of the circulation than on the right. Common examples of left to right shunt are atrial septal defect, ventricular septal defect, and patent ductus arteriosus. Anomalous return of the pulmonary veins to the right atrium instead of the left atrium is another rarer example. In all of these, arterialized (oxygenated) blood enters the venous blood.

In the *right-to-left* shunts, venous blood (deoxygenated) enters the left side of the heart, e.g., left atrium, left ventricle, or pulmonary artery. This can only occur if the pressure in the *right* heart exceeds that in the left. This may occur because of increased resistance to flow through the right heart, either because of abnormalities of the tricuspid or pulmonary valve, or because of general increase in lung resistance. Common examples of the right to left shunts are: tetralogy of Fallot (essentially a ventricular septal defect with pulmonary valve narrowing or stenosis), tricuspid atresia (where the tricuspid valve is very narrow or absent and a large atrial septal defect exists), and transposition of the great vessels, where the aorta arises from the right ventricle and transmits *venous* blood, and the pulmonary artery arises from the left ventricle. In some of these, other abnormalities such as a patent ductus arteriosus are present as compensatory devices. Many patients with these disorders are cyanosed (bluish in colour) because of the mixture of venous and arterial blood which is pumped through the systemic circulation.

The third division is congenital heart disease without shunt. These are usually abnormalities of the heart valves or of the great vessels leaving the heart. Thus pulmonary valve stenosis, aortic valve stenosis, and coarctation (narrowing) of the aorta or of the pulmonary artery can all occur. The tricuspid and mitral valves may also be stenosed, but more common perhaps is insufficiency, regurgitation, or incompetence—all names for the situation in which the valve allows blood to flow backwards as well as forwards when the atrium or ventricle contracts. In these disorders, there is no admixture of blood from either side of the heart, so that central cyanosis does not occur.

General Features of Congenital Heart Disease

Most children with significant congenital heart disease have breathlessness, frequent respiratory infections, and failure of proper growth. These occur whether the patient is cyanosed or not. Complaints which are often found in the first year of life are fatigue, undue sweating, pallor, and slowness in attaining the development milestones. The child with severe congenital heart disease is hard to rear, more pernickety in diet, and often unhappy and cross grained, even at a relatively late age. Most symptoms, physical or psychic, are aggravated in hot weather.

The child with cyanotic congenital heart disease, apart from blueness, may have complaints due to anoxia. Thus, a child with severe tetralogy of Fallot may have attacks of paroxysmal dyspnea superimposed upon his normal breathlessness. These spells may culminate in unconsciousness and twitching, occasionally progressing to a convulsion. Attacks of abdominal pain, which later are replaced by chest pain of an anginal type, are sometimes found in severe cyanotic conditions. Headache is a common symptom in them. General symptoms and signs of the type described are strikingly absent in children with isolated pulmonary stenosis, simple aortic coarctation, and isolated aortic stenosis.

Some General Signs

These afflicted children are mostly in the low growth percentiles. Chest deformity (Harrison's grooves, protuberant sternum) is common in those who have been breathless since early in life, or who have had frequent respiratory infections. The cyanosed child will show clubbing (abnormality of the size and shape) of the toes, nose, and fingers, usually in the order stated, but this sign is often delayed until the sixth month of life, even if cyanosis has appeared much earlier. Babies who are suffering from a serious lesion (cyanotic or not) often show hypotonia. Some delay in motor progress may be confirmed by examination, but true mental defect is not more common than in other groups of children. Pallor is common in children with left to right shunt.

The severely cyanosed child will show suffusion (redness) of the conjunctivae and mucous membranes. Some coldness of the skin is usual, and distention of the superficial veins is characteristic.

Specific Left-to-Right Shunts

Isolated Ventricular Septal Defect

This is a relatively common disorder, which varies greatly in severity. Often only the larger defects have the general symptoms noted above. In many patients, the condition is suspected when an abnormal cardiac noise—a murmur—is heard early in life at some routine examination. In some, the defect is associated with the presence of a *thrill*, i.e., a vibration which can be felt, and is coincident with the heart's contraction.

Figure 43 summarizes the effect of a ventricular septal defect on the circulation. From this it is seen that the *mitral* flow increases, so that left ventricular work will be augmented. Similarly, the blood flow through the lungs increases.

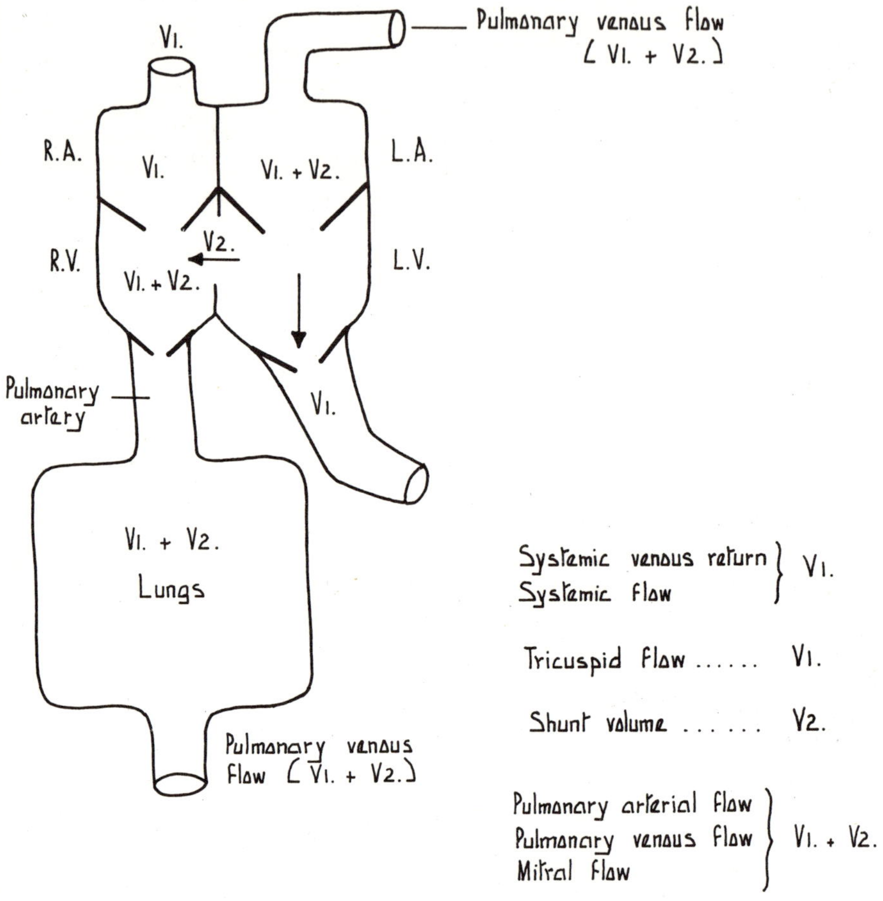

Fig. 43. Hemodynamics of ventricular septal defect. R.A.: right atrium. R.V.: right ventricle. L.A.: left atrium. L.V.: left ventricle.

Thus, on x-raying a patient with ventricular septal defect, the lung fields may show increased vascularity (plethora). Because of the increased lung flow, the left atrium may also be abnormally prominent. The left ventricle may also be seen on the electrocardiogram. However, because of the ability of the left ventricle to increase its work load with ease, evidence of its enlargement is often absent. The diagnosis is confirmed by cardiac catheterization which shows evidence of a leak of oxygenated blood into the right ventricle. Ventricular septal defects often close spontaneously in the first few years of life, usually when the child has no symptoms, there is no thrill, and the x-rays are normal. Otherwise they can be closed surgically, usually at the school-age and in patients who have a large shunt.

Patent Ductus Arteriosus

Before birth the ductus arteriosus short-circuits the blood from the pulmonary artery to the aorta. It closes within a few weeks of birth but if it persists an abnormal left to right shunt occurs (see Figure 44)

Clinical features. The general symptoms (growth failure, frequent chest infections) referred to above occur in large shunts. Otherwise the diagnosis may be made because of the presence of a cardiac murmur. Typically, this is found in both systole and diastole—it is continuous. Because of the wide pulse pressure (i.e., the difference between systolic and diastolic blood pressures), the pulses are active and bounding. The E.C.G. and x-ray signs are identical to those found in ventricular septal defect.

The disorder can be confirmed at cardiac catheterization by finding high O_2 levels in the pulmonary artery. The catheter will often enter the aorta through the *ductus*. The treatment is to divide the ductus at operation.

Atrial Septal Defect

The less serious type is called an ostium secundum defect. This means that it does not involve the mitral or tricuspid valve rings, nor the ventricular septum.

Clinical features. These usually occur after infancy; most often the condition is suspected by finding a systolic murmur and/or fine thrill in the upper left chest. In large shunts, the child may have the general features described above. Figure 45 shows the effect upon the circulation and from it follow the x-ray findings—pulmonary plethora, and right ventricular enlargement. The E.C.G. will also show the latter. Cardiac catheterization shows an abnormal increase in the O_2 content of the right atrial blood. Closure of the defect by open heart surgery is done when the shunt is large.

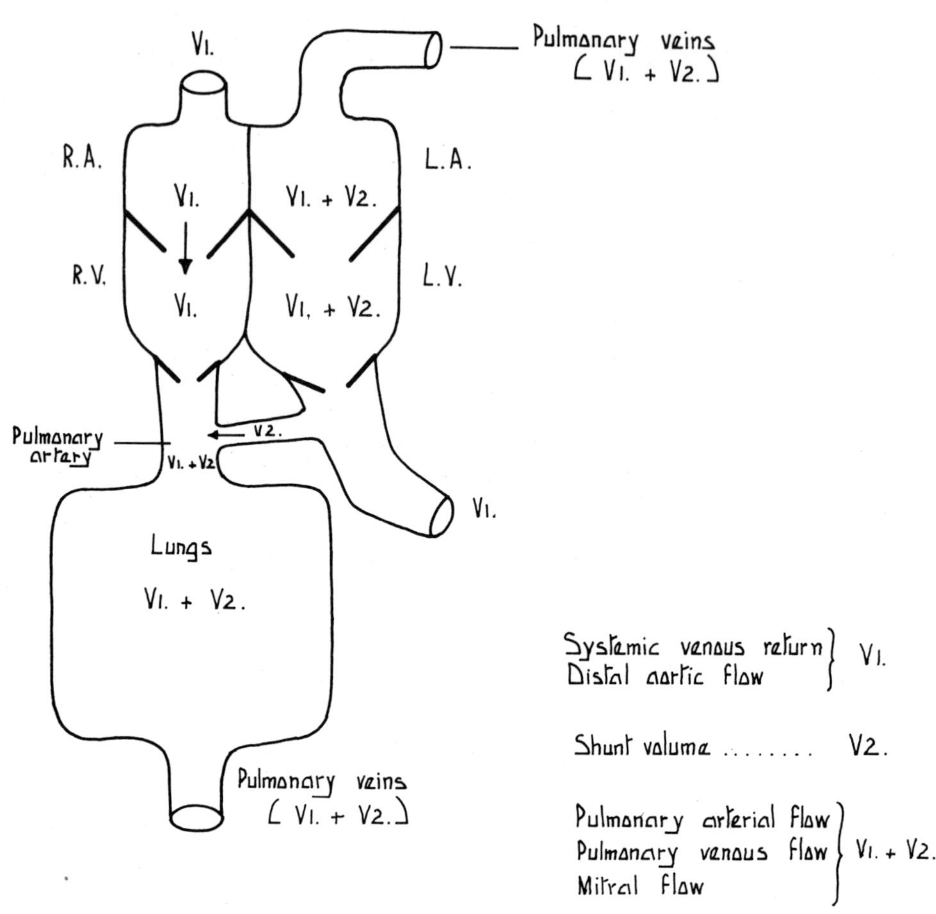

Results: Pulmonary plethora.
Left ventricular work increase.
Left atrial increase (septum intact.)

Fig. 44. Hemodynamics of patent ductus arteriosus. R.A.: right atrium. R.V.: right ventricle. L.A.: left atrium. L.V.: left ventricle.

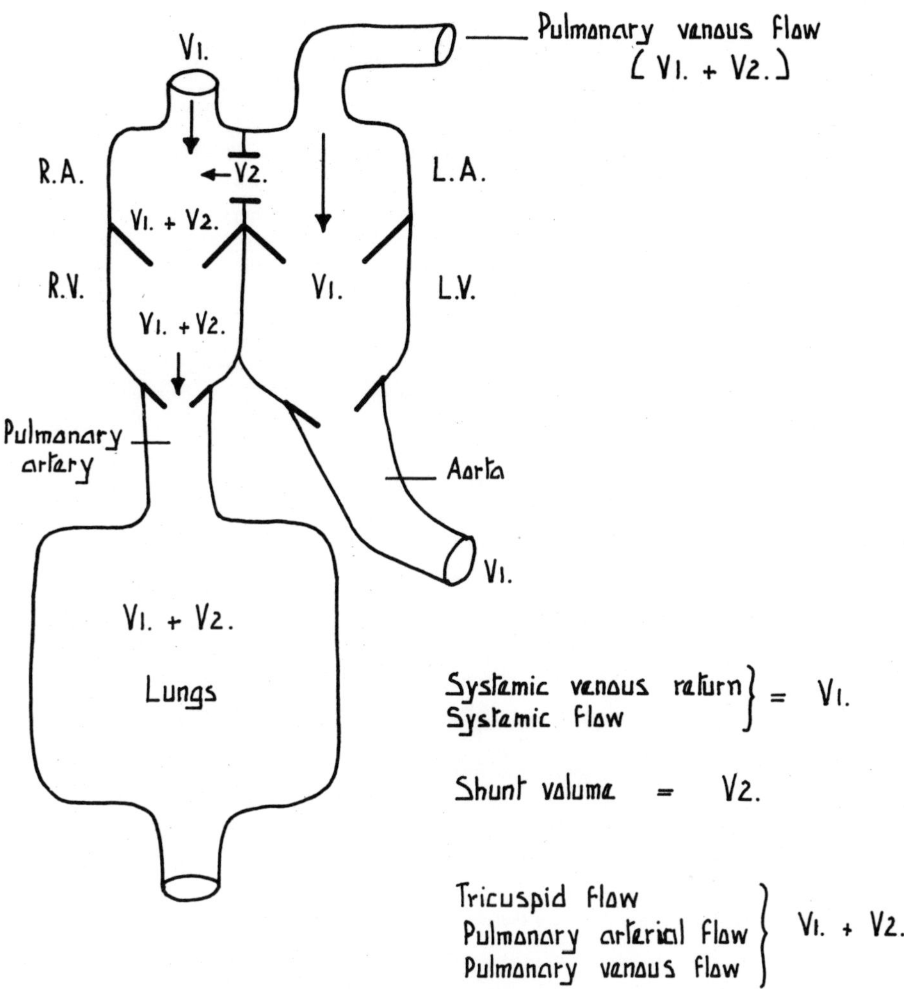

∴ Right ventricular work +
Pulmonary plethora
Atrial septum breached, so <u>NO</u> left atrial enlargement.

Fig. 45. Hemodynamics of atrial septal defect. R.A.: right atrium. R.V.: right ventricle. L.A.: left atrium. L.V.: left ventricle.

Endocardial Cushion Defects (ostium primum, atrioventricular communis)

This is the term applied to a variety of conditions involving the lower atrial septum, the tricuspid and mitral valves, and the upper ventricular septum. These are the structures which are formed by the endocardial cushions which divide the primitive single atrium and ventricle into the right and left atria and ventricles and the atrioventricular (mitral and tricuspid) valves.

Endocardial cushion defects are most commonly found in children suffering from Down's syndrome.

Clinical Features. Most of these children have growth failure, and frequent chest infections. They are also more prone to develop congestive cardiac failure, partly because of the complexity of the cardiac lesion, and partly because of the development of pulmonary hypertension which embarrasses the right ventricle (see Eisenmenger's complex below).

In ostium primum, the atrial defect has a lower edge, but the mitral valve is split. In atrioventricularis communis, there is both an atrial and ventricular septal defect, with mitral and tricuspid valve involvement. The cardiac signs will vary accordingly, from those described under atrial septal defect to those of ventricular septal defect with mitral or tricuspid insufficiency. Generally the x-rays will show pulmonary plethora and enlargement of both ventricles. The latter will also be reflected in the E.C.G.

These children require careful further examination to confirm the diagnosis. Usually this takes the form of right and left heart catheterization, together with angiography. Ostium primum defects may be readily closed at cardiac surgery. Atrioventricularis communis closure is a much more difficult procedure and is undertaken only if strictly necessary.

Anomalous Pulmonary Venous Return

Partial (1 or 2 veins) anomalous return to the right atrium is common in atrial septal defect. *Total* anomalous pulmonary venous return is a severe form of left to right shunt, which causes early symptoms and signs. The pulmonary veins can drain into the superior vena cava, coronary sinus, or right atrium (supradiaphragmatic drainage). They may also enter the inferior vena cava or even the portal veins (subdiaphragmatic drainage). This latter is the more dangerous type, associated with poor growth, dyspnea, cyanosis, and heart failure. Both systolic and diastolic murmurs are found. The diagnosis is confirmed by cardiac catheterization.

In supradiaphragmatic drainage, transfer of the abnormal veins to the left side is often possible at open heart surgery. Subdiaphragmatic lesions are often inoperable.

Eisenmenger's Complex

This is a complication which may occur in any left to right shunt, and cause the direction of shunt to reverse. This will make the patient cyanosed, and generally will aggravate his breathlessness and other symptoms. The cause of the condition is an increase in the resistance of the blood vessels in the lungs due to arteriosclerosis. This in turn increases the pressure in the pulmonary artery, right ventricle, and eventually in the right atrium.

This increase may be so great as to exceed the level in the corresponding area of the left sided circulation, causing the shunt to go the other way, e.g., from pulmonary artery to aorta in patent ductus, and right ventricle to left ventricle in ventricular septal defect.

Clinical features. Those of the primary disorder (e.g., ventricular septal defect) are present but exaggerated. Cyanosis and clubbing develop and episodes of cardiac failure occur. Hemoptysis is not uncommon. The auscultatory signs (murmurs) do not change much, but both the x-rays and E.C.G. show signs of right ventricular increase.

Treatment. Medical treatment only is advised, since surgical attempts to close any defect result in intractable failure of the right ventricle.

Conditions Associated with Right to Left Shunt

The general features found in children with this disorder include breathlessness, cyanosis, failure to grow, and frequent respiratory infections. Cyanosis and breathlessness may present in the first weeks of life, and growth failure after the first few months. In severely affected infants, paroxysms of dyspnea may culminate in loss of consciousness. Very breathless infants are often also retarded in their motor milestones. In older children, dyspnea or exertion is characteristically relieved by squatting. Abdominal or chest pain is also complained of by older children with severe right to left shunts. Clubbing (enlargement) of the toes and fingers is common in cyanosed infants. Chest deformity accompanies frequent chest infections or severe dyspnea. Polycythemia (a compensatory increase in hemoglobin level) may cause suffusion of the conjunctival vessels.

Some Specific Disorders

Tetralogy of Fallot

This consists in a ventricular septal defect and narrowing of the pulmonary valve area or the outflow tract immediately below it (the infundibulum). The aorta may communicate with the right ventricle by its relationship to the ventricular septal defect (overriding). The narrowing of the pulmonary valve area causes the right ventricular pressure to exceed that in the left ventricle, so that the right to left leak of venous blood takes place.

The general features noted above occur within a few months of birth. The physician will find evidence of an overactive right ventricle, feel a thrill in the suprasternal area, and perhaps in the precordium, and hear a systolic murmur.

At x-ray there is evidence of reduction of blood flow through the lungs (oligemia) and right ventricular enlargement. The latter is also obvious on the E.C.G. The reasons for these changes are shown in the circulatory diagram (Figure 46).

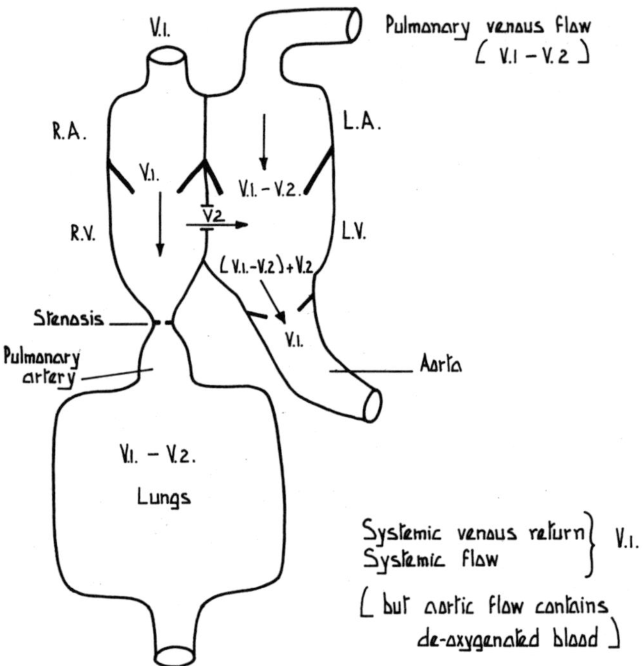

Fig. 46. Hemodynamics of tetralogy of fallot. R.A.: right atrium. R.V.: right ventricle. L.A.: left atrium. L.V.: left ventricle.

Angiocardiography will delineate the abnormal valve and the right-to-left shunt. Cardiac catheterization will demonstrate the rise in pressure in the right ventricle; often the catheter will pass through the septal defect into the aorta.

The surgical treatment of tetralogy of Fallot takes 2 forms, palliative and radical. Palliative surgery consists in increasing the blood flow to the lungs by connecting a systemic blood vessel (e.g., the subclavian artery, aorta) to the pulmonary artery or one of its branches. This procedure is mostly done in children who are too young to have a complete repair or where other abnormalities preclude it. Radical surgery is an open heart procedure at which the septal defect is closed, and the pulmonary valve repaired.

Pulmonary atresia with ventricular septal defect (pseudotruncus)

This is a more severe variant of tetralogy. The pulmonary artery has no lumen at all, so the lungs are supplied with blood either by a persisting ductus arteriosus, hypertrophied bronchial circulation, or both. The symptoms begin early in life with marked cyanosis and dyspnea. The features are otherwise as described for tetralogy. A palliative anastomosis of a systemic vessel to the pulmonary circulation is all that is surgically possible in this situation.

Pulmonary stenosis with atrial septal defect

In this condition the primary problem is the valve stenosis which increases right ventricular pressure. In turn right atrial pressure increases, and if an atrial septal defect is present, may cause a shunt of venous blood to the left atrium. It is not a very common problem, usually presenting in the early years of life with symptoms like those of mild tetralogy. The x-ray and E.C.G. signs are very similar to the latter. Confirmation of diagnosis is by angiocardiography. Open heart relief of the stenosis and closure of the septal defect is the treatment of choice.

Tricuspid atresia

This is a severe defect in which the tricuspid valve is severely malformed or absent. As a result, the right ventricle is usually tiny, and the blood supply to the lungs greatly reduced and transmitted by a tortuous course.

Clinical features. The infant often seems normal in the first weeks of life. Then cyanosis and dyspnea develop and growth and activity slow down. Paroxysmal attacks of dyspnea are common. Clubbing and chest deformity occur in the later months of life. Sudden death may occur.

Murmurs and thrills are variable in tricuspid atresia, but often resemble those described under tetralogy of Fallot. X-rays usually demonstrate reduced pulmonary blood flow and cardiac enlargement—which is almost entirely the left ventricle. The E.C.G. shows only left ventricular complexes and this is very useful guide to the diagnosis, since most cyanosis-causing disorders cause *right* ventricular overload.

The condition is treated by a palliative procedure, by anastomosis of a systemic artery, or the superior vena cava to the pulmonary circulation. The exact technique is decided at thoracotomy.

Transposition of the great vessels

This is a complex and severe defect with many variants. The commoner type is *complete* transposition, in which the aorta (supplying the systemic circulation) arises from the right ventricle, and the pulmonary artery from a left ventricle (i.e., one which receives oxygenated blood). Clearly the infant could not survive long after birth unless some opportunity is present for the venous and arterial circulations to mix, thus allowing oxygenation in the lungs. Therefore, associated defects, e.g., atrial septal, ventricular septal, and patent ductus arteriosus are usually present in those who survive birth. Severe valvular defects, e.g., atresia of the tricuspid or pulmonary valves, or mitral and aortic valve anomalies may also be found.

Clinical features. In complete transposition, the infant is breathless and cyanosed within a few hours of birth. The cyanosis is not substantially relieved by oxygen (as in respiratory distress syndrome) and congestive heart failure may be early and severe. In less severe instances, symptoms akin to those of a severe tetralogy occur within the first few months of life. Dyspnea is constant and cyanosis, clubbing, and growth failure severe.

In the newborn, murmurs may be absent. In the older child the signs of a compensatory disorder, e.g., ventricular septal defect, may be present. X-rays usually show cardiac enlargement and plethoric lungs. The diagnosis is confirmed by cardioangiography.

Treatment. This is most urgent when symptoms arise in the neonate. What is done is to increase the exchange of blood between the two circulations, usually by creating or enlarging an atrial septal defect (Rashkind procedure). This is done at the time of diagnosis, by a special cardiac catheter with an inflatable balloon at its tip. This is inserted into the left atrium, the balloon inflated with radiopaque dye, which is then pulled back into the right atrium. The atrial septum is ripped on the way. This procedure may require later repetition. In the survivors, a more radical procedure (Mustard's operation) can be done. This reroutes the systemic venous blood to the lungs and the pulmonary venous blood to the body.

Congenital heart diseases which have no shunt

Mostly these involve simple anatomical abnormalities of the heart valves, or great vessels. The commonest conditions are pulmonary valve stenosis, coarctation of the aorta, and aortic valve stenosis—more or less in that order.

These conditions are largely asymptomatic, the patients grow well, are not breathless, and are not cyanosed. In most instances the diagnosis is made because a murmur is found during an examination for some other condition such as a respiratory infection.

Pulmonary valve stenosis

In this, the valve is narrowed and distorted, causing an increase in resistance which raises the right ventricular pressure. The signs found are a thrill in the suprasternal area, a loud systolic murmur, and signs of right ventricular increase on E.C.G. and x-ray. However, the latter shows no change in the circulation of blood through the lungs, since the pulmonary blood flow is normal. The severity of the condition is measured by cardiac catheterization. If the pressure in the right ventricle is very high, the valve is refashioned to relieve the obstruction.

Aortic valve stenosis

The features of this are very similar to those described for pulmonary stenosis. Most patients are asymptomatic, and a loud murmur is the usual chief complaint. X-rays and E.C.G. show evidence of left ventricular overload and left-heart catheterization reveals a greatly increased pressure in the left ventricle. The ordinary blood pressure reading is normal. In a very tight stenosis, the valve may be refashioned at an open heart operation. This will relieve the left ventricular strain.

Isolated coarctation of the aorta

This is a narrowing of the aorta which occurs usually at the site of entrance of the ductus arteriosus.

Clinical features. The condition is usually asymptomatic, being discovered either because of a murmur heard, or because the arm blood pressure is found to be increased. In a very few infants, congestive failure may occur in the first few weeks of life.

Apart from the murmur, the characteristic sign is weak or impalpable femoral pulsations at the groin, together with low blood pressure readings in the legs as compared with the arms. A bypass (collateral) circulation develops, and this may give rise to arterial pulsations in unusual places, e.g., around the scapula, between the ribs.

As left ventricular pressure is greatly increased, the increased work load may be seen on the E.C.G. or x-ray. The latter may also show notching of the ribs due to the enlarged collateral intercostal arteries.

Special investigations are usually unnecessary. At an appropriate age (say 10 years) the narrowed area can be cut out and the aorta reconnected.

Congenital mitral valve insufficiency

This is usually associated with growth failure, dyspnea, and sometimes the early onset of heart failure. Systolic thrills and murmurs are usual signs to be found. Left atrial and ventricular enlargement may be found on x-ray or E.C.G. Most children may be treated medically for their cardiac failure. If, however, this is intractable, replacement of the defective valve may be done.

Congenital tricuspid valve insufficiency

This has the synonym of Ebstein's disease, and is due to a malposition and malformation of the valve. The main result of the subsequent insufficiency is an increase in the right atrial pressure level. If the foramen ovale is open, then a right to left shunt may follow the increase in right atrial pressure.

The condition may be suspected because a murmur is found, because growth failure and dyspnea occur, or because of the late onset of cyanosis or congestive heart failure. Surgical repair of the valve is not impossible, but seldom tried, preference being given to medical modes of control of the cardiac failure.

Special investigations in congenital heart disease

Cardiac catheterization

This investigation can be done at any age, and consists in placing a radiopaque catheter into a large vein (e.g., the femoral) and manoeuvering it into the pulmonary artery or its branches. By using a strain gauge, the pressures at various places in the heart can be measured, and by drawing samples, the oxygen content of blood at various sites can be measured. Samples for the demonstration of left to right shunts are taken in the great veins, the right atrium, the right ventricle, and the pulmonary artery. In ventricular septal defect for example, the O_2 content of the samples in the great veins and atrium would be lower than those in the right ventricle and pulmonary arteries. Some examples of oxygen contents in various defects are shown in the table 19. Using these it is possible to calculate the volume of the shunt. Occasionally shunt detection is also done by dye curve. In this technique, an injection of indocyanine green is made into the circulation and

Table 19. Example of oximetry findings at cardiac catheterization

Site	Oxygen Content (Vol %)			
	Normal	ASD	VSD	PDA
Superior vena cava	8.8	8.8	8.8	8.8
Right atrium	8.9	12.0	8.9	8.9
Inferior vena cava	9.2	9.2	9.2	9.2
Right ventricle	9.0	12.0	12.0	9.0
Pulmonary artery	9.0	12.0	12.0	12.0

ASD = Atrial septal defect.
VSD = Ventricular septal defect.
PDA = Patent ductus arteriosus.

its dilution pattern recorded by drawing arterial blood through a suitable densitometer. The shape of the curve tells whether the shunt is R→L or L→R. This technique is not often used, but can be helpful in the R→L shunt situation in which the O_2 contents in the right heart are normal.

Left heart catheterization

This may be done incidentally to right heart studies if the catheter happens to get into the left atrium or left ventricle by way of the foramen ovale, or through an atrial septal defect. Left heart catheterization is not as often done in children as in adults, principally because of the rarity of left sided lesions. Although the investigation may be done by the transeptal route, this is more difficult and perhaps more dangerous than in the adult. Accordingly, retrograde catheterization through a great vessel, e.g., a femoral or brachial artery, is usually to be preferred. By this route the condition of the aortic valve, and of the left ventricle may be determined. Left ventricular angiography will give some estimation of the degree of mitral valve insufficiency. The left atrium is not easy to enter by this route, except in the presence of mitral insufficiency. Thus, in cases of suspected mitral stenosis, the transeptal route may be preferred.

Angiocardiography

This is the method whereby an anatomical situation may be rendered visible by the injection of radiopaque substances into selected sites in the right or left heart. The patient should always be tested for sensitivity to the injectate prior to the procedure. Suitable recordings may be made, either by cinefluorography or by rapid change x-ray cassette mechanisms. The results are usually diagnostic in either case but for adequate anatomical interpretation it is essential to have views taken in two planes, viz, posteroanterior and lateral. This is particularly so in young infants where transposition syndromes are common. Angiocardiography should, as far as possible, be selective. The injection of radiopaque substances into large volume compartments, such as the right atrium, is much less likely to give satisfactory films than appropriately localized injections in the ventricle. Thus a diagnostic cardiac catheterization is done as a preliminary to angiography.

Management of the child with congenital heart disease

In infancy, if dyspnea is severe, then gavage feeding may be required. A full caloric intake is given, usually by more frequent feeds. Since these infants are more prone to chest infection than normals, protection from obvious cross-infection is helpful in the early months of life. A full course of prophylactic inoculations should be given.

Established respiratory infections should be vigorously treated by humidified air or oxygen, and antibiotics if necessary. Anemia is common and should be treated by prescription of iron.

Paroxysmal dyspnea, in cyanotic patients, is an indication for surgery. Temporary relief may be obtained by the injection of small doses of morphia. The same patients respond poorly to high environmental temperatures, so that appropriate cooling should be arranged, and the fluid intake maintained.

The parents should be warned that the child's growth may be slower than normal. Reassurance that dwarfing and mental retardation is not to be expected will often quieten their fears.

In the older child who has few symptoms, it is important that he lead as normal a life as possible. Restriction of exertion or forbidding the playing of games is to be deprecated, since it leads, in parents and child, to a preoccupation with the heart which may result in neurosis, e.g., fear of exertion.

OTHER FORMS OF HEART DISEASE

Many of these are acquired, rheumatic fever being a common cause. It is usual to describe these disorders as affecting the 3 major cardiac tissues, viz, the endocardium, myocardium, and pericardium. It should be understood, however, that all 3 tissues are frequently affected together.

Rheumatic endocarditis

This is the most important facet of rheumatic fever, complicating about 10% of first attacks, and being more common with recurrences. The inflammation and scarring of the endocardium causes abnormalities of the cardiac valves,which places a mechanical strain on the heart muscle (the myocardium). The commonest consequence of rheumatic endocarditis is mitral insufficiency alone, but combined mitral stenosis and insufficiency, or aortic insufficiency are not rare.

The consequences of mitral insufficiency or aortic valve disease are similar in that left ventricular work is increased. Mitral insufficiency or mitral stenosis also raises left atrial pressure, and this increase is reflected back via the pulmonary veins to the pulmonary circulation. Thus, right ventricular pressure, and hence right ventricular work, will increase. Clearly then, mitral insufficiency can lead to combined ventricular failure. There are of course many grades of severity, so that valvular disease may be asymptomatic for many years.

The diagnosis of valvular defects is usually suggested by auscultation of the heart. Systolic murmurs are common in insufficiency of the atrioventricular (mitral and tricuspid) valves and diastolic murmurs are characteristic of *stenosis* of these same valves. In relation to the arterial (pulmonary and aortic) valves, stenosis causes systolic murmurs and insufficiency diastolic murmurs.

In mild disorders, neither the x-rays nor E.C.G. are abnormal. The changes otherwise can be predicted from the mechanical effects of the valve abnormality. Thus, in *mitral insufficiency*, the left ventricle increases in size, as does the left atrium. Secondary pulmonary hypertension will cause increase in the right ventricular and ultimately right atrial size. In *mitral stenosis*, only the left atrium increases in size, to be followed by the effects of pulmonary hypertension. In *aortic* stenosis or insufficiency, only the left ventricle normally becomes enlarged. In *tricuspid* disease, only the right ventricle and atrium enlarge.

The E.C.G. changes follow those noted above. The P waves (which reflect atrial activity) may enlarge or split (become bifid). Ventricular overload is reflected in the appropriate leads and ventricular complexes.

In general, other special investigations are rarely used in rheumatic endocarditis. Left heart catheterization and angiography may be used to estimate the degree of mitral insufficiency.

Conservative management is usual for children with rheumatic heart disease. Only an occasional patient will require operation upon, or replacement of, a heart valve, usually because of intractable cardiac failure.

Endocardial fibroelastosis

The cause of this condition is unknown, but it is associated with the formation of a membrane on the endocardium, and by degeneration of the myocardium.

Clinical features. These come on early in life, and are those of congenital heart disease in general. Specifically there is a strong risk of congestive heart failure. The mitral valve is the usual site of trouble, and appropriate murmurs may be present. Medical management of the cardiac failure is all that is possible.

Sub-acute bacterial endocarditis

This is a rare condition until the teenage period; mostly it is implanted upon rheumatic fever. Occasionally it happens in sufferers from congenital heart disease.

Clinical features. These are superimposed upon the primary condition. The onset is usually subacute with lethargy, anorexia, general malaise, and dyspnea; fever is usual, and loss of weight almost invariable. Occasionally the sudden onset of congestive failure in a previously well-compensated lesion may be the presenting feature. Physical examination reveals an ill-looking child, with a pallid, muddy complexion, and evidence of recent weight loss. The skin may show purpuric spots (these may be a symptom) and the spleen is enlarged. Splinter hemorrhages under the nails are inconsistent. Urinalysis usually shows many red cells. Anemia, high sedimentation rates, and leucocytosis are usual. The cardiac murmurs may show changes, e.g., diastolic bruits may develop in previous mitral insufficiency, and the heart increases in size. In late cases, embolic phenomena (to the peripheral limb vessels, or to the brain) may cause appropriate symptoms and signs. Clubbing is only of significance if it was previously absent. Blood cultures (which should be repeated at least 3 times) usually reveal a growth of streptococcus viridans.

Prevention. Surgical and dental procedures should always be carried out under penicillin cover in patients with rheumatic or congenital heart disease.

Treatment. Antibiotics should be used in full dosage, according to the sensitivity pattern of the organism. Treatment should continue for 4-6 weeks. Supportive therapy, such as blood transfusion is often necessary. Congestive cardiac failure requires appropriate therapy.

Diseases of the myocardium

The heart muscle may be affected in many conditions. Direct poisoning may occur from the toxin of diphtheria, viral (coxsackie) infections may involve it, or degeneration may occur in the collagen disorders (e.g., lupus erythematosus), or, if the coronary arteries arise from an abnormal site such as the pulmonary artery. In thalassemia, iron depositions and chronic anemia cause a myocarditis. This complication also occurs in glycogen storage (Pompe's) disease, the mucopolysaccharidoses (gargoylism), and in the late stages of muscular dystrophy.

Clinical features. Those of the primary disease, e.g., diphtheria, are present. Thus the patient becomes breathless, shows rib retraction, and develops blueness of the hands, feet, and face. The pulse becomes rapid and the heart is found to be enlarged clinically, and by x-ray. Florid congestive cardiac failure may ensue, with edema and hepatomegaly. The main auscultatory sign is a loud gallop rhythm.

In the viral myocarditis of the newborn, the infant suddenly develops dyspnea, refusal to feed, and restlessness. Congestive failure soon sets in. The x-rays show marked cardiac enlargement, and pulmonary edema.

The treatment of myocarditis is confined to care of the congestive cardiac failure, or to the underlying causative disease.

Disorders of the pericardium

Pericarditis

This is rare in children. Most episodes are associated with the pancarditis of rheumatic fever. Occasional children are affected by extension of staphylococcal pneumonia to the pericardium, or by pericardial involvement in rheumatoid arthritis or disseminated lupus erythematosus.

Clinical features. The patient is restless and uncomfortable, with pain in the chest or abdomen which may be very severe. On auscultation a leathery creak can be heard. This is the so-called pericardial rub.

Treatment. Analgesics are given for the pain, and the underlying disease treated.

Pericarditis with effusion

This usually occurs in the course of rheumatic fever. Its early features are those of a simple pericarditis. If the effusion develops rapidly, tension upon the heart causes dyspnea, bulging of the neck veins, and often signs of acute cardiac failure with liver enlargement and ascites.

The treatment is to aspirate the effusion if pressure symptoms occur. Otherwise it is that of the primary disease.

Disorders of cardiac rhythm and rate

Rhythm disorders

Sinus arrhythmia, is a normal situation in which the rate increases in inspiration and decreases in expiration, The rhythm becomes perfectly regular on exercising.

Extrasystoles. These are extra interpolated beats of the heart. They may originate either from the ventricles, or from the atrial areas. Extrasystoles are of little significance, although they may occur during rheumatic fever and diphtheria. Digitalis also may cause them, and if this happens, the dosage should be reviewed.

Rate disorders

Tachycardias. This means that the heart rate is increased. The most common type which is harmless, is *sinus tachycardia*. This occurs after exercise, and if the child is frightened or anxious, or during infections, especially of the respiratory system. In little children, the rate may be as high as 200/minute. The electrocardiogram shows normal complexes. The treatment is that of the underlying state.

Paroxysmal tachycardia. This is a very rapid heart rate which originates from an abnormal focus in the atrium. In many children, the attacks last only a short time, the main symptom being a feeling of anxiety and fluttering in the chest. Prolonged attacks of tachycardia decrease cardiac efficiency, so that congestive cardiac failure can arise. The E.C.G. shows abnormal complexes and the P waves are invisible. No treatment is needed in short paroxysms. More prolonged attacks can be controlled by digitalis.

Atrial flutter. This is another variant of paroxysmal tachycardia. It can be identified only by E.C.G. Its symptoms and treatment are as described above.

In *atrial fibrillation*, the heart rate is not only fast, but it is irregular, causing considerable interference with the heart's efficiency. This disorder is not common in children, but it does occur during severe rheumatic fever, or in those with a formidable valve disorder. The pulse is rapid and irregular, the abnormality being aggravated by exertion. It is confirmed by E.C.G. The treatment is to give digitalis to slow the heart. The abnormal rhythm may be abolished by quinidine, or occasionally by controlled electric shock (cardioversion).

Ventricular fibrillation

This is a terminal phenomenon, occurring in cardiac and other types of surgery. Cardiac massage and electrical defibrillation are sometimes effective in restoring a normal heart beat.

Conditions associated with a slow heart rate

This is defined as a bradycardia, and in most children it is of no significance, a rate of around 50 being quite common in active, athletic older children. In infants, however, it may be due to neonatal cold injury or occasionally severe hypothroidism. Sinus bradycardia of this type requires no treatment, other than that of the underlying condition.

The other situation in which a slow heart rate occurs is in heart block (atrioventricular dissociation). This happens because the area which determines the basic normal heart rate of around 70/minute is situated in the atrium. If the communication to the ventricles is broken, then the intrinsic rate of the ventricles sets the speed of the heart, and this ventricular rate is of the order of 40-60/minute. The condition may be congenital and have no background of disease, or it may occur as part of a congenital anatomical defect of the heart, e.g., corrected transposition. Otherwise it is most often found in children who have been treated with digitalis. In most instances there are no specific symptoms. Rarely, if the heart is changing from slow to normal speed, and vice versa, the patient may have Stokes-Adams attacks. These are transient attacks of unconsciousness because the blood supply to the brain is interrupted. The diagnosis is made by electrocardiogram, and the treatment is usually that of the underlying disease. If the Stokes-Adams attacks are severe and intractable then a pacemaker can be implanted to maintain a more normal rhythm. It should be emphasized, however, that this is very rarely done in children.

Disorder of the systemic circulation

Arterial hypertension

High blood pressure is not common in children. Very often the hypertension is due to the child's apprehension, or to taking the blood pressure with a too narrow cuff. Apprehension is usually easily recognized and the resulting hypertension disappears when the child is calmed or asleep.

Otherwise, the commonest causes of hypertension in children are coarctation of the aorta and renal disease. In renal disease the usual cause is acute hemorrhagic glomerulonephritis, in which the hypertension is usually of short duration. Chronic renal disease, such as pyelonephritis, may result in some degree of renal failure, and one of the signs of renal failure is hypertension. If coarctation and renal disease are excluded then it is important to remember that high blood pressure may be due to raised intracranial pressure. This is usually due to cerebral tumour and there is a history of vomiting, headache, and the sign of papilledema. Lead poisoning also raises the pressure within the skull and may be the cause of the systemic hypertension. Very rare causes are the tumours in the sympathetic system, e.g., pheochromocytoma, which produce catecholamines (e.g., adrenalin) which are capable of raising the blood pressure. Steroid treatment may also cause hypertension, especially if given in excess dosage.

Another substance which can cause high blood pressure is renin, and its product, angiotensin. These are normally produced by the body but the production rate can increase if the blood supply to the kidney is reduced. This would happen in stenosis of the renal artery, but is a very unusual problem in children.

Treatment. This depends upon the underlying cause. Obviously if the condition is due to drugs or raised intracranial pressure, then it will respond to appropriate action. If the child has essential hypertension, i.e. high blood pressure without obvious precipitating cause, then antihypertensive drugs are used, as in adults. The substances in common use are chlorothiazide combined with another antihypertensive drug such as guanethidine or methyldopa.

Disorders of the pulmonary circulation

The normal pressure in the pulmonary artery and right ventricle is about 20 mm of mercury. If this is greatly increased then the condition is called pulmonary hypertension, which in turn increases the work done by the right heart which may eventually fail. High blood pressure in the pulmonary vessels may occur as part of a congenital cardiac defect (see Eisenmenger's complex above) or be due to chronic lung disease, usually mucoviscidosis, chronic bronchitis, or bronchiectasis. The clinical features are those of the primary disease so there will be cough, purulent sputum, finger clubbing, growth failure, and cyanosis. The E.C.G. and x-rays will show evidence of the increased work done by the right ventricle. Heart failure in this condition is often precipated by a respiratory infection which further increases the resistance in the lung vessels. The treatment is that of the chest condition and digitalis and diuretics for the heart failure.

Primary pulmonary hypertension is a rare condition, associated with arteriosclerosis of the lung vessels, often occurring early in life. Usually there are no clinical features until the child becomes breathless because of the cardiac embarrassment, or develops congestive cardiac failure. No specific treatment is available. Digitalis and diuretics are given for the cardiac failure.

13 Disorders of the urogenital system

ANATOMY AND PHYSIOLOGY

The principal activity of the kidney is to maintain water, electrolyte, and acid-base balance, and to excrete nitrogenous waste products. The functional unit is the nephron. This begins as the glomerulus, which is a tuft of capillaries located in the renal cortex, surrounded by Bowman's capsule, which communicates with the tubular apparatus. This is made up successively of the proximal convoluted tubule, the pars recta (straight descending limb), the hairpin-like loop of Henle, and the ascending limb which terminates in the distal convoluted tubule. The latter, placed near the glomerulus, enters the system of collecting ducts, which in turn enter the renal calyces. The glomeruli, the proximal, distal convoluted tubules and many loops of Henle lie in the renal cortex. The tubules attached to the deeper glomeruli run a long course in the medulla.

The main function of the glomerulus is to form a plasma ultra filtrate and to pass this filtrate to the tubule for further processing. Tubular function is a blend of active transport mechanisms (secretion and resorption), and of diffusion processes which do not demand energy. An example of the former is the active resorption of glucose; of the latter, the excretion of urea.

Most of the residual protein and glucose presented to the tubule is resorbed in the proximal convolution. There is, however, a limit to this process, so that glycosuria occurs over the normal renal threshold of 180 g%. The same threshold concept applies to the resorption of aminoacids which are also moved at the convoluted tubule. If an excess of aminoacid is present in the blood, aminoaciduria will occur. The proximal convoluted tubule also reabsorbs phosphate, being controlled by the action of the parathyroids, and the volume of the extracellular space.

Sodium is actively resorbed mainly in the proximal tubule, but also in the descending and ascending limbs of Henle's loop. In the distal tubule, active resorption of sodium occurs, some of it in exchange for H^+ and K^+ ion, some in association with chloride diffusion. *Water* resorption is largely brought about by passive diffusion in relation to the process of sodium resorption, and occurs in the same areas. *Potassium* is both resorbed and secreted. Almost all of the potassium in the glomerular filtrate is resorbed by the proximal tubule. Potassium is then added to the urine at the distal tubule in exchange for sodium. This is an active transport mechanism. Chloride is transported by diffusion, and largely follows the flux of sodium. Hydrogen H^+ ion is also excreted by the tubular apparatus. There are 3 modes of ion exchange, the bicarbonate method, the phosphate (PO_4) buffer system, and the formation of ammonia.

Water is reabsorbed (or the urine is concentrated) throughout the tubular system. The activity of the distal convoluted tubule and collecting duct of the tubular apparatus can be affected by the action of antidiuretic hormone (ADH) This mechanism helps the kidney to produce a concentrated or dilute urine as circumstances demand.

Urea, the main nitrogenous waste product is readily diffusible, so the kidney uses little energy in excreting it. Generally urea excretion follows water excretion, so that urea clearance will increase with increased urinary flow.

Active (energy using) tubular mechanisms exist for the secretion of substances such as creatinine and drugs which are used therapeutically.

SPECIFIC DISORDERS

Congenital Defects

Agenesis (Absence) of the Kidneys

Clinical features. These occur only when both kidneys are absent. The newborn infant is difficult to resuscitate, breathless, and soon dies from renal failure. The diagnosis, in boys, may be suggested by the appearance (Potter facies). The child looks abnormal, the nose is flat, and the ears large and underslung. The legs may also show congenital defects. There is no treatment for this condition.

Congenital Hypoplastic Kidneys

In this, the kidney is only partly developed. If both are affected, the child develops renal failure, with growth deficit, thirst (polydipsia), polyuria, and biochemical evidence of renal failure. There is usually also renal infection which may progress to septicemia.

If a single kidney is affected, the usual problem is of recurrent urinary infection.

Treatment. If only one kidney is involved, and infection is present, nephrectomy is done. If both kidneys are hypoplastic, infection is controlled if possible, otherwise treatment is as shown for chronic renal failure (see below).

Multicystic Kidney

Clinical features. This condition is usually suspected by finding an abnormal mass which turns out to be an enlarged, functionless, kidney. The treatment is surgical removal.

Polycystic Kidneys

In this, both kidneys have cysts in them. The main clinical feature is feeling the enlarged kidneys at routine examination. Otherwise, the child may present with evidence of renal failure—lethargy, slow growth, failure to feed, and dehydration. The diagnosis can usually be confirmed by pyelography, which shows the distortion of kidney structure by the cysts.

Treatment. None is available except for that of renal failure.

Fused and Ectopic Kidneys

Many of these anomalies are asymptomatic. In some, pyelonephritis, hydronephrosis, or stones may occur. There are many types; the commoner are the following.

The horse-shoe kidney. In this condition, a band of renal tissue joins the lower pole of each kidney. The renal pelvis is downward displaced and turned forward. This feature, and the inward displacement of the lower calyx, are visible on pyelography, which is the mode of recognition.

Ectopic kidneys, are usually displaced downwards, even into the pelvis. In crossed ectopia, both kidneys are on the same side.

Clinical features. These are of the complication such as pyelonephritis or stone.

Treatment. None is necessary except where complications have occurred. In these, nephrectomy is commonly necessary.

SYDNROMES OF OBSTRUCTIVE UROPATHY

In most children, these are due to some congenital abnormality which usually can be distinguished only by special investigations. The *clinical features* are rather variable, but divide themselves into several patterns. The most common is episodic urinary infection, especially in young children. Growth delay with renal failure is a rather late phenomenon, but unfortunately one which occurs regularly. Less often symptoms of urinary infection, or stone, or the palpation of an enlarged kidney or bladder may be the first sign of the condition. Enuresis is seldom a symptom of obstructive uropathy, but may be the initial complaint, either of chronic renal failure, or of retention with overflow.

High Ureteric Obstruction

This leads to hydronephrosis (dilatation of the pelvis and kidney) with variable degrees of renal destruction. It is usually associated with ureteric stenosis or kinking of the ureter in its upper part. An aberrant blood vessel may occasionally be the cause. The condition is usually unilateral.

Clinical features. The hydronephrosis may present as a palpable mass soon after birth, and may have no other symptom. In other children the condition is revealed after investigation for urinary infection.

Low Ureteric Obstruction

This must, of course, cause hydroureter (dilatation of the ureter) as well as hydronephrosis. Unilateral cases are usually due to stenosis at the ureterovesical junction. If the narrowing affects only the mucosa of the ureteral opening, a *ureterocele* is formed. In others, the stenosis is longer and involves the lower part of the ureter in its course outside the bladder.

Clinical features. Usually the child presents with a urinary infection, and the condition is confirmed by pyelography or cystography.

Treatment. In many cases, especially of ureterocele, ureteric reimplantation can be carried out to short circuit the obstruction.

Ectopic Ureters

These are rather rare conditions, the majority being extra ureters derived from the upper pelvis of a double kidney. Thus, they may open normally into the bladder, and then be symptomless. However, obstruction may occur when the opening is into some other part of the genitourinary tract.

In boys, the opening is most commonly into the posterior urethra, occasionally into some part of the seminiferous system. In these sites, obstruction and infection may occur, but urinary incontinence is absent because the abnormal opening is proximal to the sphincter. In the female, the ectopic ureter may open into the urethra below the sphincter, or into the vagina or vestibule. Such an opening is associated with incontinence, which expresses itself as dribbling in spite of normal micturition. This symptom may occur only during the day—so called vertical enuresis.

Diagnosis. This is a matter of some difficulty. In double kidney ureter, the pyelogram may be of great help in suspecting the primary condition. If cystoscopy reveals only 2 ureteric orifices, the ureter must be bifid—which may be revealed by retrograde ureterography—or completely duplicated and ectopic. The latter commonly requires surgical exploration to demonstrate the site of final drainage.

Treatment. This is surgical, and usually consists in removal of the dilated ectopic ureter and its associated renal tissue.

Ureteric Reflux

This may follow bladder outlet obstruction or occur by itself. The cause is apparently physiological rather than anatomical.

Clinical features. The child usually has a urinary infection, acute or chronic. The intravenous pyelogram may seem normal, but on cinecystography the dilated ureters are seen on micturition. A minor degree of hydronephrosis is not uncommon. If untreated, the constant urinary infections will lead to chronic renal failure.

Differential diagnosis. This must always be from chronic bladder neck obstruction, or other conditions (e.g., tuberculosis) causing cystitis. These are usually readily excluded by cystography.

Treatment. The major problem is to prevent progressive pyelonephritis. In many cases this can be achieved by medical means alone. If infection is frequent or intractable, operative procedures are indicated.

LOWER URINARY TRACT OBSTRUCTION

This is much more common in males, because of their greater urogenital complexity. In either sex, however, the obstruction may be neurogenic with paralysis of the external sphincter and subsequent urinary retention. This is perhaps most commonly due to meningomyelocele, although spinal trauma or tumours may be the cause. In these children, the neurological problem is primary, and the urinary problem a later one. Deficiency of the musculature of the abdominal wall may also cause obstruction of the lower urinary tract.

Thus, in the *megacystis megaureter syndrome*, which is of unknown etiology, there is often no true chronic retention, but the child voids infrequently, and the bladder is very large. The condition is rare and resistant to surgical repair.

An important and relatively common condition in males is that of *congenital posterior urethral valves*. In congenital bladder neck obstruction (Marion's disease), there is also an abnormality of the posterior urethra. This condition may occur in either sex.

General clinical features. Failure to empty the bladder leads to urinary infection and this is the usual problem. In other cases, the enlarged bladder is discovered at routine examination. In all too many children, chronic renal failure is the presenting feature. Chronic retention of urine is often associated with overflow incontinence, but this symptom is usually underestimated because of the age of the patient. Infrequency of micturition may be a feature of the megacystis megaureter syndrome. Most children with obstructive uropathy are undersized.

In all such children, the bladder is enlarged and does not empty completely after micturition. Dribbling of urine is common and the urinary stream may be weak. The kidneys may be palpable because of secondary hydronephrosis.

Specific diagnosis. In those children with neurogenic bladder, the underlying neurological deficits are usually readily appreciable and urine is easily expressed from the bladder. In all, evidence of urinary infection (pyuria, increased colony count) is common, even in the absence of obvious symptoms of infection.

Provided that renal function is still adequate, intravenous pyelography may show bilateral hydronephrosis and hydroureter. Cinecystogram with micturating films should always be carried out, as these will demonstrate posterior urethral valves and other causes of obstruction.

Treatment. This is surgical and should be carried out even if there is evidence of renal failure, but after treatment of any infection.

In neurogenic bladder, urinary diversion into an ileal loop may be necessary. Such procedures are followed by constant prophylaxis of urinary infection and also attention to the prevention and treatment of hypochloremic acidosis. This is a dehydrating, salt- and chloride-losing, condition, requiring treatment with fluid and alkali.

Congenital Absence of the Abdominal Muscles (prune-belly syndrome)

Clinical features. This curious condition affects males and is associated with congenital defects of the feet and arms. The most obvious feature is the wrinkled, soft, sometimes distended abdominal wall, through which can be felt the dilated bladder and the viscera. No abdominal muscles are palpable, and the testes are undescended. Many of these infants die soon after birth. In the survivors, most rapidly develop urinary infection and renal failure. Intravenous pyelogram, or cystogram, confirms the presence of an enormous bladder with hydroureter and hydronephroses.

Treatment. Nephrostomy for urinary drainage and general attention to the fluid and electrolyte situation are indicated, as well as search and treatment for urinary infection.

URINARY INFECTION

The usual type is pyelonephritis which is a common disorder, occurring principally in females, and often early in life. If not properly treated, the infection will become chronic and cause renal failure in later years.

In many instances, urinary infection is associated with an anatomical or physiological abnormality of the renal tract (see obstructive uropathy) which causes urinary stasis. This is especially so in male patients, and is common enough in females to warrant full investigation.

Clinical features. In the first 2 years of life these are often nonspecific, with fever, irritability, anorexia, and vomiting. Diarrhea may also occur. Definite urinary symptoms such as frequency, or discomfort on micturition (dysuria) are often minor features in this age group. Sometimes the diagnosis is suspected only after finding pus cells in the urine of a vaguely ill child. In the older child, frequency and dysuria are more obvious, as well as a fever, vomiting, and abdominal pain. In a few children, sudden enuresis is a feature.

The diagnosis is confirmed by finding pus cells in the urine and culturing organisms from it.

Further investigations in Children with Urinary Infections

The estimation of residual urine requires the child's cooperation. This is so uncommon in the early years, that it is, to a large extent, worthless. Intravenous pyelography is the usual screening test for anatomical abnormality. Cinefluorocystography should be carried out in order to investigate the physiological state of the urinary tract.

Differential diagnosis. Mistakes are most liable to be made in the early months of life. The preponderance of vomiting, irritability, and anorexia in these children recalls the symptom complex of meningitis. Infective gastroenteritis may be suspected if diarrhea is present. In a severely ill, dehydrated child, the clinical picture is not unlike a severe septicemia (which indeed it may have become).

Treatment. In general, treatment depends on whether or not there is an underlying anatomical or physiological abnormality. If these are present, then surgical correction should be carried out if possible. Where reflux exists without obvious anatomical abnormality, the technique of multiple voiding is used.

The drugs used for an acute attack are sulphonamides, nitrofurantoin, and nalidixic acid. These will deal with most infections due to *E. coli*. These drugs should be used only on a definite bacteriological basis. Symptomatic treatment, especially in the younger child, may include intravenous fluids for the relief of dehydration.

Follow-up. Any patient who has had a urinary infection, requires careful and prolonged follow-up, if the incidence of chronic pyelonephritis is to be reduced. Accordingly, urinary examination for pus cells should continue over at least 6 months and tests should be normal for at least 4 months before final cure is accepted.

Prevention of urinary infection. This is indicated principally in those children who have neurological abnormalities such as meningomyelocele, and in whom multiple micturition or other manoeuvres have failed to prevent urinary infection. In these and any children with inoperable anatomical abnormalities, the long-term use of small doses of sulphonamides, nitrofurantoin, or nalidixic acid is in order, but should be embarked upon with care.

DISORDERS OF THE GLOMERULUS

Acute Hemorrhagic Glomerulonephritis

This condition is rare until after the second birthday, and is related to a previous streptococcal infection, usually tonsillitis, less commonly impetigo or scarlatina.

Clinical features. The child is vaguely unwell for a day or two, then the parents notice that he is passing dark urine, and that his face is swollen with edema. Oliguria (infrequent passing of small amounts of urine) may also be a complaint. Examination shows a pallid child with a variable amount of edema, usually most marked in the face, but present also in the pretibial areas, sacrum, and occasionally in the scrotum. Hypertension is present, usually only to a moderate degree. Evidence of streptococcal infection, e.g., tonsillitis may also be present.

Rarely the hypertension may be so severe as to cause the presenting complaint. This is *hypertensive encephalopathy* in which the child becomes drowsy or comatose and may have convulsions. Papilledema confirms the raised intracranial pressure. Less common is *acute left heart failure* with breathlessness and edema of the lungs.

Urinalysis reveals many red cells, proteinuria, and the presence of red cell casts. Blood examination will reveal anemia, reflecting the urinary blood loss. The antistreptolysin titre is often increased, suggesting a previous streptococcal infection, and the blood complement (an immune factor) may be decreased. If oliguria is extreme, there is evidence of nitrogen retention.

Differential diagnosis. As the principle sign is hematuria, this is the cardinal area of differential diagnosis. Scares may arise when the urine is pigmented—commonly after beetroot ingestion or eosin dyes in sweets.

Hematuria may be due to stones in the renal tract, but these are always associated with pain; Henoch-Schönlein syndrome may present with hematuria, purpura, joint pain, and swelling and abdominal colic. In Henoch-Schönlein syndrome, hematuria signifies a nephritic process.

Progress. In most sufferers, the disease is soon over. The edema and hematuria clear, and urinary output returns to normal within a week or two. The only abnormality present may be an excess of red cells when the urine is examined by microscope. In only a few does the edema and other changes fail to clear up and the condition merge into the nephrotic syndrome (see below).

Treatment. Streptococcal infection is cleared up by giving penicillin. A normal fluid intake is usually prescribed but a careful fluid chart should be kept especially in the oliguric phase. No special dietary prescription is required in view of the short-lived nature of the disease. Prolonged bed rest is unnecessary. Hypertensive encephalopathy seldom needs vigorous treatment as spontaneous recovery is the rule. Marked hypertension and retinal changes indicate the need for antihypertensive drugs, such as hydralazine and rauwolfia products. Follow-up consists in preventing further streptococcal infection (by penicillin prophylaxis if necessary) and by ensuring that the red cell count in the urine decreases. This is a sure sign of healing. If it does not occur, and if proteinuria is also present, further investigation, e.g., by renal biopsy, may be needed. This is, unusual, however, as in general the prognosis of glomerulonephritis is very good.

NEPHROTIC SYNDROME

This is the name given to a disorder of the nephron whose main features are edema and proteinuria. The use of the term syndrome implies that the exact cause of the disease is not always known, and that its clinical features, and response to treatment, may be very variable. Nowadays it is usual to carry out renal biopsy in these patients and a classification by the microscopic examination of the biopsy has been proposed. This would include varieties of the nephrotic syndrome called *minimal-change* lesion, i.e., likely to respond well to treatment, or *membrano-proliferative*, i.e., extensive changes in the nephron implying resistance to treatment and a deteriorating course. Intermediate varieties also occur.

While in most children no cause can be found, the disorder may complicate an autoimmune condition such as lupus erythematosus, or follow exposure to heavy metals (mercury) or various drugs.

Clinical features. The sole symptoms are swelling and pallor. The edema is universal, though best seen in the soft tissues of the face, hands, legs, and feet. The abdomen is full of fluid, as may be the pleural spaces, and dyspnea may occur. The general health is little affected, although when gross fluid is accumulating observant parents will conclude that the child is not passing much urine. The pallor seen is not due to a true anemia.

The diagnosis is made upon the presence of general edema, with marked proteinuria. Renal function is unimpaired so that blood chemistry is normal. So is the urine, apart from proteinuria and some fatty casts. As this loss of protein continues, the plasma albumin fraction decreases, with a relative increase in the globulins. Cholesterol levels are usually increased. In a few cases, spontaneous remission may occur. This is preceded by a decrease in the proteinuria followed by weight loss as the fluid is excreted. With the completion of diuresis, obvious muscle wasting is seen. The same picture occurs with an induced remission. In both circumstances, the reappearance of proteinuria may herald a return of fluid accumulation. Oliguria and severe proteinuria accompany this aggravation.

At any time the child may develop infections. Mostly these are minor, such as tonsillitis, but may be associated with a return of the disease. Much less common, but more dangerous, are pneumococcal infections such as peritonitis and pneumonia. As the child may be on steroids, the usual symptoms of inflammation may be absent. Any vague illness in the edematous child who is on steroids should demand a diagnostic peritoneal or pleural tap, since, if unrecognized, the infection may progress to a state of shock and early death.

In a few cases, where acute glomerulonephritis has preceded the disease, microscopic or gross hematuria will indicate a superimposition of the original lesion. Renal failure will occur in those unfortunate children who often show no real remission (see below).

General care. Rest in bed is unnecessary unless the edema is so gross as to fatigue the child. He should be allowed his own choice in this regard. Accurate weighing will quantitate the degree of edema.

Dietary protein should be increased to maximum tolerance. Low salt diets are potentially dangerous, and should be confined to those treated in hospital.

Induction of remission. This may occur spontaneously, but cannot be relied upon. The preferred treatment is with steroids. Dosage is high, and is given in periods of 10-14 days, after which it is reduced. If diuresis does not occur in the following week high doses should begin again, and the cycle continued until diuresis occurs. A reduction in urinary protein is a good sign. When loss of weight indicates remission, it should be remembered that massive loss of sodium and potassium may occur. Dietary restriction of sodium should be abandoned at this stage and, if necessary, salt and potassium supplements given.

Transfusion with plasma, hypertonic salt-free dextran, and aminoacids are valueless in the treatment of the nephrotic syndrome. Similarly, diuretics are of limited value. A partial remission may be helped along by giving chlorothiazide (with K supplement). Aldosterone inhibitors as yet have an unknown place in therapy. In certain situations (steroid resistance, biopsy indications) the immunosuppressant azothioprin may have a place in therapy.

Management of the remission. With the dangers of sodium and potassium loss over, the long-term treatment may be planned. The mother should be taught to test the urine daily for protein (by a stick method) and should report regularly. Similarly, she should weigh the child twice weekly. Proteinuria and increasing weight are danger signs which must be taken seriously, and may indicate the need to increase the dose of steroids. Steroids may be continued for long periods in small quantities, and this may help to maintain a remission. Regular throat swabs are done and appropriate steps taken if infection is found.

Prognosis. A considerable number (30%) have a total remission. Many others have remissions and aggravations over several years. Some develop a progressive glomerulonephritis leading to ultimate renal failure.

DISORDERS OF THE RENAL TUBULE

The renal tubule reabsorbs body water which is passed from the glomerulus, as well as most of the aminoacids, glucose, sodium, potassium, bicarbonate, phosphate. It follows then that disease states may exist which represent a disorder of one or more of the above functions.

Disorders of reabsorption of aminoacids

It would appear that there are 3 principal independent mechanisms for the reabsorption of urinary amino acids. One deals with cystine, arginine, lysine and ornithine. Another reabsorbs proline and hydroxyproline, and the third absorbs 13 or 14 different amino acids.

Cystinuria

This is a genetically determined condition in which cystine, arginine, ornithine, and lysine are excreted in large quantities in the urine.

Clinical features. The urinary cystine is relatively insoluble and tends to form renal stones. Thus, the first indication is usually an attack of renal colic. Urinary infection may occur if the stone is in the bladder. Occasionally large bilateral staghorn calculi form, which could precipitate renal failure. The diagnosis is confirmed by finding amino acids in the urine and by analysis of the stone.

Treatment. The fluid intake should be increased and treatment with penicillamine may be of value in severe stone formers, since it makes the cystine more soluble.

Hartnup Disease

In this condition, the neutral amino acids are ineffectively transported by the renal tubule and the cells of the jejunum, so that tryptophan metabolism and nicotinamide synthesis are interfered with. The nicotinamide lack gives rise to the characteristic skin lesions of pellagra. Associated is episodic cerebellar ataxia. Mental retardation may coexist.

Treatment. Nicotinamide is specific for the skin lesions. The cerebellar episodes may be treated by temporary reduction of protein intake and gut sterilization with neomycin.

De Toni-Fanconi-Debré Sydnrome

This disease is associated with abnormal losses of glucose, amino acids, phosphate, and bicarbonate in the urine. Total renal failure follows, and is the usual mode of death. The phosphaturia gives rise to a resistant rickets, and the chronic acidosis may be associated with problems of fluid and electrolytes.

Clinical features. The infant usually seems normal during the first 6 months. Then there is failure to grow and gain weight, vomiting, episodes of dehydration, and unexplained fever. Polyuria and polydipsia may be noted and suggest renal failure. In other cases, the features of rickets are the first complaints. Physical examination confirms the failure of growth. Metaphyseal swelling and bone deformation denote rickets.

Biochemical features. There is glycosuria, and an abnormally high amino aciduria, and urinary phosphate. Arterial pH is low, and urinary pH is relatively high. The features of renal failure are also found.

X-rays. Initially there is evidence of decalcification followed by the features of rickets.

Differential diagnosis. This is most commonly from renal failure due to other causes such as hypoplasia of the kidneys, or chronic infection. Renal tubular acidosis (see below) may cause confusion, although in this disease there is neither glycosuria nor aminoaciduria. Other causes of vitamin D resistant rickets may be considered.

Prognosis. This condition is generally fatal, with terminal renal failure.

Treatment. This is based upon replacement of the expected losses.

There is no specific therapy. The episodes of dehydration are treated on general lines. Otherwise, treatment divides itself into the care of the rickets by high dose of vitamin D, with calcium and phosphate dietary supplements. The acidosis is difficult to treat, but may partially respond to alkali therapy.

Other Renal Tubular Problems

Cystinosis

This condition is really a variant of the de Toni-Fanconi-Debré syndrome, except that signs of renal failure are very clear indeed and hypokalemia is an important cause of clinical deterioration. Photophobia is common and growth failure marked.

Oculocerebrorenal Syndromes (Lowe's disease)

These are rare, hereditary conditions which affect males.

Clinical features. These children are mentally retarded, and have large eyes, commonly with buphthalmos. Bilateral cataracts are always present. Signs of rickets are present by the first birthday, and pathological fractures occur. Proteinuria and a generalized aminoaciduria are present, together with increased organic acids. Episodes of dehydration are common and early death from renal failure usual.

Isolated Renal Tubular Acidosis

This is a rare familiar condition in which the renal tubule is unable to excrete hydrogen ion. This exists as an isolated defect, although it may be one of a combination of disorders in the Fanconi syndrome.

Clinical features. The onset may be in infancy, with failure to grow and gain, vomiting and episodes of severe dehydration. Polyuria is sometimes a complaint.

Differential diagnosis. In infancy, the dehydration may be confused with that due to gastroenteritis, or the salt losing adrenocortical syndrome. However, the biochemical changes are different, and age of onset usually earlier. Renal failure may be clinically similar, but has demonstrable poverty of renal function. In the older patient, renal tubular acidosis may be associated with rickets or nephrocalcinosis.

Treatment. The infantile type is treated by the administration of alkali in the form of a mixture of potassium citrate and sodium bicarbonate. The dose should be adjusted to maintain arterial and urinary pH values within normal limits. The episodes of acute dehydration usually require intravenous fluid and electrolyte therapy.

Nephrogenic Diabetes Insipidus

This is a condition in which the renal tubule is unable to respond to antidiuretic hormone. The clinical features are those of the ordinary type of diabetes insipidus, e.g., polydipsia and polyuria.

In the infant, or young child, the inability to get to a source of water may cause dehydration and electrolyte imbalance. The condition is diagnosed by finding a low specific gravity urine, in the absence of supporting signs of renal failure, and by the failure of vasopressin to relieve the condition. Thiazide diuretics will usually cause some decrease in the polyuria, but in all instances the child should be given unlimited access to fluid.

ACUTE RENAL FAILURE

Etiology. Conventionally the syndrome is divided into those due to prerenal, renal, and postrenal causes. Of the 3, the prerenal one is the most important, implying poor renal perfusion, usually due to low blood volume. Gastroenteritis and other dehydrating disorders are common causes, followed by severe infections, burns and trauma.

Renal causes imply parenchymatous disease such as occasional cases of glomerulonephritis, and hemolytic-uremic syndrome, the collagen disorders, mismatched transfusions, or reactions to poisons such as heavy metals, organic solvents, ethylene glycol or drugs (sulphonamides, kanamycin). Chronic renal failure can of course be complicated by the acute variety.

Postrenal anuria may occasionally complicate renal stones, or severe crystalluria from sulphonamides or uric acid.

Clinical features. These are superimposed upon the primary disease. The cardinal feature is extreme oliguria ($<$ 100 ml urine/day) or anuria. Mild edema is also an early sign. The uremic syndrome consists in vomiting, drowsiness and coma, usually with hypertension. The bladder can neither be percussed nor palpated, and is empty on catheterization (to be avoided if possible) or suprapubic puncture.

Biochemistry. Apart from increased urea values this may be entirely normal, but hyperkalemia is common. pH and bicarbonate values are initially normal but fall as the period of anuria lengthens.

Course and prognosis. In most instances a spontaneous diuresis occurs within a week or so. The urinary output rises in an exponential fashion, and care should be taken to restore fluid and electrolyte intake to normal levels during this time. Monitoring the patient's weight is the best mode of control. Abnormalities of renal function may persist for a month or two but are seldom permanent.

Treatment. This will depend largely on the etiology. Appropriate intravenous salt solutions are in order in the prerenal type, and should, in most instances, result in a prompt diuresis. In the renal type (which may follow the prerenal variety) the child should, if dehydrated, be restored to his assessed normal weight. This done, and in the absence of any source of loss of water or electrolyte, he should be given glucose-containing fluids at a level sufficient to maintain him at his normal weight. Potassium should be completely withheld. Frequent electrolyte and B.U.N. measurements are necessary, as well as measurements of pH and plasma bicarbonate. A decrease in serum sodium values, in the absence of a source of loss, usually means that too much fluid is being given. Supporting signs that this is so are a rise in body weight, extension of edema, and hypertension. Hyperkalemia is a feared complication and the electrocardiogram is the best mode of following cellular potassium levels.

Peritoneal dialysis. This is indicated when there is evidence of hyperkalemia by E.C.G., or where the serum potassium has risen steadily to 8 or more mEq/1; blood urea values>150 mg% are also an indication, as is the presence of severe acidosis. The clinical features of uremia usually also indicate a need for dialysis.

Haemolytic Uremic Sydrome

This is a rare condition which sometimes occurs in small epidemics. The exact etiology is as yet unknown, although an autoimmune basis has been proposed. If the patient survives the acute phase, the disease is largely self-limited.

Clinical features. A precedent viral infection is usual, and may take the form of an upper respiratory tract infection, or apparent gastroenteritis. After a variable time (3-14 days) the child rapidly becomes pale, has bleeding into the skin, the onset of or aggravation of a preexisting bloody diarrhea, and suppression of urine. Stupor or coma are not unusual. The patient may be hypertensive and dehydration occurs.

Urine. This is scanty or suppressed, and shows many red and white cells and casts.

The blood. There is a severe anemia with evidence of red cell fragmentation—reticulocytes, burr cells, and normoblasts. The platelets are reduced. The Coomb's test is negative. The bone marrow shows erythroid hyperplasia, with normal megakaryocytes.

Biochemistry. The blood urea is greatly increased. Hyperkalemia is not uncommon.

Progress. The late signs are basically those of acute renal failure. Spontaneous diuresis and improvement may occur at any stage. Many of the fluid and electrolyte problems are associated with injudicious I.V. therapy.

Treatment. This essentially is as outlined for acute renal failure, together with transfusion of blood and attention to the coagulation defect.

CHRONIC RENAL FAILURE

This has a multitude of causes. Chronic pyelonephritis, with anatomical anomalies, is probably the commonest. Hypoplasia of the kidneys, usually with infection, occurs in the younger age groups. Acute glomerulonephritis and the nephrotic syndrome may progress to this unfortunate conclusion.

The clinical picture is common to all etiologies. Poor general health, with easy fatiguability, poor appetite, and failure of growth are usual. Polyuria and polydipsia are elicited more by questioning than as direct complaints. Occasionally the disease is first suspected because of coma or unexplained hypertension. Dehydration and electrolyte disturbances are occasionally the presenting symptoms. In rare cases where the chronic renal failure is due to potassium loss (aldosteronism) muscular paralysis may present.

Anemia is common in this disease, and is due not only to depression of erythropoiesis, but to a hemolytic element in the serum.

Treatment: General. As in all potentially fatal conditions, it is important that at least one of the parents be told the ultimate prognosis. The parental feelings should always be closely consulted in relation to therapy designed to prolong life. The parents are otherwise advised to give as happy life to the child as possible. This does not imply that discipline should break down completely, or that an orgy of self-indulgence is in order. Normally it is best to adhere, as far as possible, to the child's routine. Dietary control is of limited value, and the child's desires should be the criteria of the diet of choice.

Supportive. Most renal crises are due to aberrations of salt and water metabolism. The child with renal failure requires water as a diabetic requires insulin. Thus, it is essential to prescribe the minimum volume which the child should drink. This is usually equal to volume of urine passed, as the water content of food is adequate to supply the balance. The child's thirst is an unreliable control of the need for water. As in the diabetic, illness, especially a febrile one, often precedes a water and salt crisis. Therefore, it is good practice to urge the parents to seek medical attention at the earliest stage of even mild illness.

In the renal crisis of fluid and electrolyte depletion, it is wisest to give intravenous therapy. Half-normal salt solution is best, and should be given until urine is passed and blood pressure returns to normal (often hypertensive) values. Potassium is used with great caution as hyperkalemia often exists. If tables for water needs are used in the calculation, 30-50% above average values are often required to excrete the nitrogen. Acidosis is a frequent accompaniment of renal failure, but unless pH is seriously depressed, e.g., to 7.1 or less, alkaline solution should be used with caution. Calcium should always be given with alkaline infusions.

As renal failure progresses, potassium and nitrogen retention is common. The patient is tided over by peritoneal or hemodialysis. The question of renal transplant may be raised at this stage, but presently this operation is not a routine one.

The anemia of renal failure is difficult to treat except by transfusion.

Dietary Management of Chronic Renal Failure

The need for an adequate intake of fluid has already been mentioned. Additionally, when renal failure is obvious, it is necessary to consider restriction of dietary protein. In the adult, nitrogen balance can be maintained on relatively low amounts of protein. In the child, protein is necessary for growth so that a more liberal allowance is advisable. Thus, the minimum daily protein should be about 1.0 g/kg of expected body weight and larger amounts (to 1.5 g/kg) should be given in the first few months of life. In older children, say of school-age, the protein requirement may be allowed to fall to 0.5-0.75 g/kg. Low protein diets which are also deficient in first class protein have been advocated. This is the so-called Giovanetti diet in which egg is the chief source of first class protein, although the essential amino acids are added as a supplement. Second class protein, as in wheat products and vegetables, are greatly reduced. The latter gives a problem of variety in the diet. In children, therefore, it is wise to modify the Giovanetti diet in the direction of maintaining the ratio of high class:second class protein to 1:1. It should be noted that low protein diets *must* contain adequate calories.

Sodium restriction should be carried out with care in children, for fear of an intractable low salt syndrome. A daily salt intake (including that from food) is about 40 mEq/l in restricted diets. Similar levels of potassium intake are used for older children, and may be reduced pro rata for infants. The serum levels and electrocardiogram should be monitored in order to avoid hypokalemia. The hypocalcemia of renal failure does not respond to increased dietary calcium. In renal osteodystrophy additional vitamin D intake (as calciferol) and $Al(OH)_3$ therapy to bind gut phosphate may be of value.

Dialysis

This is the preliminary in most instances to renal transplant. The techniques used depend upon the exchange of urea and other ions against a semipermeable membrane, which is the interface between the body fluids, and a dialysis fluid of appropriate composition.

In *acute* renal failure, the commoner indications for dialysis are the failure of conservative therapy to control serious hyperkalemia (K>7 mEq/l with E.C.G. changes) fluid and saline excess, and urea levels which are>200mg%

The indications are essentially similar in chronic renal failure, although the technique is usually embarked upon as a preliminary to transplant operations, and especially where the symptoms of nausea, vomiting, pericarditis, and intestinal ulceration are present.

Peritoneal Dialysis

In this technique the peritoneum acts as the semipermeable membrane. Across this, diffusion of small molecules occurs in proportion to the concentration gradient. The dialysis fluid is essentially similar in its ionic composition to extracellular fluids, but potassium is usually omitted and lactate substituted for bicarbonate. The fluid instilled into the peritoneal cavity attains equilibrium with the body fluid and then is removed. Urea, potassium, and sodium are capable of removal and, by variation of the osmolality of the dialysis fluid, water may be extracted from the extracellular space. The technique basically is to place a cannula in the peritoneal cavity and through it instil the warmed dialysis fluid. The volume given in children varies from 40 ml/kg in infants to 75-100 ml/kg in older subjects. Fluid balance, body weight, and blood pressure should carefully be monitored.

Hemodialysis

In this the blood is passed through a system which allows an interface between the blood film and an appropriate dialysis fluid. It is less used in children because of the technical difficulties of establishing an arteriovenous (Scribner) shunt. The coil of the artificial kidney is interpolated between. The problem of the patient's bleeding into the dialysis coil has not yet been satisfactorily solved in the infant, so that the technique is seldom applicable at that age. In older children, arteriovenous shunts can be made and intermittent hemodialysis carried out essentially as in adults.

Renal Transplantation

The age groups in which this is carried out is steadily declining. An essential is the ability to tolerate chronic hemodialysis. Most children are

6 or more years of age. A success rate of about 40-50% can be attained in the best centres.

TUMOURS OF THE KIDNEY

These are among the more frequent tumours of childhood, the commonest is embryonal adenosarcoma. Rarer tumours are hamartoma and renal carcinoma. These are usually only diagnosable after histological examination of the removed kidney.

Embryonal Adenomyosarcoma of the Kidney (Wilm's tumour)

Clinical features. In more than half of children with this tumour, the initial complaint is of an abdominal mass. Fever, abdominal discomfort, weakness, and loss of appetite are next most common. Hematuria is relatively rare (6%).

The lump is initially smooth and rounded, but hemorrhage and necrosis may cause it to feel fluctuant. Abdominal x-rays show the mass, and pyelography shows absence of function in the affected kidney. Albuminuria and pyuria may occur. Hypertension is rare.

Differential diagnosis. The tumour is most commonly confused with other masses of renal origin, usually hydronephrosis. This, and polycystic disease of the kidneys, can usually be excluded by pyelography. Neuroblastoma may show calcification. Retroperitoneal sarcoma sometimes cannot be excluded except by laparotomy and biopsy, but pyelography however usually reveals a functional, albeit displaced, kidney. The tumour may metastasize to the lungs, giving the round cannon ball secondary.

Treatment. Prompt removal of the affected kidney and radical radiation and chemotherapy would appear to be the best treatment. Metastases can also be treated by radiotherapy and chemotherapy.

Prognosis. This is not good. Only 20% are alive 2 years after removal of the tumour.

RENAL CALCULI

These are not very common in children, but may occur as part of a metabolic disease, e.g., cystinuria, familial oxalosis. Hypercalciuria, especially associated with prolonged bed rest, or hypercorticalism may be a cause.

Clinical features. In many instances, the stone is discovered when the child comes in with a urinary tract infection; in others there may be hematuria, or renal colic, with abdominal or back pain radiating to the groin. Asymptomatic stones may be found on routine x-ray examination.

X-rays. The stone may be visible on plain x-ray although pure uric acid stones are radiolucent. Pyelography commonly reveals some evidence of obstructive uropathy, e.g., hydronephrosis, hydroureter—dependent upon the situation of the stone.

Urinalysis. Microscopic hematuria is common, as is evidence of infection. Hypercalciuria and cystinosis should always be sought for.

Differential diagnosis. If hematuria is the principal symptom, renal trauma and acute hemorrhagic glomerulonephritis may require consideration. Where pain is prominent, pyelonephritis, and appendicitis require exclusion.

Treatment. Acute renal colic will require analgesics, and metabolic defects should be corrected if possible. The treatment otherwise is surgical.

RENAL VEIN THROMBOSIS

This condition is most common in the very young, and is usually associated with some dehydrating condition such as gastroenteritis.

Clinical features. Those of the precipitating condition are present, and the infant may be found to have an enlarged kidney on routine examination. There may be hematuria, marked albuminuria, or circulatory failure in spite of adequate resuscitation. Pyelography may show a nonfunctioning kidney.

Treatment. The infarcted kidney and renal vein should be removed as soon as practicable. This will prevent spread to the opposite kidney.

Prognosis. In unilateral, early treated cases, the outlook is good. Nephrotic syndrome may occasionally complicate the untreated case.

DISORDERS OF THE BLADDER

Congenital Anomalies

Exstrophy of the Bladder

This may be partial or complete. In the latter, there is a large abdominal defect which reveals the interior of the bladder from its apex to the urethra. There is epispadias and separation of the pubic rami. In the lesser forms, a smaller part of the bladder is seen, but some of the other lesions mentioned, as well as inguinal herniae, may coincide. The bladder mucosa is pink and sensitive, although sensation is decreased after some months. In both instances, there is dribbling of urine from the bladder cavity. Secondary infection of the urinary tract is common, although the condition is compatible with long life.

Treatment. This is entirely surgical.

Patent Urachus

The urachus is a tubule remnant of the bladder formed as the latter descends from the umbilical area to the pelvis during development. On occasion it remains completely patent, so that urine dribbles at the umbilicus.

Urachal *cysts* may form anywhere along the track of bladder descent. Urinary discharge does not occur. The principal symptom is a midline swelling, which may become infected, forming an abscess.

Treatment. This is surgical.

Infections of the Bladder (cystitis)

This coincides with infection elsewhere in the urinary tract, but in females may occur as an isolated problem.

Clinical features. In the young child the features may be non-specific—fever, anorexia, vomiting—with frequency and pain obvious only on close observation.

In the older child the complaints are of frequent, painful micturition with only small amounts of urine being passed at a time. Suprapubic pain is also common. In rare instances, marked hematuria may occur, suggesting hemorrhagic cystitis (a viral disorder). Cystitis may be due to the presence of a bladder stone or other foreign body, and this possibility should always be considered.

Bladder Calculi

These may follow stone formation higher in the urinary tract, or complicate long standing urinary infection. The latter may be the first symptom. Otherwise, frequency and pain (often felt at the end of urination) are common symptoms. Acute retention is relatively rare. The stone is usually radiopaque, and hence easily seen on x-ray.

Treatment. Any precipitating condition, e.g., urinary obstruction, should be dealt with. The calculus is otherwise removed surgically, usually by cystotomy.

Tumour of the Bladder

These are relatively rare in children, most are malignant, the commonest is rhabdomyosarcoma.

Clinical features. These are somewhat protean. However, pain (dysuria), frequency, and episodes of urinary infection occur. In rare instances, acute retention may develop. Compression of the rectum will cause constipation, which may progress to intestinal obstruction. The mass may be felt on rectal examination. Cystoscopy will reveal distortion of the bladder and, on occasion, multiple polypoid tumours (sarcoma botryoides).

Treatment. This is by excision after preliminary irradiation and cytotoxic therapy. The prognosis is poor.

DISORDERS OF THE GENITALIA

The Male External Genitals

Common congenital abnormalities of the penis are hypospadias and epispadias.

Hypospadias

In this condition, the urethra opens at some site on the ventral surface of the penis. Common varities are glandular, penile, and perineal hypospadias. In the last, the scrotum is abnormal and in some cases pseudovagina may cause difficulty in determining the infant's sex. In most instances too, chordee (ventral bowing of the penis) is present, and the true terminal urinary meatus is narrowed.

Epispadias

In this the urethra opens on the dorsal top surface of the penis. The condition is relatively uncommon, but may accompany exstrophy of the bladder. In both epispadias and hypospadias, the treatment is surgical. The foreskin should be conserved for the ultimate plastic procedures.

Stenosis of the Penile Meatus

This is quite rare and occurs mainly in circumcised infants. Even a small meatus may be adequate to transmit a strong urinary stream. If observation suggests that this indeed is the case, meatotomy is unnecessary.

Phimosis

This refers to the situation in which the foreskin cannot be retracted and the preputial opening is small. Both of these situations apply in the *normal* newborn, so that overdiagnosis should be avoided. As the penis develops, both preputial opening and the ability to retract the foreskin are enhanced. Persistent balanitis, or definite evidence of urinary obstruction are the principal indications for surgical care.

Paraphimosis

In this situation, the foreskin has been forcibly retracted and will not again go forward. A constriction band forms, causing local pain and swelling of the glans. The condition is treated by anesthetizing the child and reducing the paraphimosis by manipulation or by incision of the constricting ring of tissue.

Circumcision

This procedure is frequently done but is seldom justifiable for other than ritual reasons. The newborn foreskin is normally adherent to the glans and this does not require treatment. Frequent and recurrent balanoposthitis is the main indication in the older child, but even then, surgery should be advised only after efforts to instil hygienic practices have failed.

In the newborn, if circumcision is insisted upon, it should be carried out after the 7th-10th day when blood coagulation difficulties are less common. The presence of hypospadias or epispadias is a total contra-indication to circumcision.

Balanoposthitis

This is an inflammation of the prepuce and subjacent glans. There is local pain and itching, with swelling and redness of the foreskin. Pus exudes from the preputial orifice. The condition is commonly associated with poor hygienic practices.

Treatment. Suitable cold compresses, mild analgesics, and correct hygiene will suffice to treat most cases. Antibiotics and splitting of the prepuce are necessary only in severe local inflammation.

Meatal Ulcer

This condition occurs in circumcised infants who have ammoniacal dermatitis. The mother may have failed to change the infant as frequently as desirable. The treatment is to remove the diapers, treat the dermatitis, and apply an analgesic/antiseptic water-soluble compound to the ulcer. This will result in prompt healing.

Disorders of the Testes

Cryptorchidism

This is the condition in which the testes fail to enter the scrotum. The testes may be ectopic, i.e., not in the normal path of descent through the inguinal canal. Common sites are the perineum, the suprapubic area, and the femoral area. The true *undescended* testis may be intraabdominal, or within the inguinal canal.

Perhaps the commonest cause of undescended testicle is undue retractility. In this, the testis is in the upper scrotum or in the superficial inguinal pouch. In either case, it can be readily brought down by seating the infant in a bath of warm (not hot) water and gently manipulating the inguinal areas. If the maldescent is bilateral and true, care should be taken to exclude female pseudo-hermaphrodism, or in less frequent instances, the male Turner syndrome.

The treatment of ectopic and undescended testes is surgical. There is some evidence that ectopic testes which cannot be restored to the scrotum may undergo malignant change in later life. This may constitute a reason for excision. In most instances of bilateral undescended testes, a decision concerning surgery should not be postponed much after the 5th year. A more expectant policy may be followed in unilateral cases. The fertility of the patient who has had apparently successful surgery for bilateral cryptorchidism cannot always be guaranteed.

Torsion of the Testis

This may occur at any age, but is perhaps more common in the grade school group. The patient complains of minor discomfort followed by severe pain in the testis and lower abdomen. The scrotum becomes red and swollen. Fever and vomiting are not unusual, and marked local tenderness is invariable.

In the younger child, the only sign may be a red, swollen scrotum.

Treatment. This, if infarction of the testis is to be avoided, is a matter of emergency. The scrotum is explored and the twist undone. However, if the condition has persisted for more than a few hours, testicular atrophy is relatively common.

Hydrocele

This is a collection of fluid along the course of the processus vaginalis, most commonly presenting as a hydrocele of the tunica. This is asymptomatic and presents as a soft, painless mass on the testis, which is transilluminable, and is limited above by the external inguinal ring. Hydrocele of the spermatic cord also occurs.

Treatment. Most hydroceles disappear spontaneously in the first year of life. Surgical treatment is usually indicated in those persisting longer, especially if a hernia is associated with a tunica vaginalis hydrocele.

The Female Genitals

Adhesion of the Labia

This minor problem is usually found on routine inspection of the newborn. It may be complete enough to prevent urination. Manual separation is easy.

Obstruction of the Vagina

This may be due to atresia of the vagina proper, or of the hymen. In the latter the condition may be suspected at routine neonatal examination when the bulging membrane is seen. In vaginal obstruction, the retained fluid will cause *hydrocolpos*. Pyocolpos occurs with secondary infection and hydrometrocolpos implies that both uterus and vagina are distended.

Hematocolpos

This disorder usually occurs in the second decade.

Clinical features. These depend upon the degree of fluid accumulation. In advanced situations, the condition may present as an abdominal mass, with retention of urine and constipation. The diagnosis is more readily made when the hymen is imperforate, as the fluid can readily be aspirated. In vaginal atresia, laparotomy may be necessary to reveal the condition.

Differential diagnosis. This is principally from other causes of abdominal mass such as retroperitoneal tumours, enlarged bladder, and hydronephrosis.

Treatment. In imperforate hymen, the fluid is aspirated and the membrane incised. In vaginal atresia, the surgical technique will depend upon the local situation.

Vulvovaginitis

This is a not uncommon situation. The vulva is painful and itchy, and looks red. A mucoid or purulent discharge may be present. Redness of the vulva may be due to lack of hygiene or the friction of clothing. An offensive vaginal discharge should raise the question of foreign body. This may be palpated by rectal examination, seen through an ear speculum, or, if radiopaque, visualized on x-ray. Gonococcal and other infections nowadays occur only sporadically. It should be noted that a creamy vaginal discharge, which stiffens on the underclothing, is a normal premenstrual phenomenon. Pain and evidence of inflammation are absent in this condition.

Treatment. In most instances, improved hygiene and mildly antiseptic baths are sufficient to cure the condition. Foreign bodies should of course be removed, and antibiotics used if specific organisms, e.g., gonococcus are found in the pus.

Tumours of the Vagina

These are rare. The usual one is rhabdomyosarcoma (sarcoma botryoides) which may also originate from the bladder. The principal clinical feature is of a mass protruding from the vagina. This grows rapidly and may form polypoid (grape-like) tumours. The condition responds poorly to treatment.

Conditions affecting the ovaries

These are relatively uncommon in children. Usually they are dermoids, or simple cysts.

Clinical features. Symptoms usually are caused by torsion of the pedicle, which gives rise to abdominal pain and sometimes vomiting. The condition may be confirmed only at laparatomy.

In other instances there may be a complaint of swelling of the belly, usually without much discomfort. The treatment is excision and the prognosis is good.

Intersexuality

At birth, sexing is carried out by inspection of the external genitals. Accordingly, most problems arise because this estimate of the child's sex is at variance with other modes of determining sex, i.e., chromosomal complement, and gonadal apparatus. As noted elsewhere, the possession of an XY set of chromosomes defines masculinity, and XX femininity. However, in most disorders of the sex chromosome, e.g., Turner's, Klinefelter's syndromes, the pragmatic sex—in the sense of being male or female—is seldom at variance with the external genital appearance. The principal practical problems lie in the area of pseudohermaphroditism, i.e., where the external genitals are ambiguous, and at variance with the gonadal sex. As a result, the pragmatic sex (way in which the child has been reared) is at variance with the chromosomal sex.

Male Pseudohermaphroditism

This may be due to gross abnormality of the external genitals, usually in cases of severe perineal hypospadias with incomplete fusion of the labioscrotal eminences, and undescended testes. The buccal smear shows no Barr body, and the chromosomal sex is XY

Testicular Feminization Syndrome

This condition is familial, and apparently due to an inability of the appropriate tissues to respond to androgen. The patient is phenotypically female, although the external genitals may remain infantile. Testes are also present, but are ectopic in the abdomen, labia, or inguinal canals. The complaints are usually of amenorrhea at puberty, or the ectopic testes are found at examination of the herniae which are commonly present. The genotype is male, and these children have usually been reared as females. In most instances, the patient should be left as a female and the ectopic testes may be removed surgically. Improvement of the female habitus may be obtained by appropriate estrogen therapy.

In a few instances of male adrenal hyperplasia due to 3-β- hydroxysteroid deficiency, the external genitals are ambiguous, and there is hypospadias and undescended testes. Most of these patients present with low salt syndrome.

Female Pseudohermaphroditism

The female fetus is sensitive to androgen activity so that most female newborns with marked virilization have adrenal hyperplasia. A severe salt-losing state may be the first symptom of this condition.

In other instances, the mother has been treated for threatened abortion with progesterone, testosterone, or other drugs.

The labia are usually fused, and the clitoris greatly enlarged. In very rare instances, a urethra traverses the enlarged clitoris. These children have an XX (female) chromosome complement and a uterus and vagina. The principal differential diagnosis from the causes mentioned is true hermaphroditism, which may require laparotomy for its substantiation.

True Hermaphroditism

In this rare condition, elements of both male and female gonads are present. The genitals are usually ambiguous but may be normal enough to suggest that the infant is male or female. The genotype is commonly XX, whatever the apparent phenotype. Mosaicism has been described. The diagnosis depends upon laparotomy with the demonstration of both types of gonadal tissue. Sometimes this is present in a single organ, the ovotestis. In most instances it is surgically easier to produce female external genitals and to rear the child as such.

Appendix 1: Examination of the urine

Routine Urinalysis

This is the most important method of investigation of a patient with renal disease. The tests which are done are those for specific gravity, protein, cells, and casts.

Specific Gravity

This has been mentioned above. In random samples, the S.G. will vary with the amount of water recently drunk. Accordingly, early morning samples are most reliable. The infant, with his relatively high intake of fluid, will in general excrete a less concentrated urine. He can, however, increase the S.G. of his urine to 1020 or more if stressed. The S.G. of urine will be affected by protein and glucose. For each g% of the former, 0.004 S.G. unit should be subtracted, and for the latter 0.003 S.G. unit.

Proteinuria

Up to 100 mg of protein/24 hours can be excreted by normal children. Febrile illness and heavy exercise may cause transient increases. Persistent proteinuria in excess of 200 mg/24 hours suggests renal disease. Stick tests are useful for routine urinalysis. 24-hour excretion values are best established by the Biuret method; the Esbach method has a variation of up to 25%.

Orthostatic Proteinuria

This is a not uncommon finding in older children. It is a benign exaggeration of the normal proteinuria. Albumen is the principal protein excreted, and is absent in specimens taken before the child rises in the morning, is maximal after 2-3 hours of standing activity, and lessens after going to bed.

Hematuria

This is a common symptom of renal disease, with an enormous differential diagnosis. Localization of the bleeding is more difficult than in adults, although in older children, a modified 3-glass test is of value. In this the child urinates successively into 3 specimen glasses. The amount of blood present is quantitated by inspection. Urethral bleeding gives rise to a hematuria most marked in the early sample, terminal bleeding suggests a cystic origin, bleeding from the kidney is generally distributed evenly through the specimens.

Microscopic Hematuria

This is usually assessed on the centrifuged specimen. Conventionally the highpower (45**x**) is used to quantitate the number of RBC's present. In normal children, 1-2/HPF is common, and will be increased in dehydrating conditions and febrile disease. The increase is not great (up to 15 RBC/HPF) and does not necessarily signify renal disease. Dilute urines cause rapid RBC lysis so that falsely low levels may be found unless the specimen is examined quickly.

Pyuria

Small numbers of leucocytes (0-1/HPF) may be found in the urine of normal children. Such cells may also originate from the vulva or vagina and epithelial cells may also be mistaken for leucocytes. Epithelial cells are larger and the nuclei show no lobes. Staining of the centrifuged specimen with a special stain (Sternheimer-Malbin) may be useful in differentiating the 2 types of cells.

In acute pyelitis, large numbers of leucocytes, often aggregated into clumps are usually readily seen.

Urinary casts

These are tubular in origin, and proteinaceous in content. Hyaline casts, which contain only mucoprotein, are found in small numbers in normal children. *Cellular casts* commonly imply renal disease, although they occur transiently after dehydrating illness. Red cell casts are typical of glomerular inflammation as leucocyte casts are of pyelonephritis. Epithelial casts also occur in the latter condition, whether acute or chronic. Granular casts originate from degenerate tubular cells, and occur in most types of chronic renal disease. Those which contain fat are common in the nephrotic syndrome.

The Addis count

This is a semiquantitative measure of the 12-hour excretion of cells and casts. A sample of the bulked specimen is spun, and the cell and cast number enumerated in a hemocytometer chamber. The normal numbers of RBC excreted in 12 hours is 600,000, of leucocytes 1,000,000, and of casts 10,000. A good deal of variation from normal occurs, so that only values in excess of twice or thrice those quoted are of significance.

Examination of the urine for infection

This should always be done on the freshly passed specimen. If this is translucent, and has no leucocytes in it, infection is unlikely. If it is cloudy, contains leucocytes, and mobile bacteria, then infection is probable. Culture of the urine must be done immediately as contaminants grow rapidly in what is an admirable nutrient medium. Even with the most thorough local cleaning, contamination from the skin is inevitable, and should be appreciated. In older children, a mid stream specimen can often be obtained, in the younger a sterile plastic bag, suitably secured, is the usual method of obtaining urine for culture. The latter method is subject to contamination and even colony counts are suspect in such a situation. In infants, suprapubic aspiration of the bladder is a safe method of obtaining urine for culture. Urethral catheterization should seldom be practised, as it carries a risk of introducing infection.

It is perhaps worth repeating that the best way of diagnosing urinary infection is to examine a freshly passed sample for leucocytes. Usually too, these patients have symptoms of urinary infection.

X-RAY EXAMINATION OF THE RENAL TRACT

Plain films of this are generally unrewarding, except to reveal radiopaque calculi, and occasionally to give some idea of the kidney size. The upper tract is usually examined by intravenous pyelography. The dye used is an iodine derivative, and sensitivity to this should be excluded. The medium is largely excreted by filtration so that excessive water intake, or failure of filtration from disease, will not give good contrast. In infancy, setting up a scalp vein drip is a useful technique to infuse the contrast material.

The lower renal tract is examined by cystourethrography, following the instillation of contrast medium into the bladder. Cine films are usually made, and these will give some indication of the physiological, as well as the anatomical situation, in so far as urethral reflux on micturition can be seen.

RENAL SCANS

A detector is placed externally over each kidney and the emanation from the area examined. Unilateral kidney disease may thus be suspected because of the difference in external counts. The technique is seldom applicable in children and usually only in those who have unexplained hypertension.

RENAL BIOPSY

This is not normally used where the diagnosis can be established by other methods. The findings may have prognostic value in resistant nephrotic syndrome, and be of diagnostic value in obscure cases of hematuria, proteinuria, or hypertension.

A preliminary I.V.P. is essential to establish the presence and location of both kidneys. Any bleeding tendency is a contra-indication, as is advanced renal failure, single kidney, and severe hypertension. Minor complications include hematuria and local pain. An expert can obtain adequate samples in about 80% of children studied.

TESTS OF RENAL FUNCTION

Most of these are inapplicable except in the older child, as they demand close timing of sampling, and complete emptying of the bladder.

Glomerular filtration rate

This is calculated on the assumption that the substance studied is filtered by the glomerulus to the same level as in the plasma, and is not reabsorbed or secreted by the renal tubule. In this circumstance, if the urine volume in unit time is known (V), and the urinary concentration of the substance is known (U), as well as its plasma concentration (P), then the glomerular filtration rate (GFR) (renal clearance—C) is expressed by the formula: $C = UV/P$. Academically, the polysaccharide inulin is used; clinically, *creatinine* or urea clearance is of more moment.

Other substances which can be used to measure GFR are radioactive vitamin B_{12}. Comparison of the plasma and urinary radioactivities allows the appropriate calculation to be made. The excretion of ^{131}I labelled sodium diatrozoate is used similarly. These radioactive methods are seldom indicated in children, and must not be used repeatedly in them.

Renal plasma flow (RPF)

This is based on the Fick principle (rate of removal of the substance/arteriovenous difference of the same substance). If the substance is totally removed in 1 circulation, then only the plasma concentration need be known. Para-aminohippuric acid (PAH) is so handled by the kidney, so that the mixed venous value is essentially that of the renal artery. The renal venous level is of course zero. Thus, the calculation is—$RPF = UV/P$—where urinary concentration (U) multiplied by urinary volume (V) is the rate of removal and P is the plasma concentration.

Tests of tubular activity

Vagaries of tubular function may sometimes be suspected by finding in the urine those products which are usually resorbed. Examples of such substances are glucose, and amino acids in the congenital tubular nephropathies. More specific tests of tubular function relate to studies of tubular resorption, tubular secretion, and tubular handling of water and solute.

Tubular resorption

The conventional measure of this is the tubular transport maximum (Tm). Glucose, or phosphate, can be used to establish the approximate Tm. In the case of glucose, an intravenous infusion is set up, and urine collected. The plasma and urinary glucose values are measured, and the urinary glucose excretion (which occurs at levels >180 mg%) assessed. The resorption of glucose is the difference between the amount filtered and the amount excreted.

Tubular secretion

A similar Tm can be established for the tubular secretory function. As we have already seen, the tubule can elaborate a concentrated or dilute urine as circumstances demand. The urinary concentration test is simple and reliable. It is carried out by withholding fluid overnight, or for 12 hours, after the bladder has been emptied. Subsequent urine is tested for specific gravity, which will commonly rise to 1024 or 900 mOsm/l or greater. The test must be carried out with caution in established renal disorder, or dehydration may ensue. Similarly, if the child is diuresing, as in acute glomerulonephritis or the nephrotic syndrome, renal concentrating ability is temporarily impaired.

If the child can be induced to drink a lot of water, a dilution test can conveniently follow. A urinary specific gravity of 1001 may be reached under this stimulus.

14 Disorders of the hemopoietic system

BLOOD GLOSSARY

Microcyte:	Cells of diameter $> 6.5\mu$; thin; less Hb; M.C.V. decreased.
Macrocyte:	Diameter $> 8.5\mu$; thick; full of Hb; M.C.V. increased.
Megaloblast:	Abnormal nucleated erythroid cells, with fine nuclear chromatin, but eosinophilic cytoplasm.
Heinz bodies:	Roundish granules at periphery of RBC; single or multiple; stained by cresyl blue.
Target cell:	Hb concentrated in centre and periphery of RBC.
Reticulocyte:	Normal cell, larger than RBC, containing nuclear remnants (RNA); staining with cresyl blue.
Poikilocyte:	Irregularity in shape; often pear-shaped.
Burr cells *Pyknocyte* *Acanthocyte*	Poikilocytes with spiny projections.
Howell-Jolly bodies:	Nuclear remnants presenting as fine 1μ particles eccentrically placed.
Basophilic strippling (punctate basophilia):	Coarse violet or dark blue granules in RBC cytoplasm.
Siderocytes:	RBC, containing Fe of non Hb source; stainable by prussian blue.

OUTLINE OF PHYSIOLOGY

Blood is the essential transport system of the body, carrying energy-giving substances such as glucose and fat, as well as the enzymes and protective proteins (immunoglobulins) made in the body. The red cell, which is primarily composed of hemoglobin (Hb) can take up and release oxygen and carbon dioxide without itself using much energy. As well hemoglobin and the blood proteins have an important buffering ability, i.e., they can balance the acid/base content of the body within fine limits (see also p. 522).

The origin and structure of the red cell

The mature red cell (R.B.C.) is a biconcave disc of 8.5μ diameter, which is derived from the normoblast (erythroblast) cells of the bone marrow. Intermediate forms of red cells are recognizable but the one which is of clinical importance is the *reticulocyte*, which is the immediate precursor of the red cell. In general, the more mature is a red cell precursor, the less is its ability to make energy sources such as glucose or lipid. Hemoglobin, the effective part of the red cell, is composed of 4 heme (a compound of iron and protoporphyrin) groups, to each of which is joined 4 long chains of amino acids. These are called polypeptide globin chains, and they can be further identified as α, β, γ, δ. The importance of identifying these as such lies in the fact that hemoglobin can have several forms. Thus, in health, fetal hemoglobin (HbF) is made up of α and γ chains ($\alpha_2 \gamma_2$) and the major adult hemoglobin (A_1) is $\alpha_2\beta_2$. Abnormalities of production of some Hb types (e.g., fetal) may cause disease (thalassemia). Abnormalities of the sequence of amino acids in the polypeptide chain can also cause disease by making the Hb structurally abnormal, as in sickle-cell disease.

ANEMIA

The factors needed to make red cells are protein, iron, copper, ascorbic acid, vitamin B_{12} (cyanocobalamin) and possibly thyroxin. Protein deficiency is very unusual, the commonest difficulties of supply being, in order of frequency, iron, folic acid, and vitamin B_{12}. If hemoglobin cannot be made, and if it is destroyed quickly, then anemia results, and is one of the common disorders of childhood. It is defined as insufficient hemoglobin or red cells when related to the age of the child. The age factor is important, since, as seen in table 20, hemoglobin and red cell levels are quite different at various times. This type is called absolute anemia. Relative anemia exists when the child has normal values (as shown in the table) but actually needs more red cells. This could occur, for example, in cyanotic congenital heart disease, where oxygen

Table 20. Normal values of hemoglobin and red blood cell levels

Age	Hemoglobin (g. %)	Red Blood Cells (million mm^3)
Birth	17–20	5–6
2–4 weeks	15–16	4–5
3 months	11.5	3.5–4
1 year	12	4.5–5
2–3 years	13	5
5–6 years	14	5–5.5

The values given are for infants receiving an adequate intake or iron.

carrying ability impaired by circulatory factors, can be partly compensated for by having a higher red cell count.

Classifications of anemia

A suitable subdivision is into those anemias due to *underproduction* of blood, and those due to *overdestruction*. These divisions take account of the cause (etiology) of the disorder. The pathologist may also classify anemias on *morphological* grounds, that is by the shape and size of the red cells when examined microscopically.

General clinical features of anemia

Hemoglobin levels contribute to the normal pinkness of the face, ear lobes, conjunctivae, mucous membranes of the mouth and lines in the palm, so, if there is significant anemia, then these areas seem pallid. In dark skinned people, one must examine the conjunctivae and mouth rather than the face and hands. *It must be noted that anemia can exist without blanching of the areas mentioned.*

The fall in oxygen carrying ability means that the heart must pump more blood each minute to supply the body. This increase in cardiac output gives rise to visible signs in the cardiovascular system. Thus, the heart is quick, the beat forceful, and the blood vessels at the root of the neck can be seen jumping. In other words, the resting child looks as if he has been exercising. Breathlessness at rest occurs when the anemia is severe and heart murmurs are usually heard by the pediatrician. Of course, if blood loss is rapid and large, all the above signs are exaggerated and the blood pressure falls to low levels (shock). Some signs may be related to the cause of the anemia, such as pigment in the urine in rapid blood destruction, or jaundice in less acute destruction.

General investigations of anemia

Capillary (heel stab) blood is usually examined unless there is edema, when a venous sample is used. The Hb content, the red cell number, and the proportion of red cells to serum (the hematocrit) is measured, and a film made for staining and microscopic examination. These are the routine things done; in certain circumstances the hemoglobin type is identified, and the serum examined for the presence of substances (usually proteins) which can clump and destroy the red cells.

The size and hemoglobin content of the red cells may be roughly assessed by the hematologist when he looks at the stained slide. More often they are derived from the primary measurements of Hb, RBC, and hematocrit, e.g.,

$$\text{Mean cell Hb content} = \frac{\text{Hb(gm/100ml)}}{\text{Hematocrit (\%)}} \times 100$$

The patient's red cells can be radioactively labelled, reinjected into the blood stream, and the length of their stay in the circulation measured by a radioactive detector. This will give the life span of the cell; this technique is seldom used in children because of the possible hazard of radioactivity in them.

Anemias due to impaired production (dyshemopoiesis)

Iron deficiency

This occurs in premature babies because most storage iron is laid down in the last trimester of pregnancy, so the shorter the pregnancy the greater the iron deficiency. Otherwise, the commonest cause is an iron deficient diet, occurring especially in cow's milk-fed babies who receive little else to eat. Malabsorption and chronic blood loss are other causes. The disorder is most common between 6 and 18 months of age.

Clinical features. These may be quite minor. Often pallor is the only clue, observed by the parent, nurse, or doctor. Some babies seem to be irritable and more prone to serious infections, but these are nonspecific problems. Inactivity and breathlessness occur only at low levels of hemoglobin, e.g., 4 g or less. The signs are pallor and the circulatory findings already described. Enlargement of the spleen is also common.

Investigations. There is a decrease in the Hb, RBC and hematocrit, with the film showing anisocytosis, poikilocytosis and pallid red cells. The serum iron is low and the serum binding capacity (a measure of the need for iron) is high.

Diagnosis. Recall that normal babies have Hb values lower than those of adults. Renal failure, scurvy, or hypothyroidism can all cause anemia with similar findings, but their own features are usually associated.

Prevention. Extra iron is given to prematures. Milk-fed babies are given iron-containing cereals, vegetables, and meat.

Treatment. Ferrous iron is given in a dose of 6 mg/element/day until the Hb returns to normal. Dietary adjustments are also made. Injections of iron are seldom used unless the child has malabsorption. Transfusion is reserved for those with levels of 5 g% or less, or in prematurity, 8 g% or less.

Vitamin B_{12} Deficiency (juvenile pernicious anemia)

This substance is absorbed in the presence of gastric intrinsic factor. It is not a common disorder in children, but occasionally complicates the malabsorptive states.

Clinical features. Those of any severe anemia occur, sometimes with a smooth painful tongue (glossitis) although this sign is far more common in adults. Tingling in, and weakness of the limbs, together with ataxia (difficulty in balancing) occur only in patients who have been long undiagnosed or whose treatment has been neglected.

Investigations. The Hb and RBC values are low, but the anemia is megaloblastic and macrocytic. The serum vitamin B_{12} level is low, and the Schilling test is positive. This is done by giving the patient a small dose of labelled B_{12} and checking its excretion in the urine.

Treatment. Injections of vitamin B_{12} (cyanocobalamin) are given until the blood values return to normal.

Folic acid deficiency

This may occur in malnourished children, especially those born prematurely. It may also occur in severe hemolytic anemia, complicate leukemia, or be the side effect of certain drugs, e.g., trimethoprim and the phenytoin anticonvulsants.

Clinical features. The general features of anemia are present—pallor and hemodynamic findings. The blood findings are those described under B_{12} deficiency except that the blood folic acid level is low, and that of B_{12} is normal.

Treatment. Folic acid is given by mouth until the blood is normal. In chronic hemolysis, it will be required for the duration of that disease. It is important to note that, although vitamin B_{12} and folic acid deficiencies give similar disorders, the treatment of each is *not* interchangeable. Indeed, folic acid treatment of B_{12} may cause a severe neurological disturbance. Iron is also necessary in the care of these megaloblastic anemias.

Anemias due to other vitamin deficiencies

The commonest of these occurs in scurvy (vitamin C deficiency) usually as an incidental finding. Iron deficiency due to blood loss is present but normal blood levels are not reached without giving vitamin C. Pyridoxine (vitamin B_6) deficiency is very unusual, with features resembling ordinary iron lack anemia. However, the serum iron levels are high, and the condition yields only to pyridoxine treatment.

Anemia of bone marrow depression

This may occur in chronic infections of the lung, renal tract and bones. Rheumatic fever and rheumatoid arthritis have a similar effect.

Clinical features. These are of the underlying disease, together with anemia, discovered by routine blood examination, or suspected by the presence of pallor, and the cardiovascular features already described.

Investigations. The anemia is normochromic and normocytic, although microcytosis occurs after some time. A low serum iron is found together with a *normal* iron binding capacity (cf. iron deficiency states).

Treatment. This is basically of the primary disease, with extra iron given by mouth and in the diet.

Anemias of endocrine disease

There is some evidence that hypothyroidism and suppression of adrenal function may depress the bone marrow. The findings are similar to, although often less marked than, those described for chronic infection. The treatment is that of the underlying disease.

Anemias associated with reduction of marrow cell number

In this situation, the red cell precursors are incapable of division, have been crowded out by marrow invasive disorders such as leukemia, or have been poisoned by drugs, heavy metals, or toxins of bacterial origin. The depression of the erythroid series may coincide with that of other blood cell lines. It is then part of a *pancytopenia* which is described later.

Congenital hypoplastic anemia (erythrogenesis imperfecta; Diamond-Blackfan disease).

This unusual condition may be familial. It appears to affect only the red cell precursors.

Clinical features. The infant is normal at birth but by the age of 3 months or so has the signs of a severe anemia. The child's growth is normal, and hepatosplenomegaly is absent. There is a severe anemia, but the red cells are normal in shape, and there are no changes in the other blood cells. Reticulocytes are normal or low. Bone marrow puncture (or biopsy preferably) shows a marked reduction in the early red cell series.

Treatment. Steroids should always be tried out, and may have some success. Otherwise transfusion to maintain the hemoglobin at 8g% is in order.

Prognosis. In most instances the severely affected child develops transfusion hemosiderosis, often with congestive cardiac failure. In occasional cases, spontaneous remission occurs at puberty.

Acquired red cell hypoplasia

This is clinically similar to the congenital type. It may be due to drugs, especially perhaps chloramphenicol. In such a circumstance the hypoplasia of the red cell series may precede depression of all elements of the bone marrow. The etiology is otherwise uncertain. A few cases have been found in association with thymic tumours. The examination of the blood and bone marrow is as already described.

Treatment. In some instances none is necessary, as rapid remission occurs. Otherwise, steroid (cortisone) therapy may be of value.

Anemias due to increased blood destruction

A primary division of this group is into the conditions with which are associated *intrinsic* red cell defects, i.e., of shape or metabolism. Many of these are congenital and familial.

Abnormalities of red cell shape

The most common of these is hereditary spherocytosis; elliptocytosis is very rare. Other abnormalities of red cell shape are associated with hemolytic anemias of various types, e.g., pyknocytosis in glucose-6-phosphate dehydrogenase deficiency, or with other primary diseases, e.g., acanthocytosis in hereditary abetalipoproteinemia.

Hereditary spherocytosis

This condition is transmitted as an autosomal dominant. The cells formed in the marrow are spheroidal, and this physical abnormality is associated with changes in its metabolism. The condition gives rise to clinical problems because of the extraordinary ability of the spleen to filter out and destroy abnormally shaped red cells. Splenectomy is thus usually curative.

Clinical features. The disease is usually recognized in later childhood. However, it may appear in newborns, who develop a severe hemolytic crisis, with jaundice, and increasing anemia. Severe degrees of jaundice may lead to kernicterus. The older child may show little save pallor. Occasionally *hemolytic* crisis with weakness, fever, vomiting, and abdominal pain and jaundice can take place.
The hemoglobin may fall disastrously within a few hours in such patients. The constant hemolysis increases bilirubin production so that biliary colic or bile duct obstruction may follow. In older patients, malleolar (ankle) ulcers and corneal opacities may occur.

Examination may reveal little save pallor, and the cardiovascular signs of anemia. In most cases the spleen is palpable, but marked enlargement is unusual. Icterus may be readily recognizable. In the hemolytic crisis there is tenderness in the abdomen and back.

Special examination. The red cell and hemoglobin values are reduced in parallel. The reticulocyte count is enormous (20-30% of red cells). Morphologically there is anisocytosis, and spherocytes. Prolonged hemolytic states may be associated with a leucocytosis and reduced platelet counts.

The indirect bilirubin level is raised only in the older child, in severely afflicted neonates, or those in hemolytic crisis.

Treatment. Removal of the spleen relieves the anemia, although the shape of the cells is unchanged. Leucocytosis is usual after splenectomy. The platelet count may transiently reach high levels so that daily platelet levels should be done in the first 14 postoperative days and anticoagulant measures taken if necessary.

Elliptocytosis

This is a hereditary disorder, which is transmitted as a dominant. It is rather rare.

Clinical features. The condition is often discovered on routine blood examination, e.g., for intercurrent infections. Some 25-40% of the red cells are elliptical, but the condition is asymptomatic, apart from mild anemia.

Hemolysis due to abnormal red cell metabolism

The red cell uses glucose through the Embden-Meyerhof and pentose-phosphate shunts, which have many steps, each enzyme activated. Theoretically, the enzyme for any step could be absent, thus causing disease. Practically, the commonly absent enzymes are glucose-6-phosphate dehydrogenase (G6PD) and pyruvate kinase.

The deficiency may cause no trouble until the blood is exposed to a sensitizing agent, e.g., for G6PD deficiency—bean products, antimalarial drugs, sulphonamides, after which the blood begins to break down.

Clinical features. In the newborn, the hemolysis causes jaundice with the risk of kernicterus. The other features of anemia also occur. In the older child, the problems are mainly related to the speed with which blood destruction occurs, and a common form is after exposure to broad bean products which is called *favism*. In this, a severe hemolytic reaction is shown by fever, shivering, pain in the back, pallor, and fall in blood pressure. The urine may be dark from free hemoglobin, and jaundice eventually occurs.

Laboratory studies. The specific enzyme deficiency can be found by biochemical examination. There is a marked fall in Hb with the affected red cells showing poikilocytosis, pyknocytosis, and Heinz bodies. Reticulocytes and nucleated red cells (normoblasts) are greatly increased in number.

Differential diagnosis. In the newborn, this is mainly from erythroblastosis, in the older child from severe infections (including malaria in appropriate areas), and from hemolysis due to abnormal hemoglobins as in sickle cell anemia. The major positive point is the demonstration of the specific enzyme defect.

Treatment. Any precipitating agent, such as drugs, should be avoided. In hemolysis of the newborn, an exchange transfusion may be needed to prevent kernicterus. Otherwise blood transfusion is required. Once an enzyme deficiency has been shown, the parents should be given a list of drugs which should be avoided.

Anemias associated with abnormal hemoglobin production

The process of normal hemoglobin synthesis has already been described. If the sequence of amino acids in the polypeptide chain of globin is altered then an abnormal hemoglobin is produced. Theoretically, abnormalities can occur in each of the 4 chains, α, β, γ, δ. For practical purposes, however, most abnormal hemoglobins are caused by variations in the amino acid sequence of the α or β chains.

In the cord blood of the normal newborn, hemoglobin F predominates, together with about 30% of adult hemoglobin A_1 and very small amounts of adult hemoglobin A_2. In some surveys another hemoglobin B (Bart's) has been described. In the first year of life, the ratios rapidly change until at 1 year, Hb A_1 represents 96%, Hb A_2 about 2%, and Hb F the remainder. The abnormal hemoglobins are recognized by a variety of biochemical techniques—electrophoresis, chromatography, solubility, and by immunological methods.

Disorders of the β chain of hemoglobin

The most important of these is sickle-cell (Hb.S) disease, usually called sickle-cell anemia.

Sickle-cell anemia

This disease occurs mainly in negroes and may coexist with thalassemia (see below), or G6PD deficiency. It occurs only in homozygotes.

Clinical features. Sometimes only mild hemolysis occurs giving rise to the symptoms of anemia as already described. In addition, however, there is a strong tendency to venous block (thrombosis) which causes swelling and interference with function in the drained area of the body. The whole is called a venous infarct, and the process may be set off by an infection. So then, painful swelling of the hands, feet and knees occurs when the venous drainage of a bone is blocked. If the splenic veins are involved, there is severe abdominal pain and vomiting. Rather rarely, the cerebral veins are blocked causing fits and hemiplegia. In some young children, a severe shock-like state may occur, the cause of which is unknown. Chronic anemia is followed by growth failure and a lowered resistance to infection, especially to salmonella osteomyelitis.

Special studies. The usual signs of a severe hemolytic anemia are present, and the red cells can be made to assume the typical sickle shape by treating them with sodium metabisulphate (a reducing agent). Electrophoresis will specifically identify the abnormal hemoglobin.

Treatment. Local pain and swelling are treated with rest and pain killing drugs. Blood transfusion is used for the hemolytic crises—liberally when shock is present.

Prognosis. This is not good. Most sufferers die of heart failure in the second decade of life.

Sickle-cell trait

This is the heterozygous form of the disease, i.e., only a percentage of the hemoglobin is in the S form. If both parents have the trait, the children tend to have the full-blown disease. Otherwise, the trait is of minor clinical import.

Other abnormalities of the β chain

These are called hemoglobin C, D, and E diseases, each giving rise to a mild hemolytic anemia with considerable enlargement of the spleen. They are specifically identified by electrophoresis.

Abnormalities of the γ and δ chain are of genetic and biochemical interest, but give rise to little in the way of real disease.

Thalassemia syndromes

These are conditions in which there is failure of production of one of the polypeptide chains of globin. Accordingly, no *abnormal* hemoglobin is produced, but the *proportions* of normal hemoglobins in the blood are changed. The commonest condition is Mediterranean anemia.

Mediterranean anemia

In this there is impaired synthesis of the β chains, i.e., those represented in adult Hb A ($\alpha^2\beta^2$). The major proportion of hemoglobin then is the fetal variety (Hb F;$\alpha^2\gamma^2$). In beta thalassemia major, the amount of Hb F is very large. This is the homozygous form. In the heterozygous form, thalassemia minor (or trait), the levels of Hb F are low and the levels of Hb A_2 ($\alpha^2\delta^2$) are greatly increased.

Thalassemia major

Clinical features. The severe type has its onset early in life, and is associated with pallor, anorexia, lethargy, and a tendency to infections, especially of the respiratory system. Splenomegaly and cardiac murmurs are usually present. Transfusion temporarily relieves the anemia, but the extraordinary erythroblastic activity ultimately causes changes in the bones. Thus, the thickening of the facial and skull bones may give rise to a mongolian appearance. The teeth protrude, and the hands and feet become of a broad and heavy appearance. The minor (heterozygous) type of thalassemia is largely symptom free unless an illness such as pneumonia supervenes. The hemoglobin drop is mild, and activity usually unchanged. These patients are frequently discovered when the family of the severely afflicted child is examined.

Laboratory investigations. The severe type shows a marked drop in hemoglobin value. The cell count is usually increased out of proportion to the hemoglobin level. The film shows macrocytosis and microcytosis. The cellular hemoglobin is of irregular distribution and, if centrally placed, the target cell is produced. Erythroblastic activity is shown by a reticulocytosis and the presence of nucleated red cell precursors. A moderate polymorph leucocytosis is usual. The serum iron is normal, but the bilirubin may be elevated.

Paper electrophoresis usually indicates the presence of fetal hemoglobin (hemoglobin F) and Hb A_2 in amounts disparate with the child's age. Special investigations show that there is accelerated disruption of the red cells. The bone marrow is hyperplastic, being crowded with the red cell precursors.

Complications. The severe untreated thalassemic may be the victim of congestive cardiac failure. Otherwise, the main complication is of hemosiderosis—the result of multiple transfusions. The skin becomes of a sallow, muddy colour, and the liver enlarged. Stunting of growth is usual in cases who survive the sixth year, and puberty delayed or absent. Cardiomyopathy is always present after 4-5 years.

X-ray findings. These are mainly related to the marked erythroblastic activity, and found only in the severe cases. The medullary cavities of the bone increase in size, with cortical thinning. The skull bones become greatly thickened, with radiating bony spines giving the hair-on-end appearance. The maxillae are commonly increased in size. Cardiomegaly is found in the established disorder.

Treatment. Transfusion to maintain the Hb level at about 8 g% is carried out, and chelators of iron may be given with the transfusion to delay hemosiderosis. Digitalis and diuretics are of value when congestive failure develops.

Thalassemia minor

This is the heterozygous form of the disease.

Clinical features. There is only mild anemia, so that the condition may not be suspected until infection precipitates blood examination, or pregnancy aggravates the effects of the low hemoglobin. Pallor and cardiovascular signs are minimal.

Laboratory. The red cells are microcytic and hypochromic, and occasionally show poikilocytosis and basophilic stippling. Target cells are not common. In contradistinction to iron deficiency, which is the principal differential diagnosis, the serum iron levels are high. In most instances Hb A_2 levels are increased ($>2.5\%$), Hb F levels are less frequently disturbed.

Treatment. This is normally unnecessary.

Alpha-thalassemia (Barts' hemoglobinopathy)

In this condition, the alpha chains are not synthesized so that the $\gamma^2\gamma^2(\gamma^4)$ tetramer hemoglobin Barts (Hb Barts) is formed. This condition occurs in people of Malayan or Chinese descent.

Clinical features. In the heterozygous form, the infant may have a mild hemolytic anemia, with reticulocytosis. The abnormal hemoglobin is found on electrophoresis. The disease is self-limited, with the abnormality disappearing in a few months.

The severe homozygous form has been reported only from Malaya where hydrops and intrauterine death, or early neonatal death, has been described.

Hereditary persistence of Hb F

This trait is without clinical effect. It involves negroes and those of Mediterranean origin. The Hb F level, in heterozygotes, is as high as 20-30% and is found in all red cells. Hb S disorder, when it coexists, causes only a mild anemia.

Methemoglobinemias

Methemoglobin is an oxidized form of hemoglobin in which the heme group iron is not ferrous ++, but ferric +++; thus the normal *reversible* combination of oxygen with hem cannot occur. As small amounts of methemoglobin are always formed in the body, modes for its control are present. Principally this is carried out by reduction of methemoglobin to oxyhemoglobin by methemoglobin reductase. Absence of this mechanism will give rise to the congenital disease process. Another familial mode is where there is an abnormal hemoglobin, presumably due to an amino acid substitution in the globin molecule adjacent to the hem group. Such a substitution forms a stable complex with the ferric hem group which disallows the normal enzymatic reduction to the active and reversible ferrous form. These abnormal hemoglobins—and there are several—are designated *Hb M*. The clinical features of these two are identical, and closely similar to the acquired methemoglobinemias, which are due to drugs. Commonly, the responsible substance is aniline, and the source unfixed marking dyes on napkins.

Clinical features. Soon after birth, in the congenital variety, or after appropriate exposure in the acquired type, the infant is noted to be cyanosed. This appears to be central in type, but significantly is not usually associated with dyspnea, tachycardia, or murmurs. The x-ray and E.C.G. are normal. The blood is noted to be brown in colour, and it cannot be saturated with oxygen by shaking it in air (cf. the blood from infants cyanosed by congenital heart disease). The abnormal Hb is readily detected spectroscopically, and is at least 10% of the total Hb present. In the hereditary variety, the enzyme defect can be found in the red cells, or the abnormal Hb M demonstrated by electrophoresis.

Treatment. In the acquired variety, the offending substance should be removed, and a dose of methylene blue (1-2 mg/kg as 1% solution in 0.9% saline) given. In the hereditary variety, methylene blue by mouth, with large doses (300-400 mg day) of ascorbic acid should be given.

Disorders of the heme synthesis

This molecule is an iron-protoporphyrin complex; disorders of the protoporphyrin formation—*congenital erythropoietic porphyria* can occur.

Clinical features. This is a rare condition, sometimes suggested at birth by the passage of urine or meconium which stain the nappies red. After a few months, a blistering skin rash is found, together with evidence of hemolytic anemia. The erupting teeth are red with porphyrins. If hemolysis is severe, splenomegaly occurs. The porphyrins are readily demonstrable in the urine.

In older children, a latent condition may be precipitated by exposure to drugs, usually barbiturates. There is then abdominal pain with vomiting, irritability, unreasonable behaviour, or apparent delirium.

The signs of a polyneuritis follow. Porphyrinuria is marked during these episodes.

Paroxysmal nocturnal hemoglobinuria

This is a rare condition due to some unexplained abnormality of the red cell which causes it to break down easily at normal body pH.

Clinical features. The urine is noted to be dark in the morning after sleep, and there is evidence of mild hemolytic anemia, often with thrombotic episodes, and infections. The condition may complicate or precede aplastic anemias. The susceptibility to hemolysis in an acid medium is diagnostic. Splenectomy is occasionally helpful.

Hemolysis due to extrinsic causes

The general etiology here is the effects of infections, physical agents, poisons (vegetable, animal, chemical), and the results of immunological mechanisms. The last is perhaps of primary importance in pediatrics.

Immunological affections of the red cell

In all of these, antibodies are found. The commoner causes of this type of hemolysis are mismatched transfusion, and erythroblastosis fetalis (passive immune states). The autoimmune anemias are produced by the body itself reacting against its own red cells. In some children the process is *idiopathic*, in others it is consequent to another primary disease such as the lymphomas, disseminated lupus erythematosus, neoplasms, and the collagen diseases. In these the white cells may also be involved. Infectious mononucleosis or herpes virus infections are other causes of immunological hemolysis.

Clinical features. In *primary* idiopathic autoimmune hemolysis, there is a slow onset, with pallor, fatigue, and sometimes fever. Jaundice is common, although bilirubin levels are only mildly increased. The spleen is moderately enlarged. Sudden aggravations of the process, with increased pallor and hemoglobinuria occur. In the acute episodes, blood examination shows anemia, leucocytosis, reticulocytosis, and normoblastemia. The red cells are abnormally shaped, with spherocytes, anisocytosis, and macrocytosis. The monocytes frequently show erythrophagocytosis (ingestion of RBC's).

Serology. Autoagglutinins (components clumping the RBC's) and autohemolysins (substances dissolving the red cells) can be demonstrated by special tests.

In *secondary* autoimmune hemolytic anemia, the above features are grafted upon those of the primary disease (e.g., a tumour). The red cell morphology is similar, although not so constant, and the serological findings are those described.

Differential diagnosis. This is principally between the primary and secondary autoimmune states. No child should be accepted as having the primary disease until a thorough search has been made for an underlying disorder. Other differential diagnoses include chemical toxins as a cause for the anemia. These do not have serological changes but may have a suggestive history.

Treatment. Steroids are indicated, and should be given (as prednisone) in full doses until hematological remission is obtained. Thereupon maintenance dosage is given. Transfusion is given if the hemoglobin falls below 8 g%, but care is necessary in blood cross-matching since accuracy may be interfered with by the patient's serum abnormalities. If steroids fail to control the situation, the immunosuppressive drugs should be tried.

Paroxysmal "cold" hemoglobinuria

This condition, usually associated with congenital syphilis, is nowadays rare.

Clinical features. These follow exposure to cold. They are suggestive of mismatched transfusion, e.g., fever, rigors, abdominal pain, pallor, and dark urine. The blood shows evidence of an acute hemolytic process and various serological tests, e.g., Coombs', W.R., and Kline test, and the Donath-Landsteiner antibody, are positive.

Treatment. The syphilis is treated with penicillin and the patient transfused with stored blood since complement from fresh blood may cause a fresh hemolytic crisis.

Erythroblastosis fetalis (hemolytic disease of the newborn)

This condition is usually due to isoimmunization for the Rh factor. The A and B subgroups are less commonly involved, the MNS, Kell, and Duffy reactions are curiosities.

The genetics of rhesus incompatibility. The rhesus (Rh) antigens are determined by 3 pairs of genes. These genotypes are Cc, Dd, Ee. The clinically important pair is Dd, which gives rise to the severe forms of erythroblastosis. Rh positivity is equated with D positivity, and D negativity with the Rh negative state. The children of an Rh (D) positive father and an Rh (d) negative mother will be Rh (D) positive in all cases, providing the father has a DD pattern (homozygosity). If his pattern is Dd (heterozygosity) then only 50% of the offspring will be Rh (D) positive. The Rh (d) negative groups exist in about 15% of the general white population.

Cause of the disease. There must be D(Rh) incompatibility between the father and the mother. The disease cannot appear unless the fetal red cells have sensitized the mother's agglutinin mechanism. Therefore, the first pregnancy results usually in a normal child, with the creation of sensitivity in the mother. The first child can only be affected if the mother has previously been sensitized by the injection or transfusion of Rh (D) positive blood. Clearly, if the father is heterozygous (Dd), then several pregnancies may pass before a fetus which is D positive stimulates agglutinin production in the mother. Limitation of family numbers may result, therefore, in no child of a heterozygous father being affected. Presumably this accounts for the deficiency between the observed and the expected incidence of erythroblastosis.

Clinical characteristics. These are somewhat variable, running the gamut from the stillborn, hydropic fetus, to the infant who shows no obvious abnormality. The major signs and symptoms are due to hemolysis. In most cases, the infant is normal at birth, although yellow vernix may be a warning sign. The more severe cases develop jaundice within a short interval after birth. In others this sign may be delayed for up to 12 hours. Pallor of the skin is often distinguishable, and purpuric spots not uncommon. The spleen and liver are enlarged. Gross hydrops is usually incompatible with life, but mild edema of the face and legs may occur in some infants who survive—especially if they are premature.

Kernicterus

This is due to the deposition of bile pigment in the basal ganglia and adjacent reticular substance.

Clinical features. The infant has been jaundiced, usually heavily, for a day or two. He then displays poverty of movement, refusal to feed, twitching, extensor spasms, or frank convulsions. Opisthotonos may occur in the very severely affected patient. Loss of the Moro reflex and a high-pitched cry may occur at any stage. Sudden death, with pulmonary hemorrhage is not unusual; prematurity accelerates the whole process. In the survivors there is a high risk of the cerebral palsy syndrome. Deafness and mental retardation are frequent concomitants.

Blood examination. In the typical cases, the cord blood hemoglobin and red cell levels are decreased. There is an excess of nucleated red cells, and often a leucocytosis, and thrombocytopenia. Coagulation defects occur. The bilirubin is elevated above 2-3 mg%, usually this is in the indirect form. All affected children, even those who have a normal blood picture, will have a positive Coombs' test, as evidence of sensitization.

Treatment. Clearly the infant must be cleared of cells which will be destroyed. This will avoid the kernicterus and hyperbilirubinemia. Therefore, exchange transfusion with ABO compatible, RhD negative blood is carried out.

Indication for exchange transfusion:

1. Prematurity with a positive Coombs' test.
2. The obviously affected, with high bilirubin values, and a cord hemoglobin level of 15 g% or less.
3. The clinically unaffected, with a cord hemoglobin of 15 g% or less, or a bilirubin value of more than 2.5mg%.
4. Where there is a history of disease in previous siblings, exchange transfusion is usually necessary even if the above indications are initially absent.

The child who does not have the indications for exchange transfusion at birth must be closely watched. Hemoglobin estimations are done, preferably on venous blood. If this value decreases below 15 g%, or if the bilirubin reaches 10 mg% in the first 24 hours, then exchange transfusion should be done.

Repeat exchange transfusion. Those infants who are affected and have had 1 exchange, should be followed most carefully. The hemoglobin and bilirubin should be estimated at least every 3 hours for the first 24 hours and 6-hourly thereafter. If the bilirubin level reaches 18 mg% then it should be estimated hourly. A further increase is an indication for a repeat exchange transfusion. This may be necessary (especially in the premature) on 2 or 3 occasions. Lesser rises in bilirubin may be treated by phototherapy (q.v.).

Technique of exchange transfusion. This is carried out as a sterile surgical procedure. A polythene catheter is placed in the umbilical vein, and by means of a suitable manifold arrangement, blood is withdrawn from the infant, and replaced by donor blood. Thus, aliquots of blood are withdrawn and replaced until twice the blood volume has been replaced. Blood volume is roughly calculable as the product of body weight in kg x 100 ml.

As the anticoagulant in the donor blood contains citrate, a metabolic alkalosis with tetany may occur, and is prevented by giving 2 ml of calcium gluconate with every 100 ml of transfused blood. Larger quantities of calcium are necessary if the signs of calcium deficiency develop.

A variant of technique is to catheterize both umbilical artery and umbilical vein. The systemic blood pressure drains the blood from the baby, and gravity feeds the donor blood into it. Suitable clamps ensure that the exit-entrant volumes are compatible. The catheters require flushing with heparinized saline, and calcium gluconate is given as already described.

Overloading of the right heart is avoided by frequent estimation of venous pressure and comparison with the pre-transfusion level. Increases are treated by aspiration of fetal blood until the pressure falls. The aliquots exchanged thereafter should be decreased. The infant requires to be kept warm during the procedure.

Intrauterine transfusion. This procedure is carried out in mothers who have had multiple stillbirths because of severe intrauterine erythroblastosis. Throughout the third trimester of pregnancy, amniotic samples are taken and their optical density determined spectrophotometrically. This can be related to the amount of bilirubin, and used to assess the likely outcome of the pregnancy. If in the upper zone (fetus liable to I.U. death, or hydrops) and in the face of a sinister history, intrauterine transfusion is done. Essentially this consists in placing a needle into the fetal peritoneal cavity, followed by the injection of suitable blood. This may be repeated to ensure that the baby survives. He will, however, require multiple exchange transfusions after birth. Many such infants are born in a hydropic state, and most die.

Prevention of erythroblastosis. This may be accomplished by the injection of high-titre Rh antibody (anti D) to the mother at risk. If properly used, this technic can prevent 95% of recurrences.

Hemolytic disease of A or B incompatibility

This is a much milder condition, so that jaundice rather than pallor is the major finding. The liver and spleen are not affected. There is only a mild anemia with a moderate reticulocytosis and spherocytosis. The Coombs' test is often negative.

The jaundice occurs in the first 24 hours in most cases. The possibility of AB incompatibility is usually canvassed when other causes of neonatal jaundice are being considered. The presence of such incompatibility between mother and child should lead to a search for the appropriate agglutinins. Most of these infants do not require treatment other than phototherapy, but a bilirubin of 20 or more mg% is an indication for exchange transfusion.

Other acquired hemolytic anemias

These may be due to drugs or to infections. The latter are possibly more common. A variety of organisms such as the staphylococcus, malaria, syphilis, and various viruses such as rubella, herpes virus, and possible enterovirus as in the hemolytic-uremic syndrome may be responsible. The anemia may coexist with the so-called consumption-coagulopathy (p. 351).

The drugs and poisons which cause hemolytic anemias are legion. The effect of some (e.g., antimalarials, bean products, P.A.S., vitamin

K) are really due to enzyme deficiencies in the red cells. Toxic chemicals, which can cause hemolysis are lead, benzene ring compounds, and insecticides.

Clinical features. In those hemolytic states due to infection, the primary state predominates, e.g., staphylococcal pneumonias, the neonatal viral infections (cytemegalo, rubella) which have concomitant thrombocytopenia and purpura. All of these patients may be jaundiced. The hematological features are increased bilirubin, reticulocytosis, and primitive red cell forms. Monocytic erythrophagocytosis is often seen. These conditions are not associated with agglutinin formation so that the Coombs' test is negative.

Toxic hemolytic states

Clinical features. There is a history (often obscure) of toxin exposure. The anemia is suggested by pallor, fatigue, and evidence of a high-output state, e.g., loud venous hums, functional murmurs, loud third heart sounds. There may be signs of involvement of other systems, e.g., lead encephalopathy, liver damage. The hematological examination suggests only a non specific hemolysis. Stippling of the red cells is seen in lead poisoning.

Miscellaneous causes of acquired hemolysis

Burns are commonly associated with red cell destruction, usually in the first 5-6 days after the burn. Children who have had plastic patches inserted for cardiac septal defect, or prostheses for valvular disease may develop traumatic hemolytic anemias. These are usually of only mild severity, jaundice hardly ever being seen. Conditions associated with marked splenomegaly, e.g., portal hypertension, histiocytosis X, and various storage diseases may have mild hemolytic states, sometimes combined with leucopenia.

Pancytopenia (aplastic anemia)

This may be associated with various congenital defects of the bones, heart, and palate—the Fanconi type of aplastic anemia. Some victims of the congenital rubella syndrome may similarly be affected, and other severe viral infections of the neonate (salivary gland virus, herpes virus) may cause aplasia. In many instances, the condition is due to poisons such as benzene ring compounds, heavy metals, chloramphenicol, sulphonamides, hydantoins and meprobamate.

The bone marrow may also be compromised by invasion of neoplastic tissue (leukemia, neuroblastoma, histiocytosis), or by osteopetrosis.

Clinical features. These may initially be those of the underlying disease. Thus, the child with the Fanconi syndrome has obvious congenital abnormalities. The child exposed to toxic drugs and chemicals (sulphas, chloramphenicol, anticonvulsants, organic solvents, and benzene ring compounds) may have an initial hemolytic episode with jaundice and splenomegaly.

The features otherwise depend upon which blood component shows major depression. Thus, if the *granulocytes* (nucleated white cells) are involved, the features are those of unrestrained infection, at first affecting the mouth, fauces, vagina, or rectum. Skin and lung infections follow, when septicemia also occurs.

If the *platelets* are depressed, purpura and skin bruising are found often in a cyclic fashion. Bleeding from the nose, gut, and kidney occur. Intracranial bleeding often closes the picture. Pallor, weakness, and breathlessness betoken the failure of erythropoiesis.

Blood examination. There is a severe normocytic, normochromic anemia. The platelets are markedly reduced, and the circulating white cells mostly lymphocytes. Reticulocytes are low. The *bone marrow* confirms the absence of the red and white cell precursors, and the limitation of megakaryocytes. Fatty replacement, or infiltration with foreign cellular masses may be obvious.

Treatment. Antibiotics and blood transfusions are used. The transfusion of platelets must be from siliconed plastic collection packs, but platelet survival is poor. Steroids should be tried but are of little value. Testosterone derivatives (oxymetholone) have shown some promise.

DISORDERS OF THE WHITE CELLS

The main types of white cell are the neutrophil polymorphs (granulocytes), monocytes, lymphocytes, eosinophils, and basophils. The number and proportion of each can vary considerably with age, as can the total white cell count. This is shown in Table 21.

The *neutrophil polymorphs* originate in the bone marrow from the myeloblast which is transformed sequentially into the promelocyte, myelocyte, and metamyelocyte before assuming the mature form. The latter can exist as a reserve within the bone marrow. This one can be released relatively slowly, usually under the influence of infection. Another neutrophil reserve is maintained in the small blood vessels. This is released by stimuli such as catecholamines or exercise.

The *monocytes* are large phagocytic cells principally produced in the spleen and lymph notes, possibly from a common ancestor to the myeloblast and lymphoblast.

Table 21. Normal values of white cells

Age	Average Total and Range	Average% Granulocytes	% Lymphocytes
Birth	22,000 (10,000–40,000)	60 (40–80)	30
10 days	12,000 (6,000–20,000)	40 (35–55)	50
6 months	12,000 (7,000–20,000)	30 (20–40)	60
1 year	10,000 (7,000–12,000)	30	60
4 years	10,000 (6,000–10,000)	40	55
6 years	8,000	60	35

Monocytes 5–6% throughout infancy.
Eosinophils 3% throughout infancy.

The *eosinophil* is not strongly phagoctyic and exists in the skin, gut, respiratory tract, and in tissue fluid. It may be concerned with the degradation and removal of protein complexes. Eosinophilia is common in allergic states, and the cell may have some limiting effect upon the pharmacologic effectors (bradykinin, serotonin, histamine) of this state.

The *basophil*. This cell makes up only a small proportion of the total white cell count. Its function is obscure.

The *lymphocyte*. This, and the related plasma cell, have the important function of maintaining immunological competence (see p. 143). The peripheral lymphocyte count presumably includes long surviving, immunologically committed cells, which retain the capacity for division under an appropriate antigenic stimulus. Lymphocytes are not phagocytic, and do not respond to the chemical mediators which attract other white cells. The plasma cells contain and produce antibody and mediate the humoral immune response.

There is no good evidence that any specific factor is needed for the production of white cells, although vitamin B_{12} and folic acid deficiency may be associated with leucopenia.

The white cells are metabolically active, utilizing the same pathways for energy use as does the red cell. A larger number of enzyme systems is, however, present in leucocytes, and these may reflect those of the whole cellular system. Thus, it is possible to use the white cell to demonstrate specific enzyme deficiency states, as in maple syrup urine disease.

Phagocytosis

This is the property of ingesting foreign particles, especially microorganisms. The polymorphs and monocytes are the predominant phagocytes, the monocyte being superior to the neutrophil in dealing with large particles such as protozoa or red cells. Phagocytosis occurs principally within the tissues, the leucocytes being attracted and perhaps aggregated by the process of chemotaxis (leucotaxis). The origin of the phenomenon is obscure, although the participation of the prostaglandins or the cyclic nucleotides, has been suggested.

Leucocytosis

This is the term applied to a change in the total circulating white cell count. It may be associated with a variation in the relative proportions of the white cell types. Such an increased proportion can, however, exist without any change in total white count.

Polymorph Leucocytosis

The most frequent cause of a granulocyte (polymorph) leucocytosis is, of course, infection. Leucocytosis not due to infection is found in hemolytic states after acute blood loss, burns, and as part of diabetic coma. The stress of anesthesia, cardiac arrhythmias and grand mal seizures is also associated with leucocytosis.

Lymphocytosis

An absolute lymphocytosis, with a normal total white count, is characteristic of recovery from *any* acute infection and in viral infections. Relative lymphocytosis is seen in any condition associated with granulocytopenia. A high total white count, principally lymphocytes (true lymphocytosis), is found in mononucleosis, pertussis, and in acute infectious lymphocytosis. The last is a rather rare disease, with vague clinical features of mild upper respiratory tract infection, or transient abdominal pain and diarrhea. In most cases, the condition is suspected by the hematological findings (no anemia, WBC 15,000 +, lymphocytes 65%+), and by the exclusion of other causes.

Eosinophilia

This term implies an increase in the proportion of and the total circulating eosinophils. It is perhaps most common in the allergic states and skin disorders such as dermatitis herpetiformis and erythema multiforme. Intestinal parasitism is also a common cause, although this may be present without causing eosinophilia. The collagen disorders are also causes of this change, as are occasional instances of leukemia and lymphoma.

Monocytosis

This is found in protozoal and rickettsial infections, and occasionally in tuberculosis, lymphomata, and the lipid storage diseases.

Leucopenia

This signifies a reduction in the total white cell count. If one cell (e.g., the neutrophil) is affected, the proportion of the other cells will increase. The *total* white count may be normal in spite of a drastic reduction in the proportion of any single cell type. In general, leucopenia may be defined as a level of circulating white cells which is less than 5,000 cells/mm^3. In the newborn, the arbitrary level is higher—say 7,500 cells/mm^3.

Agranulocytopenia (neutropenia)

This is the commonest form of leucopenia. Accordingly, the proportions of lymphocytes is greatly increased. Minor depression of the polymorphs is common in viral diseases, especially those affecting the upper respiratory tract. More severe depressions, especially in the newborn, are found in the rubella/herpes virus/cytomegalovirus infections. Such a change can, however, accompany severe infections of other than viral etiology. Neutropenia is a feature of the pancytopenias or can be a response to drugs, bone marrow invasion, immune processes, or splenomegaly. In many instances the neutropenia is an incidental finding in the basic (usually hematological) disease.

Agranulocytosis is the extreme form of neutropenia, in which few or no granulocytes are present. Signs of infection are almost invariable with fever, reddening, and ulceration of mucous membranes and skin, severe pulmonary infections (often staphylococcal), diarrhea, and weight loss.

Drug-induced neutropenia

Again, this may be part of a total toxic bone marrow aplasia. The leucocytes are, however, prone to assault by chloramphenicol, sulphonamides, thiouracil and its derivatives, and the tranquillizers such as chlorpromazine and meprobamate. They are indeed usually the first cells to show a toxic response, and the best cells to follow during the treatment with such drugs. In most cases, the depression gives rise to few problems, the finding being incidental to the condition requiring use of the drugs noted. In a few children, the neutrophils are so seriously depressed that the agranulocytic syndrome (see below) is precipitated.

Idiopathic neutropenias

These are rather rare pediatric entities. Perhaps the more common are the following.

Chronic benign granulocytopenia

The condition is discovered by blood examination of children who have repeated minor infections, e.g., of the skin or respiratory tract. The polymorphs are very low in number. These children are however generally well and have little trouble with infections. Spontaneous cure in late childhood is the rule.

A possible variant of the above is *infantile genetic agranulocytosis* in which a simple recessive inheritance appears to operate. The infant has agranulocytosis, usually with severe infection of the skin and areolar tissue. Raised gamma globulin levels are usual, and the bone marrow shows impaired myelopoietic activity. Some of these children do poorly even with full antibiotic therapy.

Cyclic neutropenia

This curious and rare condition is characterized by disappearance of the polymorphs about every 3-4 weeks for 7-10 days. During the agranulocytic periods, there are infections of the skin, mouth, throat. The lymph glands and spleen enlarge during these episodes. The infections demand antibiotics, and these may be given prophylactically when the cycle has been clearly defined.

Pancreatic insufficiency and neutropenia

This is rare, and the neutropenia is an incidental finding in a child with failure to thrive, malabsorption due to steatorrhea, absence of pancreatic enzymes by duodenal intubation and a *normal* sweat test. This is not mucoviscidosis, and does not have chest infections as a primary manifestation. The treatment is that of the pancreatic disorder.

Immunological disorders of the granulocyte

As in similar disorders of the red cells (with which they often coexist) the leucocytes may be depressed in tumours, collagen diseases (e.g., disseminated lupus rheumatoid arthritis), and the lymphomata. In these, an autoimmune mechanism is postulated and certainly the neutrophil count will sometimes recover under the influence of steroids, pari-passu with the red cell dysplasia. Infants born of mothers with chronic neutropenia will sometimes show a transient neutropenia, analogous to the thrombocytopenia found in the infants of mothers who have idiopathic thrombocytopenic purpura. In these an immune mechanism is adduced, sometimes more convincingly associated with the presence of leuco-agglutinins (proteins which clump the white cells). In these conditions, the treatment is that of the primary disease.

Morphological disorders of the leucocytes

These are incidental, sometimes diagnostic, findings in generalized disease processes. The principal ones, which are rare, are the following.

Chediak-Higashi syndrome

Clinical features. This autosomal recessive condition is associated with frequent infections, failure to thrive, hepatosplenomegaly, and some of the failures of albinism, viz., photophobia, nystagmus, and the lack of pigmentation. The condition is commonly lethal early in life. Wright's stain reveals greenish granules in the polymorphs, the lymphocytes often contain red-staining inclusion bodies.

Pelger Huët anomaly

This is an asymptomatic variation in the polymorphs of autosomal dominant inheritance; in the majority of cells examined, no more than 2 lobes are present. No treatment is required for this type.

Reilly bodies

These are heavily granulated, azurophilic bodies found in the polymorphs of sufferers from gargoylism, lymphocytic inclusions are also often present. Alder's anomaly is Reilly bodies occurring as a rare autosomal recessive in otherwise normal children.

Functional disorders of the leucocytes

Chronic granulomatous disease

This rare condition is an x-linked recessive in which neither the polymorphs nor the monocytes can kill ingested bacteria.

Clinical features. These are severe infections of the skin, mucous membranes, chest, and gut. Micro abscesses of the skin are characteristic. The process will yield initially to antibiotics, although cure is incomplete and flares when they are discontinued. Chronic lymphadenopathy and hepatosplenomegaly are usually present.

Differential diagnosis. This is principally from the immunological diseases such as agammaglobulinemia, and other white cell anomalies, e.g., Chediak-Higashi.

Treatment. Antibiotic treatment and prophylaxis are carried out as indicated bacteriologically. No treatment exists for the defect in the leucocyte.

Lazy-leucocyte syndrome

This familial disorder is apparently due to absence of chemotactic ability in these cells.

Clinical features. The child suffers from recurrent attacks of fever, severe mouth infection with ulceration of the gums, and otitis media. The peripheral and bone marrow counts for leucocytes are normal, as are tests of humoral and cellular immunity mechanism. There is no morphological abnormality, but *in vitro* studies show impaired migration in response to chemical or inflammatory stimuli.

Treatment. Antibiotics are of value, there is otherwise none. The prognosis for life is generally satisfactory, although recurrent infections are usual.

Lymphocytopenia

This, and its extreme form, alymphocytosis, is a feature of the immunological deficiency diseases such as thymic alymphoplasia and Swiss-type agammaglobulinemia. These conditions are described in full elsewhere, but present with severe infections, failure to thrive and malabsorption.

Otherwise reduction in the total lymphocyte count is due to overwhelming infection, irrespective of the specific etiology, or to an adverse reaction to drugs, especially the anti-mitotic agents (cyclophosphamide, busulphan, benzene ring compounds, x-rays). Normally the neutrophil series is also affected.

Eosinopenia

This may be associated with any of the causes of pancytopenia already mentioned. A finding of small moment, steroid therapy is perhaps the commoner cause.

Leukemia in childhood

This is the most common neoplasm of childhood. It is almost always acute. The difficulty of pathological interpretation means that it is usually called stem-cell leukemia.

The disease can occur at any age, but it is most common between the fourth and seventh year. Congenital leukemia is higher in incidence in those children who have Down's syndrome.

Clinical features. These are very variable, but broadly divisible into those symptoms which are due to bone marrow destruction, and those which accompany invasion of other organs.

Thus, the first complaints may be those which are characteristic of aplastic anemia. If the erythroid series is primarily affected, then pallor, fatigue, and breathlessness predominate. White cell depression causes widespread infections. Depression of platelet production causes bleeding—purpura, espistaxes, and bleeding from the gut or renal tract. Unfortunately symptoms due to depression of all 3 blood elements may coexist. Infiltration of the subperiosteum gives rise to the common complaint of bone pain. This may superficially simulate rheumatic fever by its intermittent flitting quality. Fullness or swelling of the abdomen, due to hepatosplenomegaly is rarely the presenting symptom, but occurs often in the later stages of the disease. Enlargement of the superficial lymph glands is more commonly a sign than a symptom, but observant parents may present this as the first complaint. Pressure symptoms in the mediastinum or nervous system are most commonly found later in the disease process. Fever is usual at some stage, and may be an initial complaint.

The signs are clearly protean, variable, and affected by therapy. Pallor and purpura are commonly found in the skin. Leukemic invasion giving tumour-like masses may also occur there and initially may simulate allergic spots. Lymphadenopathy is common, but often regresses with chemotherapy. The liver and spleen become enlarged sooner or later. Examination of the chest may reveal evidence of tracheobronchial compression and even evidence of great vein obstruction is found. At any stage there may be tenderness of the bones, especially the tibiae and sternum. Leukemic infiltration of the orbits may cause proptosis (eye protrusion). Central nervous system invasion may be accompanied by headache, vomiting, drowsiness, or coma. Signs of meningeal irritation may be present, and papilledema betokens the raised intracranial pressure. The spinal fluid may show a pleocytosis. Nowadays these symptoms are more prone to occur in the treated individual, often in those who have remissions. Spinal tap is the best mode of anticipating C.N.S. leukemia.

Diagnosis. This is based upon the demonstration of leukemic cells in the bone marrow. Few cases should be diagnosed without this confirmatory measure. The peripheral blood usually shows a severe anemia, with the red cells normal in shape and size. The white cells may be quite normal in number and differential count, but many patients, however, show a florid increase in the white count, the majority being primitive cells. The granulocytes and platelets are commonly greatly reduced. All of these changes may be changed by antileukemic treatment. Biopsy of superficial glands often reveals invasion with leukemic tissue.

Needle aspiration of the marrow is necessary for immediate diagnosis. It is also one method by which treatment is controlled. The marrow usually shows depression or absence of the normal blood elements, such as the erythroid series and the megakaryocytes. The majority of the cells are highly abnormal lymphocytes with deeply staining, often mitotic, nuclei.

Complications. The previous section has outlined most of those to be expected. Others which may occur are renal failure, usually after prolonged hematuria, pleural effusion, and ascites. Bleeding into the retina may cause blindness. Deafness results from hemorrhage into the auditory system. Intracranial hemorrhage is one of the common modes of death in leukemia.

Treatment. Leukemia is an invariably fatal disease, which may be remitted for a long or shorter time, by appropriate therapy. Initially, there must be no doubt about the diagnosis. With this premise it is necessary to interview the parents at some length. The ultimate prognosis must be given to one or other partner. Sometimes there is initial rejection of the diagnosis. If there is, then confirmatory consultation should immediately be arranged. This will avoid, to some extent, the distressing shopping around which occurs in this condition. The parents should be assured that a remission with treatment is usual, and urged to plan accordingly. They should be encouraged to discuss their problems at any time.

Supportive treatment is represented by judicious blood transfusion in amounts adequate to maintain the hemoglobin level around 8g%. As transfusions are often closely spaced, a skilled hand with the needle is a mercy to the child. Antibiotics are used when the granulocyte count is very low, or when actual infection is present. They should not be used as a routine.

Drug treatment. Steroids (prednisone) and a variety of antimetabolites, are used in the treatment of leukemia in childhood. Prednisone is always given and is followed by vincristine, 6-mercaptopurine, methotrexate, and cyclophosphamide. The individual drugs may be given until the remission fails, or given in sequence for periods of 4-6 weeks. The exact dosage varies from patient to patient, but is often close to toxic levels. Accordingly, a close watch upon the patient must be kept by parents and physicians. The mouth should be inspected daily for ulceration and infection, and frequent white counts and occasional bone marrow examinations are essential in controlling therapy. Side effects should be explained to the parents and, as far as possible, anticipated. Rubidomycin may be of value in myeloid leukemia and asparaginase treatment is under trial for stem-cell leukemias.

Ultimate resistance to any form of therapy occurs, but only after some years, and then a decision must be made as to the desirability (or feasibility) of further therapy. Much will depend upon the individual philosophy of the family and medical attendant. However, efforts at treatment should be abandoned only after careful consideration, especially since the median survival time (presently 5 years), can be expected to rise with new and improved therapies.

The problems of bleeding—often from all orifices—are difficult. Blood replacement is of transient help and platelet transfusion usually of little benefit. Radiotherapy is valueless except for local lesions, e.g., obstructing mediastinal glands, or for relieving local bone pain.

THE BLEEDING DISORDERS

Physiology

Hemostasis

The process of stopping bleeding is divided into 2 main parts. Firstly, when a blood vessel is injured the hole must be plugged by a collection of platelets, then this must be consolidated by the formation of a blood clot.

The formation of the platelet plug begins when the collagen of the vessel is exposed by the injury. This attracts some platelets, which act upon each other to release chemicals (e.g., adenosine diphosphate) which attracts yet more platelets. At this stage, the platelet plug releases a factor (platelet factor III), which causes the release of thrombin, a factor in the formation of the clot which consolidates the platelet plug. Simultaneously the extrinsic (tissue) thromboplastin system is also activated to release thrombin.

Coagulation

This process requires many factors, each with synonyms. These with their physiological activities, are shown in table 22. Essentially, the process consists in the activation of factor II (prothrombin) to thrombin. The conversion occurs by 2 possible routes. In the *intrinsic* system, the change in electrical charge when collagen is exposed, initiates activation of factor XII, which in turn activates factors XI, IX, VIII, and X. The last, in the presence of factor V and platelet membrane lipoprotein (PF3) generates *intrinsic* thromboplastin (prothrombin activator) which in turn catalyzes the change of prothrombin to thrombin.

In the *extrinsic* system, the platelet and factor XII form platelet tissue factor. The latter, factor VII, and tissue lipoprotein factor form the tissue factor/factor VII complex which activates factor X. In the presence of factor V, calcium (factor IV), and lipoprotein tissue factor,

Table 22. Factors involved in coagulation

Factor Number	Synonym	Definition
I	Fibrinogen	The protein, which in the presence of thrombin, forms a fibrin clot.
II	Prothrombin	An alphaglobulin which is converted to thrombin when in the presence of thromboplastin accelerators and calcium.
III	Tissue thromboplastin	Exact identity unknown; promotes conversion of prothrombin to thombin. In plasma has a multiple origin, and is transient.
IV	Calcium (ionized)	Essential in the first and second stages of coagulation.
V	Proaccelerin, accelerator globulin, labile factor	A plasma factor taking part in the first and and second stages of coagulation.
VI (Archaic)	Accelerin, serum Ac. globulin	Active form of above.
VII	Proconvertin, stable factor, SPCA, auto prothrombin I	A plasma factor needed to convert prothrombin to thombin; quantitatively increased in the clotting process.
VIII	Antihemophiliac factor (AHF), antihemophilic globulin (AHG)	A thromboplastic factor of the beta globulin factor; deficiency causes classic hemophilia.
IX	Plasma thomboplastin component (PTC), Christmas factor, autoprothrombin II	An alphaglobulin associated with thromboplastin formation.
X	Stuart-Prower factor, Stuart factor, Prower-Stuart factor	Takes part in both thromboplastin formation and prothrombin conversion
XI	Plasma thromboplastin antecedent (PTA)	Reacts with activated Hageman factor to form thromboplastic substances.
XII	Hageman factor, contact factor	Initiates, at least in part, clotting *in vitro* activated by rough, i.e., unsiliconized surfaces clinically of no importance.
XIII	Fibrin stabilizing factor	A serum factor which maintains clot stability.

the *extrinsic* thromboplastin (prothrombin activator) is formed. This final product can also catalyze the change of prothrombin to thrombin. Thrombin converts fibrinogen (factor 1) to fibrin monomer. A polymer is then formed which converts to fibrin. The latter is stabilized by factor XIII. The process is summarized in figure 47.

It should be noted that the initial stages of the formation of the platelet plug can occur in the absence of coagulation mechanism.

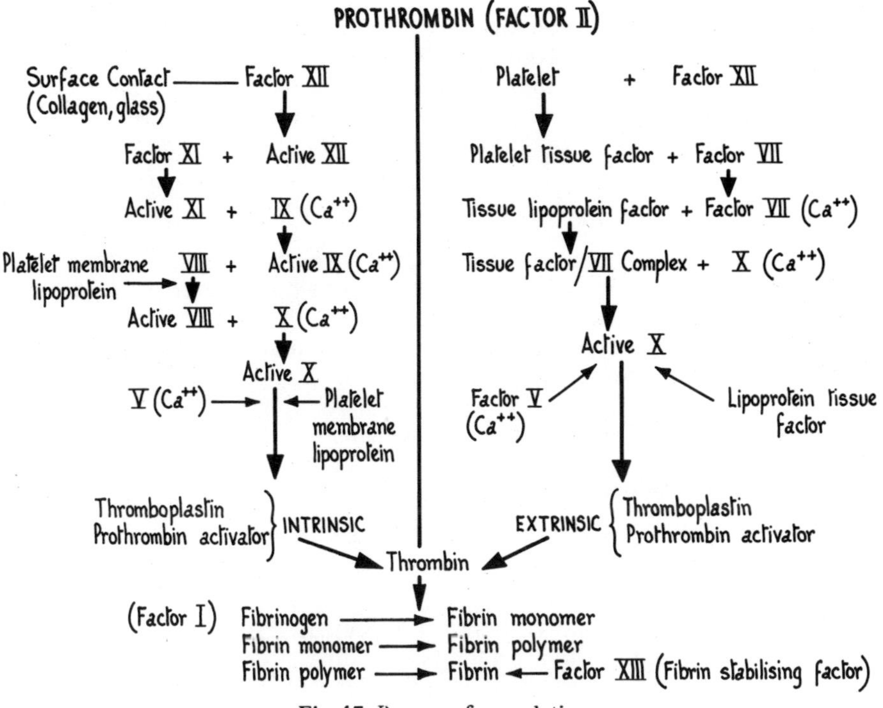

Fig. 47. Process of coagulation.

Conversely, an abnormality of platelet aggregation may lead to a deficiency in hemostasis, but not necessarily to a deficiency in coagulation.

Symptomatology of bleeding disorders

It is convenient to divide this into those features common in disorders of the platelets and/or capillaries and those found mainly in the coagulation defects. Clearly, some symptoms will be common to each.

The following are frequent in *platelet and capillary defects*. Purpura, small multiple bruises, epistaxis, menorrhagia, and spontaneous gastrointestinal bleeding. Hemorrhage from superficial abrasions is often profuse and repeated. Tooth extraction and surgical procedures cause immediate bleeding, usually controllable by local pressure, and often remitting in a short time. Deep hematomata and hemarthrosis are rare.

In *coagulation* disorders, bruises are usually single, large, spread readily to deep tissue planes, and occur after known injury. Bleeding into muscles or serous cavities *after minor injury* is particularly suggestive of a coagulation disorder.

It is important to recall that bruising is common in children, and memories are short. Accordingly, a history of spontaneous bruising should be carefully evaluated. Admission to hospital, bedrest, and close observation may be a necessary confirmation of the history. Similarly, epistaxis is common in children. The nose should always be inspected then, before this symptom is ascribed to a bleeding disorder. In relation to injury, the duration of the bleeding is of greater significance than is the amount of blood lost.

A sinister situation is a disorder which is characterized by extensive and spreading bruising and purpura, together with evidence of bleeding after intramuscular and intravenous injection. This argues a deficiency both of the coagulation mechanisms and of platelet number and function. Capillary disorder may be associated.

Some disorders of coagulation mechanism

Classic hemophilia (factor VIII deficiency)

This is the commoner disorder seen, It is familial, and caused by an X-linked recessive gene which means that only males have the disease, although females transmit it.

Clinical features. In short, these are repeated episodes of apparently spontaneous bleeding, and prolonged bleeding after minor injury. The situation may reveal itself early in life after circumcision, but the first symptoms are usually delayed until the child walks, and, therefore, liable to fall and injure himself. Then a minor fall causes a very large bruise or a small cut bleeds for a long time. Bleeding into muscles or the spaces between muscle masses (the fascial planes) is very typical and causes much pain and loss of use of the limbs.

Many symptoms depend on where the bleeding occurs; if into the abdomen or retroperitoneal space, they may resemble an abdominal catastrophe. Fortunately this is rare. A much more common event is bleeding into the knee and other joints, with pain and limping. When bleeding occurs into or between the muscles, the collection may press upon adjacent blood vessels and nerves, causing loss of sensation or actual paralysis. Occasionally a collection of blood persists to cause a blood cyst which can erode skin or bone. Low-grade inflammation of joints (osteoarthritis) is a common problem after repeated bleeds into them.

The situation described is that of the moderately severe variety of hemophilia. Mildly affected patients may not be discovered until tooth extraction or surgery causes prolonged bleeding. However, whatever the severity of the condition, periods of quiescence can occur at any age.

Diagnosis. Factor VIII is deficient, so that coagulation screening tests are abnormal.

General treatment. Since this is a familial condition, the parents feel guilty, so they must be comforted. They and the child are warned about the effects of injury, but this should not be overdone, since a big problem is to avoid undue restriction of the child's life. He must be allowed to play games and learn the skills of his own age group, and the price of this is some risk of bleeding. So the parents must accept the need for the child spending occasional periods in hospital. The child can play *supervised* games, and clearly should avoid the more dangerous sports.

Specific treatment. The coagulating mechanism can be made normal by injecting intravenously a dose of factor VIII (antihemophilic globulin). Enough is given to restore the level to about 50% of normal Whole blood is given only to replace lost blood, and not to restore coagulation power.

Many small bleeds do not need factor VIII replacement, as hemorrhage will stop with rest and immobilization of the affected part.

Factor IX deficiency (Christmas disease, hemophilia B)

Genetically and clinically this is the same as classic hemophilia, being distinguishable only by the test which reveals the identity of the missing coagulation factor. The care and treatment are as for factor VIII deficiency.

Factor XI deficiency

This is also familial (an autosomal recessive) which can affect either sex. It gives rise to minor bleeding episodes, mainly nose bleeds, or prolonged loss with dental or surgical procedures.

Treatment. The specific treatment is to give plasma, which contains the missing factor. This is necessary only as a preoperative measure, or where simple means, e.g., pressure, packing, fail to control the bleeding.

Factor V deficiency (parahemophilia)

This is again distinguishable from classic hemophilia only by special tests. The general treatment for hemophilia is followed. Specific replacement of factor V is by giving fresh plasma or blood.

Difficulties of factors II, VII, X

These clotting factors are made by the liver and require vitamin K for the process. Bleeding disorders then can occur in failure of vitamin K absorption, e.g., malabsorption; advanced liver disease; in the rare congenital deficiency of production; or after interference with these actions by drugs, e.g., aspirin, dicoumarol. However, the commonest disorder is hemorrhagic disease of the newborn.

Hemorrhagic disease of the newborn

The cardinal feature is bleeding, obvious or occult, usually as hematemesis or melena, occasionally as hematuria or in females, vaginal loss. Purpura is often present in the skin. The signs of anemia or shock are present according to the degree of blood loss. The first clue may be severe bleeding at circumcision or other neonatal operations. The mother has seldom been given prophylactic vitamin K.

Laboratory. The clotting time, one stage prothrombin, and thromboplastin tests are abnormal.

Differential diagnosis. This is mainly from other causes of acute blood loss such as ruptured spleen. Hematemesis may be due to swallowing blood from the maternal passages, In this situation the baby is not shocked, and test of the vomited blood shows its maternal origin. Vaginal bleeding due to placental hormones is not associated with the signs of anemia and shock. In all of the entities mentioned, the laboratory examination is normal.

Treatment. Resuscitate the baby by transfusion if need be, and give vitamin K.

Congenital factor I deficiency (afibrinogenemia)

This is rare, and is carried on as autosomal recessive. The blood is incoagulable, but spontaneous hemorrhage is mild, occurring mainly as epistaxes and bruising. Hemarthroses do not occur. Bleeding after tooth extraction, surgery or trauma is, however, severe and prolonged. Fibrinogen levels are low by direct measurement.

Treatment. Adequate plasma concentration is maintained by the infusion of fibrinogen. This is usually needed only if bleeding symptoms are severe, or as a preliminary to surgery.

Acquired fibrinogen deficiency is a leading abnormality in the syndrome of consumption coagulopathy (see p. 351).

Factor XIII deficiency

This is a rare congenital disorder.

Clinical features. Bleeding from the healing navel is the usual first feature. This may be the sole abnormality, or be followed in later life by a bleeding disorder resembling factor VIII deficiency, with bruising, bleeding from tooth extraction, or after surgery. Rather rarely is there hemarthrosis or extensive bruising.

Laboratory. The coagulation screening tests are all *normal*, as is quantitative fibrinogen determination. The clot is, however, abnormally soluble in 5 molar urea, and there is acceleration of euglobulin lysis.

Treatment. Fresh blood or plasma, in small volume (e.g., to 150 ml) will correct the bleeding abnormality for 3-4 days. The remainder of the therapy is as described for factor VIII hemophilia.

DISORDERS OF PLATELET FUNCTION

Primary disorders are congenital, the exact lesion reflected in a corresponding platelet function. There is a growing number of these entities, summarized in table 23.

Clinical features. These are very similar in each condition. Usually there is a history of a mild or moderate bleeding disorder, mainly purpuric spots, nose bleeds, and small multiple bruises. Prolonged oozing after dental extraction or operation is common, and minor cuts may bleed for a long time. Rarely there is bleeding into the gut or brain.

Treatment. Fresh platelet transfusion is given during acute, bleeding episodes *except* Von Willebrand's disease. In this cryoprecipitate (as used in classic hemophilia) will suffice.

Secondary disorders of platelet function

These occur in the advanced stages of uremia, cirrhosis and consumption coagulopathy (see below), and are found in Ehler-Danlos disease, osteogenesis imperfecta, and systemic lupus erythematosus. The clinical features are those described above. Aspirin, antihistamines, and some tranquilizers may cause abnormalities of the tests of platelet function, but seldom give rise to clinical disease.

Disorders of platelet number

Thrombocytopenia means a fall in the number of circulating platelets. These platelets may also be abnormal in function. Two general types can be recognized.

Thrombocytopenia due to under production of platelets. In this, the bone marrow megakaryocytes, which are the platelet precursors, are themselves reduced in number. There are many causes, mainly bone marrow aplasia, which may follow exposure to radiation or drugs, e.g., 6-mercaptopurine, folic acid antagonists, other cytotoxic agents, chloramphenicol, sulphonamide, anticonvulsants, phenylbutazone, tranquilizers, and insecticides. Extensive invasion of the bone marrow by leukemia, tumours, or the storage disorders are also possible causes.

Table 23. The common disorders of platelet function

Disorder	Genetics	Platelet Adhesion to Glass	Platelet Aggregation	PF 3 Release	Clot Retraction	Platelet Number	Platelet Morphology	Other Studies
Von Willebrand's disease	Autosomal dominant	Decreased	N	N	N	N	N	Decreased Factor VIII Prothrombin time decreased
Glanzmann's thrombasthenia	Autosomal recessive	Decreased	Decreased to collagen ADP thrombin adrenalin	Abnormal	Abnormal	N	Abnormal	–
Thrombopathia syn: Portsmouth syndrome ADP release defect	Variable	Decreased*	Decreased to collagen* Adrenaline* low ADP concentration	Decreased+	N	N	N	–
Thrombocytopathy (PF3 defect)	Autosomal dominant?	Usually N	Normal	Decreased	N	N	N	–
Thrombasthenia impaired response to ADP	Autosomal recessive	Decreased	Decreased to ADP collagen	Decreased	N	N	N	–

* Correctable by adding ADP.
N = Normal.

Normal platelet production, accelerated platelet destruction in the blood. In this the megakaryocytes are normal or increased in number, but platelet life span is reduced. An immune mechanism is likely in most cases, and this can arise after exposure to drugs (e.g. antihistamines, thiazide diuretics, barbiturates) or be a feature of severe viral infections (e.g., neonatal rubella, mononucleosis), or septicemias. Diseases is which a large spleen has developed, or where large hemangiomata are present may entrap enough platelets to cause a scarcity.

General features of thrombocytopenia

The usual problem is purpura—small widely spread areas of hemorrhage into the skin. The spots may coalesce to form bruises. Bleeding from cuts and injections is prolonged. Occasionally there is bleeding from the kidney or gut, or into the brain.

The bleeding time is prolonged, the platelet count is reduced and specific tests of platelet function may be abnormal. The 2 types noted above are eventually distinguished by bone marrow examination to count the megakaryocytes.

Some specific entities

These are the more common disorders seen in practice, and most are associated with platelet destruction by an immune process.

Neonatal thrombocytopenia

This may be due to drugs given to the mother (mainly thiazide diuretics), passive antibody transfer in material thrombocytopenic purpura, or an isoimmune state. The latter is an analogue of erythroblastosis of the Rh type, in that the baby's and mother's platelets are incompatible and maternal antibodies develop.

Clinical features. Purpura, extensive bruising of the presenting part and cephalhematoma are the usual features. The platelets are greatly reduced in number. A history of drug exposure may be obtained, or maternal platelet antibodies are demonstrable.

Treatment. None may be necessary in mild cases, especially when further drug exposure can be avoided. In the isoimmune state, with high levels of maternal antibodies to platelets, severe disease may warrant an exchange transfusion.

Idiopathic thrombocytopenic purpura

This condition is most probably due to an autoimmune mechanism, although the details remain obscure.

Clinical features. This is mostly a disease of preschool children. The condition is of sudden onset, often with a preliminary cold followed by skin purpura, bruising, nose bleeds, and occasionally hemorrhage, from the gut and kidney. Purpuric spots in the mouth and on the palate is a very suggestive finding. Minor injury causes extensive bruising.

Laboratory. The platelets are reduced, and may be abnormal in shape. The bleeding time and clot reaction are abnormal, as may be tests of capillary fragility (Hess test).

Progress. Mostly the disease clears up in a few weeks. In the remainder it may present for up to a year, but in only about 10% for longer.

Treatment. In most cases only the avoidance of injury is needed. If bleeding is marked, the loss is made up by transfusion, and steroids may be used. If the disease is chronic and unrelieved by several courses of steroids, then splenectomy is usually advised.

Wiskott-Aldrich syndrome

This is a rare, sex-linked recessive affecting boys.

Clinical features. Purpura, easy bruising, prolonged bleeding, eczema and susceptibility to infections date from infancy. The latter may be quite severe, with arthritis and septicemia being common. In addition to positive tests for abnormal platelet number and function, there is a reduction in the immunoglobulin M; only the infections of this condition are treatable. Lymphatic tumours may complicate the late stages.

Miscellaneous causes of thrombocytopenia

As already mentioned, splenic enlargement, from whatever cause, may be associated with low platelet number. So too are massive transfusions, and some episodes of extracorporeal circulation as used in open heart operations. These problems occasionally demand platelet transfusion if bleeding is severe.

Increased number of platelets

This is thrombocytosis (thrombocythemia) and is essentially a laboratory diagnosis made when the platelet count exceeds 750,000 mm^3. It has a wide etiology, principally following hemorrhage, and in hemolytic anemias. The platelet count may rise greatly after splenectomy for idiopathic thrombocytopenic purpura or for hemolytic disease. Treatment is generally unnecessary, as thrombosis is exceptionally rare.

Purpura

This is the sympton of multiple small hemorrhages into the skin and mucous membranes. These may increase in size to cause small bruises. Occasionally prolonged bleeding follows local injury, and more serious bleeding disorders may coexist. Clearly the symptom is due to a defect in local hemostasis, and all of the described platelet disorders of decreased number and function may be operative. However, a vascular component may be present in the exanthems (e.g., measles), or in scurvy. A physical rupture of the capillary may be present, as in the traumatic purpuras of pertussis, or in obstructed labour.

Specific entities

The exanthems. Purpura of mild degree is not unusual in measles and chicken pox. Normally it affects only the skin, sparing the mucous membranes. Platelet number and function are unaffected in most cases. Evidence of bleeding from the gut, kidney, or injection sites suggests consumption coagulopathy (see below). A few purpuric spots are common in meningococcal infections and in the salmonelloses. Rare causes of purpura include *Rendu-Osler-Weber* disease in which multiple skin telangiectases are associated with purpura and excessive bleeding after surgery. These symptoms are due to the local vascular abnormality. In *Ehler-Danlos* syndrome, the purpura is a minor component of a total picture of hyperelastic friable skin, pseudotumours, and hyperextensible joints. Platelet function may also be disturbed in this condition (see p. 392).

Henoch-Schönlein syndrome

This is described in full elsewhere (p. 544). In brief, however, it is a condition associated with streptococcal invasion which may present with arthropathy, abdominal pain, or a skin manifestation. The latter is most pertinent to this section. It begins as an itchy urticarial wheal which rapidly becomes petechial or frankly hemorrhagic. The lesion goes through the colour changes of a bruise, ending as a tobacco coloured stain. The skin changes are found typically on the buttocks and flexor surfaces. Bleeding from the gut or kidney may coincide.

Laboratory. The platelet count is normal, anemia will reflect the blood loss. Leucocytosis is usual, as is an increased E.S.R.

Consumption coagulopathy

This is a severe bleeding disorder, most often due to severe viral and bacterial infections. Intravascular coagulation is common and depletes the substances appropriate to normal clotting. These include factors I,

II, V, and VIII, and platelets. Excessive fibrinolysis is common, presumably due to abnormal activation of plasminogen to plasmin by thrombin or urokinase. The exact reason for the latter reaction is not fully elucidated. Hemolysis is a common associated finding. The disorders (and their synonyms) which are associated with consumption coagulopathy are shown in table 24.

Table 24. Consumption coagulopathy

SYNONYMS	Defibrination syndrome Purpura Fulminans Hemolytic-uremic syndrome ? Thrombotic thrombocytopenic purpura Waterhouse-Friedrichsen syndrome Generalized Schwartzman reactions
ETIOLOGY	
Newborn	Rubella, herpes virus, cytomegalovirus infections, congenital syphilis, gram-negative septicemias, respiratory distress syndrome
Infants and older children	Meningococcal infection, exanthems, smallpox, septicemias (usually gram-negative, occasionally staphylococcal) Acute leukemia Cyanotic congenital heart disease, mismatched blood transfusion
Older children	Advanced cirrhosis, snake bite (viperines, elapidae)

Laboratory investigations. Hemoglobin is reduced, the red cells are abnormal with spherocytes and burr cells. Erythrophagocytosis may be obvious. Hyperbilirubinemia may reflect rapid blood destruction. The platelet count is commonly reduced, often to very low levels. Platelet function is disordered, with increased bleeding time and impaired clot retraction. The screening tests of coagulation are usually abnormal, reflecting reduction in factors, I, II, V, and VIII. These cannot be corrected by vitamin K therapy. Increased fibrinolysis may be demonstrable by accelerated dissolution of the incubated clot, or by a shortened euglobulin lysis time.

Clinical features. Those of the primary disorders are present. Neonatal viral infections (rubella, herpes, cytomegalovirus), protozoal invasion, and neonatal septicemia are described elsewhere (p. 48). Additionally there is widespread purpura, multiple bruising, and oozing from mucous membranes and injection sites. The septicemias of older children display fever, shock, rapid anemia, usually without overt jaundice, and especially in pseudomonas infections, local skin necrosis, The features of the hemolytic-uremic syndrome are described on p. 295.

Thrombotic states may occur not only as a skin manifestation (necrosis) but be evidenced by the sudden onset of blindness, aphasia (loss of speech), convulsions, and various neurological signs.

Differential diagnosis. In the newborn, the principal consideration is simple vitamin K dependent hemorrhagic disease of the newborn. In this entity, the child's state, if parlous, reflects only blood loss. Transfusion will restore him to apparent normality, and vitamin K corrects the abnormality in the clotting factors. In the older child *Henoch-Schönlein* purpura is a consideration. In this disease, platelet number is normal, urticaria is, or has been, present and the purpura tends to be localized. Bleeding and clotting studies are normal. Disorders of platelet function and number are differentiated by the studies noted above, and by the fact that the tests of coagulation are normal.

Treatment. The primary disease should be treated if possible. Normally this means vigorous and appropriate antibiotic therapy for the bacterial septicemias. Fluid and electrolyte depletion are common and should receive appropriate repair, although great care is needed in the hemolytic-uremic syndrome. The latter also requires appropriate treatment for anuria and uremia (p. 297). Blood transfusion is necessary, often repeatedly, as transfused cells may have a shorter than usual survival time. Infusions of the factors found to be deficient, e.g., I, II, V, and VIII (the so-called PPSD infusion) may help stem the bleeding. Platelet transfusion is indicated in thrombocytopenia where bleeding continues after the coagulation factors are apparently increasing in quantity. Many patients will recover on these regimes alone. Heparin therapy (50-100 units/kg) is principally indicated where excessive fibrinolysis is demonstrable, platelet counts are relatively high, and infused factor I (fibrinogen) rapidly disappears. Obvious thrombotic phenomena are also an indication for heparin although less logically, since these begin as platelet plug deposition and aggregation, a process unaffected by anticoagulant activity. The use of drugs (dipyridamole) to inhibit platelet aggregation is as yet unproved, as is the use of epsilon aminocaproic acid to fibrinolytic syndromes.

Prognosis. This is not good, especially in the fulminant septicemias and the thrombotic thrombocytopenic variant. Patients with the hemolytic-uremic syndrome will recover in about 50% of cases. The finding in children with cyanotic congenital heart disease is mild, and of small moment unless open heart surgery is contemplated.

15 Disorders of the endocrine system

THE PITUITARY GLAND

Physiology. The pituitary is divisible into the anterior and posterior parts. The former, partly controlled by the nearby hypothalamus, produces thyroid stimulating hormone (T.S.H.), A.C.T.H. (regulating adrenal cortical activity), follicle stimulating hormone (F.S.H.), and L.H. (luteinizing hormone) which control some aspects of ovarian and testicular function, as well as H.G.H. (human growth hormone). The production of each of the stimulating hormones is largely controlled by a feedback mechanism, e.g., when sufficient quantities of thyroid hormone are present in the blood, this is appreciated by the pituitary, and the stimulating hormone turns off.

The posterior pituitary (neurohypophysis) releases 2 main hormones, oxytocin and vasopressin (antidiuretic hormone, A.D.H.). Each can stimulate muscular contraction, and vasopressin also inhibits urine production by increasing the reabsorption of water in the kidney tubules.

In spite of its multiple functions, disease of the pituitary is rather rare in children.

Hypopituitarism

Failure of pituitary function is usually expressed as failure of growth due to absence of H.G.H. activity. In *isolated* H.G.H. deficiency, the child is normal at birth, but gradually falls behind in height and weight until by 2-3 years of age he is recognizably shorter than his peers. The body proportions are normal and the child indeed looks quite muscular and well covered, if not obese, but he is in the low percentiles.

Apart from a delayed bone age by x-ray, clinical examination is negative. The diagnosis is confirmed by failure to show normal H.G.H. secretion.

Treatment. H.G.H. is injected in regular courses until growth velocity is normal.

If the patient is deficient in the gonadotrophins (L.H., F.S.H.) then growth failure coincides with absent sexual development. Persistence of juvenile features is common in such sufferers. Other evidences of trophic hormone deficiency (thyroid, adrenal) may be demonstrated biochemically, or suspected by the presence of features of hypothyroidism or disturbed adrenal function. Deficiency of all of the pituitary hormones (panhypopituitarism) is quite rare, occurring usually after removal of an adjacent tumour. In such patients the posterior pituitary function may be interfered with. Thus vasopressin lack will then cause diabetes insipidus (see below).

Hyperpituitarism

Gigantism is associated with high levels of H.G.H. production and accelerated linear growth. The causal tumour may be associated with symptoms and signs of raised intracranial pressure. The treatment is surgical destruction of the pituitary gland.

Cushing's syndrome. This is caused by excess production of adrenal steroids by a tumour (basophilic adenoma) of the pituitary which causes overproduction of A.C.T.H. The disorder is described in detail elsewhere (p. 361). The treatment is removal of the tumour.

Diabetes insipidus

This follows disease of the posterior pituitary (neurohypophysis) with failure of release of vasopressin (antidiuretic hormone).

It may be an isolated familial disorder, or be part of panhypopituitarism. In either case, the main symptom is the passing of large amounts of urine (polyuria) due to the failure of the kidney tubule to resorb water. The polyuria must be compensated by an equivalent thirst (polydipsia). The urine is dilute, but otherwise normal, the principal diagnostic test is resolution of the symptoms after giving vasopressin.

In *nephrogenic* diabetes insipidus, which is also familial, the symptoms and signs are identical; however, there is no response of the kidney to vasopressin. In some instances there is some relief by giving thiazide diuretics.

THE THYROID GLAND

Physiology. The thyroid hormones are required to maintain normal energy production within the cells. Specifically, they are necessary for normal growth of the body and brain. Thyroid hormone production is stimulated by the pituitary T.S.H. The main functional hormones are triiodothyronine (T_3), and thyroxin (T_4). The gland traps iodine and combines it with tyrosine, using the enzymes peroxidase and iodinase. Two products are formed. One, monoiodotyrosine (T_1) contains a single iodine atom, the other diiodotyrosine (T_2) contains 2 such atoms.

Two molecules of the latter combine to form thyroxine (T_4); 1 of each (T_1 and T_2) can combine to form triiodothyronine—each process requiring a coupling enzyme. The final products are stored in thyroglobulin from which they are released as required by a protease. Eventually broken down by metabolic activity, the iodine again enters the thyroid gland for further use.

Hypothyroidism

Failure of thyroid function can occur if the gland is congenitally absent, is deprived of sufficient dietary iodine to maintain its function, or lacks any of the enzymes necessary to T_3 and T_4 synthesis already described. The taking of drugs (goitrogens) which interfere with thyroid function is a rare cause of hypothyroidism.

Sporadic Cretinism

This is the name given to hypothyroidism emerging soon after birth.

Clinical features. Prolonged neonatal jaundice or an abnormally low body temperature (hypothermia) are occasional first symptoms. More often, a few weeks after birth, the baby is lethargic, feeds poorly, is constipated, and neither gains weight nor grows. The yellowish appearance of the baby, due to the pigment carotene, may be a parental complaint.

Occasionally the disease is recognized by the major signs—a yellowish inactive baby with a poorly sustained, hoarse cry, in the low percentiles for growth, and with swollen face, eyes, and limbs (myxedema). The baby feels cool, and the pulse is slowed, and spontaneous activity is much reduced. Smiling, sitting up, and rolling over are late or absent. In the late presenting child, all of the above are associated with marked growth failure, the retention of infantile proportions, delayed dentition, and poor head growth.

Special investigations. X-rays reveal a delayed bone age and multiple foci of epiphyseal ossification (epiphyseal dysgenesis). T_3 and T_4 blood levels are low, and T.S.H. values and thyroid binding index (T.B.I.) are increased.

Treatment. This is the permanent replacement of the absent hormone by sodium-1-thyroxine, in amounts sufficient to restore the T_3 and T_4 and T.S.H. levels to normal. This should coincide with acceleration of growth, resolution of the infantile proportions and restoration of the x-ray bone age to normal.

Juvenile hypothyroidism

This may be due to abnormal thyroid size, position, or function. Goitre may coincide or destruction of thyroid tissue can be due to an autoimmune process (Hashimoto's disease).

Clinical features. The main problem is growth failure, inactivity, slowness, and delay in achieving accomplishments. Constipation and complaints about feeling cold are common. The signs of cretinism are present although less obviously. The thyroid gland may be enlarged (goitrous). The investigation and treatment are as described for cretinism.

Hashimoto's disease

This autoimmune disorder causes a firm thyroid swelling (goitre) which may ultimately be associated with symptoms and signs of hypothyroidism. Immunological studies may be suggestive, but the diagnosis is finalized by biopsy. The treatment varies with the stage of the disease.

Where a goitre, with high T.S.H. values is present, then thyroxin may reduce the thyroid swelling by reducing pituitary activity. The same therapy is given for the hypothyroid states.

Hyperthyroidism (thyrotoxicosis)

Chronic overactivity of the thyroid gland is uncommon in children, occurring most often in school-age girls. Rarely it occurs in the infants of mothers overtreated for pregnancy *hypothyroidism*. Most patients will have an excess of long acting thyroid stimulator (L.A.T.S.).

Clinical features. Most of these are symptoms: excitability, restlessness, emotional instability, short attention span, and poor school results. Parents may note sweatiness, undue hunger, loss of weight, and thyroid swelling (goitre), as well as pop-eyes (exophthalmos). Excess thyroid stimulates the sympathetic nervous system, so that sweaty hands, skin flushing, tremor, a fast pulse, and raised systolic blood pressure are common signs. Exophthalmos is usually mild, and may be absent. The height is usually in a higher percentile than that for weight.

Laboratory studies. The T_3 and T_4 levels are high. T.B.I. and T.S.H. are low, but L.A.T.S. may be increased.

Complications. Occasional patients develop congestive cardiac failure due to the greatly increased cardiac activity. Even rarer is the hyperthyroid storm—increased body temperature, extremely fast heart rate, acute congestive failure, and death from apparent exhaustion.

Treatment. The first treatment is always with the antithyroid drugs, carbimazole or propylthiouracil. Repeated courses of these drugs are usually necessary. If there is no satisfactory response, then partial removal of the thyroid (thyroidectomy) is done.

Neonatal hyperthyroidism (thyrotoxicosis)

This occurs in the babies of women who are themselves hyperthyroid during pregnancy.

Clinical features. The infant is restless, irritable, has a fast pulse, and fails to gain weight. Dehydration or congestive failure may occur. The treatment is to give simple sedatives and iodides (potassium iodide) until spontaneous recovery takes place. This may take a few weeks to a month or two.

Goitre

This means enlargement of the thyroid gland. There are many causes, the most common being deficiency of iodine in the diet. Autoimmune disease (see p. 326) causes Hashimoto's disease discussed above. In many instances, no obvious cause can be found—as in pubertal goitre of girls.

Clinical features. These are most dramatic in the newborn, when the enlarged gland presses upon the airway, giving rise to respiratory difficulty, viz, head retraction, dyspnea, and rib and sternal retraction. Tracheal intubation, followed by removal of part of the gland is the treatment.

Simple (sporadic) goitre

This is usually seen in pubertal girls, usually without obvious cause. In a few patients there is a history of exposure to goitrogens such as cobalt, para-aminosalicylic acid (used in treating tuberculosis) or skin applications containing resorcinol.

Clinical features. The main feature is a general enlargement of the thyroid gland. There are many blood vessels within it, so listening with a stethoscope over the gland may reveal loudish murmurs. Spontaneous recovery is usual. Persisting enlargement should hasten doing a biopsy, which may reveal the changes of Hashimoto's disease. Thyroxin is occasionally given to hasten decrease in the size of the gland.

Thyroid tumour

These are usually carcinomas, and are rare in children.

Clinical features. Most are asymptomatic except for the presence of a lump in the thyroid. If the tumour spreads (metastasizes), it may cause painless enlargement of the lymph glands of the neck. If the spread is to the glands within the thorax, then pressure symptoms can occur. These are cough, difficulty in swallowing, and breathlessness. If pressure on the superior vena cava occurs, then the face head and arms may swell, with prominent superficial veins.

Treatment. The thyroid tumour is removed surgically and radioactive iodine is given to destroy the tumour remnants.

THE ADRENAL GLAND

This gland has 2 distinct parts, each with a separate function. The adrenal *medulla* secretes catecholamines (adrenaline, noradrenaline). The *cortex* is more complex, and produces several hormones. These include the glucocorticoids (21-carbon steroids), the principal member of which is hydrocortisone (alias 17-hydroxycorticosterone, cortisol), which can be converted to cortisone. These glucocorticoids promote the formation of glucose, water and salt retention in the body, and loss of potassium by the kidneys. The same compounds can be synthesized, and are used for their antiinflammatory and immunosuppressant effects. *Aldosterone* is a *mineralocorticoid* which controls sodium reabsorption by the kidney tubule. Its secretion is controlled mainly by the body sodium content, which in turn is monitored by special (juxtaglomerular) cells situated on certain blood vessels in the kidney.

Androgens (male sex hormones) and *estrogens* (female sex hormones) are also made by the adrenal cortex.

The ultimate stimulus to adrenal cortical function is the pituitary hormone A.C.T.H. The production of this pituitary hormone is controlled by feedback of the adrenal cortical hormones, i.e., if the blood hydrocortisone level rises, then pituitary A.C.T.H. production falls, and vice versa.

Disorders due to overactivity of the adrenal cortex (adrenal cortical hyperfunction: adrenogenital syndrome).

These are usually due to an abnormality in the manufacture of the adrenal hormones. This fault is usually an enzyme defect, very rarely it is due to a tumour. In most instances, hydrocortisone is not formed, so that feedback control of pituitary A.C.T.H. is impossible. High levels of A.C.T.H. further stimulate the adrenal to produce excessive normal androgens and abnormal androgen intermediates. Aldosterone deficiency is an important association since this causes loss of salt and dehydration. Many enzyme defects are possible, but in 90% of patients, 21-hydroxylase is lacking, either in part or totally. If the latter, the patient dehydrates easily. The possible enzyme deficiencies with some of the clinical results are shown in table 25.

Clinical features. The first problems are usually due to the *salt losing state*, with refusal to feed, vomiting, and loss of weight. These will rapidly progress to full scale dehydration with tachycardia, greyish cyanosis, low blood pressure, and loss of skin turgor. Occasionally diarrhea also is present. Sudden death is not unknown.

Table 25. Possible results of various enzyme deficiencies

Enzyme Defect	Possible Result
21–hydroxylase	Virilization, salt loss
11–β hydroxylase	Virilization, hypertension
3–β-hydroxysteriod dehydrogenase	Salt loss, incomplete genital development in males
17–hydroxylase	Hypertension, genital changes in females

Otherwise the baby may have changes in the genitals. These are most easily seen in girl babies in whom adrenal androgen production causes enlargement of the clitoris and fusion of the labia so that superficially they may resemble boys. This situation is called pseudohermaphroditism. If not treated these girls eventually have a muscular masculine appearance, with male type pubic and axillary hair, although a vagina, uterus, and ovaries are all present, and the chromosomes are of the female type.

In male infants, there is isosexual precocity, i.e., the genitals mature with abnormal rapidity. Mostly this takes some months to occur so that precocity is not a very helpful sign in boys in the early stages. However, by the age of 6/12, the penis is enlarged, and this is followed over a year or two by the growth of pubic hair, testicular enlargement, increased muscular development, acne, and breaking of the voice. Growth velocity is increased early, but then slows because of fusion of the bone epiphyses (the growing areas) by the androgens. In either sex, abnormal brownish pigmentation of the genitals or areolae (area around the nipples) may occur.

In summary then, the important clinical features are salt loss, and abnormal production of androgens which causes pseudohermaphroditism in females and precocious isosexual puberty in males.

Laboratory. The urine will contain abnormal intermediate products. In the common 21-hydroxylase deficiency, this is pregnanetriol. All patients with virilizing changes will have an excess of 17-ketosteroids.

In the salt losing states, serum sodium is low, and serum potassium is high. Chloride values may also decrease. Abnormalities of aldosterone levels may also be found.

Treatment. The principles are to relieve any dehydration or salt losing and to reduce adrenal function by supplying drugs (steroids) which will reduce pituitary A.C.T.H. production. The first end is achieved by intravenous saline, followed by extra salt in the diet. Salt retention is assured by giving I.M. desoxycorticosterone acetate (D.O.C.A.) until the electrolytes (Na, C1, K) are stable. Then the injections are replaced by the drug 9-α fluorocortisone given by mouth. This ensures stability of the salt/water situation. Suppression of the pituitary A.C.T.H. production is attained by giving glucocorticoids as cortisone.

The cortisone *must* be given for life, the exact dosage being controlled by keeping the child well, and his urinary pregnanetriol normal. If there is no salt-losing state, then cortisone alone is needed.

Any patient with adrenogenital syndrome will require increased drug dosage and added salt in emergencies such as infection, injury or proposed surgery.

Virilizing adrenocortical tumour

The clinical features are similar to those of adrenogenital syndrome, but females do not have genital changes at birth, and salt losing states with dehydration are relatively uncommon. The biochemical abnormalities are those already described for adrenogenital syndrome, e.g., high urinary pregnanetriol. These changes cannot, however, be suppressed by giving cortisone-like compounds, and this is the main test for the presence of a tumour rather than simple overfunction. The treatment is surgical removal of the neoplasm.

Cushing's syndrome

This disorder is due to the overproduction of hydrocortisone (cortisol). As a primary disease it is rare in children, and usually due to a tumour. Most children with Cushing's syndrome have been given an excess of cortisone or similar drugs for the treatment of some other disorder, e.g., the nephrotic syndrome.

Clinical features. The child accumulates fat, especially in the face, upper trunk, and nape of the neck (the buffalo hump). Although the weight percentile is high, the height percentile is usually low. The skin becomes a light violet in colour and excessive hair growth (hirsuties) is common, as is acne. The skin splits with the rapid accumulation of fat and this causes purplish seams (striae) in the topmost skin layer.

In females there may be premature puberty with clitoral enlargement and menstruation. Boys may show a similar acceleration of masculine characteristics. High blood pressure, and diabetes occurs in either sex. As the disease progresses, apathy and poor school performance are usual.

Laboratory. The corticosteroid content of blood and urine is increased. If the condition is due to simple overactivity of the gland, these levels can substantially be reduced by giving a drug called dexamethasone (itself a synthetic corticosteroid). This response does not occur if the overactivity is due to an adrenal tumour.

Treatment. A tumour if present, is excised, if not, control is achieved by partial or complete removal of the adrenal.

Pheochromocytoma

This is a tumour of the adrenal medulla which results in the overproduction of the catecholamines, adrenaline, and noradrenaline.

Clinical features. The usual symptoms are attacks of headache, pallor, sweating, and vomiting. The blood pressure is found to be increased. Thirst and polyuria are common later symptoms. Eventually the sustained hypertension causes congestive cardiac failure, or less often, hypertensive encephalopathy with convulsions and disturbances of consciousness.

Laboratory. The urine contains large amounts of catecholamines and their breakdown products.

Treatment. The tumour is removed after treatment with drugs designed to antagonize the effects of the catecholamines.

Aldosteronism

This means excess production of the mineralocorticoid (salt retaining) hormone, aldosterone. It is *primary* in disorders of the adrenal gland, and *secondary* when the kidney produces an excess of renin (as in some types of high blood pressure), which in turn stimulates the secretion of aldosterone. Both types are rare in childhood.

Clinical features. These suggest kidney disease, in that the patient is thirsty and passes large volumes of urine. As aldosterone causes loss of potassium, low blood levels of this element may be associated with muscular weakness or paralysis.

In secondary aldosteronism, hypertension is severe, and complications (cardiac failure, encephalopathy, renal failure) may be the first things noted.

Laboratory. Low blood potassium (hypokalemia) is usual, with high sodium levels in the primary type, and low or normal sodium values in the secondary type. The high aldosterone values can also be measured by appropriate methods.

Diseases due to underactivity of the adrenal gland (adrenal cortical insufficiency)

Acute insufficiency

This has many causes, but the same affect—acute salt loss with dehydration and shock. Temporary exhaustion of the adrenals can occur in the adrenogenital syndrome, and when steroids are rapidly stopped when high doses have been given.

In the newborn, hemorrhages into the adrenals can happen, and at any age bacterial toxins (e.g., of meningococcus) can damage the glands.

Clinical features. These are superimposed upon the primary disease, in the course of which the child suddenly deteriorates with grayish cyanosis, sweating, rapid heart, low blood pressure, and cold extremities. Vomiting and dehydration rapidly occur, with decreases in the serum sodium, chloride, and glucose values.

Treatment. This is as outlined for dehydration with the addition of large doses of hydrocortisone given intravenously. Any associated infection will also require treatment.

Chronic adrenal insufficiency (Addison's disease)

The cause of this disorder is seldom found. In most children it probably has an autoimmune basis.

Clinical features. These are at first nonspecific, viz., weakness, lack of energy, poor appetite, weight loss. Episodes of vomiting and diarrhea can occur, and may precipitate serious dehydration and acute adrenal insufficiency. Some children have an extraordinary craving for salt. Examination usually confirms loss of weight and muscle wasting, and brownish pigmentation can be present in the mouth, axillae, nipples, and genitals, as well as on the face and hands. The blood pressure is lower than normal.

Laboratory. The blood sodium and chloride levels are low, and the potassium value high. Blood and urine corticoid levels are decreased and cannot be stimulated by the injection of A.C.T.H.

Treatment. D.O.C.A. and extra dietary salt are given to ensure the maintenance of normal fluid and electrolyte values in the body. Eventually the injected D.O.C.A. can be replaced by 9-α fluorocortisone given by mouth. Hydrocortisone given by mouth is useful in increasing abnormally low blood glucose values. These replacement drugs must be increased during an acute illness, surgical operation or other stressful situation.

Adrenal neuroblastoma

This is a common malignant tumour of the sympathetic nervous system, which most commonly arises in the medulla of the adrenal. This tumour is highly invasive so its features are very variable.

Clinical features. The commoner presentation is as a large abdominal mass, with the rapid onset of pallor, fatigue, and weight loss. Sometimes the first symptoms are due to tumour spread (metastasis), especially to the areas behind the eyes (retro-orbital spread). This will cause apparent bruising of the eyelids, and pushing forward of the eye itself (proptosis). Spread to the bones causes pain, and sometimes deformity or fracture.

In a few children, the symptoms are vague—fever, anorexia, loss of activity and weight—and the tumour is found only after a prolonged search.

The diagnosis is almost certain if the abdominal mass shows calcification within it. Otherwise, surgical exploration, biopsy, and microscopical examination is done. The urine may contain end products of tumour activity—vanillomandelic acid, etc.

Treatment. If the tumour is localized, then cytotoxic (tumour-killing) drugs are given, and the mass removed. If there is much spread then cytotoxic drugs and radiotherapy are used, and surgery is employed only to relieve pressure on vital structures such as the airway.

THE PANCREAS

Endocrine disorders of the pancreas

This organ secretes 2 hormones, insulin and glucagon. Insulin is required for releasing energy from glucose and in the formation of muscle and liver glycogen. It also tends to slow the formation of fatty acids and protein by the liver. If insulin is lacking as in *diabetes mellitus*, the body cannot effectively use glucose, so fatty acids are used as an energy source. This leads to the accumulation of keto acids (acetoacetic, acetone, and β-hydroxybutyric). This acidosis is compensated by increasing excretion of H^+ ion by the kidney. Insulin, then, tends to reduce blood sugar, and increase glycogen storage. Glucagon tends to increase blood sugar, and probably acts in keeping its levels within physiological limits.

Diabetes mellitus

This is the commonest endocrine disorder of children. It is familial. Any age group may be affected, but the onset of the disease is usually between 5-10 years.

Clinical features. The principal symptoms are thirst (polydipsia) and polyuria (passing much urine). Nocturia (urination through the night) and bed wetting are other expressions of polyuria. Tiredness and rapid weight loss are usual.

About 10% of children with the disease present with acute dehydration (diabetic coma—see below). A small number are discovered by finding glucose in the child's urine.

Diabetes is the usual cause of carbohydrate in the urine (melituria). Specific tests for glucose employ reagents containing the enzyme glucose oxidase, such as clinistix or testape. Tests which are based on the copper reduction method (Clinitest tablets, Benedict's solution), will react with other sugars (galactose, fructose, pentoses) and with drugs which are excreted in the urine such as salicylates and ascorbic acid.

Glycosuria, and a high blood glucose level (hyperglycemia) make the diagnosis of diabetes mellitus almost certain.

Laboratory investigation. The glucose tolerance test is usually done when the child is suspected of having diabetes, usually because of intermittent glycosuria. It is not indicated when the disease is of acute onset. The test is carried out by obtaining fasting blood and urine samples; then a dose of glucose is given by mouth and blood and urine samples collected every 30 minutes for the next 2 hours. These are analyzed for glucose. In the diabetic, the fasting sample has a glucose content of > 200 mg%, and high levels present for at least the next hour. Glycosuria is also found, the amount being roughly proportional to the degree of hyperglycemia. Ketones (acetoacetic acid, acetone, etc.) and high blood fat (nonesterified fatty acid) are also present to excess in the untreated diabetic. A mild degree of compensated acidosis (due to the accumulation of ketones, etc.) is reflected in a reduction in the plasma bicarbonate.

Differential diagnosis. This is mainly related to the symptoms of polydipsia and polyuria. These can occur in diabetes insipidus, and in chronic renal failure. In the former, urinary specific gravity is very low, and there is no glycosuria. In the latter, the history is of a prolonged illness, the blood urea levels are high, and growth retardation is present. Also, there is seldom glycosuria except in the rare DeToni-Fanconi-Debré syndrome, in which, however, the blood sugar is normal (normoglycemia). Occasionally, compulsive water drinking is a possibility, mainly in older children.

Treatment. The principles are the life-long use of insulin, advice about diet, and teaching the child and his family to accept and assess his disorder. The end of treatment is to assure a normal life for the patient.

Insulin. This is a replacement for the natural hormone prepared from animals. Several preparations and compounds are available. The available insulins are:

i. *Short-acting insulin* (regular, soluble, insulin BP). This acts early, and for a short time (4-5 hours). The preferred type is *neutral* insulin (pH 7), which is more compatible with other insulins than the acid (pH 3-4) types of soluble insulins.
ii. *Medium duration insulins.* These have their maximum effect 8 hours after injection and some activity is present for 16 hours.

These are modified insulins (insulin zinc suspension (amorphous) B.P., Semilente, isophane (N.P.H.) and Rapitard).

iii. *Long acting insulins*. These have their greatest effect 10-12 hours after injection. Insulin zinc suspension (lente insulin) has an effect which persists for up to 25 hours. Ultra-lente (insulin zinc suspension crystalline), and protamine zinc insulin extend their maximum effect 16 hours after injection, and these effects can continue for up to 36 hours. The last two are seldom used in routine pediatric diabetes.

Diets in diabetes. The main aim is to give enough food for good growth, and to satisfy the child's appetite. The diet prescribed is unrestricted, except for caution concerning excessive intake of sweets and other foods rich in carbohydrate. The first move is to calculate the child's need for calories. This is done from a table (see Table 26), which also gives the requirement of protein. Each of these needs is based on weight for age. This is taken as the weight for the 50th percentile (since weight loss is usual in diabetes). An example then (using Table 26) would be: Age 6 years, male, 50th percentile weight = 20 kg. Total calories requirement/24 hours is 20 kg x 90 = 1,800 cal.

Table 26. Caloric and protein requirement

Age	Cal/kg/24 hours	Protein g/kg/24 hours
Infancy	110	2.5–3.0
1–3 years	100	2.5
4–6 years	90	2.0–2.5
7–9 years	80	2.0–2.5
10–12 years	70	2.0
13–15 years	60	1.5

Of this total, 50% of the calories is prescribed as carbohydrate = 900 cal. Again from table 26 this child requires 20 kg x 2g. protein. The caloric value/g. protein = 4.5, so protein contributes 180 cal. Carbohydrate and protein together now contribute 1,080 cal. of the total 24-hour need of 1,800 calories. The balance is 720 cal. which is to be supplied as fat. Since fat contains 9 cal./g., then the amount of fat is approximately 80 g. However, whatever the prescription of calories, some leeway is implicit, since satiety (the feeling of having had enough to eat) is important to children. Extra calories can, within limits, be catered for by giving extra insulin. Similarly, some children may not be able to eat all of the food prescribed. This is not a crime, and is easily dealt with by reducing the dose of insulin. The child's diet should, as far as possible, resemble that of the family as a whole. Every effort must be made to explain simple dietetics to the parents—and the child if he is old enough to understand. Many parents tend to be too rigid in their attitudes at first, so that the child's diet becomes fixed and uninteresting. The dietitian's responsibility is to explain the mixed nature of foods (as protein, carbohydrate, or fat) and lead them from the prescription to the cooking of the meals.

Clinical use of insulin. The diet should have been accepted and the carbohydrate intake made equal for each main meal. Soluble (neutral) insulin is injected subcutaneously several times a day. An approximation of the total 24-hour dose of insulin is 2 units/kg body weight, but requirements vary widely. Specific dosage is usually obtained by assessing the degree of glycosuria (by Clinitest tablets) and using a sliding scale (see table 27). If the child is unable to urinate to order, as in the very young, it may be necessary to control the insulin dosage by blood sugar assessment by Dextrostix. A careful watch must be kept for hypoglycemia (low blood sugar) as insulin requirements may decrease very rapidly. When the urine tests stabilize at 1+ glycosuria, then an attempt should be made to give the insulin by one daily injection. This degree of stabilization takes 4-5 days and the child should be as active as possible during this time. The transfer to a single injection is usually done by prescribing a morning dose of insulin consisting in 1/3 neutral soluble insulin and 2/3 medium-acting, e.g., semilente insulin. The urine testing is continued, but a morning glycosuria of 2-3+ is not regarded as a serious aberration. If the midday urine is 2-3+, then the *soluble* fraction of the combined insulin is increased. If the evening (5 p.m.) test is high in sugar, then the long-acting insulin is increased. In some children with relatively low insulin requirement, medium-acting insulins alone, or special combinations of rapid and medium insulins (e.g., Rapitard) may be used.

Parents and patient must be actively involved in the stabilization process and the reasons for each treatment explained. The parents will give the injections, and they, and the child (unless he is very young), are taught urinalysis for glucose and ketones.

After discharge from hospital, where stabilization usually occurs, the child is seen twice weekly at least for a month. This period is used to

Table 27. Example of approximate insulin needed

Degrees of Glycosuria (by clinitest tablets)	Weight (kg)		
	40 units	20 units	10 units
4+	12	8	5
3+	8	5	3
2+	4	3	0

reassure the parents, explain dietary problems (such as the exchange system) and insist on the need for changing the sites of injection. After a month or two, a child who is old enough (9+) can be taught to inject the insulin himself, and to keep his own records of urinalysis.

Assessment of control. The criteria for good control are normal growth, avoidance of complications (hypoglycemia, diabetic acidosis), acceptance of the disease by parents and patient, and the ability to lead a normal life. Immaculate urinalyses are only a part of the process of treatment and reflect only the day to day variations. A moderate (3+) morning glycosuria is compatible with good control, especially when it is associated with only minor hyperglycemia.

Normal growth is assessed by regular measurements and plotting on a percentile chart. As the child grows, his diet must be increased, or he will become discontented and uncooperative. Particular care with diet prescription is needed for the adolescent, when caloric and insulin requirements suddenly increase.

Emotional aspects of diabetes. The incidence of minor behaviour problems is slightly increased in diabetic children. This is because the need for injection and urinalysis is a constant reminder that they are different. The problems are greatly increased if the diet is too restricted, if the child has many episodes of hypoglycemia or diabetic acidosis, or if immaculate urinalyses are demanded by parents or physician. The best way to prevent emotional disturbance is to engender confidence by teaching independence in injections, testing, and diet, and by encouraging a normal social life, e.g., sports, overnight visits, and parties. Sometimes parents, knowing that diet restriction and oral hypoglycemics (tablets for diabetic control) are used in adults, feel that this should be so for their children. Again, constant explanation is the way in which parents and medical people are stopped from becoming at loggerheads, unwittingly or not.

Complications of diabetes mellitus

Diabetic coma (acidosis)

This may be the way in which the disease presents. It is a situation of prolonged ketoacidosis which culminates in a state of dehydration, or low salt syndrome. It is most often brought on by infection, especially the gastrointestinal sort, but may occur after surgery, or failure to give insulin, either wilfully or through ignorance.

Clinical features. Thirst and polyuria return, and in the early stages appetite fails, fluid intake decreases and nausea and vomiting occur. Abdominal pain is common and may be the first symptom to which attention is paid. The pain may be intermittent (colicky) or constant, and is often described as being in the lower abdomen. Observant parents may note the deeper breathing pattern of acidosis. The urine shows a heavy glycosuria and strongly positive tests for ketones. The child is inactive, becomes pale, sleepy, and may relapse into *coma*. In the latter, the child is still rousable, but confused. His memory is impaired. He has the signs of dehydration—hollow eyes, dry mouth, cold extremities, fast pulse, low blood pressure, and deep acidotic breathing. Little or no urine is passed. He smells of ketones and shows abdominal tenderness, and even muscle rigidity (guarding).

Laboratory findings in diabetic acidosis. There is hyperglycemia and ketonemia. The blood pH may be reduced. Sodium and chloride values are variable, but a reduction is common. Potassium values are usually normal. The blood urea may be increased if dehydration has been present for more than 6-8 hours. This is because the renal blood supply has been reduced. The white cell count is increased, irrespective of the presence of infection. Hemoconcentration (due to dehydration) is evidenced by high hemoglobin and hematocrit values.

Differential diagnosis. This is mainly from other causes of coma, in most instances due to accidental poisoning by antihistamines, tranquilizing drugs, or salicylates. In these, the history, and the absence of hyperglycemia suffice to make the true diagnosis. If abdominal pain is an early symptom, confusion may arise with surgical problems such as appendicitis, or with medical disorders (e.g., rheumatic fever, Henoch-Schönlein purpura) which cause abdominal pain. Again, testing for sugar in blood and urine will put the matter right.

Treatment. The principles are to relieve dehydration, give soluble insulin, and treat any underlying infection. Dehydration is treated by the methods already outlined (p. 526), usually with an intravenous solution of 0.45-0.9% saline solution. If pH reduction is marked (pH <7.2) then bicarbonate is added to the infusion. This and the effect of insulin suffice to correct the acidosis. Potassium deficiency is common in diabetic coma, so vigorous rehydration until urine is passed is followed by the addition of potassium (as KCl) to the infusion. Intravenous fluids are continued until the patient's condition has been stable for 48 hours, and he is able to take and retain a normal amount of fluid and calories.

Insulin. The soluble type is used. A common first dose is 2 units/kg body weight, of which 50% is given intravenously, the remainder intramuscularly. Higher doses may be required if hyperglycemia is extreme (>750 mg%). The soluble insulin is repeated every 4-6 hours, the dose varying according to a sliding scale if urinalysis is the mode of control. In many instances this is impracticable and then blood sugar estimation is used to control the insulin dose. When blood sugar levels reach 200 mg%, or less, then 2.5% dextrose is added to the saline solution.

As the child's condition improves, and he retains food and fluid then a stabilization routine as already described is begun.

Hypoglycemia (low blood sugar)

This generally occurs because of an excess of insulin, or a lack of carbohydrate in the diet, or increased exercise which uses up carbohydrate. With insulin excess, the symptoms occur an hour or two after a meal. The urine tests have often been negative for sugar beforehand. The main complaints are feelings of hunger, unreality, and anxiety. Small children may not, of course, express these symptoms, which are followed by sweating and faintness. Convulsions and coma are not very common, occurring usually if the early symptoms are unnoticed and therefore untreated. Children who are on long-acting insulins have less typical symptoms, with less in the way of sweating and faintness, and more in the way of confusional states, and bizarre behaviour. Hypoglycemia can be confirmed specifically by blood sugar measurement, or, indirectly, by the response to taking sugar.

Treatment. The child is taught to carry glucose sweets (or a lump of sugar), and to take this if he has hypoglycemic symptoms. If the patient is convulsing or comatose, then intravenous glucose or subcutaneous glucagon (1 mg) should be given. In every instance the child's diet and insulin dose should be reviewed.

The longer-term complications of diabetes

The main problems are abnormalities of the blood vessels supplying the *retina* and *kidney*. These give rise to the diseases called *retinopathy* and *nephropathy*.

Retinopathy. This diagnosis is made by ophthalmoscopy, which shows the abnormalities in the vessels.

Nephropathy. (Kimmelstiel-Wilson syndrome). This is suspected by finding albumin in the urine. At first this is intermittent, then it becomes constant. The plasma proteins fall, and the patient becomes edematous. Hypertension and renal failure ultimately develop. Neither of these complications occur in children, unless the disease began early in life.

THE PARATHYROID

There are several parathyroid glands, which are placed deep to the thyroid. Each produces a hormone called parathormone which can mobilize calcium from the bones, and also helps to regulate the reabsorption of phosphate from the fluid in the kidney tubules. Calcium absorption from the gut is aided by parathormone provided that vitamin D is present in the diet. Parathormone also helps balance the effects of another (thyroid) hormone, thyrocalcitonin, which tends to lower blood calcium—the opposite effect to that of parathormone. Disease of the parathyroid is a disorder of calcium metabolism.

Clinical disorders

Hypoparathyroidism

Transient hypoparathyroidism occurs in the newborn, mainly in the dysmature; coincident hypoglycemia is common. The main symptom is an increase in muscular excitability. This occurs as twitching attacks, affecting the face and limbs, occasionally as frank convulsions. Episodes of rapid eyelid blinking or waving about of the limbs can occur, as do apneic spells—usually with coincident cyanosis. The condition is diagnosed with certainty only by finding a low level of calcium in the blood.

In older (>3 weeks) babies, the problem may be dietary in origin, due to the high phosphate content of the cow's milk fed to the infant. An excess of phosphate essentially acts to reduce the calcium content, and gives rise to the same symptoms (tetany) as described for the newborn.

Permanent hypoparathyroidism in the newborn is rare. Failure to thrive, fits, and undue liability to infections are the main problems. As before, serum calcium levels are depressed.

Treatment. This is to restore calcium levels to normal. Severe and acute states are treated by giving intravenous calcium gluconate. Less dramatic varieties are treated by giving calcium gluconate and small doses (100 u) of vitamin D by mouth.

Parathyroid diseases in older children

Idiopathic hypoparathyroidism

This disease may have an autoimmune base and may rarely coincide with Addison's disease or autoimmune thyroiditis.

Clinical features. The chief complaint is of convulsions. Older children complain of pain and tingling in the limbs. Eye abnormalities (keratitis, corneal ulcers, cataracts) occur as complications or may be the presenting features. A late complication is raised intracranial pressure with headache, vomiting, and papilledema. The skin is often dry and scaly, and the hair thin. Fungal infections (monilia) of the nails and mouth are common, but are not the cause of the disease.

Albright's hereditary osteodystrophy

This is also called pseudohypoparathyroidism and, even more incredibly, pseudo-pseudohypoparathyroidism.

Clinical features. The child is stunted, mentally retarded, and has short fingers. In addition, he has convulsions and eye abnormalities, such as cataracts.

In the pseudo type, the serum calcium is low. In the pseudo-pseudo type, the calcium is normal and, although parathormone is produced, it seems not to have an effect on the tissues.

Tetany

This is really a disturbance of calcium metabolism which it is convenient to consider now. There are many causes, the main one being an increase in pH in the body (metabolic alkalosis). This results in insufficient ionization of calcium which means functional hypocalcemia although the *total* blood calcium may be normal. Alkalosis can follow the taking or the injection of alkalis such as sodium bicarbonate or citrate. Minor tetany can occur in hyperventilation which causes a respiratory alkalosis.

The symptoms of tetany have largely been described under hypoparathyroidism. They consist in twitching, tingling, and occasionally of fits; local muscular irritability may occur as spasm of the larynx or of the hands and feet (carpo pedal spasm). Latent (hidden) tetany is the name given to signs which elicit some of the features of tetany, e.g., spasm of the facial muscles on tapping the facial nerve is called Chvostek's sign.

The treatment of these hypocalcemic states is with calcium gluconate as already described.

Hyperparathyroidism

This may be primary, as in a parathormone secreting tumour, or secondary to chronic hypocalcemia as in chronic renal disease, intestinal malabsorption of calcium, or gross vitamin D deficiency.

Primary hyperparathyroidism

Clinical features. The result of a high parathormone level is a high calcium level (hypercalcemia) in the blood, and leaching of calcium from the bones. The high blood calcium damages the kidney and may cause the formation of renal stones. Thus *renal colic*, or the signs of advanced renal disease (growth failure, polyuria, polydipsia, etc.) are common features. Skeletal decalcification gives rise to bone pain, deformities, and fractures.

Laboratory. The serum calcium is greatly increased, as is the enzyme alkaline phosphatase. The blood phosphate is reduced.

Treatment. The parathyroids are explored surgically; if a tumour (adenoma) is found, it is excised. If the glands are simply overgrown and overactive (hyperplastic), then partial removal of the gland is done.

Secondary hyperparathyroidism

This has no symptoms of its own, only the features of the underlying disease (e.g., renal disorder, malabsorption) are present, and the treatment is of these primary disorders.

16 Disorders of the eye

These are common in childhood, especially in relation to minor infections, injuries, strabismus (squint), and refractive errors. The eye is also importantly involved in disease processes which affect the whole child.

SEVERE CONGENITAL ABNORMALITIES OF THE EYE

These are important in directing the attention of the clinician to more generalized disorders. Thus, anophthalmia (absence of an eye), or severe microphthalmia (small eye) may suggest the possibility of disorders of the autosome (e.g., trisomy 18), or of congenital rubella. In either case, other severe defects, such as of the heart, commonly coexist. Disorders of the cornea, or cataract, and of the retina are also associated with system disease, as in metabolic disorders. These are described in the appropriate section. *Coloboma* is due to a failure of fusion of the eye tissues. It is a variable cleft of the eye structure. In many instances, minor defects of the most anterior part of the eye go unnoticed. When the iris is deficient, the characteristic key-hole pupil is seen, but the cleft may extend through the choroid to the optic nerve. *Aniridia*, is absence of the iris, which may be familial.

Minor congenital deformities mostly involve the eyelids. Thus, epicanthic fold—a ridge of skin from brow to nose, obscuring the inner canthus, is racial, often bilateral, and is also found in Down's syndrome. Another common lesion is congenital ptosis, due to a defect in the levator palpebrae superioris.

DISORDERS OF THE LACRIMAL SYSTEM

The commonest of these is blockage of the nasolacrimal duct, so that the tears cannot reach the nasopharynx. Canalization of the duct may be incomplete, or blockage by epithelial debris occur. The chief complaint is of tearing (epiphora) of the eye. Secondary infection is common, usually as conjunctivitis (q.v.) occasionally as *dacryocystitis*. The latter presents as a red, brawny swelling of the lower lid and adjacent nose, pus can sometimes be expressed from the nasal punctum. If treatment is delayed, bursting of the abscess may cause a fistula.

Treatment. In many instances the duct will open spontaneously. If this does not occur, gentle irrigation of the nasolacrimal duct with 0.9%

saline is in order. Expert probing of the duct may be necessary in a minority of children, and is preceded by the treatment of any infection.

Infection of the lacrimal gland (Dacryoadenitis)

The symptoms are pain and swelling external to the upper eyelid. Resolution usually takes place without specific treatment. In few cases abscess or orbital cellulitis may occur, and require appropriate antibiotic and surgical treatment. Chronic enlargement of the lacrimal glands is occasionally seen in leukemia or lymphosarcoma, or it may be part of the sarcoid syndrome. In these the treatment is of the primary disease.

DISORDERS OF THE EYELIDS

Edema of the lids

This is common in conditions such as congestive cardiac failure, acute glomerulonephritis, nephrotic syndrome, serum sickness, and the urticarial diseases. In either, the edema may be unilateral if the infant has been lying with the affected eye downwards. Edema of the eye lids is also common in severe conjunctivitis.

Congenital ptosis

This is a not unusual congenital deficit, which may be unilateral or bilateral. It is due to maldevelopment of the levator palpebrae superioris or, more probably, its nerve supply, since a superior rectus palsy is often associated.

Treatment. This is only indicated in the severe case where visual difficulty causes the child to cock his head backwards, when plastic surgery procedures are done.

INFECTIONS OF THE EYELIDS

Blepharitis marginalis

This is inflammation of the eyelid edges. It is common in seborrheic dermatitis and atopic eczemas, and acutely in measles. Otherwise it is usually staphylococcal in origin, and may be persistent. The principal sign is redness and minor swelling of the lid margins, together with the formation of yellowish crusts. Complicating styes are common.

Treatment. The crusts are soaked off with normal saline compresses and a suitable antibiotic ointment applied. Associated skin disease will require appropriate care.

Stye (hordeolum)

This is an inflammation of the gland (of Zeiss), at the base of a lash. There is pain and local redness and swelling which may progress to edema of the whole eyelid. The cause is usually the staphylococcus.

Treatment. Specific treatment is seldom necessary, as the abscess ruptures readily. Warm compresses are comforting and may accelerate the healing process.

Chalazion

This is a mild granuloma of the Meibomian gland and adjacent tarsal plate. It is painless, and the complaint is of a lump in the eyelid—usually the upper one. The overlying skin is mobile but the consistency, and sometimes the colour of the overlying conjunctiva, is abnormal, and in some instances, is eroded by granulation tissue.

Treatment. The cyst is excised and a short course of antibiotic eye ointment given.

DISORDERS OF THE CONJUNCTIVA

These are common in children. The staphylococcus has replaced the gonococcus as the usual cause of severe infantile conjunctivitis. Mixed organismal (e.g., *E. coli*) and viral infections (e.g., measles) are not uncommon. Chemical conjunctivitis may follow the instillation of prophylactic silver nitrate eyedrops. The appearance of infective conjunctivitis may be mimicked in the allergic state of hay fever.

Clinical features. These are quite variable. In the milder cases there is no great discomfort, although a scratchy sensation may be reported by older children. Examination reveals redness and increased vascularity of the conjunctiva. The vessels are easily seen, and stop short of the cornea (pinkeye). Beads of pus can usually be seen in the inner canthus, or the eye lids are reported to be stuck together in the morning.

In the more severe case, and especially in infants, pus exudes from the eye, and swelling of the eyelids may be a prominent sign. Edema (chemosis) of the conjunctiva is present as well as intense hyperemia. There is nothing very specific in the early appearances of gonococcal, staphylococcal, or viral conjunctivitis. Accordingly, culture should always be made. As already noted, neonatal conjunctivitis may be associated with blockage of the nasolacrimal duct. In older children, chronic blepharitis may have been causal.

Treatment. Once the bacteriological samples have been obtained, the eye is irrigated gently with 0.9% sterile saline solution, and a broad-spectrum antibiotic eye ointment instilled.

Prophylaxis. This is principally against gonococcal infection, and may be necessary where the disease is rife and antenatal care wanting. The introduction of 1 drop of 1% *aqueous* silver nitrate solution and holding the lids open for a minute or so is usually sufficient, not only to prevent gonococcal infection, but to produce a mild chemical conjunctivitis.

Special forms of conjunctivitis

Trachoma

This is a widespread, chronic, viral induced infection. There are few early symptoms, the condition frequently being found on routine examination.

In the early stage, there is local conjunctival redness, this extends to give rise to follicular excrescenses. The process may only be present on the sub palpebral conjunctiva, so that this area must be examined in at-risk children. Eventually the process of vascularization involves the cornea, the thickening being called the pannus. At this stage, pain, epiphora, and photophobia are common. Scarring of the palpebral conjunctiva (usually the upper lid) causes entropion (turning in of the eyelid margins) and the displaced eyelashes aggravate the siuation by causing trauma and infection. In neglected cases, corneal scarring causes partial or total blindness. The diagnosis can be confirmed by finding the viral inclusion bodies in conjunctival scrapings.

Treatment. Sulphonamide eye ointment, occasionally supplemented by oral therapy, is the treatment which is generally used. Keratitis is treated as discussed below, and grafting may be required if corneal scarring is extensive.

Phlyctenular conjunctivitis

This is an allergic manifestation of tuberculous infection, and accordingly may be found in areas where this disease is ill-controlled. The usual sign is a localized yellow blob, with a surrounding conjunctival redness found near the limbus. This is the phlyctenule which may rupture and spread to the cornea causing iritis. Resolution with scarring is usual.

Treatment. The child should be investigated and treated for tuberculosis. The iritis is treated as discussed below.

THE CORNEA

Simple corneal opacity

This is not very uncommon in premature infants and consists in a greyish appearance of the cornea without inflammation. It may be patchy or involve most of the cornea. The condition clears spontaneously within a week or two.

Corneal opacity in systemic disease

Quite severe and permanent corneal opacity is seen in a variety of pediatric disease. At birth, the commoner disorders are the chromosomal syndromes and ectodermal dysplasia. Corneal opacities are seen at a later age in mucopolysaccharidoses (gargoylism), incontinentia pigmenti (Bloch-Sulzberger syndrome), and Marfan's syndrome.

Edema of the cornea

This gives rise to a steamy, semi-transparent opacity involving the whole cornea, and is seen in infection (keratitis) and glaucoma.

Inflammation of the cornea (keratitis)

This may follow bacterial or viral infections, or complicate chemical or physical injury. It may complicate a severe conjunctivitis.

Clinical features. In the acute type, there are complaints of photophobia and lacrimation. In young children, photophobia (pain on iris movement) may be expressed by irritability and refusal to open the eye. Inspection reveals an edematous, steamy cornea, with circumcorneal (ciliary) and subconjunctival vascular injection. The vessels, being relatively deep, cannot be individually distinguished. The appearance then is of a general redness. This, and the fact that the inflammation extends to the corneal edge and does not produce purulent exudate, are the principal differentiating points from a severe conjunctivitis.

So called *interstitial keratitis* involves the deep layer of the cornea and may be associated with uveitis. The symptoms and signs are those described above, except that the corneal discolouration is greater and more prolonged.

DISORDERS OF THE LENS

Cataract

This is often found in very abnormal eyes, e.g., microphthalmia. Cataract is also common in such disorders as the rubella syndrome, galactosemia, ectodermal dysplasia, mucopolysaccharidosis, incontinentia pigmenti, Lowe's syndrome (hypotonia, mental retardation, tubular aminoaciduria), and parathyroid disorders. It also occurs in chromosomal defects, e.g., Turner's syndrome, Down's syndrome, trisomy D.

Drug induced cataracts are uncommon in children. They have followed the use of triparanol, and busulfan, and from the topical use of powerful cholinesterase inhibitors (e.g., phosphine iodide) in glaucoma or strabismus.

Clinical features. In the most severe instances, the condition is discovered on routine examination at neonatal follow-up. The cataract presents as an opaque mass occupying all or part of the pupil, sometimes best seen by side-lighting. A useful test is to elicit the red reflex which is dimmed or absent in cataract.

On finding a cataract, the pediatrician's responsibility is to exclude a metabolic or syndromal cause. The details of specific treatment can be decided only by an expert ophthalmologist.

Ectopia lentis (dislocated lens)

This may reflect a general disorder, as in Marfan's syndrome and homocystinuria. Another common cause of dislocation is injury, in which there are complaints of acute visual loss. In the other situations, the dislocation may be found because of deliberate search, or because other eye defects are present. Inspection may show the edge of the lens stretching across the pupil, and readily shifting its position. Acute glaucoma is the principal complication, although retinal detachment also occurs. Treatment is principally of the complicating glaucoma. Lens extraction may be tried if medical methods of controlling the glaucoma fail.

Glaucoma

This is the name given to the condition of elevated intraocular pressure, usually in the anterior chamber of the eye. The relationships of this area are shown in figure 48. From this it will be seen that affections and injuries of the lens, cornea, and adjacent structures (ciliary muscle, iris—the anterior uveal tract) may all interfere with the circulation of the aqueous humour. This is secreted by the ciliary processes in the posterior chamber and filters out in the angle of the anterior chamber into the canal of Schlemm. As already noted, glaucoma can complicate dislocation of the lens, as clearly could marked corneal abnormality, either congenital or following keratitis. Abnormalities of the iris, congenital or acquired from uveitis, may also be causal. Trauma directly, or by subsequent hemorrhage, may disrupt the filtration tissues in the anterior chamber.

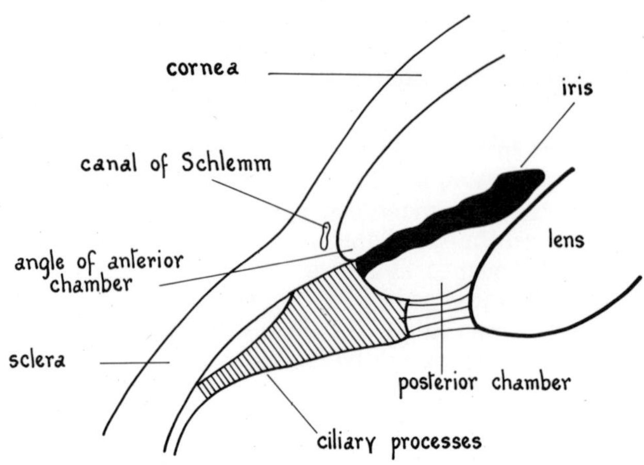

Fig. 48. Causes of glaucoma.

Congenital glaucoma

This may be familial, and is due to an abnormality in the filtration angle. Although relatively rare, it is important because of the blindness which can follow delayed treatment.

Symptoms. These commonly occur in the first year of life, sometimes as early as the newborn period. The principal symptom is photophobia. The infant is delayed in opening his eyes, or does so only in shade. Irritability and crying are common. In some instances this phase does not occur, or is not observed and the main complaint is of an enlarged eye, which may seem to be dislocated forwards.

Signs. The cornea becomes edematous and steamy because of the blockage of aqueous filtration. Hyperemia is not uncommon and eyeball tension is increased.

Treatment. Medical treatment is unrewarding. The patient requires expert surgery.

Acute glaucoma in older children

There is considerable pain, lacrimation, sometimes nausea and vomiting, and much loss of vision. All of the eye vessels are congested, the cornea hazy, and the pupil dilated, often oval, and sluggish in its reaction.

The principal differential diagnosis is from acute iritis, in which visual loss is slight and only the ciliary vessels are injected. The cornea is clear and the affected pupil constricted and often irregular. The differentiation is important since giving a cycloplegic (sometimes indicated in iritis) may be disastrous to the child with glaucoma.

DISORDERS OF THE UVEAL TRACT

This is the vascular layer of the eye. The iris and ciliary body make up the anterior uveal tract, and the choroid the posterior tract. Disorders of either division occur in some general pediatric disorders.

Acute iridocyclitis (anterior uveitis)

In most primary types the cause is unknown. The syndrome may complicate pediatric rheumatoid disease, ulcerative colitis, and sarcoidosis. Syphilis is nowadays an unusual cause. Secondary iridocyclitis spreads from conditions which cause corneal ulcers which rupture into the anterior chamber. There is some evidence for an autoimmune process in those cases of dubious etiology.

Clinical features. In *acute iritis*, the eye is painful, both subjectively and on palpation. Lacrimation and blurring of vision are usual. Inspection shows marked circumcorneal (ciliary) hyperemia and a small, sometimes irregularly shaped, pupil which moves poorly. The clear cornea and difference in pupil shape and size, are the main differentiating points from acute glaucoma. In children with involvement, principally of the ciliary tract, the onset is not acute and indeed may be discovered at routine examination, or when there is visual blurring or a complaint of spots in the visual field (floaters). Such a patient requires special ophthalmological opinion to confirm the diagnosis, as external signs such as hyperemia are absent.

The course of iridocyclitis is a prolonged one, with the possibility of corneal and lenticular changes, or secondary glaucoma.

Treatment. This is a matter for the expert ophthalmologist.

Posterior uveitis

This is a problem which regularly comes to the pediatrician's attention, usually because of the unknown relationship of inflammation of the choroid and retina to such conditions as rubella syndrome, neonatal cytomegalovirus, and herpes virus infection, and in toxoplasmosis.

In infants, the diagnosis is usually suspected at ophthalmoscopy. In active disease, there are white raised areas, sometimes with associated areas of hemorrhage. Healed choreoretinitis is characterized by the appearance of white areas (the subjacent choroid) surrounded by hyperpigmented retinal tissue. In older children, the symptoms are related to visual difficulty. Thus, if the child has bilateral involvement of the macula, visual loss is severe, and the child has searching eye movements and other characteristics of the blind. In unilateral cases, a squint may be the first symptom. Difficulty in seeing school work is an occasional primary complaint.

THE RETINA AND ITS DISORDERS

Many of these have been mentioned elsewhere, as complications of disorders which present primarily as pediatric central nervous system disease. Thus, *macular* and other central degenerative processes may be congenital and isolated (e.g., Best's, Stargardt's macular disorders) or form part of the syndromes of the infantile lipidoses (Tay-Sach's, Gaucher's, Nieman-Pick). The more peripheral retinal lesions also tend to be familial and usually show pigmentary change. Disease states (described in details elsewhere) in which such changes are found include Friedreich's ataxia, the cerebellar ataxia of Marie Leber's optic atrophy, and the Laurence-Moon-Biedl syndrome.

In the macular and other central degenerative disease, the vision is early affected, with the emergence of searching eye movements, knuckling of the eyes, and failure to respond to visual cues. These signs may be overlooked in children with other severe manifestations, such as intellectual deterioration and advanced neurological disorder.

In the peripheral lesions, vision is maintained into childhood. The first difficulties may be night blindness, usually followed by progressive diminution of the visual fields. The speed of visual loss is variable.

No treatment is available for these disorders.

Retrolental fibroplasia

This entity, formerly not uncommon in premature infants, is due apparently to the exposure to high (>40%) ambient oxygen levels. The response is primarily a retinopathy, often with folding and detachment of its substance. In severe cases, the cornea is cloudy, the eye fails to grow, and widespread fibrosis affects the retrolental area. The condition is bilateral.

Clinical signs. These should be sought in any infant appropriately at risk. The first sign is the presence of constricted vessels. This is followed by the development of a dilated, tortuous retinal vascular pattern, often with dull white, raised areas in the retinal periphery. The vitreous becomes vascularized, and fibrosis causes retinal detachment. Little can be done to treat the process. Careful monitoring of ambient oxygen levels and avoidance of O_2 therapy, except when really indicated, are essential prophylactic measures. Especially at risk are prematures treated by aided respiration.

Retinal detachment

This may occur as a congenital disorder, or be also associated with other anomalies of the eye, e.g., retrolental fibroplasia. It may follow uveitis from any cause, or be a late complication of diabetes mellitus, or follow trauma to the eye.

Symptoms. Pain is absent, and visual difficulties take various forms. If the break is near the macula, visual loss is severe. In the young infant unable to complain, the first sign of sight loss may be strabismus. Older children may complain of flashing lights and loss of peripheral vision.

Signs. Ophthalmoscopy may reveal an obvious edge, or retinal elevation.

Treatment. This is a matter for the expert ophthalmologist. The principles are to close any retinal defect, thus sealing off the entry of vitreous. Efforts are then made to return the retina to its proper position.

Retinoblastoma

This is the commoner tumour affecting the eye, and is a congenital lesion, occurring in up to 50% of the children of a previously affected parent. The neoplasm is often bilateral.

Clinical features. The condition should deliberately be sought in the children of affected parents, or in the siblings of an affected child. On ophthalmoscopy, the tumour appears first as a small yellow nodule. The red reflex becomes yellowish, and clearly different from that of a normal eye. This is often a presenting complaint from the parents. In other instances, and especially if the tumour invades the macula, loss of sight and squint may be the first signs. In some instances the first problem follows invasion of the brain, giving rise to focal neurological signs.

Treatment. In those in whom the condition is diagnosed early, the combination of linear accelerator radiation with triethylene melamine administration seems very satisfactory. In advanced cases enucleation is necessary. The use of phototherapy and cryosurgery in this tumour is still experimental.

Genetic counselling. In the situation where one parent has had the disease, further pregnancies should be avoided. Retinoblastoma in the collaterals of unaffected parents who produce an affected child is probably also an indication for family restriction.

STRABISMUS (SQUINT)

This is a common problem, affecting perhaps 1-2% of children.

General clinical features

Subjective. These are not very common, and are unreliable for diagnosis at a stage at which effective treatment is possible. In most instances, complaints come from older children, often in those with a paralyzed eye muscle. Thus, diplopia and clumsiness may be features. In many, however, this stage does not occur, and suppression of one image occurs and may become severe and permanent. Then poor vision (amblyopia or anopsia) is complained of by the patient, or deduced by the parent.

Objective. The usual parental complaint is that the child has a squint, or that the eye deviates unnaturally. Often this is noted when the child is tired, or about to go to sleep. The parents may have noted that the abnormality is more obvious when the child gazes in a certain direction. Another mode in which squint presents, is through the presence of some compensatory manoeuvre, usually head tilting or face rotation. The former may be so constant as to cause confusion with torticollis.

Types of strabismus

Pseudostrabismus

In this there are no subjective symptoms. The complaint is of a squint towards the nose. This is an artefact due to epicanthic folds, almond-shaped (oriental) eyes, a broadly based nose, or a combination of each factor. The result is that less of the white of the eye is seen on the nasal aspect of one eye than the other and this conveys the impression of a squint. Eye movement is, however, normal.

True strabismus

The importance of these conditions lies in the fact that uncorrected squint, giving rise to imperfect image fusion, will lead to progressive disuse of one eye with resulting amblyopia. Late discovery may also render effective treatment impossible if the child has learned abnormal retinal correspondence, i.e., fixing with the fovea of one eye, and with another area of the retina with the other. Such difficulties are most likely to arise with convergent squints, which make up the majority of serious squints in childhood. (See figure 49.)

Latent strabismus (heterophoria)

In this condition, the desire and ability for image fusion is sufficient to overcome the tendency to squint. This condition is usually delayed in its recognition for some years, often appearing in the school-age groups. Some children may complain of tired eyes after lessons. In most instances the tendency is for the eyeball to deviate outwards (exophoria).

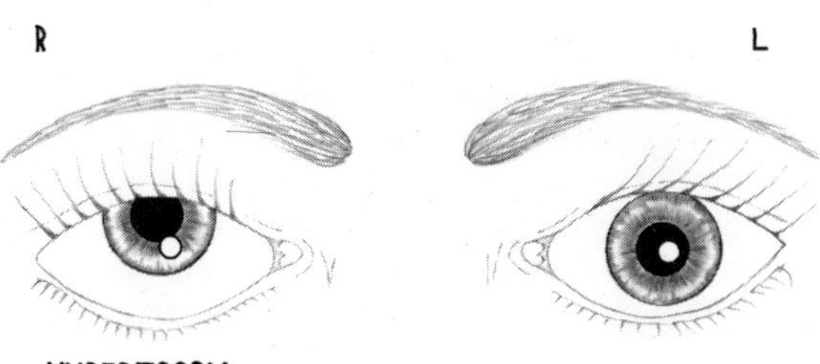

HYPERTROPIA............
Right eye turned upward.

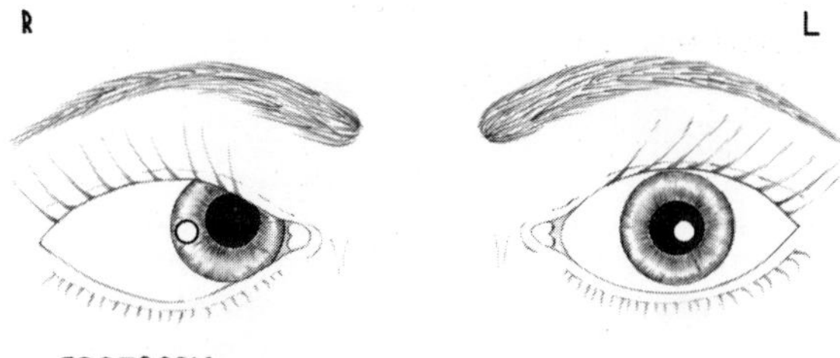

ESOTROPIA............
Right eye turned in toward the nose.

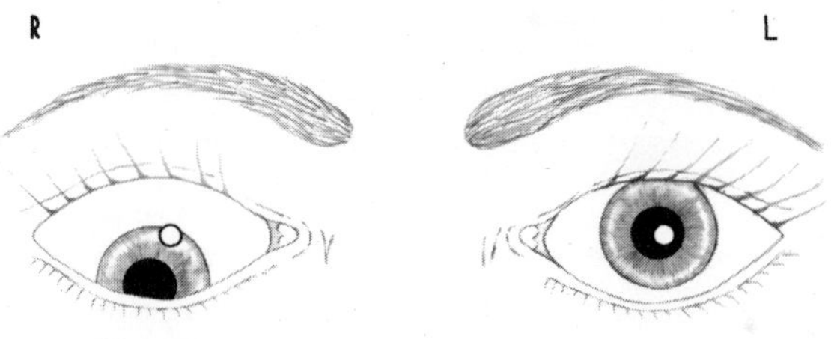

HYPOTROPIA............
Right eye turned downward.

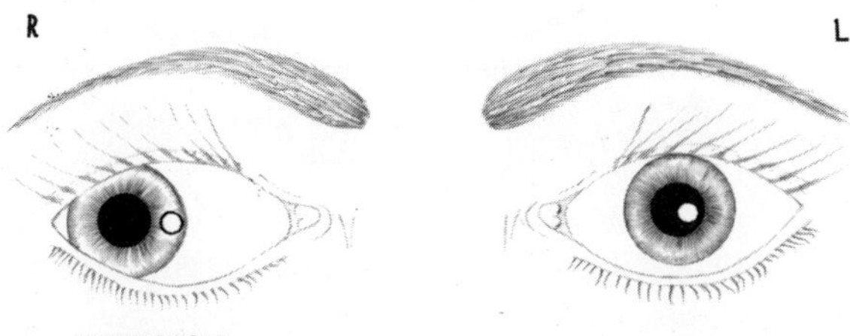

EXOTROPIA............
Right eye turned out toward the temple.

Fig. 49. Types of strabismus.

Esophoria (tendency to inward deviation) or hyperphoria (tendency to vertical deviation) are much less common.

The condition is confirmed by varying the cover test—usually by rapidly alternating the cover/uncover technique from eye to eye. If the alternation is done slowly, little abnormality is present, but deviation of the axes occurs when alternation is rapid. The degree of deviation can further be assessed only by special ophthalmological techniques.

Overt strabismus (heterotropia)

This may be diagnosed by simple inspection, or be revealed when the cover/uncover alternation is done slowly.

The common types are *concomitant* strabismus in which the muscle power is normal in each eye, and the deviation of the squinting eye is similar in all directions of gaze.

In *paralytic* strabismus, there is a squint only in the visual field to which the eyeball would be turned by the affected muscle. Diplopia is common in paralytic strabismus, and an uncommon complaint in concomitant strabismus. *Paralytic squints should always be considered as due to C.N.S. disease until otherwise proven.* The general causes of such squints are considered elsewhere.

Concomitant strabismus

A common variety is *intermittent convergent strabismus*. This variety is usually due to hyperopia of one eye; thus, as the child interests himself in near objects, he makes a severe effort at accommodation in order to see clearly. This exaggerates the normal converging effort of accommodation. Thus the squint is usually absent in the first year, and becomes increasingly obvious thereafter. Initially it may be seen only when the child is tired or looking at near objects. In time, it will become more constant. There is deterioration of vision (due to suppression) in the deviating eye.

Examination will usually confirm the refractive lesion in one eye, and the above tests for squint are positive. So too is the *binocular* uncovering test. In this, the suspected strabismic eye is covered and uncovered while the other eye fixes. In concomitant strabismus, no movement occurs in the squinting eye, as it is covered and uncovered. If the good eye is uncovered or covered, both eyes move.

Treatment. Primarily this is to preserve sight by forcing the use of the squinting eye. The good eye is accordingly covered. Surgery is not often indicated in this condition.

Congenital convergent strabismus

This condition is usually the object of parental concern from an early age. The degree of squint may seem quite alarming. Refractive errors are less common in such patients. Early surgery is often advisable.

Divergent strabismus

This is a rather less common variety of squint, often of later onset, and sometimes associated with acquired blindness of one eye. One eye deviates outward on fixation by the other. The condition is usually intermittent and refractive errors (except occasional myopia) are unusual. Surgery is the usual treatment.

Summary

The reason for early case finding and treatment of strabismus is the conservation of sight. Amblyopia ex anopsia is a common cause of poor vision in adults. The suppressive agencies which cause the poor vision are very readily learned, and continue to operate essentially at a subconscious level. Correction of any visual defect, orthoptic exercises, and operations may each play a part.

REFRACTIVE ERRORS IN CHILDREN

These are common. Their importance in the causation of strabismus is discussed elsewhere.

Case finding. There is a clear case for the routine survey of all children for refractive error, preferably before they enter school; while retinoscopy can be used at any age, this technique is seldom within the powers of the average physician. Accordingly, he is usually obliged to use confrontation tests of various types. In the older, literate child, the use of test types (Snellen) presents little difficulty. In the younger (or illiterate) child the use of the E chart, in which the subject indicates the direction in which the limbs of the E point, is conventional, but sometimes inaccurate. It is not applicable to the older infants (say up to the age of 3½ or so), largely because of their inattentiveness or boredom. The older children of this group may be tested by matching the Snellen letters to a comparison chart held by the child and supervised by the mother; for the younger child, the problem of maintaining the subject's attention in the usual range of vision testing (3m) is overcome by watching his response to a white ball rolled across his visual field at various ranges. This method is useful as a screen, and will prevent much unnecessary retinoscopy.

Definitions

Hyperopia

In this condition, the eyeball is relatively short so that the point of focus is behind the eye. Some degree of this is physiological in young children whose superior powers of accommodation serve to correct the focusing defect; in severe hyperopia, plus lenses are prescribed.

Myopia

In this, the focal point is in front of the retina. Minus lenses are corrective.

Astigmatism

In this condition, the lens shape is abnormal in that its spherical curves are dissimilar in the two meridians, i.e., it tends to be spoon shaped. This causes unequal refraction of transmitted light which may blur the vision. Minor degrees of astigmatism are common and asymptomatic. The condition may coexist with other refractive errors.

Symptomatology

As discussed elsewhere, the most important problem is squint with amblyopia as a possible consequence. In many children, there are no subjective symptoms of refractive error, and complaints of headache, or tired eyes are heard often enough in children with normal findings on refraction. Most problems arise at school because the teacher deduces difficulty in vision, or because the child himself begins to realize that he cannot see as well as his peers. This is especially so with myopia.

Treatment. This consists in the prescription of spectacles after suitable refraction.

INJURIES TO THE EYE

These are relatively common in children, and all except the most minor and obvious require an expert's opinion, if not his attention. Common causes of trauma include blows from moving objects—stones, sticks, arrows, and ricocheting objects of various shapes. Direct injury in road accident is an increasing problem.

Extraocular foreign body

In most instances this is mobile and affects only the *conjunctiva*. The child complains of irritation, tearing, and bloodshot eyes rapidly follow. In young children only the last two may occur. Most objects are washed out by the tears, or deliberately removed after anesthetizing the conjunctiva.

Corneal foreign body

This is static so the pain is in the same place, but the signs are essentially the same as those described above. Superficial objects may be irrigated out; deeply seated objects require removal by an expert. Anesthetic and antibiotic eyedrops with *protection of the eye* are usual first aid methods. Chemical burns of the eye may occur from a wide variety of agents, but especially lime, lye, and acids. The eye should immediately be washed with water in large quantities after the lids have been pressed apart. No effort should be made to neutralize the acid or alkali but cycloplegic drops are usually in order. Powder burns of the eye are firecracker injuries which deposit gun powder and other chemicals in the conjunctiva and cornea. All of these demand expert opinion and attention.

Penetrating eye injuries

These vary greatly in their severity. Gross eyeball disorganization may be evident. Most troublesome are those with small entry wounds. Corneal perforations will show early opacification and distortion of the pupil, and in many instances there is loss of aqueous, with pain, redness, and prolapse of the iris. X-rays should always be done to locate possible radiopaque fragments. The care of all penetrating injuries is the field of the expert. The worst complication is infection with a sympathetic ophthalmia of the other eye.

CARE OF THE VISUALLY HANDICAPPED CHILD

In general, the care of the child begins with a full, adequate, and repeated explanation to the parents. Especially should care be taken to foster acceptance of the situation, and to heal parental feelings of guilt.

In the details of care, much will depend upon the presence of associated defects, and these should be diligently sought for. In the infant, blindness may coexist with cerebral palsy, or intellectual retardation. Similarly, in the postrubella syndrome, deafness and visual difficulty may be present, together. In all circumstances, an effort should be made to assess the child's intellect. In early days, the best objective evidence is the steady increase of head circumference. If this is present, and the increase itself is within normal percentiles, then an assumption may be made that the child is intellectually capable. This assumption should frequently be tested, allowing for slowness in motor milestones (e.g., standing, walking) in which vision plays an important part. The ability to communicate is a valuable parameter in the assessment of the blind child. If total blindness is clearly present on anatomical grounds, the intelligence seems fair, and associated defects are not severe, then arrangements should be made for an early examination of the child by the authorities of the local school for the blind. If other sensory difficulties are present, e.g., deafness, an early study must be made as to whether this association is partly, or wholly, remediable. This is because it is essential that the blind child has some mode of perception which will help compensate his visual difficulties. The whole aim of treatment is to make the child as independent as possible. Accordingly, it is essential that this be explained to parents, so that they may, at all stages in the child's life, avoid the overprotection which inhibits this primary aim. Children who have never had vision are usually reasonably content with their lot and, in the ordinary way, are no more likely to be troublesome than their normal peers. This does not of course exempt them from the usual tantrums of childhood, nor the rebellious behaviour of adolescence.

The partially sighted child

These require special aid in ordinary schools, e.g., a favoured class position, large print books, the use of tape recorded material as compensation for educational aids, such as T.V. programmes which they cannot distinguish. Visual acuity which is <10/200 (Snellen 6/60) commonly means that they are best educated in special schools for the blind. Partially sighted children whose condition is likely to deteriorate should be introduced to the techniques used by the totally blind (e.g., Braille) at a reasonably early stage.

In the end however, educational efforts are only partly successful if they do not lead to reasonable economic independence. Accordingly, the pediatrician will support every effort, moral or legal, which will aid the blind child's acceptance into gainful employment

17 Disorders of the skin

Skin disorders are common in children, the usual being infantile eczema, bacterial infections, and fungal invasions. However, even the less common disorders are important in that they may reflect a more generalized disease process.

GENETIC DISORDERS

Epidermolysis bullosa

This is an uncommon condition which exists in 2 forms, dominant and recessive. The latter starts earlier and is more severe.

Clinical features. The infant develops severe blistering with the most minor injury. In the recessive form, this may occur at birth, affecting most of the skin and mucous membranes. In the dominant form (simplex), the onset is later and the resistance to trauma greater; thus blister formation may be delayed until the child begins to crawl, and then affect only the weight bearing areas.

Dysphagia may occur in the severer types, due to enormous fragile blisters in the mouth. Esophageal and pharyngeal lesions may be complicated by scarring. As in burns (to which the lesions bear a close resemblance) considerable protein and gamma globulin loss is usual, so that infections (sometimes fatal) are commonplace.

Treatment. This is similar to that of burns. In the severe recessive form, the infant should be isolated, sedated if irritable, and protected from trauma. Large blisters may be aseptically aspirated, but the skin should not be removed. Vaseline gauze dressings are employed as a local protection, and antibiotics administered as the local condition and bacteriology demands. In the late onset dominant type, protection from trauma, and local vaseline gauze dressings are useful.

Ichthyosis

This usually presents as a simple dominant.

Clinical features. There is scaling of the skin, usually affecting the extensor surfaces. The scales are greyish or fawn in colour and are painless except in cold weather when cracking occurs. Itching is common.

Treatment. No specific cure is available. The scales are easier to remove if soaked in water, and given an occlusive dressing of ung. aequosum B.P.

Ichthyosis neonatorum (congenital ichthyosiform erythema)

This is a severe, and often lethal, variant in which the skin is not only scaly but erythematous. The child may seem to be coated with collodion. Associated congenital defects are common, and may be the major problem.

Refsum's disease

This is ichthyosis with polyneuritis, cerebellar ataxia, muscular weakness and sensory loss. Retinitis pigmentosa is common, as is progressive nerve deafness. No effective treatment is known and death occurs a few years after the appearance of the florid disease.

Mongolian blue spots

These are mentioned because, although entirely physiological, they may cause difficulty in diagnosis; the lesions are bluish areas, not raised, and having no symptomatology (except in the parents' minds). They occur principally on the sacral area near the midline, but may extend upwards along the line of the lumbar and thoracic vertebrae.

The condition occurs in children of Chinese, Indian, Malayan, American Indian, African, and Australian Aboriginal origin, and are not unusual in those from the Mediterranean littoral. The principal differential diagnosis is from bruising, as in the battered baby syndrome. There is however *no* local swelling, and the expected colour change of the usual bruise does not occur. Treatment is confined to reassurance.

Ehlers-Danlos syndrome (cutis hyperelastica)

This is inherited as an autosomal dominant. The principal features are purpuric spots, an easily injured skin, which is readily stretched, and which heals with a thin scar. Hyperextensible joints also occur. The sole treatment is to protect the child from injury.

Ectodermal dysplasia

This may be anhydrotic, in which the lack of sweating ability may cause the child to present with heat exhaustion. The hair is sparse, and the dentition delayed and defective. Disorders of the lenses are often found.

In the hydrotic form, sparse hair, dystrophic nails, and hyperkeratosis of the palms and soles occurs, with patchy areas of darkened skin elsewhere.

PIGMENTARY DISORDERS

These are all related to failure of normal melanin production, and present early in life.

Albinism

This may be partial or total. In the latter, the hair is silky and white, and in the Caucasian the skin is pale pink. In other races, widespread white macules are seen. The condition is often associated with eye difficulties—photophobic, nystagmus, cataracts, and retinitis pigmentosa. These patients suffer severe sunburn with minor actinic exposure and the prevention of this is the principal treatment.

Vitiligo

This is a much less severe and local form of albinism in which depigmented spots are found all over the body. The condition is more obvious when tanning occurs. There is no specific treatment. Cosmetic disguise may be used if the patient is embarrassed by the skin appearance.

Peutz-Jegher syndrome

In this condition deeply pigmented areas occur on the buccal mucosa, lips, and occasionally on the hands and feet. There are associated multiple gut polyps which may bleed, or cause intussusception. The last are the only features requiring treatment.

Incontinentia pigmenti

This is described under the neurocutaneous syndromes (p. 475).

TUMOURS OF THE SKIN

The usual type is the hemangioma. The simple variety, found on the eyelids and occipital area, is very common in infants. Those on the face fade, the others are hidden by hair. They require no treatment.

Cavernous (strawberry) hemangioma

This is the so called port-wine stain, which is purplish in colour, and usually present at birth. It may be associated with intracranial vascular abnormalities (Sturge-Weber syndrome) or be complicated by an arteriovenous aneurysm of the limb. These hemangiomata do not disappear spontaneously, and no treatment is curative. Cosmetic disguise should be used in patients who have facial lesions.

Moles (benign juvenile melanoma)

These are pigmented areas formed from the melanocyte layer of the epidermis. They are very common in children, and vary in colour from light brown to near black. They are not present at birth, but appear in the school-age group. The size is variable, but few are larger than 1-2 cm in diameter. The lesions may be smooth, rough, or hairy. The chance of malignant change is very small, and this never occurs before puberty. Excision is warranted for cosmetic reasons, and biopsy is in order if the mole increases in size, becomes darker in colour, bleeds, or infiltrates the surrounding skin. These are changes suggestive of neoplastic transformation.

SKIN INFESTATIONS

Scabies (the itch)

This condition is due to a mite, *Sarcoptes scabei*, which is of endemic, and occasionally epidemic, distribution. It is perhaps more common in children who live in crowded conditions.

Clinical features. The principal complaint is of itching, especially after the child has gone to bed. Secondary infection (impetigo) is frequent. Two types of skin lesion can be found—burrows, which have a vesicle and communicating track, seen as an elevation of the skin. These contain the mature female mites and their eggs. The follicular eruption contains immature mites. Scratch marks are also present—their absence makes the diagnosis suspect. The sites of the rash are the nipples, navel, genitals, palms, interdigital areas, ventral wrist areas, and inner elbows. The face and scalp are spared, unless the mother is also a sufferer and the patient a baby. Urticarial lesions may occur.

The mite may be extracted from the burrow by a sharp needle inserted just beyond the vesicle.

Treatment. Secondary infection is appropriately treated. The child is then bathed, scrubbed, and given a general application of a 25% solution of benzyl-benzoate; this is repeated after 24 hours. The bedding and clothes are then heat sterilized and a final benzyl benzoate application given. Other members of the family should be examined and treated as necessary.

Pediculosis

The usual forms of louse infection are of the scalp, body, or pubis. The latter (crab lice) is uncommon in children. The principal clinical features are itching and secondary infection. The last is particularly common in *pediculosis capitis*, in which a fine tooth comb may reveal the parasites. Usually, however, the whitish nits which are attached to the hair are the diagnostic feature.

In *pediculosis corporis*, bites and scratch marks are the usual finding, the lice being present in the clothing; pyogenic secondary infection (impetigo) is usual. In *pediculosis pubis*, the louse is found attached to the axillary or pubic hair.

Treatment. Benzyl benzoate emulsion will clear up most cases of pediculosis. It may be combined with dicophane if necessary. Normally all persons living in the same house should be treated. Chlorhexidine baths and hexachlorophene soap will control any secondary infection.

BACTERIAL INFECTIONS

Impetigo

This is a common skin problem of children which may complicate infestations, urticarial lesions, insect bites, and seborrheic dermatitis. The responsible organisms are the staphylococcus or streptococcus, usually the former. The exposed or abradable areas (face, hands, knees) are principally affected. Erythema is followed by small vesicles which rapidly burst. Crusting and a yellowish exudate follow. The edge of the lesion may spread but with central healing, a circinate appearance occurs. The lesions may appear in crops, the older ones often showing extensive crusting. In streptococcal impetigo, pericrustal redness is common, as is associated lymphadenitis.

Treatment. The child should be kept from school, as the condition is contagious. He should use his own towels. In most instances washing with hexachlorophene soap is sufficient to soften and remove the crusts. Systemic antibiotics are given if the infection is widespread.

Bullous impetigo of the newborn

This occurs in the newborn (pemphigus neonatorum). The staphyloccus causes large pus-filled blisters, mainly on the face, hands, and skin folds (axillae, groins). These rupture leaving raw areas. Crusting is not prominent; the condition should be vigorously treated with an antibiotic.

Furunculosis (boils)

These are rather uncommon until puberty, when they may complicate acne vulgaris. The lesion begins as a folliculitis, which spreads to the base of the hair follicle to cause the true boil. This is swollen, painful, and causes some edema of the surrounding skin. The pain persists until the abscess softens and discharges. Common sites for boils are the neck, face, axillae, and perineum, and they seem to be predisposed by local friction. Occasionally there is regional lymphadenitis.

Treatment. Hexachlorophene baths will reduce the staphylococcal skin flora, and if a nasal carrier state is present, antibiotic ointment is of value. Local treatment should be kept to a minimum, avoiding poultices and occlusive dressings. A simple gauze dressing is all that is necessary. Incision is reserved for large fluctuant abscesses, usually in the axilla. Systemic antibiotics are not always necessary.

Erysipelas

The organism (*streptococcus*) gains access to the skin through a cut or crack, usually on the face. A hot, red, painful swelling, with a definite edge appears, and spreads rapidly. There is much skin edema. Blisters sometimes occur. There are fever, rigors, and marked malaise.

Treatment. The patient is given large doses of parenteral penicillin.

Cellulitis

This is common in children, usually affects the lower limbs, and originates from some injury or infection (e.g., tinea pedis) which allows the entrance of the organism (usually streptococcus, sometimes staphylococcus). As in erysipelas, general upset with fever is usual. Locally, there is a red swollen edematous area without any well-defined edge. The inguinal nodes are enlarged and painful.

Treatment. A systemic antibiotic (usually penicillin) is given and the precipitating condition, e.g., tinea, is treated.

Lupus vulgaris

This tuberculous skin disease is nowadays a curiosity in children. The lesion is usually on the face or neck, and consists in a painless, dull-red, slightly scaly patch in which the capillaries are readily seen. Lymphadenitis is usual. Biopsy will establish the diagnosis. Isoniazid is the treatment of choice.

Leprosy

This is a not uncommon problem in tropical and semitropical countries. The neurological aspects are discussed elsewhere (p. 425). The skin lesions are very varied, but 2 extremes are described, the tuberculoid and the lepromatous. In the former, the principal finding is an area of bleaching in the skin, sometimes with a scaly surface and red edges. Hypoaesthesia and loss of sweating is usual, but the surrounding skin sweats excessively in compensation.

In the lepromatous form, the skin lesion is a reddish, shiny macule, with subcutaneous thickening. These are multiple and may coalesce to form nodules and plaques. In either type, the thickened peripheral nerves may be palpable. Biopsy of the skin lesion is diagnostic. The treatment is not only of the skin problem, but of the associated neurological difficulties. Sulphones are the usual chemotherapeutic agents.

Congenital syphilis

Skin manifestations are nowadays rare unless the maternal disease has been untreated. The rash appears on the palms and soles a few days after birth. It is bullous and reddish brown in color. Other manifestations of syphilis (hepatomegaly, jaundice, anemia, snuffles) may be associated. The treatment is to give large doses of penicillin for 2-3 weeks.

FUNGAL SKIN DISORDERS

These are common in children; they are principally due to *Candida* and *Trichophyton* species.

Candidiasis

Skin involvement usually follows infection of the mouth (thrush, p. 190). The lesions are usually perianal in distribution, and erythematous macules in form. Partial coalescence is frequent. In some instances the condition affects the leg skin folds, causing a reddish, moist intertrigo with scattered papules. The diagnosis is readily confirmed by culture. The disease may be precipitated by injudicious antibiotic therapy, or occur as part of a general disease, e.g., agammaglobulinemia, leukemia, or hypoparathyroidism.

Treatment. Thrush, if present, should be treated with nystatin solution (100,000 units/ml) put in the mouth 3-4 times daily; the skin lesions may be treated with nystatin ointment, or, if very widespread, with 1% aqueous gentian violet.

Candidal paronychia

This is rare in children, usually occurring in accomplished thumb suckers. The nail is painful and swollen at the base. Pus may form. If the nail plate is involved, the nail becomes ridged and thickened.

Treatment. Sucking the thumb should be discouraged, the area kept dry, and anointed with nystatin ointment. Systemic antifungal agents may also be necessary.

Tinea

This fungal infection may affect the hair, body, or feet. Hair and body infections are commoner in those in poor and crowded social circumstances. Animals are an important source of infection for such patients. Tinea pedis (athlete's foot) is mostly found in the older child and adolescent.

Tinea capitis

This is usually without symptoms, and may be detectable only by scanning the hair with a Wood's light. This will cause a turquoise fluorescence in infections by *Microsporum canis* or *Microsporum*. Microscopy of the hair (in 10% KOH) will also reveal the fungi. Obvious scalp involvement consists in round bald areas in which hair stumps can be seen. Some scaling may be present. Redness and a few pustules are common in the ring worm due to *M. canis*.

Treatment. The source of infection (animals) should be sought and treated. Griseofulvin is given by mouth for a week. Combs, hair brushes, and head gear should be sterilized. The Wood's light is used as a test of cure. Occasionally, a longer course of griseofulvin therapy, perhaps of 4-8 weeks, is required.

Tinea corporis

This can also be acquired from animals. There are multiple circular areas which, initially red and scaly, may acquire small vesicles. They grow outwards while at times healing centrally. The peripheral area has most vesicles (tinea circinata). The fungus is readily identified in skin scrapings. The treatment is to apply Whitfield's ointment; in resistant cases, griseofulvin is given.

Tinea pedis

This usually presents with maceration and scaling between the toes. Characteristically it improves in cool weather and is aggravated by sweating. In severe cases, the underside of the toes, or sole of the foot, becomes desquamated, and may show vesicles. Secondary infection is not uncommon and may cause cellulitis. The mycelia may be seen by microscopy.

Treatment. In mild cases, with only interdigital involvement, Whitfield's ointment is sufficient; severer cases may yield to Castellani's paint. In all instances, foot hygiene should be improved, and the sodden interdigital scales removed. In institutional outbreaks, the usual source is the shower room. This should be disinfected, kept as dry as possible, and the use of protective footwear insisted upon.

VIRAL DISORDERS OF THE SKIN

Warts (verruca vulgaris)

These are very common in school-age children. The warts are clearly transmissible but have a strong tendency to spontaneous cure.

Clinical features. The appearance is well known, most lesions resembling a miniature dried out cauliflower. Common sites are the hands, knees, and feet. Plane warts are papular in form, and flesh or light brown in colour. These are usually found on the face and backs of the hands. Most fungating fresh-cauliflower-like warts on the genitals and anal areas are called condylomata acuminata, but these are relatively rare in children.

Plantar warts

As the name implies, these are found on the sole of the foot and may follow local trauma. Pressure from their growth into the sole causes variable degrees of local pain.

Treatment of warts

Small warts may be treated by physical methods (CO_2 snow, liquid nitrogen). The silver nitrate stick applied to the wart (surrounded by a protective ring of Vaseline) is also of value, although unsightly staining is a temporary problem. Extensive warts should be locally anesthetized and curetted.

Plantar warts should be superficially scraped and soaked once a day for 20 minutes in 3% formalin solution. The soaking must be local. This is achieved by placing the affected area in a tin lid containing the formalin solution. This regime is continued for about 6 weeks.

Rarely large plantar warts may require local surgical excision. Podophyllin (25% in spirit or in collodion) is useful for genital warts.

Molluscum contagiosum

This viral infection gives rise to crops of small, pearly papules with an umbilicated centre, which are usually situated on the trunk. When squeezed they exude a white curd-like material. Spontaneous cure occurs, but the lesions disappear more rapidly if pierced with a sharpened applicator dipped in phenol.

Herpes simplex

This is a common disorder of children. In rare instances it gives rise to a fatal disseminated infection of the newborn (see p. 53). The usual complaint is of cold sores affecting the lips and adjacent skin. Stomatitis may be a complication, especially in the first 3 years of life. The genitals and skin of the trunk are occasionally affected.

The lesion is a small vesicle which coalesces with its congeners, bursts, and leaves a crusted area. Itching and some pain are usual. In herpetic stomatitis, dysphagia, fever, and regional adenopathy are common.

Treatment. No specific treatment is known. A simple antiseptic application (e.g., chlorhexidine cream) may be applied locally. Stomatitis demands analgesic mouthwash (e.g., nupercaine/chlorhexidine paint), and if dysphagia is severe, a short period of intravenous fluid may be necessary.

Kaposi's varicelliform eruption (eczema herpeticum)

This is the condition in which infantile eczema is secondarily infected by the herpes simplex virus.

Clinical features. The child *always* has had infantile eczema for some time. The rash spreads, and areas of vesiculation appear, followed by crusting, umbilication, and shallow ulceration. A pyogenic superinfection may occur. Fever, vomiting, and dehydration are not uncommon, and circulatory failure may supervene.

A similar, occasionally more severe, situation arises when the eczematous infant has been deliberately or accidentally vaccinated. In vaccinal superinfection, the lesions are larger, and more prone to give rise to local necrosis.

Treatment. Dehydration should be anticipated or treated by appropriate intravenous therapy. A broad-spectrum antibiotic (e.g., ampicillin) should be given, and the infant isolated.

Herpes zoster

This is described under diseases of the posterior roots (p. 425).

ENDOGENOUS DERMATITIS

Seborrhoeic dermatitis

In infants, this begins on the scalp between 4-6 weeks of age. A usual first complaint is cradle cap which is a thick, yellowish brown collection of scales of varying size. It feels greasy, and does not itch. Patchy red areas with a lesser load of scales may be found elsewhere, usually on the brow and eyebrows, behind the ears, and in any of the skin flexures. The lesions show no vesiculation or true exudate. Secondary infection with *Candida* or pyogenic organisms can occur.

Treatment. Cradle cap is treated by softening the scales with vegetable oil, and shampooing regularly. Lesions on the body persist only for a few months, and mild cases require no treatment. Otherwise, steroid cream is used alone, or combined with antibiotic treatments if secondary infection has occurred.

Drug eruptions

The skin can react to almost any drug. However, certain of these are more liable to cause trouble, including penicillin, phenobarbitone, sulphonamides, and tranquillizers. Common findings are erythematous or morbilliform rashes, as in responses to anticonvulsants. An itching urticarial reaction is common with penicillin allergy. Purpuric rashes may complicate treatment with thiazide diuretics and some anticonvulsants.

Light sensitivity reactions

These are seen on the exposed areas such as the face, hands, and knees, and may follow treatment with dimethyl chlortetracycline, sulphonamides, penicillins, and the phenothiazine tranquillizers. The rash may vary from a sunburn-like erythema, to the formation of papules.

Erythema multiforme may follow the more minor manifestations of drug sensitivity. Lesions resembling those of lupus erythematosus have followed hydralazine and procainamide therapy, but are relatively uncommon in children. Erythema nodosum is seldom due to drugs, but has followed the use of the now archaic sulphathiazole, and may complicate the sulphone therapy of leprosy.

Exfoliative dermatitis

This is not very common in children, but can follow any of the earlier signs of drug sensitivity. Stomatitis and glossitis are early complaints; the skin shows a generalized scarlatiniform rash, with edema of the subcuticular tissues. The lymph glands are usually enlarged. Fever and vomiting may occur.

Lyell's toxic necrolysis

This condition may be a reaction to drugs, although a staphylococcal etiology has been suspected in some children.

Clinical features. The condition begins with a local reddish rash which rapidly becomes generalized. The latter is red, moist, and crusts, and resembles scalding of the skin. It is acutely painful, and exfoliation follows in a few days. The child is fevered, and may develop dehydration and shock.

General treatment of drug reactions

The offending agent should be withdrawn, the case notes suitably annotated, and the parents warned concerning the avoidance of the drug and its congeners. In mild cases, the skin reaction subsides rapidly. In urticarial reactions, the antihistamines may help in reducing the itch. If uncontrolled by this, oral steroids are of value. In exfoliative dermatitis, steroids and attention to the patient's general state by intravenous fluids are usually necessary, with systemic antibiotics as the bacteriology indicates. Potentially toxic applications, e.g., silver nitrate, should not be applied to widely exfoliated skins.

Erythema multiforme

This condition is commonly due to drug-sensitivity, or reflects a viral infection, e.g., herpes simplex. The streptococcus has also been held responsible.

The eruption is of sudden onset, usually beginning on the face, hands, forearms, and knees and mucous membranes. The lesions are variable, but pale red papules are common. Red annular spots, with a purplish centre which later goes through the colour changes of a bruise (erythema iris), are characteristic. Vesicles or bullae may form within the erythema iris. The mucous membrane of the mouth is cast off leaving a raw, painful surface. Fever, vomiting, and joint pains may occur. The skin lesions may occur in crops over a few weeks, after which the condition spontaneously disappears.

Stevens-Johnson syndrome is a more severe variety of erythema multiforme, and in addition to the mouth condition, lesions occur in the vulva, urethra, and conjunctiva.

Treatment. General nursing care is the main mode of treatment, with intravenous fluids if vomiting is present. Simple local applications (e.g., calamine lotion B.P.) aid the local discomfort. In the Stevens-Johnson syndrome, steroid therapy is indicated.

Atopic dermatitis (eczema)

This is thought to be an allergic disorder.

Clinical features. The infantile variety begins between the third and sixth month of life, with redness of the skin, papule formation, and weeping. It is itchy, sometimes intensely so. The usual place where eczema starts is on the face, whence it involves the extensor areas of the limbs, and often becomes generalized. Thickening of the skin (lichenification) develops, and secondary infection (impetigo, herpetic) is common. The disease usually abates spontaneously by 2-3 years of age, but residual lichenified areas in the flexures are common.

Diagnosis. This is mainly from seborrheic dermatitis which develops in the scalp with a greasy, scaling exudate (cradle cap), and involves principally the brow and upper face. Care should also be taken to exclude systemic disease such as Wiskott-Aldrich syndrome, of which eczema may be only a symptom.

Treatment. Sedation is of value in the early stages of the disease. Pyogenic superinfection should be controlled and topical therapy begun. This is almost invariably with steroid creams which rapidly relieve the itching, and return the skin to normal structure. If weeping is widespread, simple lotions may precede the steroid applications.

Prognosis. Infantile eczema may precede frank asthma. In other patients, the skin condition may regularly recur, though usually in a localized area.

Urticaria

This is common allergic phenomenon in children. The local condition is an itchy wheal of varying size with a surrounding red area which, in some children, coalesce to form a large lesion. The eruption may be local or generalized, but the individual lesions are usually transient, persisting in some instances for only a few hours. In most children, the urticarial hive will last a considerably shorter time. Angioneurotic edema may occur at the same time.

Etiology. Ingested allergens (foods) and drug reactions are not unusual causes. Generalized urticaria occurs in serum sickness, and may be a feature of conditions such as Henoch-Schönlein disease, and disseminated lupus erythematosus.

Investigations. Care should be taken to exclude the more dangerous diseases noted, and also the possibility of drug reaction. A most careful search should be made for the possibility of insect bites which may, in children, cause a much more generalized response than in the adult.

Treatment. If the allergen can be identified and avoided, the skin disorder will disappear in a day or two. Local treatment is of little avail, although cool alkaline baths may be comforting. Antihistamines are of some value, especially where angioneurotic edema is also present.

EXOGENOUS DERMATITIS

Napkin (diaper) dermatitis

This is a common pediatric problem. Usually it is a chemical dermatitis, due to splitting of the urine-urea into ammonia by various napkin organisms. In a few instances, it is due to laundry agents, or to constant saturation of the skin from infrequent changing. The disorder occurs in all of the age groups which are incontinent.

Clinical features. The napkins usually smell of ammonia, and the local sign is redness of the buttocks, genitals, convexities of the thighs, and sometimes the anterior abdominal wall. Papules, vesicles, and small ulcers occur. Thickening of the scrotal skin, and meatal ulcer may occur in boy babies. The skin folds are spared in true napkin dermatitis. Secondary pyogenic infection can occur.

Differential diagnosis. This is principally from candidiasis, which affects the perianal area and folds of the groins.

Treatment. Eradication of the ammonia-forming organism is carried out by collecting *all* of the napkins and boiling them. Any container used for storing the napkins should be sterilized at the same time. The boiled napkins are carefully rinsed, and the mother instructed that further washing is to be done with a mild soap.

Local treatment. The napkins should be changed frequently and occlusive plastic pants forbidden. Laying the bare-bottomed infant on an absorbent area for most of the day will aid healing. Zinc and castor oil cream is a safe local unguent. In secondary infection, antibiotic ointment is of value.

Papular urticaria

This is a common disorder which is almost always due to insect bites.

Clinical features. There are clusters of firm papules, usually on the limbs and face. These crop out at varying intervals, and are associated with intense itching, then they die down to form transient pigmented macules. Excoriation from scratching is usual, and secondary infection common. In other words, the lesion is characteristic of a mosquito bite.

Treatment. This consists in finding the offending parasite. If mosquitoes have been excluded, the usual insects to be considered are cat, dog, bird, and human fleas, the bed bug, rat mites, and dog lice. If animals are possible vectors, they, and their bedding, should thoroughly be disinfested. In warmer climates carpets should be examined for fleas and appropriately treated. The patient's own lesions will respond to time and calamine lotion.

Contact dermatitis

This is more common in the older child and adolescent. The first feature is reddening of the skin, followed by thickening and then the formation of vesicles. In chronic conditions, the skin thickens, scales, and becomes lichenified. Itching is always present. The lesions tend to be most marked on exposed areas such as the backs of the hands, face, neck and eyelids. The distribution may however be more generalized if the patient is allergic to some component in the clothing. Common etiological factors are allergens of plant origin, cosmetics, ointments, or substances (e.g., glues) used in the child's hobbies. Clothing dyes are more likely allergens than the fibre itself.

Investigations. Patch testing with the suspected allergen will give a delayed response reaction which mimicks the disease state.

Treatment. The allergen should be avoided, and the local lesion treated as described under allergic dermatitis.

SKIN REACTIONS TO HEAT AND HUMIDITY

Sweat rash

This is not uncommon in infants. It is due to excessive sweating and presents as a vesicular red eruption, which may become secondarily infected. The usual sites are the face, neck folds, and waist area, although a generalized rash may occur. The condition occurs in warm weather on in infants kept too hot, and wearing clothes (e.g., nylon) which are non-absorbent. The treatment is to cool the child by removal of the excess clothing, or by environmental adjustment. Secondary infection will yield to simple antiseptic (e.g., chlorhexidine) applications.

Prickly heat (miliaria rubra)

This is a more severe variety of the above, which occurs in hot, humid climates. It is especially common in new arrivals. It is an itchy, papulovesicular red rash most marked around the waist and in the bends of the elbows and knees. The skin is also often macerated. The treatment consists in reducing sweating, and allowing its ready evaporation. This essentially means adjusting the environment. Of the methods available, air-conditioning is the only effective one in severe cases.

SKIN REACTIONS TO COLD

Chilblains (pernio)

These are a common reaction to damp cold in children. They consist in itchy, dark red swellings, mostly found on the fingers and toes, but occurring also on the nose, ears, and occasionally on the backs of the legs and buttocks. The itching is often worst in warmer surroundings such as bed. Cracking and secondary infection sometimes occur.

Prevention. This lies in the provision of warm clothing and surroundings. Little can be done for the established lesions, except to apply calamine lotion for the itchiness.

Acrocyanosis

This is a bluish colour of the hands and feet which develops in response to cold. It is common in the newborn. *Erythrocyanosis* is a more marked cyanotic change usually seen over the lower third of the legs. Scaling may be associated, as are chilblains.

Cutis marmorata (marble skin)

This is a common and normal skin response of the infant when exposed to cold. There are areas of pale skin with bluish streaks between. The condition rapidly disappears when the infant is wrapped, and no treatment is necessary.

Neonatal cold injury

This is described elsewhere (p. 46).

DISORDERS OF THE SEBACEOUS GLANDS

Acne vulgaris

This is a common condition affecting adolescents. The usual age of onset for females is 13-16, and for males 15-18 years. In most instances, the condition is mild, and requires little treatment. The characteristic lesion is the comedo (whitehead, blackhead) found on the face, chest, back, and upper arms. A red papule may follow, which later may form a pustule. In most children, only comedones and a few papules are present. In those seeking medical help, all 3 lesions are present. In severe cases, cysts form in the areas of pustule activity. The condition varies somewhat with the seasons, and may be aggravated in climates with high humidity and temperature.

Treatment. The principal need of the patient is reassurance that he will not permanently be scarred—as is true in the vast majority of patients. Dietary restrictions are of little value. Close attention should be paid to the hygiene of the skin, including, for girls, careful removal of cosmetics. Soap and water is usually sufficient for washing. The patient should be discouraged from squeezing the blackheads and pustules.

Application to the skin. These conventionally are employed to produce some desquamation. Those most readily accepted by the patient are proprietary sulphur containing compounds with a cosmetic base. Ultraviolet exposure will also produce mild sunburn and scaling, and may be indicated in appropriate climates. In severe instances, the nocturnal application of a steroid/antibiotic cream may be of value. Systemic antibiotics and estrogen are seldom indicated.

MISCELLANEOUS

Mastocytosis

This is the condition in which mast cells accumulate in the skin. They are capable of histamine release, which is the mechanism for the symptomatology. The commonest form (and this is rare) is *urticaria pigmentosa*. In this condition, the child occasionally itches, and develops macules which show a brownish staining. Minor degrees of trauma cause these to form an urticarial lesion, and blisters and bullae are sometimes found. Dermographia may be associated. Flushing episodes may occur in older children, sometimes after taking aspirin or codeine. In very rare instances, there is involvement of the bones (seen by x-ray) or hepatosplenomegaly.

The principal differential diagnosis is from papular urticaria, in which the lesions occur in clusters on the limbs and do not show permanent pigmentation.

Pityriasis rosea

This is a common disorder of the older child. It is of unknown etiology, but may be due to a virus. It is a self-limited disease which gives rise to little trouble. The first sign is the so-called herald patch—a largish red, scaling macule found on the chest or abdominal wall. After a variable time (usually 3-4 days, rarely up to 4 weeks) a rash appears on the trunk, upper arms, and thighs (the vest and pants area). There are 2 components to the eruption—pink papules and rosy macules. The latter predominate, and have a brownish scaling centre.

The principal differential diagnosis is from measles, or from morbilliform drug reactions. In neither is a herald patch present. In the former the other symptoms, and in the latter a history of drug exposure is helpful.

Treatment. Generally none is necessary. Calamine lotion is comforting where itching is troublesome. Ultraviolet light may cause more rapid disappearance of the lesions.

Psoriasis

This is an unusual skin problem in the young child. In most instances the onset is at puberty.

Clinical features. The essential lesion is rich red with superimposed scaling. The latter is white, and may need to be scraped off to reveal the underlying red patch. The edge is well-defined, and the intervening skin is perfectly normal. A vast number of variants have been described. In children, the commoner variety is guttate psoriasis, in which many small patches are scattered over the body. This type shows rather less scaling than other varieties. Nummular psoriasis is where there are larger discs and plaques over the limbs and trunk. Itching is absent except occasionally in scalp involvement.

Treatment. In mild cases, with few patches, the application of crude coal tar ointment may help. If the response is slow, fluorinated steroid ointment under an occlusive dressing (polyethylene) is indicated. Widespread occlusive dressings should be avoided in young subjects because of the possibility of marked sweating causing undue salt loss. Sunlight (or ultra violet lamp) exposure is also helpful. Cytotoxic drugs are seldom used except in very acute and widespread lesions, and must be administered with the most careful hematological control.

HAIR DISORDERS IN CHILDREN

In chronic illness, e.g., mucoviscidosis, severe congenital heart disease, the hair is characteristically fine and silky. This finding normally coincides with growth failure. The dyspigmentation of kwashiorkor and the aminoacidopathies are described elsewhere (p. 104).

Alopecia (diffuse toxic)

Loss of hair is common in children treated with cytotoxic drugs, particularly vincristine, cyclophosphamide, methotrexate, and azothioprine. The principal offenders are vincristine and cyclophosphamide, after which alopecia almost always occurs. The hair is fully shed, and regrowth does not occur until the drug is stopped. Even then hair growth may take some time to be re-established. Poisoning with rat poisons (thallium, warfarin) may also be causal.

Hypotrichosis and alopecia of syndromal origin

Severe degrees of alopecia are seen in the ectodermal dysplasia syndromes, progeria, and occasionally as an isolated defect (atrichia congenita). Sparse, fine, brittle hair is found in Marinesco-Sjögren syndrome and the Hallermann-Streiff syndrome of bird-headed dwarfism with mandibular aplasia.

Alopecia areata

The symptom is a bald patch of varying size, at the edge of which the hair is easily pulled out and may be of exclamation mark type, i.e., with an atrophic tip which lacks the bulbous termination of normal hair. The condition may spread to involve all of the scalp, but this is not very common. The bald patch may remain unchanged for several months, normal regrowth being preceded by fine, infantile hair, which is paler than normal.

Treatment. This is difficult, since topical steroids may induce a regrowth which is rapidly shed Patience and placebo are indicated in minor lesions. A wig should be used in total alopecia, especially in girls. Recurrences are not unusual and alopecia may be permanent.

Hirsutism

This means an apparent excess of body hair. In most instances this is constitutional and racial, but it also occurs in adrenogenital syndromes.

Iatrogenic hirsutism is found in children given steroids (e.g., for nephrotic syndrome) or androgens for growth failure. Diphenyl streptomycin and anticonvulsants are other drugs which can be responsible.

Treatment. This is of the underlying condition.

18 Disorders of the central nervous system

GENERAL ORGANIZATION

The basic subdivisions are those of the neuromuscular apparatus, the sensory apparatus, the coordinating and modulating apparatus, and the higher centres. The latter coordinate the whole into willed movements and actions consequent upon the integration of intelligence, memory, and learning into logical thought. The background to the whole of willed movement are the activities which seldom enter our consciousness. Thus, the autonomic nervous system helps regulate our blood pressure, heart rate, and gastrointestinal function. Similarly, we retain our upright position or the tone (degree of stretch) of our muscles without making any conscious effort. Failure of function of these mechanisms, however, soon makes us aware of a defect.

BRIEF OUTLINES

The neuromuscular (motor) system

The first major subdivision of this is the *upper motor neurone*. There are 2 of these, 1 for each side of the body. Each begins in the cerebral cortex, in the area called the precentral gyrus, runs down to the midbrain, and pons, crosses at the medulla, and continues down the spinal cord without crossing again, as the corticospinal tracts.

These give off connecting neurones which meet the anterior horn cells. The lower motor neurone begins at the anterior horn cell, traverses the peripheral motor nerves and terminates so as to cause muscular contraction (the myoneural junction). The description given refers to the spinal nerves, but it should be remembered that the *cranial* nerves, whose origin is within the skull, are organized in the same way, viz., connected to and under the control of the upper motor neurone, and giving out a lower motor neurone. Figure 50 summarizes the situation.

The sensory system

This begins in the outlying parts of our body, and consists in cell structures which are sensitive to various stimuli such as touch, pain, and temperature. There are other organs which are sensitive to gravity and

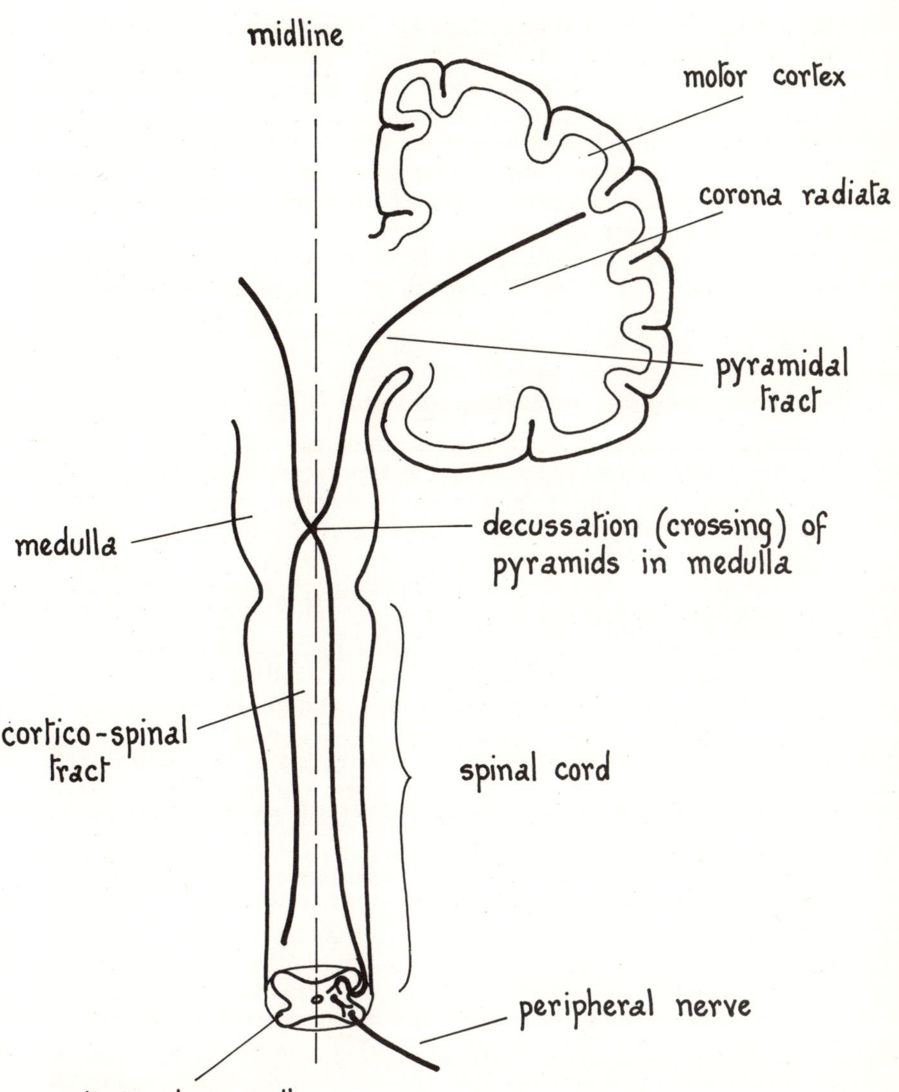

Fig. 50. The motor pathway: the upper motor neurone terminates at the anterior horn cell.

the position of limbs, and specialized cells which detect changes of position by the vestibular mechanism which is situated in the inner ear. The major special senses (hearing, vision, taste, and smell), set up impulses which flow directly to the brain. In general, sensation is supplied from one side of the body, and crosses in the cord or lower brainstem to terminate in the thalamus. Thence new fibres originate, and run upwards to terminate in the post central gyrus of the cerebral cortex. A general outline of the sensory pathway is shown in the Figure 51.

The special senses (smell, vision, hearing) are arranged in a similar way. Crossing of impulse is retained, as is connection with the thalamus. The central terminations are in appropriate special areas of the cortex, viz., the auditory cortex, visual cortex.

The coordinating and modulating apparatus

Essentially, this consists in the areas which connect the sensory and motor divisions. These can scan incoming information (sensation) and within limits make a decision as to whether such information should be transmitted to, or acted upon by the cerebral cortex. They can also receive information about outgoing motor activity, and modulate it (i.e., superimpose another pattern of behaviour). Accordingly this apparatus receives impressions from sensory supply, and from the cortical motor areas, and generally connects with the outgoing upper motor neurone. The 2 major components of the coordinating and modulating apparatus are the cerebellum and extrapyramidal system.

The *cerebellum* receives information from the skin, muscles and tendons, the vestibular apparatus, and the eyes and ears, and rapidly and continuously sorts it into patterns. These can be used to maintain basic muscular mechanisms such as posture, and be transmitted to the cortex as a preliminary to a willed movement. Thus the cerebellum is a sorter and is a short-term store of information. By its connections to the motor cortex, the cerebellum not only transmits information, but meters the level. Within limits, this level determines the speed and degree of motor activity at the time of its initiation by the motor cortex.

Damage to the cerebellum does not cause either loss of sensation or of the primary power of movement. But the integration of information is impaired, and the initiation and regulation of movement slowed and incoordinate. The more complex the movement (e.g., speech) the greater the interference.

The *extrapyramidal system* is mainly comprised of the basal nuclei which lie deep in the cerebral hemisphere near the thalamus. The main nuclei are the lentiform, caudate, amygdaloid, and the claustrum. They receive nerve fibres from the cortex, thalamus, and cerebellum, and give out fibres to the cortex and others which descend in the spinal cord. Thus both corticospinal and anterior horn cell function can be

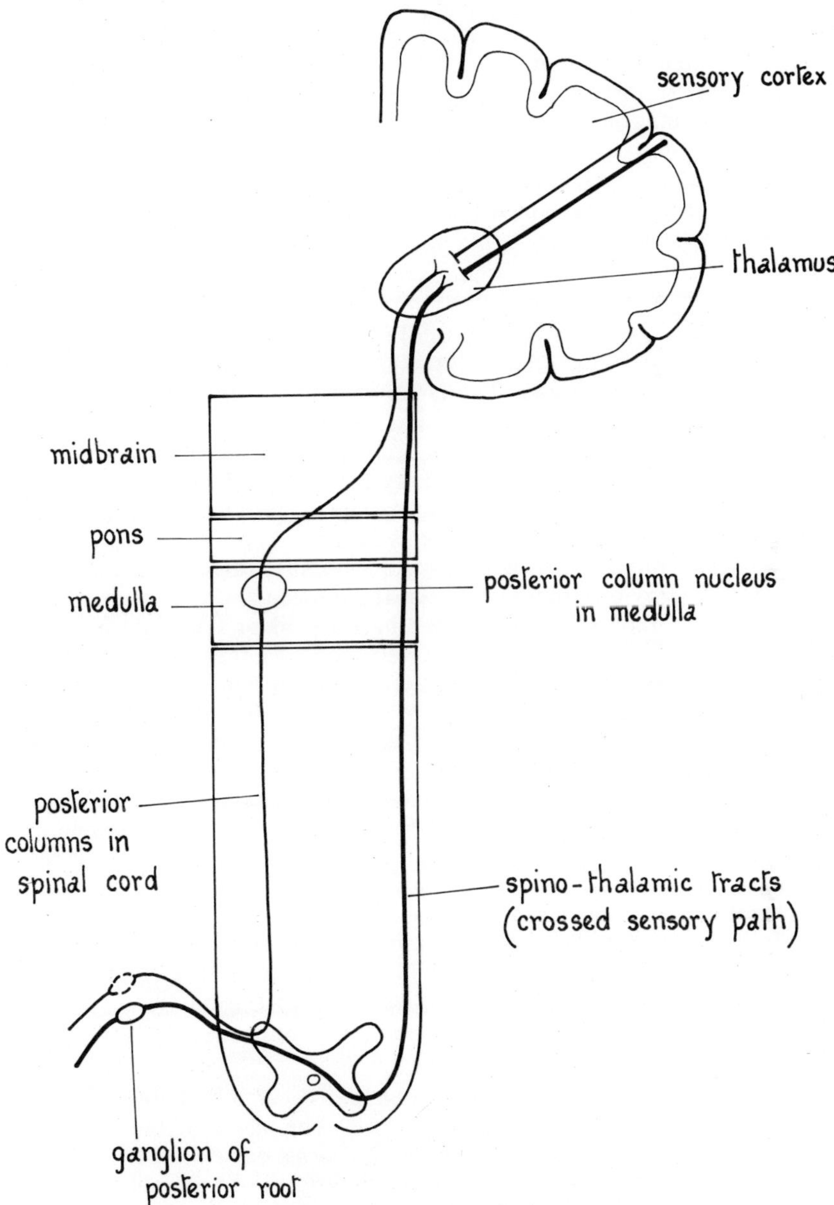

Fig. 51. The sensory pathway.

modified. Some parts of the extra-pyramidal system are probably able to initiate certain movements, but the major function of the system is to modify or suppress them.

In simple summary then, the nervous system is organized so as to receive information, process it,and deliver appropriate messages to the body which initiate and integrate movements. The sensory supply in many cases may, eventually initiate movements. In man, ideational capacity, which is independent of sensory supply will also initiate purposeful movements.

Transmission of the nervous impulse

This brings us into a consideration of microanatomy and microphysiology. The 2 basic types of individual nerve cells are the *neurone* and the *neuroglia*. The latter is thought only to support and nourish the neurone, which itself has a cell body, projections called dendrites, and a transmitting line called the axon. The neurone is designed to transmit electrical activity from one region to another of the nervous system, and to the muscles. The place at which one neurone connects with another is called the synapse.

The nerve impulse can be transmitted because there is an electrical potential (energy difference) between the outside and the inside of the axon. That is, the axon is, in the resting state, like a flashlight battery; the switch is applied by chemical stimuli (chemical transmitters), which induce an electrical change in the dendrites and body of the neurone. This in turn causes a brief shift of positively changed sodium ions from the exterior to the interior of the axon. The concomitant shift of electrons causes the impulse to pass along the axon as the sodium ions shift in and out sequentially. Not only are there transmitters (e.g., acetylcholine), but there are agents for the destruction of the transmitter (e.g., acetylcholinesterase), which prevents its accumulation at the synapse. There are also other substances which can *inhibit* the neurone transmitters.

Many drugs act upon neurotransmission, and knowledge of these allows us to design medicines which will affect the nervous system. A few diseases are also due to abnormalities of neurotransmission.

THE UPPER MOTOR NEURONE (U.M.N.)

Disorders of the upper motor neurone can occur anywhere from the cerebral cortex to the anterior horn cell. The cause of the disorder varies a good deal with age. Thus, in newborns, congenital absence of neural tissue (e.g., hydranencephaly), the effects of metabolic disturbance (hypoglycemia, aminoacidopathies, hyperammonemia) and intracranial bleeding are each important causes. Meningomyelocele is the commonest cause if corticospinal tracts are involved within the spinal cord. In early childhood, degenerative neurological conditions begin to contribute, as do cerebrovascular accidents, which may follow intracranial infection, or occur with impaired cerebral circulation, as in severe dehydration. At any age, accidental head injury may be a cause.

General features

Motor neurone disorders interfere with patterns of movement, they do not paralyze individual muscles. If a pattern of movement is represented on both sides of the brain, then such movements (breathing, frowning, crying, laughing) are retained. If the disease is in any area above the crossing of the corticospinal tracts in the medulla, then the movements of the opposite half of the body are affected. At, or below the crossing, the paralysis is on the same side as the disease, If the primary disorder is in the motor cortex, then only 1 limb may be affected (a monoplegia). This is because movement representation is spread out in the cortical area. Below the motor cortex, in the corona radiata, or cortico-spinal tracts proper, function is lost in one half of the body (hemiplegia). As the cranial nerve nuclei are adjacent, these may also be involved, causing an appropriate paralysis on the side opposite to the hemiplegia. The ascending sensory tracts and areas for control of eye movements are also nearby. Accordingly, loss of sensation (anesthesia) or loss of coordinated eye movement may be associated with motor disorders.

If both corticospinal tracts are involved, then *quadriplegia* (paralysis of all 4 limbs) will occur. *Paraplegia* exists when the lower limbs alone are affected. This must represent some problem within the spinal part of the corticospinal tracts.

Clinical findings in hemiplegia

The main finding is loss of function on the affected side. *In infancy*, this presents as poverty of movement with an absent Moro response on one side. In the early stages the limbs are flaccid, but become spastic (hypertonic) after a few months. As time goes on, a reasonable amount of gross movement may return, but fine movements of the fingers or toes do not appear. Wasting of the limbs is common in this age group, so that the hand or foot on the affected side is smaller than its fellow. Clearly the loss of function will cause delay in achieving the normal milestones of motor development, and this may be the first complaint. The degree of involvement is very variable in infancy, so that in mildly affected children, the condition may not be suspected until difficulties with walking or hand movements occur towards the end of the first year of life.

Apart from loss of function the main neurological findings are initial flaccidity (hypotonia), often with normal deep tendon (e.g., knee) reflexes, followed by spasticity with increased deep tendon reflexes. The superficial (abdominal) and plantar reflexes are of little value at this age.

In the *older child*, who has achieved normal activity, the complaint is of a sudden loss of function on one side. A convulsion and loss of consciousness may coincide. The limbs are flaccid at first, and then become spastic, with increased deep reflexes, loss of superficial reflexes, and the development of an extensor plantar response. Gross movements usually return, but clumsiness and loss of fine movement is often permanent. Muscle wasting occurs after a few months, but failure of limb growth is much less common than in the young infant.

Localizing the problem (see figure 50)

Some clue can often be found by considering the symptoms. Thus, if the UMN difficulty involves the *cerebral* (*motor*) *cortex*, then the hemiplegia is incomplete, and loss of sensation very unusual. The power of speech may be lost, because the speech centre can be affected. This is said to be in the left cortex in right-handed persons, and vice versa in the left-handed. Loss of speech of this type is called *motor aphasia*, and is seldom total, so that "yes" and "no" are preserved. As recovery sets in, the speech improves, but is hesitant, with incomplete sentence formation. If the child has learned to write, this faculty is also affected, giving rise to agraphia (inability to express oneself in writing).

If the lesion is below the cortex, e.g., in the *corona radiata* the hemiplegia may be accompanied by sensory loss, because the adjacent thalamocortical pathways are affected. In conditions involving the upper midbrain, there is paralysis of the 3rd cranial nerve, which causes loss of some eye movements on the same side (the hemiplegia is on the opposite side). If the *lower midbrain* is involved, the face may be paralyzed on the same side as the hemiplegia (a supranuclear facial paralysis). In conditions involving the pons, the 5th, 6th, and 7th cranial nerves are paralyzed, causing impaired jaw, eye and facial movement respectively. Deep pontine lesions may also involve the sensory pathways for postural sense, and less commonly those for pain and temperature. This sensory disability affects the side of the body opposite to the hemiplegia.

If the *medulla* is involved, there is a crossed hemiplegia, often with tongue paralysis (12th cranial nerve) and if the midline medulla is affected there is loss of postural sense on the hemiplegic side. In lateral medullary involvement the 9th and 10th motor cranial nerves (pharyngeal movement, swallowing) and 5th (sensory) cranial nerve, are involved on the same side as the injury, with an opposite hemiplegia and opposite loss of pain and temperature sense.

The pattern of disorder with *spinal cord* involvement is very varied. In complete transection (as in infantile myelomeningocele, or traffic accident) there is total loss of motor and sensory function. The urinary and anal sphincters are also paralyzed, causing incontinence of feces and urinary retention with overflow incontinence from the distended bladder.

In conditions which cause external pressure on the cord, involvement of the corticospinal tracts causes difficulty in walking, with the signs of a U.M.N. lesion (increased reflexes, etc.) in both legs. As the condition progresses, total paraplegia sets in. The posterior (sensory) roots of the spinal cord are often affected in such conditions. This causes painful burning and tingling sensations (root pains) in the area of the body supplied by the posterior root. If the disorder is *within* the spinal cord, sensory loss and asymmetric motor paralysis occur. Involvement of the anal and bladder sphincters is a late problem.

In disorders of the *cauda equina* (the lowest part of the spinal cord), there is a below knee motor paralysis, sensory loss mainly in the perineal (saddle) area, as well as bladder and anal paralysis.

It should be noted that localization by clinical methods is only approximate. Spinal cord lesions are usually investigated by outlining the cord with air or contrast medium (myelography). Conditions within the skull are investigated by outlining the ventricles with air (ventriculography), or by following the course of injected contrast material in the blood vessels (cerebral angiography). Shifts of brain structure may be defined by sonar (echoencephalography), or by introducing some short-lived radioactive material into the brain and checking where it goes by appropriate counting gear (cerebral scintillography).

THE LOWER MOTOR NEURONE

Diseases of this segment can occur in the anterior horn cell, the peripheral motor nerve, and at the neuromuscular junction.

Diseases of the anterior horn cell

The commonest variety is *spinal muscular atrophy*. There are several distinct forms. The cause of each remains unknown, but there is always destruction of the anterior horn cells. Some are autosomal recessives.

Werdnig-Hoffmann disease (amyotonia congenita syndrome; spinal muscular atrophy, type 1)

Clinical features. This is a serious disease which presents in the first 3 months of life. The major findings are floppiness (hypotonia), and marked weakness of all voluntary muscles. The parents may observe the latter as poverty of movement, or note the baby's floppiness when handled. If the breathing muscles are involved, a severe respiratory infection may be the first complaint. Examination confirms the infant's lack of movement and the hypotonia—which allows the limbs to be placed in bizarre positions. Reflex movement is lost. The weakness of the intercostal muscles leads to the chest becoming square in shape. Since diaphragmatic power at first is preserved, rib retraction and Harrison's groove formation is usual. The muscles supplied by the cranial nerves are less affected in the early stages, but weakness of the tongue, with difficulty in sucking and swallowing eventually appear. An important sign of anterior horn cell disease is muscular fibrillation (fasciculation). This causes irregular muscle contractions, best seen in the tongue. An *electromyogram* can be used to record fibrillation in the other muscles.

These children do not survive long, death usually following chest infection or massive lung collapse. Both complications are due to the baby's inability to cough.

Treatment. This is confined to vigorous treatment of chest infection, and tube feeding if the infant cannot swallow.

Chronic generalized spinal muscular atrophy

This is a much less severe form, which does not present until some time between the ages of 6 months and 2 years. The main complaint is of delayed motor development. Thus, the infant seldom learns to hold his head up, sit unsupported, or to roll over, and never crawls, stands, or walks. Chest infections, however, are well tolerated, and the infant survives, albeit with eventual scoliosis, joint contractures and other orthopedic deformities. Many victims live until the early teens.

Treatment. Physiotherapy is given to prevent joint contractures and to prevent and treat respiratory infections. As in all chronic diseases, the parents require help in accepting the implications of the disease, and in getting rid of their guilty feelings.

Another variety of the chronic form of spinal muscular atrophy has its onset in the preschool period, is much slower in its progression, and affects the muscles of the lower leg, feet, arms, and hands. Respiratory problems do not occur. Deformities should be prevented by physiotherapy.

General differential diagnosis of spinal muscular atrophy

This is most relevant in these patients who have an early onset of symptoms. In them, other causes of flaccidity must be considered, mainly cerebral palsy with hypotonia. Such patients do not show fibrillation of the tongue, and usually have definite U.M.N. signs. Hypotonia occurs also in idiopathic hypercalcemia, Tay-Sachs disease and Präder-Willi syndrome (obesity, mental retardation, and hypotonia). In none is muscular weakness so marked as in spinal muscular atrophy, and in none is muscle fibrillation present. Each also has particular features (see individual disease descriptions) which facilitates diagnosis.

Other disorders involving the spinal anterior horn cells

These are excessively rare: *progressive muscular atrophy* and *amyotrophic lateral sclerosis* occur as familial disorders. The clinical features are of weakness of the hands, forearms, and shoulders together with difficulty in walking. The latter is due to disease of the corticospinal (pyramidal) tract. The muscles supplied by cranial nerves 9, 10, and 11 also become involved, causing a lower motor neurone paralysis of speech and swallowing.

The upper limb muscles show wasting and fibrillation, the lower limbs are spastic, and the plantar responses are extensor. Ultimately a spastic paraplegia may be present.

No specific treatment exists for these conditions. Physiotherapy is useful in maintaining function and preventing joint contracture.

Anterior poliomyelitis

This previously common disorder of the anterior horn cell is discussed elsewhere (p. 468).

Disorders of the motor cranial nerves

General. These can be affected in diseases of the corticospinal tract, more commonly, however, they occur in children as lower motor neurone disorders, e.g., in spinal muscular atrophy (Werdnig-Hoffmann disease), poliomyelitis, or Guillain-Barré syndrome (see below), and in the late stages of the cerebral degenerative states. Temporary paralysis is usually due to a disorder at the neuromuscular junction, as in diphtheria, myasthenia gravis, and after poisoning with organophosphorus insecticides, botulism, and snake or insect bite.

Some specific disorders

Abnormalities of eye movement

The eye muscles are supplied by the 3rd, 4th, and 6th cranial nerves and act together to give smooth eye movements. Symmetric movements of both eyes (as in looking sideways) are called conjugate movements, and can occur in the vertical and horizontal planes. These are complex actions and are coordinated generally by pathways in the midbrain and internal capsule as well as by connections between the individual nerve nuclei; thus we can coordinate head and eye movement in many situations, e.g., when turning and looking at a source of sound.

Disorders of conjugate movement

Repeated forced conjugate movements (in any plane) occur in grand mal epilepsy, and in encephalitis and the cerebral degenerative disorders (leucodystrophies).

A fixed conjugate deviation may occur in acute hemiplegia, the direction of gaze being away from the side on which the disease is present. Forced conjugate deviation upwards (oculogyric crisis) in children is most often due to poisoning by the phenothiazine tranquillizers. It may occasionally be found in disorders involving the extrapyramidal tracts.

Convergence occurs when we focus upon an object, and involves conjugate adjustment of the eyes towards the midline (adduction). Paralysis of convergence is common after head injury, and occurs occasionally in disease of the midbrain and extrapyramidal system.

Paralysis of the eye muscles

3rd nerve disorder

This causes paralysis of the superior rectus, inferior rectus, internal rectus, and inferior oblique muscles of the eye. The unopposed lateral rectus muscle causes an outward squint, and the other eye movements are lost. The patient then sees 2 images (diplopia), and he cannot accommodate (shift his focus from a near to a distant object). The pupil of the affected eye is dilated because of interruption to the nerve supply of the iris, the muscle which controls pupil size.

4th nerve disorder

This paralyzes the superior oblique muscle, so that the child cannot properly look in the downwards and outwards direction. Diplopia also occurs.

6th nerve disorder

This paralyzes the external rectus muscle (which moves the eyeball in the lateral direction), so that the eye squints towards the nose. Double vision is also present.

Combined paralysis of the 3rd, 4th, and 6th nerves

In this situation all eye movements are lost. Permanent paralysis occurs when there is greatly increased intracranial pressure as in brain tumour or unrelieved hydrocephalus. Temporary paralysis is most often due to poisoning of some sort.

7th nerve paralysis: facial palsy

Causes. In the newborn, the nerve may be injured by the pressure of obstetric forceps. Occasionally the facial nerve nucleus is congenitally absent, causing a permanent lesion. In older children the nerve may be secondarily affected by mastoid infections as it courses through the skull. Bell's palsy is of unknown cause, but may represent a response to infection. Poliomyelitis is now a rare cause.

Clinical features. The affected side of the face is immobile, and this lack of movement is readily seen when crying occurs in the newborn. The eye cannot close fully, and sucking may be impaired because of the weakness of the muscles around the mouth.

In *Bell's palsy* the onset is sudden, often with pain, stiffness and numbness of the face, together with watering of the eye. Speech and mastication may also be interfered with. If the chorda tympani nerve (a branch of the facial) is also involved there is loss of taste sense in the forward two-thirds of the tongue.

Investigations. Electrophysiological studies should be done if paralysis continues for more than 5 days. The facial nerve is stimulated electrically. If a muscular twitch occurs with the normal latent period, then full recovery is usual. If no response occurs, then recovery is slow and often incomplete.

Treatment. The eye is protected, and simple massage given to the face. This is usually all that is necessary in the forceps paralysis of the newborn, and most cases of Bell's palsy. If, in the latter, nerve conduction is greatly impaired, then injections of A.C.T.H. or surgical decompression of the nerve within the facial canal should be considered.

Prognosis. Complete recovery is usual; rarely, the paralysis persists causing contracture of the facial muscle, distortion of the face, and permanent difficulties with speech and chewing.

Facial diplegia (Möbius' syndrome)

This is due to congenital absence of both 7th nerve nuclei. The face of the newborn is completely immobile, and neither eye can be closed properly. Sucking is difficult, but swallowing is normal. No treatment is possible except later plastic surgery for cosmetic reasons.

Paralysis of the 10th cranial nerve

This is a serious and life threatening disorder. Saliva cannot be swallowed, and, with food and vomit can easily enter the air passages. Thus serious respiratory infections are common, and, at worst, suffocation from tracheal blocking can occur. Additionally, since swallowing may be impossible, hydration and nutrition can be maintained only by tube feeding.

Causes. In the newborn, the condition may follow anoxia, prolonged hypoglycemia or be the earliest symptom of cerebral palsy. In older children, the cause may be anterior horn cell disease (as in amyotonia congenita), or follow poliomyelitis or tumour of the posterior fossa.

Clinical features. In the newborn, the first few sucks are followed by coughing, choking, and return of the feed. Drooling of saliva is not a great problem, but intermittent respiratory difficulty is common.

In older children, the first sign of trouble is often a change in the voice, which may become weak or nasal (the latter due to paralysis of the palate). Dribbling of saliva and difficulty in swallowing are present, and coughing is ineffective although explosive. Obvious respiratory difficulty—tachypnea and rib retraction soon follow, often with evidence of anoxia—restlessness, anxiety, and tachycardia. X-rays commonly show areas of lung collapse. If the obstruction is not relieved, dyspnea increases, cyanosis sets in, and death occurs from asphyxia. Weight loss and dehydration accompany the loss of saliva and inability to swallow.

Treatment. The principles are to drain the secretions, keep the airway open, and prevent dehydration and starvation. Turning the patient face down will allow the saliva to trickle out, and regular deep suction will remove secretions in the pharynx. If this is insufficient, an endotracheal tube is passed. This clears the airway and prevents secretions entering the lung. Food and fluid intake may be assured by passing a nasogastric tube. Feeds should be given frequently and in small quantities to reduce the risk of regurgitation.

The muscles of respiration may also be involved in conditions causing 10th cranial nerve paralysis (e.g., poliomyelitis, Guillain-Barré syndrome). Accordingly facilities for aided respiration should be available.

MOTOR DISORDERS OF THE PERIPHERAL NERVES

General remarks. These are occasionally noted in children. The causes of peripheral neuritis are many, varying from a probable viral infection (Guillain-Barré syndrome), to the toxin of diphtheria, or occurring as a rare complication of severe scarlatina, dysentery, or salmonella infection. Poisoning by lead, mercury, or arsenic may be the cause, and, in underdeveloped countries, beriberi (lack of aneurin) may be relevant.

General clinical features. These are rather similar, whatever the cause of the disease. Weakness and clumsiness of leg movement is a common early complaint, sometimes associated with feelings of numbness or tingling. Complete paralysis follows and the process may spread to involve the trunk, upper limbs, and cranial nerves.

The muscles supplied by the diseased nerves are tender, soon waste and lose their reflexes. Lack of sensation may also be present. Fasciculation or fibrillation are not seen in the muscle, and changes in electrical nerve condition tests are not constant. Spontaneous recovery from neuritis is usual, the main problems being related to treating respiratory paralysis, or the difficulty of swallowing due to 10th nerve involvement.

Specific entities

Guillain-Barré syndrome

This disease is characterized by a symmetrical, usually ascending, motor paralysis, with a variable degree of sensory disturbance. Its cause is unknown, although a virus is suspected.

Clinical features. The disease occurs in children between the ages of 3 and 10 years, and may begin with a mild respiratory infection. Clumsiness and difficulty in walking then set in, often with complaints of pain in the muscles. Weakness then spreads to the trunk, arms, muscles of swallowing and those of facial expression. Respiratory muscle weakness is common and may be severe. The full picture is of a flaccid symmetrical weakness, with muscle tenderness and impairment of vibration and positional sensory ability. The spinal fluid is normal apart from an increase in the protein content.

Diagnosis. This is mainly from poisoning by organophosphorus insecticide, in which a history of exposure is available, or from poliomyelitis in which the paralysis is patchy, and the spinal fluid contains many lymphocytes.

Treatment. If the respiratory muscles and swallowing mechanisms are impaired, then aided respiration and endotracheal intubation are necessary to prevent asphyxia and keep the airway clear of secretions. In the milder cases, splinting of the limbs in the portion of function, and physiotherapy are the main treatments.

Progress. Most patients, even the most severely affected, will ultimately recover, although full function may not return for many months.

Other forms of polyneuritis include those due to *diphtheria toxin*, or poisoning by *heavy metals*. Each follows the primary disease. In the diphtheritic type the cranial nerves are first affected, causing paralysis of the palate and eye muscles. Occasionally the 10th nerve is also affected. Further spread is rare, and full recovery is usual. In *heavy metal* poisoning there is a history of exposure, and for lead, generally a primary complaint of encephalopathy with focal neurological signs and papilledema. In arsenical and mercury poisoning vomiting, diarrhea and kidney disease are primary. In all varieties the clinical features of the polyneuritis are those already described.

THE NEUROMUSCULAR JUNCTION

Diseases of the neuromuscular junction are essentially aberrations of the neurotransmitter mechanism. In most instances the disease is intermittent, as in myasthenia gravis. Neurotransmitter interfering agents are used in anesthesia, e.g., succinylcholine, curare derivatives, and paralyze only motor function, without causing sensory loss.

A large variety of toxins can cause disease at this level, e.g., botulinus toxin, organophosphorus insecticide, certain snake and insect venoms, especially the scrub tick (*Ixodes holocyclus*).

Specific entities

Myasthenia gravis

This is a rare disorder. It can present in the infant of the mother with myasthenia, or begin of itself in middle childhood.

Myasthenia neonatorum

The mother has the disease. At birth the baby is noted to have paralysis of the eye and facial muscles, and may have difficulty in sucking and swallowing. Generalized weakness is common, but the baby can breathe effectively. All of the symptoms are relieved by giving neostigmine methylsulphate, which maintains the acetylcholine level at the neuromuscular junction.

Juvenile myasthenia

This usually begins after the second year of life with bulbar symptoms. The first sign is drooping of the eyelids (ptosis) with facial weakness. Difficulty in speaking and swallowing follow. Involvement of the limb and respiratory muscles is late and unusual. Characteristically, all of these symptoms wax and wane, and interference with every day activities is not great. The diagnosis is established by improvement with neostigmine methylsulphate.

Treatment. The acute disorder is treated by injections of neostigmine methylsulphate; then pyridostigmine bromide is substituted by mouth, in a dose large enough and frequent enough to relieve the symptoms.

Disorders due to low potassium levels

Familial periodic paralysis

This rare disorder of the neuromuscular junction causes intermittent transient weakness of the legs, which spreads to involve the trunk and arms, but is never so severe as to affect breathing. The serum potassium is low. The paralysis varies in duration, sometimes lasting several days.

Treatment. Extra potassium salts are given by mouth.

THE SENSORY SYSTEM

Since sensory impulse originates in the peripheral parts of the body, and travel to the sensory cortex of the brain, disorders of this system will be considered in the same way.

The peripheral nerve

Sensory loss usually is associated with loss of motor power, and often with disorders of the autonomic supply. The latter leads to changes in skin colour and coldness of the part. The commonest cause is peripheral neuritis as already described. Conditions which cause pressure on the nerve give rise to paresthesia (a sensation of tingling), or a burning feeling—both in the distribution of the affected nerve. Permanent loss of sensation leads to injury of the anesthetised part, which infects easily, and may ultimately cause much mutilation. This is what occurs in leprosy when there is extensive loss of sensation.

The posterior roots

These are close to the spinal cord, and receive sensory impulses from the peripheral nerves. They may be affected by leprosy, syphilis (as in taboparesis), or be compressed by tumours. Older children will complain of pain in the segment of the body from which the sensory impulses come. At first sensation in that area is perceived more acutely—as are painful stimuli. This acuteness of sensation is called *hyperesthesia* and of pain *hyperalgesia*. Loss of all forms of sensation soon follows, however.

Herpes zoster

This is a viral infection affecting the posterior roots. The first symptoms are itching and pain in the area of skin whose sensory supply is affected. Then a rash develops—small pimples which develop into vesicles and then heal, crust, and scar, leaving an area of anesthesia. This condition is a minor one unless the eye is involved, when the infection may lead to corneal scarring and visual difficulties.

The spinal sensory tracts

These receive impulses from the posterior root, and take up 2 main forms. These are the *dorsal* columns, which transmit information about the position of the limbs and muscles, together with superficial sensation, and the *ventrolateral* columns, which carry pain and temperature information. Obviously these tracts will be damaged in spinal cord interruption, as in meningomyelocele or after spinal injury. Tumours within, or pressing upon the spinal cord, will also involve the spinal sensory tracts. Degeneration of the dorsal column may occur also in congenital syphilis (taboparesis), Friedreich's ataxia, and the congenital spastic paraplegics.

Symptomatology. The main symptom is clumsiness in walking because of the loss of positional sense. Some children may note numbness of the feet or other parts and, if the ventrolateral columns are involved, there is inability to perceive pain and temperature stimuli. Testing of the various tracts is difficult except in the older child, and related mainly to postural sensibility. A typical test of the latter is the heel-toe test in which the child, with his eyes closed. is asked to place his right foot on his left knee and pass it smoothly down to his left toes. If his positional sense is disturbed he cannot do so.

The sensory cranial nerves

The 1st, 2nd, and 8th cranial nerves are those of the special senses of smell, vision, and hearing and will be considered separately. 5, 9, and 10 have a substantial sensory function and will now be considered.

The 5th (trigeminal) nerve

This nerve receives sensation from the head, face, and part of the neck and eyes. The major peripheral nerves are the mandibular (lower face and neck), maxillary (upper face, part of head), and ophthalmic (eye, brow, and part of head). Each of these must enter the skull to form a common sensory root which enters a large relay area (the trigeminal or Gasserian ganglion) and then enters a long sensory nucleus which traverses the brain stem from the pons to the spinal cord.

With such a course, the 5th cranial nerve can be affected in many disorders within and without the skull. Thus the sensory nucleus may be involved in tumours or vascular disorders of the pons, medulla, and upper spinal cord. The first (ophthalmic) division runs in the wall of the cavernous sinus and will be affected by infections or thrombosis of that area. All 3 divisions may be involved in disease of the posterior fossa of the skull which affects the trigeminal ganglion.

Ophthalmic division signs

The eye, brow, and top of the skull and nose are anesthetic. The cornea readily becomes infected (keratitis) and visual loss may follow.

Maxillary division

The upper face, upper lip, upper teeth, roof of the mouth, and lower nose lose sensation.

Mandibular division

There is loss of sensation in the lower teeth, side of the cheek, lower lip and chin, and front part of the tongue.

Trigeminal neuralgia (tic douloureux)

This is rare in children. It occurs as paroxysms of pain in one or more of the divisions of the trigeminal nerve. There is no loss of sensation during or after the attack.

Herpes virus may also involve the trigeminal nerve distribution, but is of importance only as it affects corneal sensation.

The 9th (glossopharyngeal) nerve

Disorders of this is usually associated with those of the 10th nerve. The 9th nerve supplies sensory and taste fibres to the posterior third of the tongue, the tonsils, and pharynx, and disease or damage, while unusual in children, will give rise to anesthesia in the above areas often combined with some difficulty in swallowing.

The 10th (vagus) nerve

This gives sensation to the larynx, and a branch from its jugular ganglion supplies the back of the ear and part of the external meatus. Lesions of this nerve are rare in children, but anesthesia of the larynx will cause choking, and difficulty in clearing the secretions.

THE SPECIAL SENSES

Smell

The sense of smell (olfaction) also allows us to sense flavour as opposed to taste. The nerves traverse the cribriform plate of the skull and reach the olfactory bulb; from there fibres reach the olfactory tract whence they are relayed to the olfactory areas of the posterior cerebral cortex. Disturbances of the sense of smell can only be discovered in the older cooperative child, and are tested by exposing him to odours such as peppermint, cloves, and so on. Loss of the olfactory sense (anosmia) occurs after head injury, especially when it involves the anterior fossa, but may occasionally be due to tumour of the olfactory tract. Meningitis may cause anosmia. A few children suffer from a congenital type of anosmia.

Olfactory hallucinations (usually with apparent foul odours), occur in lesions of the uncinate gyrus; in uncinate fits (rare in children), the mouth also twitches and loss of consciousness occurs.

Vision

Visual impressions reach the retina, those of the left field of vision being received by the opposite (right) retina. The impulses then run in the optic nerves to enter the skull and the part of the visual tract called the chiasma. In the latter cross occurs, so that impulses from the nasal half of each retina cross to run in the opposite optic tract, which terminates mainly in the lateral corpus quadrigeminum in the midbrain. Fibres also run to the adjacent superior geniculate body. From the corpus quadrigeminum the visual path enters the posterior limb of the internal capsule then spreads out to form the optic radiation which terminates in the visual cortex of the occipital lobe of the brain. From there, association fibres run to the sensory and motor cortex of the five-brain.

Disorders of the visual pathway (see figure 52)

These are numerous because of the long and complex route to the visual cortex. The *retina* may be affected by *optic atrophy* (degeneration of the retinal nerve cells). Most often this is secondary to some other disease, e.g., anoxia, hypoglycemia or kernicterus at birth, or raised intracranial pressure. Optic atrophy may be isolated, primary, and familial as in Leber's optic atrophy. It also is a part of the degenerative disease of the central nervous system such as the leucodystrophies in which the white matter of the nervous system is affected. Primary inflammation (optic neuritis) is rare in children, but may follow syphilis, meningo-encephalitis or lead poisoning. Optic atrophy may follow optic neuritis.

Clinical features. In infancy, optic atrophy often commences with other evidence of severe motor disorder—the baby has cerebral palsy. The child is more or less blind, so he does not respond to visual cues. Irregular, searching eye movements are common if vision is affected on both sides, and constant knuckling of the eyes is a usual finding.

The older child will complain of blindness. At first there is a central area of loss of vision (a scotoma). This extends outwards in the field of vision until blindness is complete. The ophthalmoscope is used to examine the retina. In optic atrophy, the pinkish disc becomes paler until it may become quite white. In optic neuritis the disc is swollen and the adjacent retina shows exudates and abnormality of the retinal blood vessels.

Treatment. None is possible once vision has been lost. If the condition is thought to be progressive, and if the child is of normal intelligence, Braille reading and the other skills needed for a blind child should be taught while some sight remains.

Disorders at the chiasma

The commonest cause of visual loss in the area is pressure by a tumour in the region of the pituitary gland. The result is a loss of the half-field which scans the temporal part of the visual field. This is called a bitemporal hemianopia. The defect can be marked in detail in older, cooperative children by using a technique called perimetry. This tests the vision in each quadrant of vision of the separate eyes.

The optic tracts

As figure 52 shows, these transmit impulses from the homonymous (same-sided) temporal field, and also from the opposite nasal field. This will cause a crossed homonymous field defect, i.e., if the right optic tract is damaged, there is visual loss in both left half-fields, i.e., the right nasal field, and the left temporal field. Incomplete loss is usual in the early stages so that at first only one quarter of the field is affected (quadrantic loss). Spontaneous complaint of field loss is found only in older children, in the others it must be deduced by failure to respond to visual stimuli in the appropriate half-fields of vision. The optic tracts may be involved by pituitary and other tumours at the brain base, and also in meningitis.

Disorders of the optic radiation and visual cortex

Complete interruption of either of these gives rise to a crossed homonymous hemianopia (see figure 52). In practice, however, the loss of vision is usually incomplete—upper quadrantic loss being usual, because in the radiation, the impulses from the lower retina (which scans the *upper* visual field) are more exposed to damage. In the visual cortex, central vision (impulses from all visual fields) are relatively more represented, so that a scotoma may be found. Again, visual loss can only be localized in older cooperative children.

Disorders of the visual associative areas

These cause visual *agnosia*—loss of the ability to recognize and name objects seen. A variant of this is alexia or dyslexia, in which the

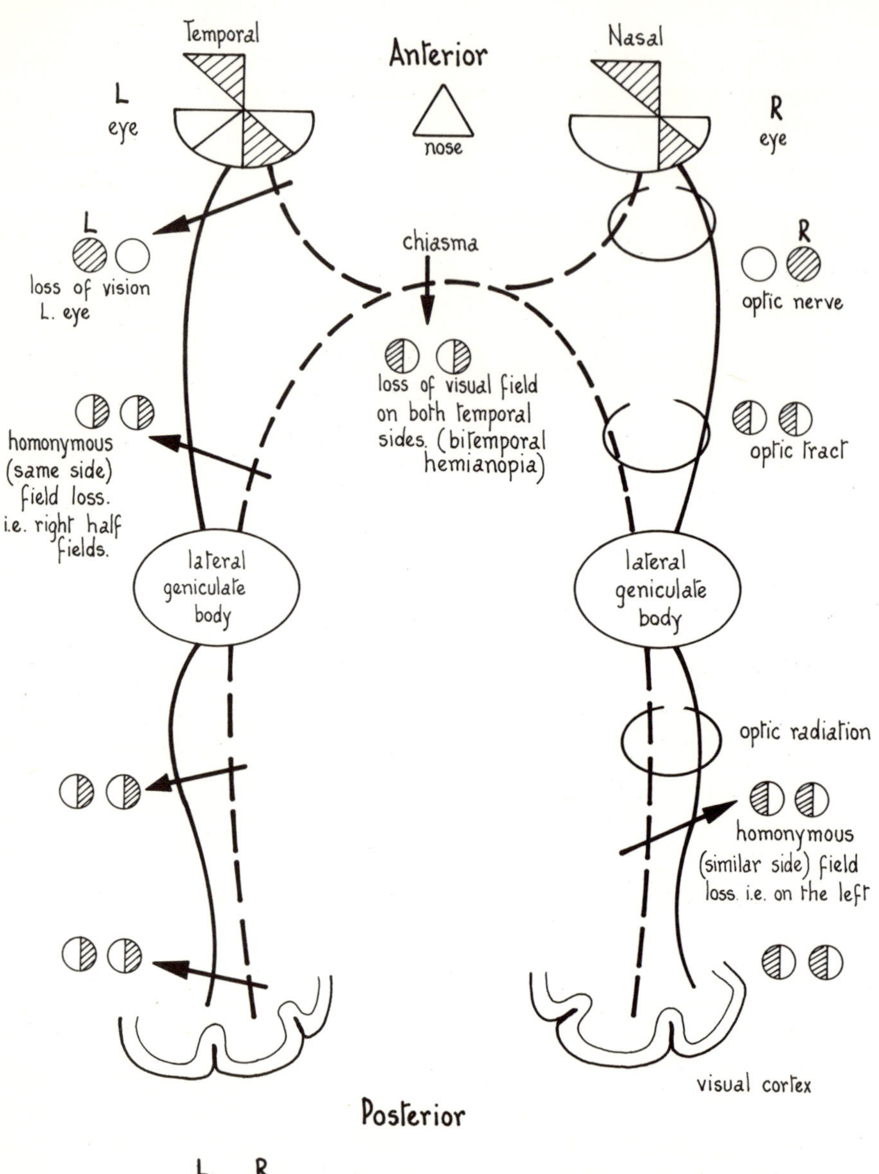

Fig. 52. Diagram of visual pathway, as seen from above. Effects of interruption of visual pathway at various levels.

significance of written symbols is lost to the child. This condition is usually quite rare, although it is often used to explain poor school performance.

Hearing

Disorders of hearing and balance

These two are considered together since each has its origin in the ear and the associated 8th (acoustic) cranial nerve.

Sound is appreciated in the cochlea, and balance in the semicircular canals. The impulses from each stimulus run in the 8th nerve into the skull. The *vestibular* (balance) impulses terminate in the nuclei of the pons, and in the cerebellum, to which they run in the inferior peduncle. Connections are also established with eye muscle nuclei and with the cerebrum.

The *auditory* (hearing) impulses relay in the cochlear nuclei of the pons, and pass to the other side of the brain stem in their ascent to the nuclei known as the inferior colliculus and medial geniculate body; from there, relays are distributed to the cortical auditory areas in the temporal lobe of the brain.

Disorders of the auditory pathway

These may originate in the inner ear, e.g., otitis media. Such causes are considered elsewhere (p. 240). The *acoustic nerve* may be affected by a wide variety of diseases such as congenital rubella, kernicterus, meningitis, syphilis, and drugs such as streptomycin, salicylates, and quinine. Congenital nerve deafness and tumour of the 8th nerve are other possible causes.

Symptoms. If the child is partially deaf, the deficiency may not be noted until he goes to school and is obviously inattentive or fails to understand. In the more complete types of deafness, of early onset, the infant fails to respond to verbal cues, and speech may not progress beyond the babbling stage. In intermediate degrees of deafness, inattentiveness is common, and speech is slowly acquired and usually imperfect. The voice may be monotonous and metallic in quality. The degree of hearing loss is measured by an *audiogram* which is obtained by observing the child's response to carefully measured amounts of sound which span the frequencies which the human ear can appreciate. Loss of midfrequency hearing is clinically of greater importance, since this is the range used in speech.

Treatment. This should begin as early as possible. Hearing aids should be used if indicated. Otherwise the child is taught lip reading, and his own speech development carefully maintained by special techniques, e.g., using his sense of touch to aid education in articulation and pronunciation.

Disorders of the auditory cortex

Hearing has strong bilateral representation in the auditory cortex, so central deafness can only occur if both temporal lobes are extensively damaged. Lesions of the *auditory associative area* (which connects with the sensory cortex and speech areas) may cause *auditory agnosia*; that is, the patient can hear, but cannot interpret what is said. It is as if he is spoken to in a foreign language. There is a response to noise, but the patient cannot follow any instructions. In the congenital type, the child does not learn normal speech, since he cannot learn to associate sounds with objects or ideas. Thus he speaks in his own language, as jargon or in unusual words representing objects or ideas (neologisms). In acquired auditory agnosia (usually the result of head injury), speech is retained, but verbal cuing is absent. No specific treatment is possible. The patient is trained to compensate for his defect by using visual cues, e.g., written instruction.

Vestibular disorders

The commonest disorder affecting children is motion sickness. This expresses itself most commonly as car sickness, but many children will develop symptoms with such simple activities as swinging. The condition seldom persists into adult life except perhaps in those who suffer from mal de mer.

Acute labyrinthitis usually follows infections of the middle ear, mastoids, or the meninges. The symptoms consist in vomiting, vertigo, deafness, and fever. Spontaneous rotary and horizontal nystagmus is present, with the slow phase directed towards the affected side. (Nystagmus is flicking of both eyeballs in the same direction).

Congenital absence of the labyrinths is rare, and gives rise to deafness. Disorders of the vestibule and its connections are sometimes seen in brain damaged children (e.g., following meningitis), and causes lack of coordination between head and eye movements, as well as truncal incoordination. Commonly, however, these vestibular disorders are overshadowed by the other neurological defects found in cerebral palsy.

Vestibular function may also be disturbed by drugs; streptomycin was formerly the commonest cause, but acute disturbances may be associated with overdosage with kanamycin and neomycin. Some patients overdosed with tranquilizers, phenobarbitone, or Dilantin, may show abnormalities of balance.

Lesions of the subcortical sensory tracts

These may follow trauma or be a complication of tumour. Lesions in the medulla are associated with contralateral sensory loss in the trunk and limbs; homolateral loss of sensation occurs in the face and occasionally in the mouth. Deep lesions cause sensory loss of the type characteristic of dorsal column function. Lateral lesions may cause loss of pain and temperature alone. Higher lesions in the pons, may cause contralateral loss of all forms of sensation and thalamic disease has the same effect.

Other disorders of the central sensory tracts

As has been described, all of the sensory impulses from the body gather together in the brain stem (medulla, pons, midbrain) and run upwards to relay in the thalamus on their way to the sensory cortex in the prefrontal area of the brain. Since the sensory and motor tracts are closely related, both may be involved in diseases of the areas mentioned (see figure 51).

Medullary lesions cause loss of sensation in the opposite trunk and limbs, with sensory loss in the face and mouth on the same side. Disease deep in the medulla gives a picture similar to that of disorder of the posterior columns of the spinal cord.

Disorders high in the *pons* or in the *thalamus* may cause loss of all form of sensation on the opposite side of the body. Disorders of the *sensory cortex* usually follow head injury, anoxia, or degenerative disorder; associated motor defects are common. Specific sensory deficits are patchy, and affect mainly the appreciation of positive and passive movement, light touch, and the ability accurately to localize. Size, shape, and form are poorly interpreted in sensory cortex disorders, but tests for these are useful only in the older child. Once such a deficit is established, nothing can be done to ensure a return of function.

THE COORDINATING AND MODULATING APPARATUS

The cerebellum and its connections

The cerebellum is concerned in maintaining normal posture, muscle tone, and in coordinating limb, trunk, head, and eye movements.

Diseases of the cerebellum

General clinical features. In infancy, the first signs are seen when rolling over is tried. Then it is seen that the head, trunk, and limb movements are incoordinate. Later there is difficulty in sitting up, with failure of the head to respond to trunk position and vice versa. Standing becomes possible only with support, and walking is impossible without parental help, since the trunk and head sway out of kilter with the limbs. The whole process of incoordination is called *ataxia*. Deliberate movements are clumsy, and the hand may overshoot when trying to pick up something. This difficulty in approximating a desired position from rest is called past pointing. Lack of vestibular information to the head/eye coordinating process is confirmed by the presence of *nystagmus* (regularly repeating flicking of the eyeball to one side). The voice is monotonous, and articulation jerky and explosive. The muscles are hypotonic, but true muscular weakness is absent.

If the child has learned to walk normally and then develops a cerebellar disorder, the main symptom is ataxia, with difficulty in walking except on a wide rolling base, with the eyes fixed downward to help him compensate. Tremor, and past pointing occur when he tries to pick up objects, and nystagmus and voice change is common.

Etiology of cerebellar disorders

The commonest cause is drugs, mainly phenobarbitone, Dilantin, antidepressants, antihistamines, and alcohol (as sweet fortified wines). In these the history is diagnostic. Other causes include the following.

Congenital cerebellar ataxia

The child is asymptomatic until he is due to stand and walk. Then the signs of cerebellar defect appear, especially affecting gait and voice.

Acute cerebellar ataxia

This occurs in the preschool child. Frequently no specific cause is found, but it can follow chicken pox, measles, or coxsackie viral infection. The signs are as described above, with refusal to walk, because the child knows he is likely to fall. Recovery is rapid and spontaneous.

Friedreich's ataxia

This is a familial degeneration of the spinocerebellar, corticospinal tracts, and of the posterior columns. The mode of transmission is dubious. The disease affects either sex.

Clinical features. The onset is insidious, and the first symptoms are often realized only in retrospect; in a few instances, the child is slow to walk, and clumsy in his movements, developing a typical staggering gait. He may have great difficulty in feeding himself because of his clumsiness with eating utensils. The same difficulty inhibits him from learning to write at school. These are phenomena of upper limb ataxia. The cerebellar control of the voice is lost, so that dysarthria, with explosive irregular speech occur. This difficulty may progress until nothing can be understood by the hearers.

In most instances, things progress more slowly and the difficulties described become obvious only in later childhood. At this stage, bulbar disturbances may occur, and nystagmus is often present. Later, deformities occur, which involve the spine (scoliosis) and the feet (pes cavus). Muscular hypotonia is followed by muscular weakness, and irregular choreiform movements occur.

Signs. Apart from the functional disturbances described, objective examination confirms the more specific signs of cerebellar disturbance. Thus, there is a wide-based gait, and Rombergism; ataxia is less marked in the arms, although the finger-nose test is usually positive. Degeneration of the posterior columns is evidenced by lack of position sense in the legs. The knee jerks are soon lost, as eventually are the upper limb reflexes. The plantar response becomes extensor, reflecting some pyramidal tract involvement.

Progress. In most instances the deformities progress, with increasing difficulty in walking. Eventually the patient is bedridden, cannot speak, becomes demented, incontinent and sometimes blind from optic atrophy. In a few children the disease stops spontaneously.

The electrocardiogram shows flattening of inversion of the T waves, implying involvement of the myocardium, but actual cardiac failure is rare.

Differential diagnosis. In the younger child, cerebral palsy may require consideration, as may Hartnup disease (see p. 292); usually, however, the difficulties in walking require that muscular dystrophy also be excluded.

Otherwise, the principal problems are other cerebellar conditions; thus acute cerebellitis has a relatively short course, and cerebellar tumour has vomiting and papilledema. The difference between Friedreich's ataxia and *Behr's* syndrome is largely academic. In the latter, spasticity and optic atrophy are early associations of the ataxia, and there is early and severe bulbar involvement.

Familial *cerebellar degeneration* is recognizable by the history, and the strong association with intellectual retardation. More common perhaps is *ataxia-telangiectasia* (Louis-Bar syndrome) in which conjunctival and facial telangiectasia coexist with progressive intellectual detioration and immunoglobulin (IgA) deficiency.

In *acanthyocytosis* (abetalipoproteinemia), the child has a history of intestinal malabsorption akin to celiac disease, and after some years, ataxia and tremor appear, sometimes with involuntary movements of an extrapyramidal type. The beta-lipoproteins are absent, cholesterol is low, and the red cells have characteristic spiny projections.

Treatment. No specific curative measures are known; general supportive care is in order.

THE BASAL GANGLIA AND EXTRAPYRAMIDAL TRACTS

Disorders of these seldom exist in children as pure entities. The symptomatology (involuntary movements, altered muscle tone), tends to shade in with disease processes involving the pyramidal tracts or the cerebellum and its connections.

Basal ganglia disorders can complicate such acquired diseases as kernicterus, or neonatal viral infections such as rubella. They may follow prolonged neonatal hypoglycemia or anoxia. At an early age head injury, and the aftermath of severe meningoencephalitis, or abnormal degenerative conditions, may cause extrapyramidal symptoms.

Acute and transient extrapyramidal disorders are usually the result of poisoning by tricyclic antidepressants (e.g., fluphenazine), or antihistaminics.

General features of extrapyramidal disease

These are abnormal involuntary movements which are usually defined as *choreiform* or *athetotic*; both types may occur in the same patient, together with muscular rigidity. Such abnormalities are not recognizable much before the sixth month of age. Recognition may further be delayed if pyramidal tract disease (as in cerebral palsy), is also present. Characteristically, however, the symptom complex is superimposed upon a pattern of delayed motor milestones.

Athetosis

Most muscle groups are involved, the first involuntary movement noted is often facial grimacing, which is aggravated if the child is under pressure, as in clinical examination. There is much difficulty with swallowing, so choking and vomiting occur. Efforts at feeding may cause anticipatory facial grimacing. The mother also notes that the child may assume curious postures, and that the muscles at times feel rigid. As motor activity advances, coarse involuntary movements appear in the arms and legs, especially when the child attempts to make a purposive movement. Twisting and extension movements of the trunk appear when the child is learning to stand and to walk. Comprehensible speech is often never attained, although the child may be observed to attempt speech movements in the appropriate situation.

If the child learns to walk a little, or to stand with some competence, certain postures are characteristic. Thus, the head is angled to one or other side, often with a forced repetitive movement. The trunk tends to be extended on the pelvis, the arms are abducted, with flexed elbows and wrists, and hyperextended fingers. The feet are plantar flexed and turned in, with extended toes. The whole appearance is somewhat reminiscent of the gait of a higher primate. All of the involuntary movements cease during sleep but can be exaggerated by voluntary effort or excitement. The tone of the various muscle groups continually varies between rigidity, normal tone, and flaccidity. Accordingly, poverty of functional movement is characteristic, the range of movement is limited, and all voluntary efforts are clumsy.

Choreiform movements

These are much less common than athetosis, with which, however, they may coexist. In general, the movements are relatively fine, impede voluntary effort far less, and, as in athetosis, are exaggerated by psychic pressure but disappear during sleep. Unusual facial movement may be the first sign, although these partake more of exaggeration of normal facial expression than the gross movements of athetosis. The child can usually walk, as his legs are less involved than the arms, and the trunk is usually spared. The muscles tend to be hypotonic rather than rigid. Speech and swallowing are reasonably normal, although feeding may be difficult because of interference with fine hand movement.

Some specific disorders

Kernicterus

This condition is due to the deposition of bile salts in the basal ganglia. This can occur only in the neonate, especially the dysmature, and follows untreated hemolytic disease.

Clinical features. The features of erythroblastosis fetalis (q.v.) are present. In affected babies, after the 48th hour of life, central nervous system symptoms appear. In the most severely affected, pallor, refusal to feed, convulsions, and rigidity, are quickly followed by death. In other children, the same symptoms are followed by an opisthotonic (arched back) posture, poverty of movement, and convulsions. A few of these children may survive to show extrapyramidal involuntary movements.

In many children no neurological signs are seen in the perinatal period, but the infant fails to thrive, attains the motor milestones slowly, and develops abnormal movements and muscle tonus. Mental retardation is often present, and may be associated with a small head circumference. Deafness is also a frequent concomitant.

Differential diagnosis. This is seldom difficult if a hemolytic situation exists. This is usually consequent to Rh and ABO incompatibility, or neonatal viral infections.

Treatment. Exchange transfusion is carried out repeatedly if need be, to keep the bilirubin level low. No other treatment is of value.

Dystonia musculorum deformans

This condition begins about the tenth year, may be familial, and has no particular sex predilection.

Clinical features. The lower limbs are first affected, with an unusual posturing of the legs, first one and then the other. The foot is first affected, being held in extension, with toe flexion. Pes cavus (high arch) then develops, followed by flexion and adduction of the thigh, and flexion at the knee. Eventually the child can walk with difficulty only on tiptoe and he compensates this by a severe lordosis. The arms are involved later, with elbow extension, wrist flexion, and internal rotation and adduction at the shoulder joint. Sooner or later the child develops severe torsion spasms, involving the trunk and limbs. These cause remarkable writhing movements, which are exaggerated by emotion or on attempting voluntary movement. As in other extrapyramidal disorders, they are abolished by sleep. The muscles are resistant to passive movement and tend to spring back to their previous positions. Ultimately the patient becomes unable to move and becomes bedridden, but the muscles of speech and swallowing are spared.

Treatment. Neurosurgical section of the basal gangliar connections may help in selected individuals. No other treatment is of value.

Wilson's disease (hepatolenticular degeneration)

This is a familial disease due to an abnormal mode of copper handling. This results in deposition of copper in the liver and in the basal ganglia. The condition is transmitted as an autosomal recessive.

Clinical features. These usually occur around puberty. The child may present with symptoms of hepatic cirrhosis (q.v.) The extrapyramidal symptoms consist in an increasing degree of tremor on voluntary movement, with impairment of walking and other movements. Speech becomes explosive and often limited. The child develops evidence of behaviour disorder, with emotional lability, and ultimately deterioration of intellectual function. The face may become mask-like, and drooling is common. Epilepsy is often found.

Copper deposition may be seen in the eyes (Descemet's membrane) by slit lamp microscopy. This is the so-called Keyser-Fleischer ring.

Biochemical investigations. The serum ceruloplasmin levels are low and urinary copper excretion is high. There is a general aminoaciduria.

Prognosis. The central nervous system lesion may remit for some time, and apparent spontaneous improvement has occurred. The hepatic component is largely untreatable, and cirrhosis the principal cause of death.

Treatment. Penicillamine may be of some value in reducing tissue copper content. This does not, however, guarantee a cure of the symptoms.

Huntington's chorea

This disease is dominantly transmissible and affects the frontal lobes as well as the extrapyramidal tracts.

Clinical features. The age at onset is variable, and progressive rigidity may be the first appreciable sign. This is associated with behaviour disorders, intellectual deterioration, and choreiform movements. Seizures are fairly common. Dementia is progressive and often associated with widespread bulbar palsies and uncontrollable involuntary movements.

Differential diagnosis. This is principally from hepatolenticular degeneration, in which the biochemical findings are characteristic. Other conditions causing dementia, such as late onset Schilder's disease will require consideration, although in such conditions, the characteristic family history of Huntington's chorea is absent.

Treatment. None is possible; the dementia usually requires that the patient be institutionalized.

Sydenham's chorea

This is discussed elsewhere (see p. 541).

Hereditary tremor

This condition, of unknown etiology, has a dominant transmission. It is not very unusual in children, and carries a good prognosis.

Clinical features. These appear between 5 and 10 years and at first one arm is affected by a fine tremor at rest and on movement. The symptoms progressively involve the other limbs. In the latter stage the condition is much worse. The signs are aggravated by emotion and embarrassment. The condition usually stabilizes in the second and third decade without affecting motor function.

THE AUTONOMIC SYSTEM

In children, most of the disorders of this system are secondary to some other disease process. Thus, the vascular phenomena in advanced muscular dystrophy, and destruction of peripheral nerves, is a relatively minor part of the primary disease process. So too is the disorder of sweating seen in leprosy. Many children develop autonomic disorders as part of poisoning by various drugs. Typical of these is the reaction to atropine (particularly common in Down's syndrome), in which fever, a red rash, delirium, and dilated pupils coexist. The reaction to the organophosphorus insecticides is described elsewhere. The anti-hypertensive drugs (rauwolfia derivatives, guanethidine, ganglion blockers) are unusual causes of juvenile poisoning although their effects should be anticipated in the baby of the mother treated for eclampsia.

Riley-Day syndrome

This condition is probably an autosomal recessive trait. It has been found most commonly in Jews, but occurs in other ethnic groups.

The onset is usually in the first 6 months of life, with difficulty in swallowing, excessive sweating, and failure to thrive and delayed motor milestones as the main complaints. Defective lacrimation may occur, as may transient blotchy rashes. The child shows poverty of movement and has the features of cerebral palsy, with hypotonia and impaired reflexes. Hypertension and hypotension, and failure of normal temperature regulation occur.

Treatment. Tube feeding is usually necessary and frequent suction is required to clear mucus.

Prognosis. The child generally develops a fatal respiratory infection.

Erythedema polyneuritica (pink disease)

This condition, nowadays of only sporadic occurrence, is due to chronic ingestion of mercury in teething powders.

Clinical features. The infant fails to thrive, becomes intensely anorexic and miserable and develops a red rash which is itchy. The skin of the hands and feet becomes moist, soggy, and cold, and the superficial layer may desquamate. Loss of finger and toenails is not unusual. Tachycardia and mild hypertension are common and photophobia a characteristic sign. Severe respiratory infection may occur.

Treatment. The source of mercury should be traced and excluded. Mercury excretion may be increased by the use of chelating agents such as B.A.L., although devoted general nursing care is the mainstay of treatment.

TOPICS RELATED TO CENTRAL NERVOUS SYSTEM DISEASE

These are introduced after the general review of nervous system disease because they are important in pediatrics, lend themselves to grouping, and encompass a wide variety of disorders under a single heading. Study of each topic will be facilitated by revision of the physiology of the nervous system as outlined previously.

Cerebral palsy

This is the name given to a collection of deficits of central nervous function which become apparent in the first months of life. Most of the major divisions of function can be affected (cerebrum, upper motor neurone, cerebellum, extrapyramidal tract, sensory system), but disorders of the upper motor neurone (corticospinal tracts) are usually the main problem. Slow progression is characteristic.

Causes. These are very varied. Before birth, viral infections (rubella, cytomegalovirus, etc.) and congenital absence of nervous tissue predominate. At birth, anoxia, hypoglycemia, kernicterus, and neonatal meningitis are common precedents. Soon after birth, the metabolic diseases (phenylketonuria and other aminoacidurias, the lipid storage diseases, and late onset hypoglycemias such as are found in the glycogen storage diseases) may all be causal. In later life severe head injury, meningoencephalitis and transient stoppage of cerebral circulation (asystole) as can occur in drowning are all relevant.

Clinical features. Clearly a very wide variety can exist, only the more common will be described.

1. In those infants who are severely affected early in life, the history is often of difficult resuscitation in a dysmature infant, who has obvious muscle flaccidity or twitching attacks in the first few days of life. Such babies have poverty of movement, are slow in learning to suck, and have difficulty in swallowing. All of these problems are out of proportion to the degree of dysmaturity if this has been a factor. The Moro reflex is incomplete, momentary weight-bearing may be absent, and persistent hypotonia is usual. Slowness in attaining the normal motor milestones is inevitable and failure of normal head growth is common.

2. In other babies the perinatal period is unremarkable, and progress is normal for a month or two, with good feeding ability, normal weight gain, and even the ability to smile at the usual time. Then the parents note poverty of movement of one or both sides of the body, undue floppiness (which reflects muscular hypotonia), or occasionally, a convulsion of the incomplete type known as a myoclonic jerk. Observant mothers may also note that the baby becomes very stiff, i.e., adopts an attitude of extension of all muscles—especially when he is cradled to be fed. These actions are called extensor spasms, and are common in babies who have widespread upper motor neurone disease. Sometimes the baby is regarded by parents as normal, but the physician notes failure of proper head growth, visual or hearing deficits, or slowness of the motor milestones.

The signs of nervous system disease in the first year of life are variable. Most of these children with cerebral palsy have upper motor neurone disease (single or double hemiplegia) as their main problem. The main signs are poverty of movement, together with muscular flaccidity, and failure to roll over, attain head control, or sit up. The Landau and protective (parachute) reflexes fail to appear. Sooner or later the muscular flaccidity is replaced by increased tonus, with exaggerated deep tendon (e.g., knee jerk) reflexes. As hypertonia advances, the legs are seen to scissor when the baby is held up. Failure of the infants hands to open up (extension of finger) is often found. Abnormal persistence of the Moro or tonic neck reflexes are unusual, but grave signs. As time goes on, signs of cerebellar or extrapyramidal tract disease may also emerge (see below).

3. In some children, apart from rather slow motor progress, little abnormality is seen until after the first birthday. If the cerebellum is permanently involved, ataxia may not be diagnosed until the age at which deliberate movements such as grasping, self-feeding, walking, and throwing are attempted. Then it is seen that the infant is more than usually clumsy, does not improve with time, and has definite past pointing, inability to judge distance and walks on a wider than normal base. Nystagmus is not always found in young children with cerebellar disease.

4. Similarly, the *basal gangliar* syndromes are seldom confidently diagnosed until the second year of life. At first there are fine wandering movements of the fingers. The limbs and trunk are progressively involved, with growing coarseness and incoordination of movement. Attempts to move—crawling and walking—are vitiated by the abnormal movement, which often involves the trunk as much as the limbs. Grimacing, drooling, and unsuccessful efforts at speech are common in these *choreoathetotic* children. All of the abnormal movements are increased if the patient is excited, fearful, or pushed beyond his physical limitations. Muscular rigidity is not common in this age group.

It must be emphasized again that all of the above patterns may occur in varying degrees in the same patient. Equally, the physical signs vary with age and the emergence of unsuspected damage.

Certain associated problems are common in all children with cerebral palsy, whatever the cause or major disorder pattern present. These are intellectual retardation, visual difficulties, and hearing difficulties. They must be sought for whenever a diagnosis of cerebral palsy is considered. The diagnosis of visual difficulties and hearing difficulties have been considered elsewhere (p. 428), and these sections should be consulted. Intellectual retardation is difficult to diagnose during the first year of life, largely because intellectual attributes at the time are geared mainly to the attainment of motor abilities. Thus, if a child cannot move to respond, he may be considered to be intellectually retarded. An objective assessment of intellectual potential lies in the measurement of head circumference. If this is significantly below normal, then the intellect is suspect. A normal head circumference is, however, no guarantee of intellectual ability, only a sign that further investigation is worthwhile.

Facial appearance may be of some help, but the expression may be immobile in the spastic, although intellectually normal, infant. A criterion of intellect, which may be independent of motor ability, is the power to communicate. This may take the usual forms in a spastic child and if speech, for example, occurs at the expected age, with appropriate content, the prognosis for intellect is reasonable. In the *dysarthric* child, especially the athetotic, the most subtle search for communicative ability should be made. Common forms consist in pulling the mother's skirt, pointing, and grunting. Children with very severe motor disorders can occasionally communicate by facial grimacing or eye movements.

Special investigations in cerebral palsy

In general, it is usual to exclude some of the causes such as aminoacidopathy by suitable biochemical tests. The power and function of various muscle groups are assessed by the pediatrician and physiotherapist, and, if necessary, vision and hearing are explored by experts in these fields. An E.E.G. is routinely done to explore the general pattern of brain activity, particularly of concern is an unduly silent record, or the presence of abnormal (epileptogenic) foci. Pneumoencephalography (the examination of the brain by injecting air into the ventricle) is only carried out if some localized lesion is suspected; where lower limb spasticity is severe, the hips should be x-rayed to see if dislocation has occurred.

Treatment: General. Much time and care must be taken to explain to the parents the nature and permanence of the condition. They should be relieved of unreasonable guilt feelings, and instructed to write down all of the questions to which they require answers. Several explanatory sessions are usually needed, and, although the treatment of cerebral palsy is a team effort they should know of *one* person whom they will regard as their primary contact. In general, a vaguely optimistic outlook should be maintained for all except the obviously disastrously affected children. The parents must be told that progress will be slow, but that progress will occur. They should be encouraged to take an active part in any treatment and educated in simple physiotherapeutic skills. Above all, attainable objectives should be set for the parents, and the problems considered as a series of 3-year plans.

Specific. As spasticity emerges, the mother is taught the techniques which prevent contractures. Emphasis is placed upon the attainment of effective food handling, attainment of balance, and the preparation for walking. During the first year, vision, hearing, and speech function are regularly checked. Splints may be necessary to maintain functional limb positions if physiotherapy alone is insufficient. Severe scissoring of the lower limbs in the second year of life may require corrective surgery, but only if the child has the intellectual capacity to cooperate postoperatively. Hip dislocation may also require orthopedic help at this stage.

At 3 years of age, the intellectual potential should again be carefully measured, and the progress of motor ability assessed. Even for special schools, some mobility, and fair visual and hearing ability is necessary. Toilet training need not yet be complete. Those who have reasonable intellect may now have more intensive educational physiotherapy and speech therapy. The child is now old enough in some instances to benefit from special orthopedic gear. A few children will ultimately be able to attend a normal school. Those with severe intellectual retardation should remain at home until institutionalization seems warranted. The moderate spastic, and the athetotic need special schooling, often on a semiresidential basis. It should be appreciated that facilities for treating the child with cerebral palsy are limited. The process of weeding out the retarded should be continuous and ruthless, although support for the family, and general pediatric care for the patient, should never be withheld.

The care of such children is continuous and arduous. The need of the parents (and the child) for a holiday from each other is too little appreciated. The understanding physician will see that facilities for this are made available or improvised. In those children unsuitable for special schooling, a little ingenuity, e.g., standing boxes, crash helmets, wide-based utensils, and suitable clothing will make a great difference to the parents. Drugs are useless in cerebral palsy, except for epilepsy, and surgery has little to commend it except in those who have an obviously remediable defect, and whose intellect is sufficient to allow them to cooperate in the convalescent phase.

Intellectual retardation

This section should be read in association with the section on normal growth and development (p. 9).

This may be defined as failure of development of the mind. The degree of failure, and the incidence within a community, will depend upon the educational demands of that community. Thus mental retardation will be better tolerated in the more primitive, but will have a higher incidence in the more technically advanced societies; in any event, the problem is a widespread one, when one considers that up to 40% of any Western community has a measured intelligence quotient of less than 100. Estimation of intelligence quotient, which can be reliably done after the second or third year, gives a useful guide to the educational future of the child. Thus, children who have an intelligence quotient of less than 70 normally require special (sometimes custodial) care; those who are in the division 70-90 are educationally subnormal and require the use of opportunity classes or other special facilities. Intellectual retardation of the more serious sort is usually found during the first year of life, a fair proportion of children, however, is confirmed as being retarded only after failure to make adequate progress at school.

Children who are specially at risk in developing mental defect are those born with a strong family history, extremely premature and dysmature infants, and the victims of severe birth anoxia, or when the mother has had an antepartum hemorrhage. Similarly, infants who develop viral or other infections in the perinatal period (rubella, cytomegalovirus, herpes virus, histoplasmosis, and neonatal meningitis) may, if they survive, be intellectually retarded.

Intellectual retardation is usually divisible into primary and secondary types. The primary type simply means that as yet no clear cut cause has been established; overall, this type of intellectual retardation is most common, and is often discovered in the preschool or early school periods.

Secondary intellectual retardation may be due, as already stated, to perinatal infections or may be part of a specific syndrome. There is a large variety of the latter, but certain groups are fairly readily recognizable. A particularly important group are the infants who suffer from metabolic disorders such as aminoacidopathies. As described elsewhere, there are many varieties of these; the classical example is phenylketonuria. Most of these, and the hyperammonemic syndromes, present primarily, with fits in the early months of life. These fits may be myoclonic jerks or *salaam* attacks. In such patients eventual mental retardation is to be expected unless suitable dietary measures can be taken; they are then the only treatable forms of mental retardation. The other metabolic abnormalities which may cause mental retardation are those in which there is interference with cerebral glucose metabolism. These will occur in untreated infantile hypoglycemia, galactosemia, and in certain of the glycogen storage diseases. Prolonged hypoglycemia from other causes later in life may also cause mental deterioration. The rarer syndromes (Lowe's disease) present primarily with hypotonia, cataracts, and renal problems. Mental retardation becomes obvious later. Other inborn errors of metabolism, which are associated with mental retardation are the sphingolipidoses, the disorders of mucopolysaccharide metabolism (gargoylism), and tuberous sclerosis.

Mental retardation and skeletal defects, commonly with obesity, occur in Albright's osteodystrophy, Präder-Willi syndrome, and Lawrence-Moon-Biedl disease. In each of these, however, other symptoms are usually primary.

Chromosome disorders are classically associated with mental retardation and the most common example of these, and indeed a usual cause of mental retardation, is Down's syndrome (mongolism). Intellectual retardation is found also in other chromosomal conditions such as cri du chat syndrome and the 17-18 trisomies and sex chromosome disorders of either sex. Intellectual retardation is common in the syndromes of cerebral palsy, which itself may have its origin in metabolic error, anoxic disaster at birth, or kernicterus.

Intellectual retardation in first year of life

Clinical features. Motor and mental development are closely correlated at this time; thus in the ordinary way, it is usual to suspect mental retardation if the child fails to attain motor milestones. Such normal criteria are described in detail elsewhere (p. 9). It should, however, always be recalled that there is an innate variation in the achievement of milestones and that the width of variation increases with the age of the child. It is also possible for a child to be unable to achieve normal motor milestones, e.g., head control, sitting up, standing, although he is of normal intellect. This is the characteristic situation in cerebral palsy or in severe muscle disorders, e.g., the amyotonia congenita syndrome. In the latter, however, the diagnosis is usually obvious enough. The principal problem arises in relation to children who have cerebral palsy and in whom there is a question of associated mental defect. In such children, and indeed in any mentally retarded child in the first 3 years of life, the most useful objective measurement is that of head circumference. The head circumference which significantly follows the chest circumference or the crown-rump length, is often reduced in mental retardation. A mentally retarded infant may show very little in the way of obvious neurological abnormality, other than lateness in achieving normal motor behaviour. The suspicion of mental retardation is usually confirmed by increasing failure to communicate. This may be obvious early in life as the incapacity to respond emotionally to the mother. The child does not smile or laugh in the circumstances which normally bring these about. The mother notices little differentiation in the cry, although most infants can express hunger, pain, or mere loneliness. This differentiation is unusual in severely retarded infants, but the value of this sign is somewhat decreased by the difficulty in obtaining a clear history from an inexperienced mother. Persistent failure to communicate by one method or another is very strong evidence of intellectual retardation. This is usually shown by failure to develop speech at the proper time. Even a deaf child with normal intelligence may not speak, but will communicate by pointing, pulling at the mother's skirt, or developing his own language. The intellectually retarded child develops these speech equivalents late and continues to use them years after they are appropriate.

Mental retardation presenting after the first birthday

Clinical features. The principal complaints are now of failure to speak, and general disquiet by the mother concerning the child's progress. Abnormal behaviour may now be a complaint: this includes restlessness, teeth grinding, irrelevant overactivity, slobbering, and the persistence of infantile habits such as putting everything into the mouth and much posturing of the hands before the eyes. Failure to achieve toilet training and persistence of infantile bowel habits is also common. In this age group also, the head is often small and the history is one of developmental delay.

Mental retardation presenting at school entry

Clinical features. Severe cases seldom present at this time. The child may have a problem with speech, specifically in relation to its limited content, although faulty execution is common. Soon after school entry, the first complaint is usually of difficulty in reading, but this is never isolated. The reading failure is usually quite complete, although the higher grade of mentally retarded child may memorize, and parrot parts of the reading material. This is common enough in normal children in the first months of school, but in the mentally retarded, all the parroting persists into the later school grades. There is also failure in all the other educational aspects. The concept of number remains a total mystery, and the ability to write or print progresses little beyond the simplest copying efforts. Pathological distractibility and inattention are characteristic of the mentally retarded schoolchild.

Such children rapidly become aware of their inferiority at school; accordingly secondary phenomena may be the presenting symptoms. These usually take the form of obvious anxiety states, such as refusal to go to school, unhappiness in the class, and persistent truancy. Negativism at home and school emerge, and the rages of frustration exceed in violence and number those which are acceptable as normal in the intellectually able child.

Other symptoms often found in retarded children

These may be the major complaints of the parents: negativism with food and toilet training are common, and may progress to autism where the child pays no attention to the environment and the persons in it. Otherwise aggressive behaviour towards other children and animals, destruction of property, lying, and stealing are not uncommon. Such symptoms of course occur in the normal child, and may be delayed until school frustrations occur. Immoral and antisocial activities are not unusual in the older defective who is not supervised.

The behavioural disorders such as head banging, repetitive trunk movements, hair pulling, pica (dirt eating), all occur in the intellectually retarded, usually in those in whom it is of a fairly severe degree. A particularly distressing symptom is self-mutilation—biting the fingers, tongue, toes, and lips until permanent injury occurs. This is particularly found in severely retarded children with a disorder of uric acid metabolism (Lesch-Nyhan syndrome).

General differential diagnosis of intellectual retardation

In the first year of life, the main problem is that of *cerebral palsy*, since children with this disorder will show delay in achieving the motor milestones. In these, abnormal limb tone, unusual movements—extensor spasms, a differentiating cry, and the acquisition of some method of communication independent of the neuromuscular defect are all guides to the true diagnosis.

Severe *system disease*, as congenital heart disease, mucoviscidosis, and other conditions requiring the infant to spend long periods in hospital are also associated with delay in motor achievement. In these there is a patchy achievement. Thus the infant smiles, can roll over, but cannot sit up. He can communicate, and may even speak before he can walk. His head growth is proportional to his other measurements.

Disorders causing *sensory defect* may also be troublesome. These are mainly blindness and deafness. The blind child responds to verbal cues, learns to communicate, and often progresses well to the stage of standing and walking. Speech is normally acquired. The deaf child is normal apart from verbal abilities, but he explores his environment and responds to visual cuing. Communication is often by gesture, or by a form of speech (neologism) specific to the child himself.

In the child who presents near the first birthday, consideration must be given to the possibility of late maturation. In this, the child's progress is slow, but steady, and the main problem is usually one of delayed speech. The child explores the environment, and has some ability to communicate. This situation is not uncommonly met with in children who have lacked the normal degree of social and emotional stimulus. It is most frequent then in children who have spent long periods in hospital or institutions, and may be found in families where both parents work and the infant is put in a baby care centre. The child looks normal, has a normal head size, and characteristically responds rapidly to individual attention. Simple game playing shows that the infant can learn rapidly. If he can do so, he is probably intellectually normal.

Autism

This is a peculiar psychosis of childhood in which the child retreats into himself, failing to make or maintain emotional or physical contact with the mother. The milestones of development have been normal, and speech may have appeared. The child then regresses to a more infantile state, rejects social contacts, and often is preoccupied with repetitive games. Emotional disorders are constant in these patients.

Treatment of the mentally retarded child

Specific treatment for the retarded child is usually impossible, accordingly every effort should be made to support the family, and to rid them of guilt feelings. Repeated discussions and explanations are necessary to prevent rejection of the child. Every effort should be made to keep the child at home. This is usually necessary anyway as institutions can seldom accept such children until 8 years of age. It is proper to tell the family that the ultimate abilities of a mentally retarded child cannot be foretold in detail. All that can be said is that the child will be slow in achievement, and that his ultimate abilities will be substantially below normal. Only when a gross defect is obvious should a more detailed prognosis be given.

The child maintained at home has a greater opportunity for stimulation than in an institution, so he is more likely to learn walking, talking, toilet training, and other simple skills. These will serve him in good stead if custodial care is needed. Such skills should be the principal ends of care in the first 5 years of life. As time goes on, it is usually possible to assess the intelligence, and on the subdivision already described, to consider whether he will require permanent care or be suitable for special education. Where it is obvious that the child is severely mentally retarded, then there is a strong probability that custodial care will ultimately be required. It is sensible, therefore, to consider the child's problem with the parents and to withstand, as far as possible, premature institutionalization. With this in mind, it is wise to attempt to educate the child in toilet training and to assess closely his modes of communication. Toilet training is a late skill in mental defectives but may be achieved by a continued process of conditioning. This skill makes it much easier to place a child in a day school or in occupational classes, and this should be explained to the parents, so that they will be encouraged to persist in their efforts.

Institutionalization may be requested because of aggressive, overactive, and destructive tendencies, all of which may make the domestic situation well nigh intolerable. Some requests may arise because the family has rejected the child. In such circumstances, removal from the home environment is inevitable. If, however, there is some parental insight and acceptance of the situation, and especially if there is evidence that efforts at education have been perhaps overenthusiastic, reducing the pressure on the child, and the prescription of a tranquilizer may help. When the parents are older, as is common in Down's syndrome, the family situation may require that the child be put into an institution. It is, however, important that this decision be made with some delicacy, otherwise guilt feelings may again arise and plague the mother and father.

It is important to realize the immense amount of time and effort which parents must put into the care of mentally retarded children and to understand that their social life is negligible. Relief is hard to get. The physician can do much to maintain morale so a timely admission to hospital is a great help in allowing parents to catch up on themselves. It is also important to point out to the parents that this can be arranged in circumstances such as illness in the mother. Inability to look after the child because of parental illness is a deep, and recurrent fear in the parents.

The educational care of the mentally retarded is a subject for the specialist. In general, however, efforts are directed towards giving the child some self-sufficiency, e.g., in clothing himself, in toilet training, and in gaining simple forms of amusement. Combined with these, is a lot of occupational therapy, since these children are distractable and easily bored. The same approaches are used in the mobile institutionalized child. A percentage of severely retarded children remain completely bedfast. For these, nursing care and simple physiotherapy are the only treatments.

CONVULSIVE DISORDERS (EPILEPSY: FITS OR CONVULSIONS)

This is defined as a sudden, transient, often recurring, disturbance of brain function. Loss of consciousness is frequent but not invariable, and inappropriate contraction of muscle groups is usual. The fit then is a symptom of brain disturbance, not necessarily a disease in itself. If a cause is found, epilepsy is then called *symptomatic*, if not, it is called *idiopathic*.

Etiology. The causes are very varied. In the newborn, anatomical abnormalities (brain cysts), the effects of anoxia, intracranial hemorrhage, hypoglycemia and hypocalemia all are relevant. So too are neonatal viral and bacterial infections such as rubella, herpes virus, and neonatal meningitis.

Soon after birth, other metabolic abnormalities such as kernicterus, aminoacidopathies, the hyperammonemias occur, with a continuance of intracranial infections, and those conditions such as hydrocephalus which raise intracranial pressure. In later childhood the effects of injury, hypoglycemia from various causes, and the cerebral degenerations are relevant. Between 6 months and 5 years, epilepsy due to a reduced seizure threshold occur. This is mainly expressed as *febrile convulsions* and the convulsions following breath-holding spells. Many of the disorders mentioned continue in one form or another from school-age until adolescence, but an increasing percentage of patients have no obvious cause, i.e., they are suffering from idiopathic convulsive disorders, many due to polygenic inheritable factors. At any age convulsions may reflect poisoning by drugs, especially amphetamines, antihistamines and tricyclic antidepressants. Drugs which paralyze respiration (e.g., organophosphorus insecticides) may cause convulsions because of cerebral anoxia.

Convulsive equivalents are rare, and consist in episodes of headache, nausea, pain in the abdomen and occasional vomiting. Such attacks are often associated with true grand mal or psychomotor attacks.

Clinical types of convulsive disorder

Myoclonic seizures

These are most common in mentally retarded infants. The usual pattern is oft-repeated, short-lived jerks of the head, body, and limbs. If head control is present, constant drop attacks in which the head falls forward may be the principal feature. In some infants the attack is stylized as a *salaam* spell, i.e., the head and trunk fall forward and the arms jerk upwards. Extensor spasms, with transient opisthotonic (back arching) attacks are a variant, and grand mal attacks may occur. The E.E.G. is often chaotic, with high voltage irregular spike and wave patterns. This is called hypsarrhythmia.

Grand mal epilepsy

In this the patient often has a warning, called an aura which precedes the fit. The aura is commonly a sinking feeling in the stomach, or flashing lights, or an unpleasant taste or smell. If present, this is followed by sudden loss of consciousness, pallor, upward rolling of the eyes, extension of the legs, flexion of the arms and arching of the trunk; the respiratory muscles are in spasm, so cyanosis occurs, occasionally the tongue is caught between the clenched teeth. Within a few seconds this *tonic* stage is followed by the *clonic* stage in which the trunk and limbs rhythmically flex and extend. Incontinence of urine and feces occurs; after a few minutes the colour improves, the jerking ceases, and the patient wakes up, often in a confused state. He then usually falls into the postictal sleep. Older children may complain of headache after the fit. In nocturnal epilepsy, these signs may not be seen, and a wet bed or bitten tongue may be the only clue. In a few children, but not those with febrile convulsions, a transient hemiplegia (Todd's paralysis) is found after a grand mal attack. The weakness may persist for a few days after the attack, especially if a Jacksonian seizure (see below) has preceded the grand mal episode.

Akinetic seizures

These are usually found as part of the grand mal fit, and are common in retarded children. The child suddenly rolls the eyes upwards, and falls to the ground. He is stiff and unconscious but true tonic/clonic convulsions do not occur. Postictal confusion and sleep are usual, as in true grand mal attacks.

Psychomotor seizures

These are rather rare in children, but may be associated with disease of the temporal lobe. The manifestations are variable, aura is common, and is followed by repetitive purposeless movements, such as blinking, eyelid fluttering, chewing movements, hand fumbling, and staring: running fits with confusion, are a rare type of psychomotor seizure. Dreamy states with hallucinations of sight and smell occur, the patient may feel that he is somewhere familiar and is looking at a scene he has viewed before (déja vu phenomenon). Postictal sleep, and lack of recollection of the event (amnesia), are common in psychomotor attacks.

Jacksonian seizures

These are fits which begin in one part of the body, usually the face, hand, mouth, or arm and spread until one half, or the whole body, is involved in a grand mal fit following loss of consciousness. *Sensory* Jacksonian attacks are rare in children. In these, cold or hot feelings in the various parts of the body progress as described above, and may be followed by motor convulsions.

Petit mal epilepsy

In this condition, which is unusual before the age of 2-3 years, there are short spells of loss of consciousness. These are so transient that the patient seldom falls, but the eyes may roll up, the head nod, or the patient drop whatever he is holding. Speech, writing, or any other activity transiently ceases. The whole cycle takes only a few seconds, and the patient is normal between attacks. The number of spells is very variable, in some children they occur at intervals of some months, in others, hundreds of daily attacks may occur (pyknolepsy). Education suffers in the latter group. Petit mal status is rare, and clinically resembles a prolonged psychomotor seizure.

Screening for convulsive disorders

In the newborn, the dextrose and calcium levels should immediately be estimated. Blood culture and lumbar puncture should follow, and if the fontanelle is bulging, subdural tap should be considered. In the absence of positive results to these, or of an obvious cause such as kernicterus, a full scale biochemical screen for the aminoacidopathies should be carried out. This commonly commences with the Guthrie test for phenylketonuria, with urine and blood scan for the amino- and organic acidurias.

In the first 3 months of life, seizures without obvious cause, and especially if myoclonic should again precipitate a scan for the aminoacidopathies, hypoglycemias and hyperammonemias. Neurological signs, and failure to attain the motor milestones, should prompt a consideration of the sphingolipidoses and other degenerative brain conditions. Cerebral palsy is, however, the usual cause of neurological signs and fits at this age, due usually to anoxia or injury at birth.

In the preschool child, hypocalcemic and hypoglycemic states occasionally still occur. The former are easily diagnosed by calcium estimation; the latter may require a close history to uncover such suggestive symptoms as sweating, pallor, and occurrence in the morning or after fasting. Every effort should be made to obtain a blood sugar level during the fit, as in such cases, the ordinary fasting levels of glucose are often normal. Accidental poisoning with antihistamines and antidepressant drugs should always be considered. Febrile convulsions are accepted only if an obvious cause for fever exists.

An electroencephalogram is warranted at any age. In febrile convulsions this test may show changes for 10-14 days after the fit, and should not be overinterpreted.

The electroencephalogram (E.E.G.)

This is a record obtained by amplifying the electric currents present during brain activity. These may become abnormal in the various forms of convulsive disorder. However, obvious epilepsy may be present in a patient whose E.E.G. is normal. The E.E.G. changes found in the various convulsive disorders are summarized in table 28.

Persistent localization of E.E.G. abnormality may be an indication for a brain scan. This is a method in which a radioactive material is injected or inhaled, and the resultant radioactive skull emanation measured in an instrument called a gamma camera (i.e., it records gamma rays). This technique is used mainly in symptomatic seizure where a tumour or abscess is suspected.

Table 28. E.E.G. changes with various convulsive disorders

Type of Convulsion	E. E. G. Pattern
Myoclonic	Irregular frequent spike and waves; chaotic hypsarrhythmia
Grand mal	Bilateral; spikes and slow waves
Psychomotor	Temporal focus; spike or slow waves
Jacksonian	Focal spikes, slow waves or spike/wave formation
Petit mal	Bilateral source; spike and wave form

Differential diagnosis of convulsions

Young children usually have fits because of disease, and this must always be sought, particularly the treatable infections and injuries, and the metabolic conditions which respond to dietary restrictions. In the older child, poisoning, with lead or drugs must always be kept in mind. If the fit sounds atypical, is not witnessed, and is allegedly recurrent, 2 conditions may require exclusion. These are *breath holding* and *masturbation*. The latter is rather rare, occurs in infants, and is characterized by repetitive movements of the extended legs, preoccupation, redness of the face and grunting, followed by sleep. There is no true tonic/clonic movement. Breath holding spells are described elsewhere (p. 492) but essentially consist in attacks of loud crying, forced expiration, cyanosis, and transient stiffening. These always have a precipitating cause, e.g., pain, frustration, rage, and there is no postictal state.

General aspects of treatment

These will vary with the cause and type of convulsion. However, the parents always require explanation and reassurance, thus in the true idiopathic epilepsy, without associated intellectual defect, the relatively benign course should be explained, and a definite statement made that the child's brain is unlikely to suffer. All epileptics should be protected from common dangers, such as fire, heights, and traffic, but every effort should be made to ensure that they receive adequate education, and lead as normal a social life as is possible. Failure to achieve this, and undue restrictions are causes of the psychological overlay which is not uncommon in those suffering from convulsive disorders.

Treatment of specific situations

Myoclonic jerks in infancy

These are very resistant to drug therapy, and since the infant is unlikely to suffer damage from falling, tongue biting, etc., heavy anticonvulsant treatment is not usually recommended. Steroids may occasionally reduce the frequency of the attacks, but they have side effects,some of which are dangerous, and cannot do anything for the intellectual retardation which is usually also present.

Grand mal seizures

The initial episode often passes off without any specific treatment. In a continuing attack, intravenous diazepam or intramuscular phenobarbitone are commonly used. Each is given with care if it is suspected that the fits are due to poisoning. This is because these drugs may enhance the action (and therefore the risk of death) in children poisoned by antihistamines or antidepressants. In recurrent grand mal attacks, the usual treatment is phenobarbitone, with or without a phenytoin (Dilantin). Each may cause a measles-like skin rash, sleepiness, or ataxia. The parents must be warned to report these possibilities. In addition, the phenytoin causes overgrowth of the gums, although this may be partly prevented by good dental hygiene. If these drugs do not control the seizures, primidone (Mysoline) or sulthiam (Ospolot) may be tried.

Psychomotor epilepsy

is treated by the same drugs used in the grand mal type.

Petit mal seizures

Drug treatment is only undertaken if the attacks are so frequent as to interfere with ordinary living and education. A few patients respond to phenobarbitone, which should always be tried first. If there is no response then ethosuximide (Zarontin) is given, largely because it gives rise to fewer side effects (light intolerance, depression of red and white blood cell elements) than troxidone (Tridione).

Duration of therapy

In idiopathic epilepsy, the parents should be told that treatment will continue for at least 3 years, and possibly for life. If the patient is free of seizures for 3 years, the drugs should be discontinued over the following 6 months; observation should, however, continue for another 3 years at least, and protection against common dangers (traffic, heights, unaccompanied swimming, and so on) insisted upon for at least 5 years.

Febrile convulsions

Clinical features. These are very unusual before the age of 6 months, and rare after 4 years. Most occur between 1½ and 2 years, often in a family with a history of similar episodes.

Such a fit is *always* superimposed upon a condition causing fever, especially if the temperature rises rapidly. Most commonly this is an upper respiratory tract infection, often viral, usually with red tonsils, frequently with otitis media. The fever is usually greater than 39 degrees C. The fit may take the form of a full scale grand mal attack, or the child may be found stiff and frothing with the eyes rolled up. A postictal sleep is usual. It is usually a single fit, at the onset of the illness. Prolonged fits are very unusual in febrile convulsions, as are Jacksonian attacks and Todd's paralysis. In every case, fever and an objective explanation for it must be present before the diagnosis can be accepted. Lumbar puncture must never be neglected in case of doubt. Febrile convulsions may recur 2 or 3 times without permanent ill-effect. In a few instances, they are the forerunners of an idiopathic epilepsy.

The treatment is to lower the fever by tepid sponging, and to treat the primary infection. Anticonvulsants may be necessary in the acute state. If recurrent febrile convulsions occur, the mother should give phenobarbitone if a fever occurs—but she should also always seek medical attention.

Status epilepticus

This is the term applied to seizures which persist for more than an hour or two. It is a potentially dangerous condition which requires vigorous but careful therapy.

Clinical features. There is a grand mal seizure which does not completely wear off. The patient tends to remain in the tonic phase, with focal twitchings of the eyes, mouth, and face. The breathing is jerky and ineffective and cyanosis is common. Purpuric spots appear on the face if the spasms do not cease quickly. At first incontinence of urine is common, but retention may occur later. The patient sweats and the temperature may rise. Leucocytosis and tachycardia are commonly found after an hour or two. Dehydration soon occurs because no fluid can be taken and if the condition persists for 12 hours or more, low blood pressure and edema of the lungs can set in.

Differential diagnosis. This is easy in the known epileptic. Otherwise tetanus, or poisoning by strychnine, the tricyclic antidepressants, or antihistamines all require consideration.

Treatment. An intravenous infusion of 0.18% saline in 5% dextrose should be set up, and pharyngeal suction instituted. The safest anticonvulsant is probably paraldehyde given intramuscularly in a dose of 0.15 ml/kg wt. Phenytoin is also of value, if these are ineffective diazepam (Valium) may be given intravenously. If drugs are unavailing and signs of exhaustion are present, the patient (in suitable circumstances) may be given a general anesthetic, intubated, paralyzed, and artifically ventilated.

Prognosis. This is guarded in prolonged, unrelieved status, since death from respiratory failure is not unusual. Punctate brain hemorrhages are found at autopsy in such patients.

RAISED INTRACRANIAL PRESSURE

Physiology

The brain and spinal cord are enclosed with a case which is relatively rigid in infants, and totally rigid when the sutures close. Within the nervous tissue are cavities (ventricles) and their connections which produce and circulate the cerebrospinal fluid (CSF). The pressure of the CSF reflects the general intracranial pressure. CSF is formed in the 4 ventricles by the choroid plexuses, traverses the tube known as the aqueduct to enter the subarachnoid space, through the openings called the foramina of Luschka & Magendie. Thus it bathes the spinal cord and brain proper, and is reabsorbed by the arachnoid process of the sinuses (veins) of the pia and by the cerebral veins. The circulation is summarized in figure 53.

Intracranial pressure will increase if the circulation or reabsorption of CSF is blocked (obstructive hydrocephalus). A small swelling within the skull will displace normal brain tissue, thus raising pressure, and may also block normal CSF circulation. Swelling of the brain cells proper (cerebral edema) will have the same effect. The rise in pressure can be compensated in the young child by widening of the sutures and head enlargement. In the older child this is not possible, so symptoms are earlier and more severe. The end result of unrelieved pressure is loss of function of neural tissue, and reduction of cerebral blood flow.

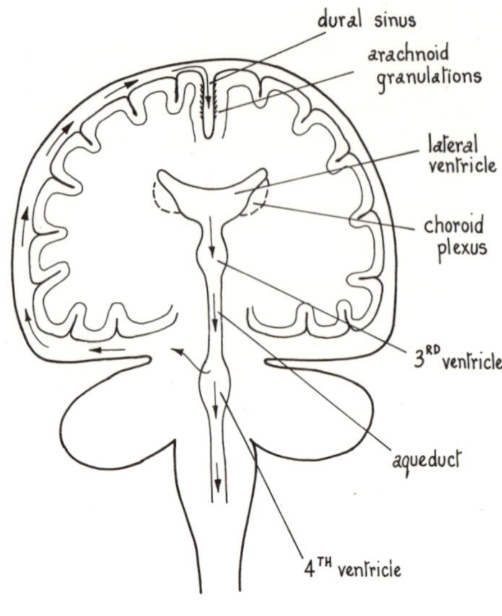

Fig. 53. Ventricular system and CSF circulation.

General features of raised intracranial pressure

In the young child, fretfulness, irritability, vomiting, and increase in head size are usual. In the older child, headache and vomiting occur. At first these occur mainly in the morning, later they are constant. Visual problems (diplopia—seeing double), and paralysis of the eye muscles because of stretching of the 3rd and 6th cranial nerves all occur. At any age, an important sign is *papilledema*. This is the swelling of the optic nerve head which can be seen by ophthalmoscopy. Hemorrhages and exudates into the retina also occur.

At any stage, sleepiness or coma, high blood pressure, slowing of the heart rate (bradycardia), severe vomiting, and convulsions mean severe intracranial hypertension.

X-ray signs of raised intracranial pressure

In infancy these are an increased head size and widening of the sutures. In older children the suture lines also widen and the normal convolutional (beaten copper) markings of the skull are exaggerated. In cases of long standing, the pituitary fossa and the adjacent bony clinoid processes may be eroded.

Special investigations

The size and position of the ventricles may be roughly determined by echogram. This is a record of the absorption of ultrasonic waves by the skull and its contents. Local masses (abscess, tumours) show characteristic appearances when radionuclides are injected or inhaled and the skull emanations measured. Direct visualization of the ventricles is done by injecting air into them and taking skull x-rays (pneumoencephalography). Angiography is the injection of contact media into a carotid artery, followed by cine-x-ray photography. Thus malformations of vessels, or their displacement by tumour or abscess can be seen.

Some specific disorders

Hydrocephalus

This means an increase in the size of the ventricles, and can be due to a block at any point in the CSF circulation.(figure 53). In young infants, the condition is most commonly associated with meningomyelocele, which although a spinal deformity, causes downward displacement of the cerebellum to block CSF circulation (Arnold-Chiari malformation). The aqueduct, 3rd and 4th ventricles may fail to canalize before birth, or be blocked by cysts, tumours, or the results of infection or hemorrhage. The two last are the common causes of blocking of the foramina of Luschka and Magendie.

Clinical features. In infants there are few early symptoms other than vomiting. The earliest feature may be unusually rapid head growth, with prominent skull veins and wide separation of the sutures. The brow begins to bulge, the upper eyelids retract and the infant appears to gaze downwards, showing excess sclera. This is called the setting sun sign. The fontanelle bulges, and the skull, if percussed, gives a dull note (cracked pot sound). Delayed motor development and retarded intellect occur. Cranial nerve palsies (of 3, 6, 10) are especially liable to occur if the Arnold-Chiari malformation is present. In older children, the symptoms are headache, vomiting, and visual difficulties. Papilledema is found in all age groups.

Diagnosis. The site of block is accurately localized by *pneumoencephalography*.

Treatment. If the block (e.g., a tumour) can be removed then this is done. Otherwise it is relieved by connecting the ventricular system to the right atrium of the heart by way of a plastic tube. This alternative route for CSF flow is called a ventriculoatrial shunt.

Chronic subdural hematoma

This is a collection of blood in the subdural space. It is due to injury, rarely as a result of labour, often as a result of violence, particularly as part of the battered baby syndrome. It is commonest between 2 and 12 months of age. The clot of blood may be small at first, but because it is not reabsorbed, it acts as a sponge to attract more fluid to it, thus increasing its size, and causing further blood vessel rupture.

Clinical features. The complaints are restlessness, irritability, vomiting, and failure to thrive. The latter may partly be due to parental neglect if the child has been subjected to violence. The head increases in size and the fontanelle bulges. Drowsiness, convulsions, and signs of hemiplegia are common. Ophthalmoscopy often shows retinal hemorrhages, and occasionally papilledema. The scalp is often tight and glossy looking.

Diagnosis. This is made by putting a needle into the subdural space and aspirating blood or blood-stained serum.

Treatment. The fluid is aspirated frequently by needle. The subsequent protein and blood loss is made up by appropriate transfusion. When the intracranial pressure has been reduced, the skull is opened by the neurosurgeon and the hematoma removed. If persistent reaccumulation occurs, a shunt may be required.

Chronic subdural effusion

This is a complication of meningitis. The effusion is usually sterile, but may be purulent.

Symptoms. These are loss of appetite, irritability, sleepiness and vomiting, together with papilledema, and often focal neurological problems such as convulsions, hemiplegia, or eye paralysis.

Treatment. This is as for subdural hematoma.

Acute epidural hematoma

This follows head injury with rupture of a meningeal artery. The shed blood causes an acute rise in intracranial pressure, which may be rapidly fatal.

Features. There is a history of injury. The child may seem well for a short time, and then complains of headache, vomits, and becomes comatose. Convulsions are common, and hemiplegia frequent. Eye paralysis, with unilateral dilated pupil are characteristic. The whole process occupies a very short time, and death is frequent unless the pressure is relieved and the bleeding point secured by the neurosurgeon.

Brain abscess

This may follow infection of the sinuses and inner ear, or be metastatic from infections of the lung (bronchiectasis) or heart (endocarditis).

The clinical features. are those of any space-occupying condition: in infancy, fever, enlarging head, vomiting, failure to thrive, convulsions, and focal signs such as hemiplegia. In the older child, fever, headache, vomiting, personality change, visual disturbances, ataxia and papilledema are characteristic. If the abscess ruptures into the ventricle, the symptoms of a severe meningitis develop. The abscess is located by the techniques mentioned—echogram, cerebral radionuclide scan, pneumoencephalogram, etc.

Treatment. Antibiotics are given, and the abscess cavity drained, filled with antibiotic solution and allowed to heal.

Benign intracranial hypertension (pseudotumour cerebri)

This is found in older children, and is most commonly due to overdosage with steroids, or occasionally with Vitamin A or tetracyclines. It may, however, occur without obvious cause.

The symptoms are the expected ones, headache, vomiting, visual disturbance, and papilledema. Special investigations (echogram, pneumoencephalogram) are normal and the condition subsides spontaneously. *This condition, however, must never be diagnosed until extensive investigations have excluded a true tumour.*

Craniosynostosis

This means abnormally early fusion of the skull sutures so that normal head growth is impaired. The longitudinal (sagittal) or transverse (coronal) sutures may be affected separately or together.

Clinical features. The main one is abnormality of the shape of the head. In obliteration of the sagittal suture, the head becomes long and narrow (scaphocephaly) and a bony ridge may be felt along the suture line. In coronal suture closure, the skull becomes fore-shortened (brachycephaly) and may look pointed (oxycephaly). Facial deformity is common, with protrusion of the eyes (exophthalmos). Squints, papilledema, and blindness may occur. Severe increase in intracranial pressure is rare unless both sagittal and coronal sutures are fusing. This gives rise to the symptoms described above.

Treatment. Surgery is indicated if the pressure is raised, and consists in separating the suture, and maintaining the gap by inserting a plastic barrier to refusion.

Intracranial tumours

The main age group with these is 2-10 years, and most of them occur in the infratentorial region, i.e., in the medulla, cerebellum, midbrain, and pons.
The *clinical features* are those of raised intracranial pressure, viz., headache, vomiting, visual problems, and papilledema. In younger patients irritability and increase in head size may occur.

Specific tumours

Medulloblastoma

This is the commonest neoplasm, with early symptoms of raised pressure. The tumour invades the cerebellum, causing ataxia and staggering, and involves the brain stem giving paralysis of the 5th, 7th, and 8th cranial nerves, and ultimately bilateral upper motor neurone (pyramidal) defects. Meningeal involvement causes irritability, neck stiffness, and painful arching of the back and neck (opisthotonos).

Cerebellar astrocytoma

The general features resemble those of medulloblastoma. The onset is usually less acute, and true cerebellar signs (nystagmus, dysmetria, truncal ataxia) predominate. Cranial nerve paralysis is a later complication.

Midbrain glioma

This causes rapid symptoms of raised intracranial pressure. Since the areas of eye control are in the midbrain, then loss of upward gaze and light reflex takes place. The pathways from the cerebellum are interrupted, as are the pyramidal tracts, so that incoordination, nystagmus, and spastic paralysis occur. Occasionally extrapyramidal syndromes are found.

Glioma of the pons

Intracranial hypertension is later in this tumour, so that the first signs are paralysis of the 5th, 6th, 7th, and 8th cranial nerves. Cerebellar and pyramidal tract involvement are common late signs, which may coincide with the first symptoms of intracranial hypertension.

Tumours of the medulla

Again, signs of raised pressure are delayed, the main early features being paralysis of the lower cranial nerves (9th, 10th, 11th, 12th), characteristically giving rise to difficulty in eating and swallowing. Vomiting, vertigo, and pyramidal tract involvement eventually occur.

Supratentorial tumours

The commonest area where these are found is above the pituitary (suprasellar) and the closely related optic chiasma.

Craniopharyngioma. This gives rise to the general features of raised intracranial pressure. In addition it causes a visual defect (bitemporal hemianopia, see p. 429) because of pressure on the optic chiasma. Pituitary and hypothalamic functions are affected, so that growth ceases because of failure of growth hormone production. Similarly, thyroid and adrenal function may be affected because of deletion of the corresponding trophic hormone. Destruction of the posterior pituitary causes lack of vasopressin and the passing of large quantities of dilute urine (diabetes insipidus). Skull x-rays usually show calcification in the suprasellar area.

Tumour of the chiasma. In addition to the general features of cerebral tumours, these interfere with vision (bitemporal hemanopia) and may cause optic atrophy. Extension into the hypothalamic area is slow, ultimately giving the features of a craniopharyngioma.

Tumour of the 3rd ventricle. Pinealoma or cysts are the typical problem in this area. Acute blockage of CSF circulation occurs early, so that signs of intracranial hypertension are rapid and severe. Midbrain syndromes (paralysis of upward gaze, constriction of the pupils) are typical. Rarely hypothalamic involvement leads to precocious sexual development.

General differential diagnosis of intracranial tumours

The principal problems to consider are brain abscess, subdural hematoma, and lead poisoning, all of which give rise to the general symptoms of intracranial hypertension. Air studies may be necessary to localize the two former, stippling of the red cells, bone lead line, and heavy metal levels in the urine will establish the latter. Papilledema without other symptoms of raised intracranial pressure may follow steroid treatments. It may also occur in so-called benign intracranial hypertension (see above). In children with widespread cranial nerve palsies, poisoning by drugs or insecticides may require consideration. These situations usually have a short history, opportunity of ingestion, and no papilledema. In all cases where a brain tumour seems definitely to be present, a search should be made for some extracranial primary source. This is commonly leukemia or neuroblastoma. Cerebellar tumours may require exclusion of acute cerebellar ataxia, muscular dystrophy and Friedrich's ataxia, but none of these have symptoms or signs of raised intracranial pressure.

Specific diagnosis

This should be left to the skilled neurosurgeon; it may require the use of echoencephalography, air encephalography, and cerebral angiography.

Treatment

This is singularly unrewarding except perhaps in the well-localized cerebellar astrocytomata in suprasellar tumours which may sometimes be relieved by drainage. If internal hydrocephalus is severe, and curative procedures are impossible, ventriculoatrial shunt may afford some symptomatic relief.

The general prognosis is in keeping with the general failure of treatment; it is particularly gloomy in medulloblastoma and brain stem tumours.

INJURIES OF THE SKULL AND BRAIN IN CHILDREN

At any age, car accidents are a common cause. In infancy, the battered baby syndrome is important. Penetrating head injuries are relatively rare, and usually due to gun shot.

Cerebral concussion

This is defined as an impairment of consciousness and brain function following a head injury. In most instances the child is unconscious for a relatively short time, wakens up and then is confused for a variable time. Amnesia is common, as are vomiting and headache.

In more severe cases, the patient is deeply unconscious, has flaccid limbs, breathes stertorously, has dilated fixed pupils, and may have a low blood pressure and rapid pulse. Death may occur because of interference with medullary function. More commonly the unconsciousness lightens to stupor, respiration and blood pressure return to normal, and the child slowly wakes up with headache and vomiting. His mood varies from irritability to a violent confused state.

Traumatic encephalopathy

This is the situation in which violence has permanently damaged many brain cells. The initial state is of concussion, but the patient stays stuporose, lies in a flexed attitude, and does not respond except to painful stimuli. This condition may last for days or weeks. As the stupor clears, signs of local neurological damage appear—as convulsions, hemiplegia, eye paralysis, and speech disorders (aphasia). Confusional states, irritability, and headaches are common in these children, and ultimate mental retardation not uncommon.

Perforating injuries of the skull and brain if not immediately fatal, cause loss of consciousness and extensive loss of function. The clinical features are those of a severe concussion, with the added risks of infective meningitis or cerebral abscess. Extensive tissue destruction may be complicated by cerebral swelling which may cause death after a few days.

Injury can give rise to space-occupying lesions, e.g., acute and chronic subdural hematoma, as already described. Skull fracture is not always present in any of the injuries described, and is relevant only if it is of the depressed type which is more liable to be associated with vessel rupture or cerebral contusion.

Treatment of head injury

The general principles are:

1. To exclude injury elsewhere, and to treat it if necessary,
2. Clear the pharyngeal secretions and maintain the airway by intubation if need be,
3. Maintain hydration by intravenous infusion,
4. Observe for signs of raised intracranial pressure, viz,
   increased restlessness
   inequality of pupils
   slowing pulse, rise and then fall of blood pressure,
5. If the intracranial pressure rises, neurosurgical exploration to remove local blood collections is warranted. If cerebral edema is present, then the use of intravenous mannitol or systemic steroids may prevent interference with medullary function.

CEREBROSPINAL INFECTIONS

These are common and important childhood conditions. Conventionally such infections are divided into meningitis (inflammation of the cerebral membranes) and encephalitis (inflammation of nervous tissue). Generally, however, they coexist as meningoencephalitis, the symptoms alone determining the clinical description.

Etiology

Where meningeal symptoms predominate, pyogenic (pus forming) organisms are most frequently responsible. In the newborn *E.coli* and *P.pyocyaneus* predominate. In older children *H.influenzae*, meningococcal, pneumococcal and streptococcal infections occur. Occasionally tuberculosis, salmonella, and fungus infection (torula) are responsible. Viral meningitis may follow infection by polio virus, Coxsackie, mumps, ECHO, and the virus of lymphocytic chromomeningitis. When an encephalitis picture predominates, a viral cause is usual. This may be one which causes a simple exanthem, e.g., measles, chicken pox, rubella, or more exotic, viz, encephalitis virus A & B, and the arbovirus of dengue fever, etc.

Pyogenic meningitis (see p. 49 for neonatal meningitis)

This is a disease of the first 2-3 years of age, with 50% of the patients being aged less than 1 year. It usually occurs in the winter months, but is rarely epidemic unless of the meningococcal variety.

Clinical features. The child may have had a mild upper respiratory infection, then he develops fever, irritability, loss of appetite, vomits, and becomes drowsy or comatose. The last 4 complaints are almost invariable; older children may additionally complain of headache and stiff neck. Convulsions are not inevitable, but tend to occur in the younger child.

In infants, the signs of meningitis may be unremarkable, and the diagnosis made following lumbar puncture on the basis of the history. Bulging of the fontanelle is an important sign, but may be slight if vomiting has caused dehydration. Neck stiffness may be absent or minimal among infants, although neck retraction is not uncommon.

In older children, neck stiffness and pain when the extended leg is bent towards the chest (Kernig's sign), are evidence of meningeal irritation. A few infants present with a nonspecific picture of gross dehydration, shock, and subnormal temperature. In these, a discordant bulging fontanelle or head retraction may provide a clue.

In meningococcal infections, a purpuric rash is often found, this may coalesce into massive bruising, evidence usually of a complicating Waterhouse-Friedrichsen's syndrome (see below).

Diagnosis. This can only be made by lumbar puncture. The spinal fluid is under pressure and is usually turbid. Microscopy will reveal large numbers of polymorph cells, and appropriate staining will usually identify the responsible organism.

Complications:

1. Waterhouse-Friedrichsen syndrome. This is an early, often fatal complication of meningococcal infections. Apart from the signs of meningitis, the patient develops extensive purpura, bruising, hypotension, and evidence of failing circulation. It is due to destruction of the adrenals by the meningococcal endotoxin.

2. Subdural effusion. This begins 7-10 days after the onset of the illness and is marked by a return of the original symptoms (fever, anorexia, drowsiness, vomiting, restlessness), together with focal neurological disorder such as convulsions or paralysis.

3. Cranial nerve palsies. (usually affecting the eye muscles), nerve deafness, speech disorders, and hydrocephalus are late complications, occurring with delayed diagnosis and treatment.

Treatment of pyogenic meningitis

Dehydration is relieved by an intravenous infusion, and an appropriate antibiotic given in large doses. Ampicillin (given intravenously) is the drug of first choice in *H.influenzae*, meningococcal and pneumococcal infections. If the organisms prove to be resistant then chloramphenicol penicillin and sulphadiazine are given together. Antibiotic therapy is continued for at least 2 weeks.

Treatment of complications

Subdural effusion is drained by needle puncture, and antibiotic therapy is reassessed and continued for at least 2 more weeks.

Waterhouse-Friedrichsen syndrome. The infant is rehydrated, given hydrocortisone intravenously, and blood transfusion if necessary. There is no specific treatment for cranial nerve palsies. Hydrocephalus may require ventriculoatrial shunt.

Tuberculous meningitis

This occurs in infants, and is part of disseminated (miliary) tuberculosis. The symptoms are as discussed, viz, irritability, fever, anorexia, vomiting, and drowsiness. However, these extend over a week or two, in contrast to the day or two of pyogenic meningitis. The patient then develops deepening coma with cranial nerve palsies, convulsions, general rigidity and severe signs of meningeal irritation. Papilledema is usual, and tubercles may be seen on the choroid of the eye. Obstructive hydrocephalus is the terminal event.

The diagnosis may be suspected because of a history of contact, a positive Mantoux test, or from the examination of the CSF. The latter contains lymphocytes, and excess globulin, which settles as a cobweb clot if left undisturbed. The mycobacteria tuberculosis can be seen after suitable staining.

Treatment. This is in general that outlined for pyogenic meningitis. The specific antibiotics are streptomycin, isoniazid and para-aminosalicylic acid (PAS). They must be given for at least 6 months. Obstructive hydrocephalus requires neurosurgical attention, often by frequent ventricular tap with the injection of streptomycin at the same time. Cure of the infection with persistent hydrocephalus indicates the need for a ventriculoatrial shunt.

Torula meningitis

This is due to a fungus (*cryptococcus neoformans*), the features resemble those of tuberculous meningitis. Occasionally a brain abscess forms. The fungus can be seen in the spinal fluid. The infection is treated with amphotericin.

Amebic meningitis

This is an acute infection due to invasion of the meninges by a waterborne ameba. The symptoms are similar to those of a fulminant pyogenic meningitis, with the rapid onset of coma, generalized rigidity, and evidence of severe intracranial hypertension. The condition is confirmed by finding the ameba in the CSF. Treatment is with amphotericin, but the mortality is high.

Viral (aseptic) meningitis

The types of viruses which cause this disease have already been mentioned.

Clinical features (except polio, Coxsackie). The older child (2-5 years) is usually affected. A preliminary upper respiratory tract infection is followed by headache, nausea, vomiting, loss of appetite, and drowsiness which may deepen to stupor. Younger patients do not complain of headache but are irritable. Neck stiffness is usual and complaints of muscular ache are frequent.

Lumbar puncture. The fluid is clear but contains a few hundred cells. In early disease polymorphs predominate over lymphocytes. In the later stage, only lymphocytes are found. The protein may be raised slightly but the glucose levels are normal; organisms are absent from the smear. The specific virus is identified by serological studies.

Poliomyelitis and Coxsackie (Types A and B)

The infection caused by these organisms may stop short at the aseptic meningitis stage already described. However, these viruses can also invade the anterior horn cells, giving rise to a lower motor neurone paralysis (see p. 417). Such a paralysis may dominate the clinical picture; a suspicious preliminary is undue stiffness of the back, so that the seated child cannot kiss his knees. Similarly, he protects himself against pain by holding the trunk rigid, but supported by his outstretched hand—the tripod sign. These signs are, however, common to all meningeal infections.

The cranial nerve nuclei which are liable to attack are those of the 9th and 10th nerves. This leads to difficulty in swallowing saliva, so that respiratory difficulty may ensue. The cells of the spinal cord may also be affected, causing limb paralysis, and more importantly, interference with the respiratory muscles. The muscles so involved may be permanently paralyzed.

Treatment of aseptic meningitis

This follows general lines—relief of dehydration if vomiting has been severe, and relief of headache or respiratory paralysis as in polio or Coxsackie infections, the principles of care are those detailed for the care of Guillain-Barré syndrome (p. 423). Essentially this means sucking out the pharyngeal secretions, endotracheal intubation, and assisted respiration if intercostal and diaphragmatic paralysis is extensive.

Encephalomyelitis

This is the term applied to a disease process of multiple etiology, in which preliminary meningeal symptoms and signs, and all of the causes mentioned under aseptic meningitis can also be associated with encephalomyelitis. Others may have an insect vector. This group will include Australian X disease, Murray Valley encephalitis, and the Japanese and St. Louis types. The encephalitis of rabies is happily unknown in Australia. The exanthems (measles, rubella, chicken pox and small pox), not only may be associated with an early meningo-encephalitis, but may give rise to an encephalitic state in the convalescent period.

Clinical features. The onset is often subacute, and characterized by a history suggestive of meningitis, viz, anorexia, vomiting, irritability, and drowsiness. In many cases the latter predominates and progresses to coma. Convulsions may herald the condition, or occur at any time during it. In those who are not stuporose, confusion, excitement and abnormal behaviour occur.

The neurological deficits are protean. Most commonly these are paralyses of the eye muscles or of speech. Ataxia and upper motor neurone disturbances occur, but each may be fleeting. Lower motor neurone paralysis does not occur. In a few patients, the course is fulminant with deepening coma, a decerebrate state, failure of respiration, hypotension, and death.

The spinal fluid usually reveals a lymphocytosis and increased protein content. Virological and antigen studies may be of value in establishing the exact cause.

Differential diagnosis. This is usually from other causes of coma, confusional states, and focal neurological problems. Principal among the conditions to be considered is poisoning, especially by barbiturates, phenothiazine derivatives, and the tricyclic antidepressants (desipramine, nortryptiline, and amitryptiline). Where confusional and manic states predominate, amphetamine ingestions may be a possibility. Lead encephalopathy may mimic all of the features noted, and stippling of the red cells should be sought, and the urine examined for heavy metals.

In children with meningeal symptoms, tuberculous meningitis will require consideration. A history of exposure, a positive Mantoux reaction, and the CSF signs already described should be sufficient to exclude this and the other pyogenic meningitides. If patchy neurological signs are predominant, poisoning with the organophosphate insecticides may again require exclusion. Central nervous system leukemia usually occurs in the treated leukemic and is seldom a presenting situation.

Treatment. This is largely symptomatic. Most patients require intravenous fluids for several days. When vomiting, or confusional states decrease, nasogastric feeding should begin. Bulbar paralysis or interference with respiration demand pharyngeal suction and nasotracheal intubation. Steroids are of dubious value in any of the encephalomyelitic states.

Progress. Death may occur rapidly from failure of the respiratory centre. Survivors often have mild mental retardation, or learning and behaviour problems.

DEVELOPMENTAL DISORDERS OF THE NERVOUS SYSTEM

Normal development

An ectodermal thickening gives rise to the neural plate, which folds upon itself to form the neural tube which develops in the middle of the embryo and extends in opposite directions (headward and tailward). The neuropores are the points of final closure, and are the areas at which most abnormalities occur. The neural tube becomes surrounded by mesodermal elements. These give rise to the meninges, spine, skull, and the connective fatty and muscle tissues which surround the brain and spinal cord. Congenital defects may involve the tissues developing from the neural tube, or from the mesodermal elements which give rise to its surroundings. Abnormalities from each division may coexist.

Conditions characterized by absence of nervous tissue,

Anencephaly

In this the forebrain, cranium, and part of the scalp are absent. Other lesions, such as meningomyelocele may also be present. The condition is incompatible with life.

Hydranencephaly

In this the cerebral cortex is absent, but the skull is intact. Obstructive hydrocephalus may develop. The infant usually seems normal at birth and the head circumference may then be normal. The sutures are wide open, but the fontanelle does not bulge. Sooner or later, the infant shows poverty of movement, feeds poorly, and may cry a great deal. Hypotonia followed by spasticity is often found—features suggestive of severe cerebral palsy. The head growth fails and a typical cracked pot sound is present on percussion. Transillumination of the skull fails to demonstrate normal cerebral contents. The infant seldom survives more than a few weeks.

Porencephaly

This consists in local defect of the cerebral substance, usually communicating with the ventricle, occasionally with the subdural space. The infant has evidence of hemiplegia, and sometimes focal (Jacksonian) convulsions. The condition can be proved by pneumoencephalography. No specific therapy is available.

Microcephaly

In this condition the brain is markedly underdeveloped. In the *primary* type, the infant appears normal, but the head is noticeably small, its circumference being much less than the chest or crown-rump measurements. The infant fails to attain motor milestones, and shows signs of cerebral palsy. In other babies, the only signs are those of severe intellectual retardation.

Secondary microcephaly follows a variety of insults to the brain, such as fetal anoxia, hypoglycemia, and the aminoacidopathies. Meningitis, intracranial venous thrombosis, and severe malnutrition are relevant in older children. The first 2 may have focal neurological signs; all are associated with varying degrees of intellectual retardation.

Agenesis of the corpus callosum

This is associated with grand mal seizures and evidence of motor and mental retardation. Hydrocephalus may coexist. The condition is demonstrated by pneumoencephalography. No treatment is indicated except for the hydrocephalus.

Absence of other parts of the nervous system, e.g., *arrhinencephaly*, may occur as part of more extensive syndromes (q.v.)

Defects of the structures surrounding the neural tube

Encephalocele

In this condition there is an opening in the skull—cranium bifidum—through which the brain can herniate. The defect is always central and most frequently in the occipital area. Examination shows a midline mass which is usually covered by normal scalp. In some instances, the cranial defect can be repaired.

Meningocele and myelomeningocele

These are the most common serious defects affecting the nervous system. They occur once in every 400-500 births. The lumbar site is the usual one (85%) but the lesion may occur anywhere along the spine. In *meningocele*, there is *spina bifida* through which the membranes of the cord protrude. The fluctuant mass is covered with normal skin, and the cord is in the proper position. There may be no associated neurological problems. Surgical repair is usually quite easy.

In *myelomeningocele*, the spinal cord is adherent to the meningocele, is spread out, and usually abnormal. The sac is covered by a thin membrane, which readily ruptures. Neurological deficit is variable. In many instances there is a complete paraplegia. In others a cauda equina lesion is present, with bladder and bowel paralysis, and perineal anesthesia. There are many with intermediate stages. Most sufferers, however, have paralysis of the bladder and bowels. The former is evidenced by continual dribbling of urine, usually with urinary retention, and the latter by a patulous anus and incontinence of feces. Spontaneous movement of the lower limbs is absent and the Moro reflex is appropriately impaired.

The Arnold-Chiari malformation often coexists with a myelomeningocele. It consists in a projection of the cerebellum, choroid plexus, and 4th ventricle, into a distended cervical canal. The cerebellar tonsils adhere to the foramen magnum. The circulation of spinal fluid is blocked and the malformation is one cause of the hydrocephalus of myelomeningocele. Other causes include aqueductal stenosis and atresia of the foramina of Luschka and Magendie (Dandy-Walker syndrome)

The longer term problems of myelomeningocele are due to the hydrocephalus, the problems of the neurogenic bladder, as well as to the specific neurological deficits. Each will demand its own form of treatment, but a complete cure is seldom if ever attained.

Treatment. The first 24 hours is critical for the avoidance of a fatal meningitis. The thin, neurodermal tissue overlying the defect is easily perforated. Every effort should be made to close the breach as soon as possible. If this is successful the head circumference should carefully be followed because of the likelihood of hydrocephalus. If this develops, it is treated by a ventriculoatrial shunt.

The mother should be taught simple physiotherapy, and instructed in expressing the bladder. She must also be taught the nursing skills necessary to avoid bedsores. The child will require careful orthopedic care, as abnormal muscle action not infrequently causes dislocation of the hips and other ailments. Urinary infection is a constant danger and dilatation of the urinary tract a usual precursor. Intravenous pyelography and cine-cystography are routine investigations early in life. Urinary infection is treated by appropriate chemotherapy, and continuous chemoprophylaxis may be necessary. Dilatation of the ureters or kidney pelvis may require transplantation of the former into an ileal loop, which drains on to the skin. This procedure is done after mature consideration, and by a skilled surgeon. Ileal loops may induce a renal acidosis (q.v.).

The family needs much support and relief of their guilt feelings. The reasons for the frequent surgical manoeuvres should carefully be explained, and the need for occasional placement in hospital to rest the family should be recognized.

Prognosis. This is still guarded. Renal failure due to chronic pyelonephritis is the usual cause of death; in some of these children, respiratory infections are poorly tolerated.

Minor defects

Congenital dermal sinus

These are not very uncommon and consist of skin-lined tubes extending to a variable depth from the surface. A few reach the meningeal layer. In these, the track may provide a route for recurrent meningitis, smaller sinuses may develop superficial infection. The usual site of a dermal sinus is in the lumbosacral or occipital regions.

Spina bifida occulta

This is a common but minor vertebral defect. It causes no symptoms and requires no treatment.

Spinal lipomata

These may coexist with myelomeningocele, or occur alone. Most are subcutaneous, a few are intraspinal and cause a compressive cord lesion.

Congenital arteriovenous fistula

These may occur anywhere in the nervous system, and consist in 1 or 2 large arteries which enter a mass of vessels, which may contain aneurysms, and drain arterialized blood to the veins.

Clinical features. In some infants, the abnormal flow of blood may be so great as to cause cardiac failure, with dyspnea, edema, and cardiomegaly. In others there are localized neurological signs, e.g., hemiplegia, seizures, or raised intracranial pressure. A loud intracranial murmur is readily heard, and the scalp veins are dilated. The condition is confirmed by cerebral arteriography. The treatment is neurosurgical.

Saccular aneurysm of the cerebral vessels

These may be asymptomatic, or cause trouble by enlarging or rupturing. As most aneurysms are in the anterior part of the circle of Willis, enlargement will commonly cause a cavernous sinus syndrome—interference with the function of 3rd and 6th motor and ophthalmic division of 5th sensory cranial nerve. Rupture of the aneurysm is associated with headache, vomiting, meningeal signs, coma, bloody spinal fluid, and retinal hemorrhages. Local neurological signs are also found. Neurosurgical treatment may help, but the prognosis is, in general, not good.

NEUROCUTANEOUS SYNDROMES

These are familial developmental abnormalities of both skin and nervous tissue. There are many of them, but only a few, discussed below, are of clinical importance.

Neurofibromatosis (Von Recklinghausen's disease)

The skin shows café au lait spots and fibromata (simple tumours of connective tissue) which are felt along the subcutaneous nerves. However, common neurological problems are acoustic nerve tumours and 6th and 7th cranial nerve palsies. Lesions within the spine can cause cord compression with associated root pains and paraplegia. A small percentage of sufferers are mentally retarded.

Prognosis. This depends on the site of the tumours since malignant change does not occur. Excision is indicated when local pressure causes symptoms.

Tuberous sclerosis

The usual story is of developmental retardation, progressing to frank mental defect, together with grand mal seizures. By the age of 2, the skin lesions appear. These are yellowish red angiomas (like stork marks in the newborn), which surround the hair follicle. They appear first in the nasolabial folds, and spread to the nose, cheeks, and forehead. Brown (café au lait) patches and pale, unpigmented areas of skin may often also present. The finger- and toe-nails grow slowly and may be deformed. Flat tumours (phakomas) are present in the fundus, and can be seen by ophthalmoscopy. Often the skin problems exist without mental retardation or fits.

Sturge-Weber syndrome

This is a rare congenital disorder. The main feature is a large birth mark on one side of the face (portwine nevus). It is found in the distribution of 1 of the divisions of the trigeminal (5th cranial) nerve. Mental retardation is common, and a hemiplegia on the side opposite to the nevus occurs in 50% of the children. Jacksonian fits are common on the same side as the hemiplegia, with appropriate E.E.G. findings. X-rays will show calcification of the intracranial portion of the nevus. No specific treatment is possible for this condition. Neurosurgery is to be avoided. Anticonvulsants and physiotherapy are prescribed for the fits and hemiplegia.

Incontinentia pigmenti (Block-Sulzberger syndrome)

This rare condition is associated with fits and mental retardation. The skin lesion begins in infancy as red vesicles and bullae, which are followed by wart-like areas in the same distribution. The final stage is a bizarre patterning of brownish pigmentation on the arms, legs and trunk. The nails and teeth are often poorly developed. Grand mal epilepsy is invariable, and moderate mental retardation is usual.

Albinism

In this condition, pigmentation is absent in the skin, hair and other organs. The eyes are pink, and nystagmus, deafness, and mental retardation may occur.

Sjögren-Larsson syndrome

In this, spastic paraplegia coexists with congenital ichthyosis and mental retardation.

PROGRESSIVE DEGENERATIVE DISEASES

These are serious untreatable disorders, mostly due to accumulation of a normal body product because of enzyme deficiency. Common to these disorders is failure of mental development, a cerebral palsy-like state, blindness and dementia.

Table 29 shows some of the possibilities together with an example from each division. These examples will now be described. Refer also to p. 111, 112 for a more detailed consideration of the metabolic disorder.

Table 29. Storage diseases involving the nervous system

Type		Disease Example
A.	Gangliosides	Tay-Sach's disease (amaurotic family idiocy)
B.	Sphingolipids	Gaucher's disease
		Niemann-Pick disease
		Fabry's disease
		Metachromatic leucodystrophy
C.	Miscellaneous:	
	Mucopolysaccharides	Mucopolysaccharidosis (Gargoylism)
	Glycogen	Pompe's disease

Tay-Sachs disease

This is only 1 of 6 possible disorders due to ganglioside accumulation. The disease involves the retina as well as the brain, so it is called a cerebromacular degeneration.

Clinical features. The baby is normal at birth, but within a few months develops poverty of movement, difficulty in feeding and obvious blindness with searching eye movements. At first hypotonic, he becomes increasingly spastic, and soon develops the picture of a severe double hemiplegia, often with bulbar palsy. Ophthalmoscopy reveals a cherry red spot at the macula. Death usually occurs from respiratory infection. A few children survive into the early years of childhood, blind, spastic, and demented.

Gaucher's disease

This is due to a storage of a sphingolipid. The acute infantile form has most of the clinical features of Tay-Sach's disease, including on occasion, the macular cherry red spot. In addition, the liver and spleen are enlarged.

Niemann-Pick disease

This is due to the storage of sphingomyelin. The child deteriorates at the end of the first year, with intellectual regression, progressive upper motor neurone paralysis, and sometimes diabetes insipidus. The liver and spleen are enlarged, and the sphingomyelin can be seen in cells obtained by bone marrow aspiration. There are many variants of the Niemann-Pick disorder, not all of them include central nervous system disease.

Metachromatic Leucodystrophy

This is due to a storage of a lipid derivative called a sulfatide. The symptoms begin in infancy, generally with the onset of clumsiness and ataxia in walking, slurring of speech, and failure of vision. Convulsions and a progressive motor neurone paralysis develop with intellectual deterioration and dementia.

Pompe's disease

This is due to the accumulation of glycogen. The main features are of enlargement of the heart, liver, and spleen, but the brain is damaged by the persistent low blood sugar found in the condition. This causes failure to attain the normal milestones of development and a spastic quadriplegia. Death occurs because of cardiac failure.

Mucopolysaccharidosis

There are many variants of these (see pp. 109, 110). The condition usually presents with failure of normal progress in a child with coarse features. Mental retardation is always present. After a few years the child loses interest in his surroundings, becomes progressively immobile, and ends up as a bedfast dement. Diseases of the heart valves, causing congestive cardiac failure occurs in some of these patients.

OTHER CONDITIONS

Schilder's disease (encephalitis periaxialis diffusa)

This is associated with destruction of the myelin sheath around the nerve fibres.

Clinical features. An early complaint is of deterioration of school performance. The quality and content of speech deteriorate, and emotional upset is common. The child becomes lethargic and develops weakness or paralysis of the limbs. Visual failure is usual and the motor cranial nerves lose function. Convulsions may occur at any stage. Ultimately the child is demented and bedridden, unable to see or swallow and often in a state of decerebrate rigidity. Death soon occurs from respiratory infection.

Treatment. There is no specific help for these children apart from general nursing care.

Subacute sclerosing panencephalitis

This disease appears to be due to a reaction to the virus of measles. Most of the children affected are in the age group 7-10, and measles may have preceded the onset by several years.

Clinical features. The first evidence is of intellectual deterioration, failure of memory, judgment, inattention, and impaired school work. Behaviour problems are common, often with rage reaction and antisocial acts. Characteristically the child develops repetitive stereotyped movements, which usually resemble myoclonic jerks. These recur at regular intervals on the dot. Rapid disintegration of the personality occurs, with intellectual failure, disorientation, and a retreat to inactivity. Sometimes upper motor neurone disorders (spastic hemiplegia) occur, more often poverty of movement, rigidity, and choreoathetotic movements imply involvement of the extrapyramidal system. Eventually the child is bedfast in a state of decerebrate rigidity. Death occurs from respiratory infection.

Special tests. The blood shows high measles antibody titres, and brain biopsy may show inclusion bodies in the cells; this is evidence of viral infection. The E.E.G. shows high voltage waves which are regularly repeated and coincide with the stereotyped myoclonic jerks which occur in the patient.

Treatment. None is possible.

19 Disorders of speech

These are common in childhood, and must always be taken seriously. The development of speech is as follows. The crying of the infant begins at birth, and is a primitive, almost reflex action, which has little emotional content. At the age of 8 weeks, on the average, the infant coos, again with the simplest of emotional content—usually pleasure, and without any sense of communication. Babbling begins by the age of 6 months, and some precocious infants are able to parrot single words by 8 or 9 months. There is little doubt that meaning is absent from their utterances at this age. At 1 year, single words are distinctly spoken in the correct context—speech is no longer mere imitation. However, communication is less reliant upon speech in the adult sense, and gesture and intelligent anticipation are still largely relied upon. By the age of 18 months, or 2 years (the variation is noteworthy), the child is capable of simple sentences of 2- or 3-word content, sufficient usually to fill his needs, though not his emotional fulfilment. Most normal children have 2-3-word speech by 2½ years at the latest. By the age of 2, the child's vocabulary is used entirely for self, in the widest sense of the word and without purpose of influencing others. This "selfishness" is shortlived in normal children, and as his ideas increase in complexity, so too does his vocabulary. The 3-year old, in a sense, becomes a politician. He no longer holds his breath in protest against society, he expresses his protest verbally. Between the ages of 4 and 6 years, the vocabulary has increased, skill in expressing ideas is gained, and emotion is less and less the sole mode of self-expression. At school-age and later the ability to communicate verbally is consolidated, and becomes more complex.

It is clear from the above that speech difficulties may have a variety of causes. Since speech is the expression of ideational capacity, it will fail when such capacity is wanting. Thus, the child who is *mentally defective* will be slow to speak, and the content of his speech will always be limited. More subtle perhaps is the problem of the child who, while possessing ideational capacity, does not have the motor ability to express his ideas. This is epitomized by the patient who has *cerebral palsy*. This child, characterized perhaps by poverty of movement, and delayed motor development, may yet be able to communicate, although speech may be not only delayed, but imperfect and difficult to understand.

In this situation, the problem may be one of *dysarthria*—the patient has imperfect motor control or poor feedback to his motor centres from the larynx. If he has essentially a *cerebellar defect*, his speech is monotonous and devoid of the normal emotional overtones; if he is spastic, his speech may be initiated by obvious effort, be explosive and dysrhythmic, be swallowed or come to a convulsive halt. The content of the speech is, however, sensible and directed to some purpose.

In the early stages of development, speech is purely imitative, and this, as far as accent is concerned remains a powerful influence until well into adult life. Therefore, the *deaf* child will manifest a speech defect. He will coo, and babble, but, if his hearing loss is more than about 60 decibels he will seldom achieve single-word speech. It is important to realize that the deaf child must be found early. His sole hope of achieving normal speech is early lip reading and skilled speech instruction. Typically the deaf child is of normal intelligence, active, inquisitive, and self-sufficient for his age. He pays no attention to spoken commands *if he cannot see the lips of the speaker*. If he can, his degree of insight into what is expected of him may be extraordinary and may baffle the innocent examiner. Audiometry reveals the true state of affairs. Above all, the deaf child, albeit sometimes emotionally disturbed, can communicate; this ability distinguishes him from his mentally defective peer. If his hearing loss is partial, the deaf child has a monotonous metallic voice with little emotional overtone. Speech, to him, is strictly a mode of ideational communication, not necessarily an emotional one. Deafness may be more subtle than merely the absence of adequate auditory equipment, thus the child, apparently of normal intelligence, and possessed of communicative ability in modes other than speech may be suffering from *auditory* (*sensory*) *aphasia*; such a child hears what is said (as audiomentry proves), he does not, however, recognize the significance of what is said to him. Accordingly, he may be capable, as is a parrot, of repeating words (more rarely 2 or 3 words), but he is to all intents and purposes suffering from a speech defect. Equally he may recognize the significance of voices, but since he does not recognize ideas from verbal expression from others, he does not in turn generate the ability to communicate his ideas by normal speech. He does so in some other way, usually by a speech variant (*idioglossia*) which is often like baby talk, with imperfect formation of the consonants. These are the keys to the diagnosis. He is not deaf, he is not unintelligent, he has motor verbal capacity; he does not use it, except at best to parrot the interrogator; if he can do so, it is likely that he has indeed a sensory aphasia. Such a child performs well in intelligence tests of the nonverbal type. He may learn spontaneously to lip read.

The child with *expressive aphasia* of the inborn type has normal milestones of development. His speech is delayed, and may consist of a few words, often with consonantal difficulties. This child responds to spoken commands. He cannot, however, return in speech any ideational cue, verbal or otherwise, of the examiner. He seeks another mode of expression, but except in those who have learned to write, ideational expression is limited. Expressive aphasia is often the result of infections of, or injuries to, the central nervous system.

The child, however, may have none of the disorders mentioned and yet his speech may be imperfect and socially unacceptable. Thus, a sufferer from *cleft palate*, especially one which has been neglected as far as speech therapy is concerned, has a voice which is monotonous, nasal, and unpleasing. The history is clear, and the local examination diagnostic. *Cluttering* of speech is common enough in early school life, and is epitomized by spoonerisms. These usually clear up spontaneously as the child learns adequately to monitor his speech. *Stuttering* and *stammering* are clearly due to faulty feedback and monitoring of speech. However, although the mode of faulty control is obvious enough, the cause of this faulty mode is not fully understood. Clearly enough, stuttering is more common in the nervous child, although whether the nervousness is primary or secondary to the speech defect is obscure. In any case, stuttering and stammering are the commonest speech defects occurring in children of normal intelligence and capacity. The problem is too well known to deserve clinical description.

The child who has demonstrated both intellectual and verbal capacity and then ceases so to do presents a not unusual problem. In most cases this is the result of an emotional impasse. The child is too shocked or terrified to speak. This is not unusual after hospitalization, especially for relatively painful procedures, e.g., tonsillectomy. More subtle is the schizophrenic (autistic) child, who has communicated normally and then withdraws from society. The failure of speech parallels this withdrawal. This child is alone, has little or no commerce with anyone, although he may for some time satisfactorily carry out the more negative functions of life—he may demand food, comfort, and general attention. His progress is, however, a withdrawal from normal life, and often a preoccupation with skills which are useless in a general context. He may ultimately resemble a mentally defective child.

All of the syndromes mentioned have been given equal importance. They should, however, be weighted in the diagnostic balance. Thus, mental defect is common, and infantile autism (schizophrenia) is rarer. Deafness is relatively common, and expressive aphasia unusual. Transient refusal to speak after hospitalization is not unusual; and unrecognized cerebral palsy presenting with a speech defect *is* unusual. How then does the pediatrician investigate the child with a speech difficulty; he recognizes first of all that there is a wide variation in individual achievement of speech. He does not, however, send the mother away totally reassured. He recognizes that speech defects may occasionally be subtle. He recognizes that a child who does not speak by the age of 2½ is abnormal. Local problems, e.g., cleft palate, are obvious enough, as are stammering and stuttering. More difficult is the problem of the deaf child whose acquired sharpness demands equally demanding clinical cunning. A basic question is, can this child communicate by means other than verbal? If he can, and if the rest of the examination is in keeping, then he probably does not suffer from mental defect. This is a critical diagnostic watershed, and should stimulate the examiner to fresh effort. Has the child *ever* normally used speech? If he has, then emotional insult, or autism should be sought for. Is the child intelligent (by nonverbal criteria), but yet does not speak? If so, he may again be deaf, or he may be aphasic, or has he had a recent cerebrovascular accident? Is the child deprived of normal opportunities for speech? These are the main approaches which are helpful.

TREATMENT AND PROGNOSIS

These are clearly dependent upon the cause. The most soluble of the problems described are those occurring in the normally intelligent, with fundamental motor ability. Thus the deaf will respond well to lip reading and speech therapy. The sensory aphasic can be taught to appreciate nonverbal cues so that they may appear normal. The expressive aphasic, although apparently taciturn, will learn (or be taught) other methods of intellectual intercourse, even including, perhaps at a third-hand level, the ability to speak; the institutionalized child, to whom no-one has talked will respond rapidly to schooling. The child who maintains infantile speech under the influence of doting parents will respond to parental discipline. In the cerebral palsied child, the outlook is less propitious. Here innate intelligence is the *sine qua non*, and may partially overcome dysarthria, or provide the drive for the acquisition of verbal trick movements.

20 Educational difficulties

Difficulties with education are important problems in children, because of the preoccupation of parents with the child's results at school, and the difficulty of placing unsuccessful students in the jobs of an industrialized society.

In infancy, the process of learning begins by imitating the rest of the family. Thus is acquired speech and certain behaviour patterns. Motor skills, especially fine manipulative movements, are similarly achieved, and constant practice and play are important components of success. So too is praise for achievement—given almost subconsciously by most mothers. The family also determines the child's acceptance of discipline and inculcates certain modes of social behaviour such as toilet training. In the early years, the orientation of the child is entirely towards the family, but by the fourth year he begins to look outside it for stimulation. At the sixth year, the child's interests are well diffused beyond the family and he will readily accept a new environment and wider variety of experience, thus he is ready for conventional schooling. There are, however, certain prerequisites which are necessary for educational success. These are the ability to receive information, ideational capacity, and the ability to express information. Success at school may then be denied those who have imperfect vision or hearing. Intellectual retardation will affect primarily the ability to relate facts, although reception and expression are usually also impaired. Lack of adequate expressive abilities may be general or specific. The latter relates more commonly to the required feats of reading and writing. Psychological factors act potently for educational success. These imply a willingness to receive the educational process, to see in it something of value for the individual, and to accept the changed social and interpersonal relationships which occur in school.

From these general statements, it is possible to predict, and sometimes to prevent, difficulties with education. Ideally, each child should be examined before he enters school, thus visual and hearing difficulties may be found and corrected.

If the child has actually gone to school, and the parents are concerned, the first thing is to assess their expectations. Some parents set unattainable goals for normal children. Failure to achieve these is not an educational difficulty. If however the complaint is genuine, then the facts should be confirmed with the school teacher. If the history suggests that the child is deficient in all areas of achievement, then mental retardation is a possibility, or a general immaturity of a degree which prevents the child from taking advantage of school. In the latter instance, the ability to communicate is usually appropriate to age, but the child is shy, distractible, or too readily moved to tears. In the former, milestones of development are usually slowed, the ability to communicate has emerged late, and speech is imperfect in mode and content. Distractibility and anxiety are common in retarded pupils, and may be the presenting complaints. If further testing reveals the I.Q. to be 75 or less, the child is usually unacceptable for conventional schooling and should be tried in ungraded opportunity classes.

The examination should include specific assessment of vision and hearing as well as a search for organic disease. The latter is not always directly relevant in school failure unless the central nervous system is involved. Thus sufferers from disorders such as congenital heart disease often do well enough at school, their principal problem being inability to keep up through frequent absence.

It is important to assess the child's ability to speak intelligibly since this is an essential in modern education. The child may be intelligent enough but the retention of an infantile speech pattern does not favour education. Such patients generally have no organic basis for their disorder, although consideration may have to be given to aphasia. Children with speech disorders are rather prone also to have reading difficulties.

SOME SPECIFIC PROBLEMS

Reading disability

This is common, being more frequent in boys than in girls. It is of relatively small importance in first grade, except as it may reflect a general level of underachievement. Many first graders memorize parts of the reading book and may not really learn to recognize words until near the end of the first school year. Reading disability is generally present if the child is 2 years below his nominal grade. The common findings are persistence of the errors of the first grader. Thus reversals (strephrosymbolia) are common such as "saw" for "was" and "ton" for "not"; equally common are misinterpretations of words having a different meaning but a superficially similar spelling, e.g., "roof" and "rough". Specific tests of reading comprehension are usually also impaired, although occasionally poor readers may perform quite well in these.

Dyslexia

This is the name applied to significant reading disability which is present after 4-5 years of conventional education. Basic reading skills are absent, but other educational areas have been mastered. These children have normal I.Q's and do well on the performance items of intelligence tests, but poorly on the verbal items.

True dyslexia is not a common cause of reading disability. Often enough the child so labelled is mildly retarded, or has behaviour problems inimical to education. Clumsiness, insecurity about right/left orientations, and minor anxiety states are found in the dyslexic child—but also in successful readers.

Treatment of reading disability

If this is an isolated difficulty, special classes are indicated. These usually allow a degree of individual attention to the pupil, with careful correction of his errors, and drilling in specific recognition procedures. Thus, there is an opportunity for praise to be given, which builds the child's confidence in a way unlikely to be achieved in the open class.

If the reading disability is superimposed upon a speech difficulty, the latter should be treated first, and remedial reading classes should follow. A switch from the look-and-say, to the older fashioned phonetic methods of learning to read will often be of benefit.

Difficulties with writing

These are closely allied to speech difficulties. In the ordinary way, however, much less is made of them. This is perhaps because early writing skills are the formation of symbols by copying. In the early school grades, confusion between similarly shaped letters (d,b) is common, as are more complex perversions such as mirror writing. The dyslexic child may show the same errors at a late stage. In older children, inability to express ideation or integration of knowledge in writing usually reflects the same disability in the verbal mode. Each may be a complication of an acquired disorder such as encephalitis or head injury. Rarely, writing difficulties reflect minor mental retardation. Children who stammer or clutter may show minor writing errors but these do not interfere with the ability to *communicate* by writing.

Arithmetical difficulties

These also may coincide with reading difficulties. Particularly common in early grades are the arithmetical analogs of strephosymbolia, i.e., failure to recognize that some verbal equivalents of numbers read left to right (as in 55), and some from right to left (as in 17). This leads to confusion in the cardinal concept of numbers, and hence to difficulties in arithmetical handling.

A total lack of ability in arithmetical handling may raise the suspicion of intellectual retardation, especially if there is evidence that the parents have drilled the child in the other more conventional skills of reading (usually by memorizing), and verbal expression. Arithmetical disabilities are perhaps more common in children with cerebral palsy, who may otherwise perform fairly well. In the intellectually normal, individual attention at school, and extra assignments supervised by the parents, is commonly helpful.

Lack of acceptance of the school situation

This is a fairly common problem in the early school years. It frequently (though not invariably) is associated with poor progress in learning. Characteristically the child has a low attention span, interrupts the routine by inappropriate talking, or may wander about the class interfering with the education of others. Others may react with ready tears or silent withdrawal from the education system. The distractible interrupters may be intellectually retarded and often have a previous history suggestive of this. The withdrawn weeper is in general more likely to have emotional rather than intellectual problems. These are generalizations. Intellectually retarded children also have emotional problems when under normal school pressures. In the absence of retardation, a history of inappropriate dependence on the mother is often found. Shyness and stunting of social initiative often coincide. Such children take time to identify with the teacher, and may benefit from going to school a few months later than their peers. In persistent problems, reassurance of the parents, explanation to the teacher, and discussion with the child about school routines and situations usually suffice to make education acceptable.

The overactive, noisy, interrupting behaviour problem child is much more difficult to treat, primarily because he disrupts the school routine and exasperates teachers. If the intellect is normal, removal from grade school and placement in the less demanding kindergarten situation is often beneficial. If the behaviour disorder is persistent, psychiatric help is necessary. The frequency of the problem is such that many education authorities organize special classes for its treatment. Full use of these should be made.

There are many other conditions which may interrupt the acceptance of school. Undoubtedly the teasing of a child by his mates may cause considerable distress. Sometimes this is related to a physical peculiarity (e.g., obesity, hair colour, nevus) or to an antisocial habit such as enuresis or encopresis. Children vary in their acceptance of teachers, and vice versa. While these factors are perhaps more commonly a cause of school phobia, they also, in aggregate, interfere substantially with schooling. The treatment is that of the primary condition if this is possible, together with appropriate reassurance. In the case of an insoluble antipathy between child and teacher, a change of class (or even of school) is usually curative.

Learning difficulties in the later years

These are not very uncommon, and generally are reflected as a poor *comparative* performance, rather than as specific problems. The complaint is frequently parental—"He is bottom of the class". This situation reflects essentially the child's innate intellectual abilities, whatever the results of the formal I.Q. tests. Some children undoubtedly reach their ceiling at the end of the primary school career and have difficulty in approaching the standards needed for secondary education. This situation must be looked at realistically by both physician and parents, especially if the latter are ambitious for their children. Usually the school authority has a good idea of the educational prognosis for secondary education, and its opinion should always be sought. A pupil without talent for an academic type of education should be guided towards a school which is less demanding intellectually. Failure to do so often will result in later anxiety states, and exaggeration of the normal difficulties of adolescents.

A child who has previously done well at school and who suddenly deteriorates, is a diagnostic challenge. Such a complaint demands a full history and physical examination. Most children so afflicted have an emotional disorder, although physical illness such as diabetes, renal disease, and so on, are occasionally found. In most instances the upset is temporary and reflects some disturbance within the family. In the adolescent, boredom in the talented, or reaction to an academically hostile family environment may be the root of the problem. Discussion may reveal that the child no longer sees any motivation for passing examinations. This is particularly common in groups against whom job discrimination is practised. The lack of motivation then becomes logical, and is curable only by a change in society.

Sudden failure at school, together with a change in the pattern of social activity and withdrawal from the family is a pattern always to be taken seriously. A deep emotional problem may be present, or the child may have been introduced to habituating drugs. Close enquiry should always be made into the latter possibility.

In the later years of secondary education a not uncommon problem is a variance between the child's abilities and desires and the ambitions of the parents. Thus we find a parent determined that the child will go to university, often at some sacrifice to the family. The child tries to please the parents in the earlier years of secondary schooling. This desire may break down as the school pressures increase and as the child emerges as a separate personality. The impasse may be met by school failure. The physician has an important role in resolving such conflicts of interest, although the resolution is usually a matter of some delicacy.

Essentially similar types of problems occur in the first year of tertiary education. The change from the discipline of secondary education to the freedom of a university may be too great for relatively immature students. Study habits become faulty, and anxiety/depressive states coincide with the stresses of examinations or with failure.

21 Mental and emotional problems

BEHAVIOUR AND ITS DISORDERS

There is much variation in the behaviour of children, as well as considerable differences in the acceptance of behaviour in the various cultures and social classes. In considering behaviour disorders, it is then necessary to have some idea of what parents believe to be acceptable, since their ideas of abnormality may represent undue conservatism, or unreasonable fears.

PROBLEMS IN INFANCY AND EARLY CHILDHOOD

Repetitive movements

These are common, and are frequent, stereotyped, voluntary actions. The usual variants are head rolling; head banging; and, in the older infant, rocking movements of the body. In normal children these repetitive movements are usually seen just before sleep. If of short duration, they are of little moment. Persistent repetitive movements are seen in lonely, often hospitalized, children, and also in older, retarded children. These movements clearly give the child a feeling of security. Many other movements such as hair curling or ear tweaking do the same thing.

Binkie syndrome

This is where the child, usually before going to sleep, plays with the edge of a blanket, and simultaneously sucks the thumb, strokes the hair, or makes some other repetitive movement. Most normal children grow out of it by the age of 2 or 3 years. It perhaps becomes pathological only if the child refuses to leave the house without the blanket, or goes out to play with a bit of it tied to his sleeve. However, even these actions should not be overemphasized. They are perhaps only a stimulus to enquire into any disturbing situation in the environment. Reversion to the binkie syndrome in the older child is common enough in conditions of stress such as changing homes or on first going to school.

Thumb sucking

This is normal and usually stops spontaneously by the age of 5 or 6 years. There is no known treatment for this condition. It is usual for the skin of the thumb to become thickened in the accomplished thumb sucker. Parents should be reassured concerning this habit. Reversion to thumb sucking in older children may occasionally indicate some anxiety-producing factor.

Nail biting

This is almost as universal as thumb sucking, although it usually does not appear until the child is 3 or more years of age. The habit is often learned either from the parents or other children. The older preoccupied nail biter usually reflects an anxiety-producing situation. The symptom reflects the child's struggle to come to terms with his environment and disappears as the child achieves an appropriate level of confidence.

Night terrors

There are few children who do not show evidence of anxiety. Even the child who is most phlegmatic during the day, may have night terrors. A typical attack is where a 2- or 3-year old wakes up screaming and is found in an obvious state of terror, with widely dilated pupils, sweating, and tachycardia. The most distressing thing to the parents is that he is quite oblivious of their presence, or their attempts to comfort him. The attack may last for 10 or 15 minutes. The child will then suddenly go back to bed and wakes up without any memory of the incident. Such episodes are usually quite normal, sometimes they appear to be induced by a memory of external incidents, in other cases there is no obvious cause. Reassurance of the parents is all the treatment that is necessary.

Somnambulism

In this the child, as part of his night terror, is found wandering about the house, often in a confused state, and sometimes carrying out well-known movements such as trying to get to the toilet. He cannot be readily aroused. Normally these children readily return to bed and wake without memory of the incident. Again, only reassurance is needed.

Pica (dirt eating)

This is not very uncommon in normal children, and early in life it is part of the exploration of his environment. Most children, however, learn from the mother that dirt eating is unacceptable, and stop doing it after a week or two. Continued dirt eating may reflect loneliness, or emotional deprivation. The importance of the condition lies in the possibility of ingesting noxious materials. Pica is a common cause of lead poisoning, usually by flaking paint. Pica may also occur in the mentally retarded. Treatment is difficult in the established disorder but definite efforts on the part of the mother to keep him company and to distract him with toys or by the company of other children is usually sufficient to break the cycle.

Negativism

This means persistent refusal of the child to do what the parents want him to do, especially in relation to such matters as food, toilet training, and general behaviour. Negativism seems to be a fairly normal part of behavioural development, but complaints about it usually emerge about the age of 2 years, sooner if the child has been an early walker. It seems not very uncommon that some mothers are quite incapable of jollying along, or distracting their children, and tend to achieve parental ends by premature punishment. This in most instances aggravates the situation. *Refusal to eat* is the most common form of negativism and, characteristically begins after the first birthday, usually in association with the child's initial efforts at self-feeding. It is common in first children, perhaps because the mother has not been made to realize that the child's appetite suffers a normal decline from the age of 9 months. Many mothers are brainwashed into believing that a good appetite is a sign of absolute health, and will spend many hours in forcing the child to achieve a food intake which is entirely unreasonable. Thus meals become battlefields of emotion, with the bowels of each party rumbling in discord. Some parents become so obsessed about the child's appetite that they will devise extraordinary punishment or rewards for a satisfactory performance. The treatment of this condition lies principally in finding out what are the parents criteria of their own success in rearing the child. Frequently enough it will be found that these are unreasonable and undesirable. If this is pointed out firmly enough, the whole situation will amend itself. Many parents fear that their children are not growing properly, and this may be the real reason for the mealtime battle. The most effective method of dealing with this fallacy is to examine the child thoroughly, weigh it, measure it, and demonstrate the normal percentiles to the parents. Otherwise, the food should be put down in front of the child, and he should be left to eat it, or not. Some respect, however, should be maintained for the child's food preferences, otherwise no other action is necessary. The physician should refuse parental requests for an appetite stimulant. Such a prescription weakens the main therapeutic endeavour which is to change the attitudes of the parents and the child towards food, and to break the impasse which has developed between them.

Other forms of negativism may reflect merely the child's desire to be left alone to do something for himself, rather than to live in an atmosphere of permanent regimentation. Frequently the complaints of negativism are associated with undue amounts and levels of punishment for the child, and it is wise always to discuss this aspect with the parents. Reasonable parents will punish children seldom and most realize that it is a last resort and that the child should receive the punishment as close as possible to the crime.

Refusal to go to bed or to sleep is a form of negativism which may reflect worry. Little children are readily affected by their peers or by older children, with fear of the dark. Their imagination can see in harmless shadows on the bedroom wall, a monster which terrifies them. They are sometimes very reticent about their problems, especially if fear has been put to them as something which is shameful rather than natural. The physician, nurse, and the parents, should try and enquire into what can be causing fear of bed and sleep. If the cause is not obvious, then a night light, the company of another child, or a favourite dog, may be all that is necessary to effect the cure.

Breath-holding spells

This is a common functional disorder of children. It is well recognized by mothers, and most children with them probably never seek help. The condition may begin in the first few weeks of life, but more commonly it begins between 6 and 12 months.

Clinical features. Breath-holding spells, unlike epilepsy, have a specific precipitating factor. Usually this is frustration by the parent or sibling of some desired activity, or pain, e.g., catching a finger in a door. In the usual case, immediately following the cause, the child sobs briefly takes a few deep breaths, and then ceases to breathe. He becomes cyanosed but in most cases recovers quickly. The children who reach medical care are those who proceed to fall and to stiffen—often assuming an opisthotonic posture. The eyes roll up and twitching may occur. There is no postictal sleep, and the child is normal within a few minutes. In most children where trauma is the precipitating cause, crying may be absent, and pallor more common than cyanosis. Neither variety ever occurs during sleep.

Progress. The condition is self-limited, usually disappearing with the acquisition of verbal facility. When the child can answer back the breath holding stops.

Treatment. Reassurance is all that is necessary. If the mother wishes, the attack can usually be terminated by sprinkling cold water on the child's face.

CONDITIONS IN THE OLDER CHILD

Trichotillomania

This means that the child constantly plays with the hair, pulls it out, and very often chews it. Areas of baldness result. Trichotillomania is probably an extension of the earlier repetitive habits which have been referred to, but occurs at a much later age, e.g., up to 8 years. It may reflect emotional deprivation and loneliness, or may be the product of a specific anxiety-producing situation such as change of school, or home, or differences between the parents. Trichotillomania is not easy to cure, and demands fairly searching review of the child's whole environment, both at school and at home. Treatment should consist in removing, if possible, sources of anxiety and in diverting the child from the habit.

Other problems

Other anxiety states and minor phobias are common in children; most are transient. Common examples are fear of the dark, fear of dogs, and other large animals, and fear of driving in cars. The latter may be associated with motion sickness or relate to previous involvement in a traffic accident. Much patience is necessary in overcoming these phobias if they are deeply seated enough to interfere with the child's ordinary activity or process of education. Nothing can be achieved by the equivalent of throwing them in at the deep end. The child's fears should be respected and he should be introduced to the objective of the phobia with the greatest care and delicacy.

Undifferentiated anxiety states such as sweating, tachycardia, and pain over the heart, occur most commonly in the schoolchild, and in the adolescent. Occasionally these are traceable to the death of a relative, with injudicious parental discussion. More commonly they reflect differences at school or in the home. Psychic and physical symptoms may coexist, of which the commonest are habit spasms, and the syndrome of pain in the limbs or pain in the belly (see below).

Habit spasms (tic)

These are repetitive responses to tension, the pattern of movement being variable. Common movements are grimacing, blinking, head tossing, shoulder shrugging, and limb movements. Each of these can voluntarily be stopped, or disappear if the child is diverted. They do not occur during sleep. The principal differential diagnosis is from Sydenham's chorea, in which the movements are involuntary and aggravated by directions to cease them.

Treatment. As far as possible the action should be ignored and the child reassured. Tension-producing situations should be relieved if possible.

Pain-in-the-limbs syndrome

This most commonly occurs between 2 and 10 years of age. The child is otherwise well, but the parents may note that the condition precedes psychic strain, e.g., examinations. The pains are not severe enough to cause limping, may last only a few minutes, and seldom occur at night. The joints are never involved, and fever is absent.

Characteristically, the symptom is relieved by parental attention such as rubbing the painful areas. This is the leading clue to the functional nature of the disorder.

Differential diagnosis. This is mainly from trauma and unaccustomed exercise.

Treatment. This is mostly reassurance, and may require to be preceded by some laboratory investigations, especially to quiet the fears of some parents concerning rheumatic fever. The fact that the child is seeking attention and reassurance is usually quite acceptable to parents. In most instances, search of the environment for precipitating causes is unrewarding. The prognosis is good.

Pain-in-the-belly syndrome

This also is a common functional disorder of children, and is found from early childhood to adolescence.

Clinical features. The onset of pain is irregular, and may occur in the day or evening. It seldom, however, wakens the child from sleep, although a wakeful child may experience the symptoms. The location is vague, and usually described as near the belly button; the severity is variable, normally it is of mild degree. The attack may last a few minutes and seldom exceeds an hour. The child may go for weeks without symptoms. Sometimes the pains are clearly relatable to stressing circumstances, or are part of refusal to go to school. Other complaints such as anorexia and vomiting are distinctly unusual.

Physical examination is usually negative, although epigastric tenderness, *without rigidity* may occasionally be present. The child is usually in the normal percentiles for growth; occasionally individual characteristics which distinguish him from the herd are present—obesity, unusual height for age, or other physical peculiarity.

Differential diagnosis. This is very wide. The principal lesion suspected or worried about by the parents is appendicitis. This latter is usually, however, associated with vomiting and pain, which, although initially umbilical, invariably shifts from it.

Another common differential diagnosis is an active *gastrocolic reflex*. This is not very uncommon in the younger child, who develops mild colicky pain after eating. This is often followed by defecation. This last, and the close relationship to eating, suffice to make the diagnosis.

Treatment. Both parents and child should be reassured that true disease is absent. The patient should not, however, be labelled as neurotic. As many children have had their symptoms for many months, some parents can only be convinced by investigations. In the nature of things, stool examination and urinalysis may be all that is necessary. The family and school environment should be explored for problems which unduly worry the child. Inevitably the question as to when medical attention should be sought will be brought up by the parents. To this it is wise to answer that help should be obtained if the pain is different in site or character, or is associated with vomiting.

Cyclical vomiting

This condition is not a very common problem. It is characterized by recurrent attacks of vomiting which may last for several days, and for which no organic cause can be found. There is anorexia, but no abdominal pain, except the muscular variety due to the vomiting. Ketosis is constant, and clinical dehydration not uncommon. Between attacks the child seems perfectly normal.

Differential diagnosis. Care must be taken to exclude the ingestion of toxic substances, and conditions causing a rise in intracranial pressure.

Treatment. The attacks are most readily aborted by giving the child a prompt intravenous drip. Antiemetics (given by rectum) are of varying utility.

Masturbation

This is common in children, and is very common in adolescent males. It is much less common in females. The process may begin in early infancy (around 6-8 months) and takes many patterns; obviously, however, the activity must be one which causes genital stimulation and a pleasurable response.

In infants and young children, manual manipulation is unusual. Sexual excitation is commonly obtained by rhythmic leg and thigh movements. The child is preoccupied during these, resents interference, and becomes red in the face. The process is terminated by a general somatic relaxation and sometimes by sleep. In older children, the practice is usually carried out in private, since the child early becomes aware of the social disapproval of masturbation. Public masturbation is usually found to be associated with intellectual retardation.

Treatment. In infants, diversion to some other activity is all that is necessary. Public masturbation in the older child should actively be discouraged, and should stimulate a search for neurotic and/or intellectual disorder. Reassurance is otherwise all that is necessary, especially for the adolescent.

THE HYPERKINETIC (HYPERACTIVE) CHILD

This is a not uncommon functional disorder in children.

Clinical features. The child may have been restless, irritable, and sleepless as an infant. When he learns to walk he has boundless energy, is always in mischief, and refuses the afternoon nap characteristic of his age group. The child is impatient, and often wilful and destructive of toys. His efforts tend to have few goals and as he is easily distractible, his primary school progress is poor. Indeed his overactivity may totally disrupt discipline in his class.

Etiology. Some sufferers are found to be mildly intellectually retarded, in others the hyperactivity is associated with epilepsy. Children who have had encephalitis (especially perhaps that of measles) may also suffer similarly. In many instances however, the child is found to be physically and intellectually normal. Hyperactivity is occasionally a sign of intolerance of drugs, especially phenobarbitone.

Treatment. The parents should be told that the child is not malevolent, but has, so to speak, an illness. In general stimulating situations involving much exposure to other children or strange adults, should be kept to a minimum. Discipline is not abandoned but should be consistent. Special attention, or on occasion special classes, is necessary at school. Drug therapy may be indicated.

SERIOUS ANTISOCIAL BEHAVIOUR

This is a common problem in older children, especially boys. Theft is the most common error, but cruelty to animals or other children, arson, and wilful destruction of property are also not unusual.

In some instances the child is found to be moderately or marginally mentally retarded. In most the school performance is poor, and truancy common. The child may be neglected, be the product of a broken home, or in some instances, have suffered physical abuse from the parents. In many situations, however, no particular precipitating factor is found. Antisocial behaviour is, however, a warning to enquire into the possibilities outlined above, and may coexist with addiction.

In stealing, a major problem is the stimulation of the child's desire to own property at a level beyond his financial ability. This, and envy of his wealthier peers, can lead to shoplifting, car stripping, and so on. In many such instances, police action is necessary, and often he becomes a recidivist, the prognosis then becomes gloomier and the possibility of rehabilitation more difficult.

Treatment. Such children should always be given a thorough social and psychological evaluation. In this way, treatable situations may be uncovered, and faulty parental attitudes corrected.

DRUG ADDICTION IN CHILDREN

This is a growing problem especially in adolescents. Occasional drug taking may be reckoned with occasional smoking—as a further exploration of the process of growing up. Persistent addiction may reflect the insecurities of a broken home, accompany strongly antisocial activities, or merely be a reflection of a psychopathic personality. It is clear that some forms of drug addiction are essentially iatrogenic; that is, in a suitable circumstance or personality, a drug used originally for a therapeutic effect leads to dependence, and finally to addiction. The line between dependence and addiction is a fine one.

The commoner forms of addiction are the inhalation of hydrocarbons (petrol, glue solvents, cleaning fluid), the ingestion of amphetamines, barbiturates, and the hallucinogens (e.g., L.S.D.); the use of marihuana and opiates is more commonly found in the older adolescent, although exploratory experiences are not infrequent in younger children.

Addiction to solvents

The commoner agents employed are petrol, toluene (in polystyrene glues) and cleaning fluids. The child may initially have accidentally inhaled the product, or may have been introduced to it by others.

Clinical features. In a few instances, the first sign is that the patient is found dead beside the container. In others, the symptoms resemble acute alcoholic intoxication with reckless and psychotic behaviour. Hallucination may be a spontaneous complaint. Tolerance and dependence occur fairly rapidly, but there are no specific withdrawal symptoms.

Amphetamine addiction

This may be a difficult diagnosis to make. The condition occurs in the older adolescent, and occasionally in younger children given amphetamines for therapeutic purposes. The signs are those of sympathetic stimulation, i.e., dilated pupils, dry mouth, tachycardia, finger tremor, and talkativeness. All of these of course are found in genuine mild anxiety states. However, examination of the urine for amphetamine end products will indicate whether the patient has actually taken these drugs. Occasionally such a patient will present with withdrawal symptoms, principally sleepiness and depression. Coexistent barbiturate habituation may accompany amphetamine addiction.

The hallucinogens

The principal of these is L.S.D. (lysergic diethylamide), a synthetic product. Vegetable products, e.g., laburnum seeds, may also produce similar effects. The features are rather similar to those found in glue sniffing, e.g., acute hallucinosis; paranoid symptoms occur, and efforts at self-destruction are not uncommon. Relatively few children have been reported to be addicted, but many must have had at least a single experience of the drug.

General casefinding

Addiction is more common in antisocial children. Accordingly, special care should be taken to screen admissions to remand homes for evidence of drug addiction.

General care of drug addiction

Prevention. This largely lies in the hands of parents who should at least normally expect to know where their children are and who their friends are. Similarly, the prescription of potentially addictive drugs, especially the anorectics, should be avoided in children. A placebo (e.g., calcium lactate tablet) is often adequate suggestive therapy in obesity. If an addicted child is found he should be admitted to hospital and *carefully watched* so that he does not obtain access to any drugs (especially barbiturates prescribed for other patients). A complete pediatric work up for possible side effects, e.g., anemia in petrol sniffing, should be followed by urgent referral to the child psychiatric service. The therapy thereafter is on an individual basis, with especial reference to the social circumstances.

NEUROSES OF CHILDHOOD

The most common of these are anxiety states. Some aspects of these have already been touched upon, especially as they affect the younger child. Florid anxiety states are more common in the adolescent, who may have somatic symptoms such as sweating, tachycardia, and diarrhea. These children admit usually to a general sense of fear concerning many things—examinations, school progress, relationships with the opposite sex, masturbation, and so on. Restlessness and difficulty in falling asleep, or early wakefulness are also common. Poor progress at school, hostility to his peers, and withdrawal to a narrow stereotyped life are less common, but perhaps more serious symptoms. There may be historical evidence of earlier anxiety symptoms.

In many, the anxiety reaction is an exaggeration of the normal inquietude of the adolescent. This may have occurred through undue parental pressure concerning school progress, some unfortunate social contretemps, or a misunderstanding of a normal bodily function.

In any case, the treatment begins with a separate interview with the child and parents. A searching examination follows, with laboratory studies if need be, to exclude physical disease.

The physiological basis of the bodily symptoms, and their association with normal fear reactions should be explained to both parties. This, with a confident statement of the absence of physical disease, may be curative. In most instances, however, it is necessary to see the patient on several occasions so that explanations and reassurance can be reinforced. A simple sedative (e.g., chloral hydrate) may be prescribed for a short period in the sleepless. An adjustment of parental attitudes and standards may be necessary, but this need not extend to an attitude of total *laissez faire*.

In many instances, the neurosis is short-lived and of good prognosis. Where anxiety symptoms extend back several years. reference to a child psychiatrist may be necessary.

ANOREXIA NERVOSA

This is almost always found in girls. While occurring principally in the adolescent, it may be seen as early as 8-10 years of age.

Symptomatology. The child does not eat, and develops an alarming weight loss. This may be so severe that she looks like a living skeleton. Threats and promises have no effect upon the food intake, and anxiety symptoms are often associated.

Background. The child may previously have been obese, and had a need to diet. In other cases, there may be concern by the child about her puberty characteristics—breast growth, pelvic broadening, and so on. The feelings of self-consciousness concerning these are dealt with by dieting which becomes permanent and pathological.

Differential diagnosis. This is from serious organic disease such as diabetes, renal failure, and thyrotoxicosis.

Treatment. The child's general health, need for intravenous therapy, and so on, will be prescribed for by the pediatrician. The services of the psychiatrist should be sought as soon as the diagnosis is suspected. The patient must closely be supervised, as many have a great ability to conceal or dispose of food uneaten.

DEPRESSION

This is rather unusual in young children, but feelings of melancholy and unhappiness are common in the adolescent, and anxiety states often coexist. Understandable depression is often found in children with a severe somatic disability, e.g., muscular dystrophy. Somatic symptoms are less common than in the adult, but school progress and social intercourse may be impaired. The child will usually readily admit his feelings of unhappiness, and commonly has good insight. In rare cases, the situation goes unnoticed until the child makes a determined (but usually unsuccessful) suicide effort.

A variant which may occur at almost any age is the *mourning reaction*. In this, the precipitating cause is the loss of a family member. In the resulting emotional response, the child is the victim of imperfectly understood explanations or concepts. Thus, anxiety may be engendered because the child feels that he himself may contract the disease from which the loved one died. An example is the belief that leukemia is infectious. Especially in the younger child, pseudocomforting phrases such as "soon we'll all be together again", may, with the child's imperfect sense of time, imply for him an early demise. Melancholy and anxiety are an almost logical result.

OBSESSIVE-COMPULSIVE STATES

Minor variants of these are common in young children who frequently indulge in ritualized activities which give feelings of confidence. Readily recognizable are the overly careful, prim children, who cannot bear dirt on their clothing, or the child who resents a disturbance of a carefully arranged set of dolls. These characteristics may, however, not outlast the later years of childhood.

The severer types of disorders, interfering with ordinary living, occur in an older, usually adolescent, age group. These people are often overconscientious, shy and punctilious—features which in themselves are not abnormal. Such children, apart from their specific obsession, tend not to mix well and to resent the intrusion of others into their activities.

The obsessions may take many forms, e.g., persistent and recurrent thoughts, often of a tormenting nature, or the drive repeatedly to do certain actions in a certain manner. The latter may refer to daily activities such as eating, walking, or the preliminaries to sleep. Preoccupation with cleanliness is common, as are hypochondriacal feelings. The child may force his obsessions upon his parents, and resent their refusal to comply. Parental obsessions or perfectionism is a common background to the disturbance.

HYSTERIA

In general, this condition is not very common in children. Essentially there is a nonorganic suspension of function. The sensory or motor systems may be involved. The former often involves loss of vision, or various anesthesias. A characteristic motor phenomenon of hysteria is astasia-abasia. In this the child will not stand or walk, although other voluntary limb movements are perfect. Many other forms of hysterical paralysis occur, especially aphonia and mutism. Much less common are trembling states of the limbs, with impaired function.

All of these disabilities are patchy, and coincide with other situations of normal function. The symptom is absent during sleep, and is almost always episodic.

Treatment. Depression, compulsive states and hysteria generally require treatment by a skilled child psychiatrist.

SCHOOL REFUSAL

This is not very uncommon in children. The principal symptom is self-evident. The child does not want to go to school. The reasons may be equally evident upon superficial enquiry. Common associations are that the child is teased because of some physical peculiarity, dislikes his teacher, fears to use the school toilet facilities, is being bullied, or is doing poorly in his school work. Another major cause which operates in the younger child is simple unwillingness to be separated from the mother. The latter may indeed have made every effort to hold on to the child.

Symptomatology. The child needs an excuse not to go to school. He develops one; it is usually somatic. Common problems are pains in the stomach; nausea; and, less commonly, vomiting. They do not occur at the weekend or during school holidays. There is rapid improvement if the mother agrees that the child remain at home. Physical examination is normal.

Treatment. If the child has a genuine grievance concerning school, this should be exorcized. Otherwise, it is necessary to insist firmly, and without mention of penalty, that he goes to school. As the mother may be herself ambivalent, it is necessary, on occasion, to reorientate her concerning the importance of school attendance.

PSYCHOSES OF CHILDHOOD

True psychoses are happily rare in childhood, although psychotic symptoms may accompany cerebral degenerative states, or complicate the course of poisoning by various drugs.

Perhaps the most characteristic syndrome is infantile autism.

Infantile autism

Clinical features. As the name suggests, the child is pathologically preoccupied with self. Early in life (to the first year) he does not react emotionally to his mother. When hugged he will stiffen or cling limply. Smiling and laughter are inappropriate or absent, and motor progress, especially that related to exploring the environment—walking and skilled hand movements—are delayed or absent. Repetitive useless movements such as head banging, finger tapping, and toe tapping, are common. The child does not relate normally to people, either his parents or other children, and characteristically looks past or turns away from those who address him. He has little reaction to noises, and may be regarded as deaf. Speech may be absent or delayed, and often nonsensical when it does appear. Communication is usually mostly by gesture. Physical overactivity, by day and night, is a distressing symptom to the parents. Play is weird, obsessive, and repetitive. Twirling, twisting, and clicking activities are preferred, and preoccupy the patient intensely. The child is pathologically conservative in eating habits, and new foods and situations are difficult to introduce and many cause a prolonged anxiety state. So too does an effort to teach the child any new motor, verbal, or social skill. The child may be pathologically reckless, deliberately walking into traffic, the sea, or other dangerous situations.

Clinical examination. The child does not have the facies of mental defect. He does not, however, pay the slightest attention to the examiner or his apparatus, has limited motor skills, and his speech may seem aphasic. Yet, the physical examination and neurological survey are normal.

Treatment. There is no specific treatment, and the parents require much support to exorcise their guilt feelings. Group therapy in special units is desirable, and treatment is based on finding an avenue of response in the child. If this is done, he may be able to be taught to appreciate himself, as the integrated sum of his members—his eyes, nose, hands, head. The exploration of environment is taught deliberately, and in general much as a mother teaches her infant.

Prognosis. If recognized early, some may be rehabilitated. In many, however, treatment is too late, or to no avail.

PSYCHOSES IN THE OLDER CHILD

These usually begin at puberty and are relatively rare.

Clinical features. A common feature is withdrawal from the parents and peer group, frequently with refusal to go to school or engage in normal activities. Deterioration in behaviour is common, and antisocial activity occurs. There is difficulty in appreciating reality and disorders of thought with delusion and hallucination may occur. All of this may coincide with a regression to infantile practices, e.g., enuresis, soiling, deterioration of eating habits; aggressive behaviour is a constant danger.

Differential diagnosis. This is principally from the degenerative brain conditions, and from such entities as intracranial tumour, or chronic poisoning from drugs or heavy metals. Withdrawal may be a feature of simple depression.

22 Disorders of bone

CONGENITAL DEFECTS

There are many of these, only the more common will be considered.

Generalized congenital defects: the chondrodystrophies

Achondroplasia

This is a genetically determined disorder which is transmitted as a dominant. The principal upset consists in failure of longitudinal growth of the long bones, because of an abnormality of cartilage formation at the epiphyseal plate. The condition is well known in animals, e.g. the Dachshund.

Clinical features. These are readily seen at birth. The limbs are short in relation to the trunk. As the infant grows the head may look relatively large, but its circumference is usually within normal limits. The brow bulges, the nose is snub, and the jaw protrudes. The shortened limbs are usually bowed. Although the trunk is of normal size, the chest shows flaring of the rib margins, and sometimes costochondral beading. Kyphosis and lordosis develop when the child walks. The fingers are short and fat, and excessive skin folds are present over the arms and legs. Intellectual development is usually normal.

Progress. Some infants die soon after birth. In the survivors, growth continues, but normal proportions are never reached and dwarfing is inevitable.

Treatment. None is effective.

Chondroectodermal Dysplasia (Ellis-Van Creveld syndrome)

This is inherited by a recessive mode and is rather rare.

Clinical features. In addition to the external features of achondroplasia, these children have polydactyly, and frequently, congenital heart disease. The nails are dystrophic, and dental abnormalities coexist. The prognosis is basically that of the cardiac defect; no treatment is available for the skeletal disorder.

Osteogenesis imperfecta (fragilitas ossium)

This condition is frequently familial, and consists in an inability to produce mature collagen, so that the fetal pattern of bone production persists.

Clinical features. These vary in severity. Some infants are stillborn, others born alive, show clinical and x-ray evidence of multiple fractures. There are palpable spaces in the skull bones, and an egg shell like crackling may be felt. The sclerae are often distinctly blue, and the eyes prominent. Some of these live-born children survive only a short time. The others fracture their bones with the most minor injury.

In the less severe form (osteopsathyrosis, osteogenesis imperfecta tarda) the infant appears normal at birth, and for up to a year afterward. He then develops fractures with minor injury. These are often in the legs, and relate to walking activities. Any of the bones may, however, be injured. Healing occurs readily, but deformity is liable to take place. Deafness and eye disorders may occur in these children.

Treatment. In the severe infantile form, little can be done except to shield the baby from injury. In the older child, expert orthopedic care is necessary to prevent severe deformity.

Prognosis. This is poor except in the late onset type; in these patients, fractures may be relatively infrequent, readily treatable, and may cease toward the time of puberty.

Osteopetrosis (Albers-Schönberg disease)

This is an autosomal recessive disease with invasion of the bone marrow cavity by excessively thickened and brittle bone.

Clinical features. The patient presents early in life with progressive loss of vision (cataracts and optic atrophy) and deafness. The encroachment upon the bone marrow gives rise to a progressively severe anemia, initially hypochromic, terminally aplastic. The brittle bones are liable to fracture, and indeed this may be the first complaint. In the late stages, the liver and spleen enlarge. Growth is soon retarded and deformities of the chest and spine are common.

Treatment. Transfusion for the anemia is necessary. The fractures heal well but careful orthopedic care is indicated. There is no specific treatment for this metabolic disorder.

LOCAL OSSEOUS DISEASE

A few of these conditions are associated with disease of another system, e.g., pes cavus, and central nervous system disease. Most, however, are primary.

Conditions involving the lower limbs

Congenital dislocation of the hip

This condition is due to delayed ossification of the femoral head and the acetabulum; in infancy, the hip is not always dislocated, but can be made to do so. It is important that it be recognized at this stage so that appropriate treatment can begin.

Clinical features. It occurs principally in females, and is relatively common. In most instances, the condition is recognized following a deliberate effort to dislocate the hip. This is done by laying the infant on his back, fixing the pelvis, holding the femur in the semi-abducted position, and lifting the limb up and down. A characteristic click is present. This is often better felt than heard. This sign persists for only 1-2 months. In some babies there is also limitation of abduction, but this sign may be absent in the first weeks.

Treatment. The limbs should be fixed in abduction for 6 months or so (initially with double napkins). This will restore normal hip anatomy and function.

Dislocation of the hip in the older child

This may be congenital, or occur in cerebral palsy where muscle spasm is severe.

Clinical features. The earliest sign is limitation of abduction, with evidence of shortening of the femoral section of the lower limb. This may be suggested by abnormal skin crease formation, persistent external rotation of the limb, and apparent widening of the perineum. In the child who has learned to walk, there is a limp, and in bilateral dislocations, a waddling gait.

X-rays. The dislocation is visible, and the acetabulum is shallow and the femoral head underdeveloped.

Treatment. At this stage, slow reduction is the usual treatment, followed by maintenance in the reduced position for many months. In spite of expert orthopedic care, the ultimate result may not be fully satisfactory.

Perthe's Disease

This condition is probably an avascular necrosis of the femoral head. It occurs mainly in the primary school child and presents with features similar to those for acute synovitis of the hip, from which it is to be differentiated by the persistence of symptoms and by the x-ray changes. In the early stage, these may show little except an increase in joint space.

Later there is sclerosis of the femoral head, followed after some time by apparent break-up of the capital epiphyses. Thereafter, the femoral head is reformed, often in an abnormal flattened form, (mushroom head), if weight bearing has been allowed.

Treatment. Weight bearing is avoided until there is reformation of the femoral head.

Slipped capital epiphysis

This occurs mostly, but not invariably, in tall, heavy, adolescent children. The symptoms may appear after apparent injury and consist in pain, usually in the hip but sometimes in the knee. A limp is invariable. These signs persist in contrast to the transient complaints of acute synovitis of the hip. X-rays show widening and irregularity of the epiphyses, and in more severe instances, a slip backwards and downwards.

Treatment. Prolonged traction is needed to restore normal anatomy.

DISORDERS OF THE FEET

Pes planus (flat foot)

The longitudinal arch is seldom completely formed until the child is 3-4 years of age, accordingly, flat foot should not be overdiagnosed in early life.

In those who have developed a reasonable arch, prolonged bedrest, or the onset of obesity may cause symptoms of early fatiguability and pain in the feet. In most instances, however, complaints are made because of parental observation, or difficulty in shoe fitting.

In the few instances where treatment is needed, the provision of shoes with a straight inside edge, occasionally with wedging, is usually sufficient.

Pes cavus (high arch)

Again this is commonly asymptomatic, most complaints relating to parental dissatisfaction or shoe fitting difficulties. The condition may of course complicate or initiate the course of peroneal muscular atrophy, or Friedreich's ataxia.

In advanced cases, where no associated disease exists, appropriate night splints and corrective exercises may be indicated.

Talipes (club foot)

In the equinovarus type, the foot is plantar flexed and inclined medially. In the calcaneovarus there is dorsiflexion with lateral deviation. The condition is readily recognized at birth, and is probably associated with the fetal position in utero. The same deformities may occur in children with meningomyelocele or arthrogryposis.

In most instances, the foot can be put into the normal position, and then overcorrected. This is an important sign which means that simple manipulative treatment will suffice. Otherwise extensive orthopedic treatment may be needed.

Metatarsus adductus

As the name implies, there is adduction of the forefoot. The condition is quite common, is mobile and readily correctable by manipulation. If neglected, it may lead to a severe case of hen toes (pigeon toes) with its characteristic gait.

DISORDERS OF THE LOWER LIMBS

Bow legs

The infant may appear to be bow legged because of an exaggeration of the normal tibial curve, and the fat distribution on the legs. However, the knees and ankles, when approximated, will fail to show any significant gap between. Severe bow leg deformity may occur in rickets, hypophosphatasia, and other metabolic bone disorders. Unilateral bow leg is unusual, and due, commonly, to an osteochondrosis of medial aspect of the upper tibial metaphysis.

Treatment. This is seldom necessary, except in advanced deformity.

Knock knees

A minor degree of this is common, especially in the overweight child. Extreme degrees are however unusual except in bone disease, such as rickets or in homocystinuria. Limb function is preserved, the complaints being cosmetic ones, from the patient or parents. In most instances, little need be done, except perhaps to reduce the overweight patient. Marked deformity requires skilled orthopedic care.

Genu recurvatum

This is found in babies who have been in the extended breech position. The knee is readily dislocatable (or is dislocated) posteriorly. A severe degree of deformity may exist, but spontaneous cure within a few weeks is usual, provided active movement is allowed.

OTHER DISORDERS OF THE LIMBS

Extensive suppression of part or all of limb formation may occur spontaneously, or be the result of drugs given the mother, e.g., thalidomide.

Such deformities may coexist with severe disorders elsewhere. *Hemimelia* is the term given to the absence of distal parts of the limbs, i.e., a hand or foot. *Phocomelia* is where the proximal limb is absent, but the distal limb present. Thus, in extreme cases, the hand will arise directly from the trunk. Many intermediate stages are described. In the thalidomide induced types, deafness, cardiac, and intellectual defects coexist. These largely decide the prognosis and types of treatment. Specialized units are necessary for the provision of appliances and education for suitable patients.

CONDITIONS ABOUT THE SHOULDER

Craniocleidodysostosis

In this the clavicles are partly or totally absent so that the shoulders can meet in front. No treatment is necessary.

Congenital scapular elevation (Sprengel's deformity)

In this the scapulae are raised and may be connected to the spine. The principal difficulty is that the arm cannot be raised beyond a right angle. Treatment is not indicated.

DISORDERS OF THE SPINE

Most of these are aberrations of the normal spinal curvature, which become obvious when the child has learned to walk.

Kyphosis is an exaggeration of the curvature of the spine which is concave forwards; *lordosis* has a convex forward curvature. In *scoliosis*, the spine is curved in the coronal plane. Each may be due to vertebral abnormality, or to muscle weakness causing imbalance in the forces acting upon the spine. This may follow disorders of the muscles which directly act upon the vertebrae, or follow disorders of the hip and lower limbs. In the latter, the deformity (usually lordosis) tends to maintain a more or less normal centre of gravity.

The presence of a spinal deformity should initiate a search for neurological abnormality, and for local spinal disorders. The latter may be congenital vertebral abnormalities. Often however, in scoliosis, no obvious cause can be found. In certain cases, splinting will be required to arrest the condition. Surgery (straightening and fusion) is carried out when spinal growth has ceased.

Scheuermann's disease

This resembles the osteochondritic diseases, and may involve 1 or more vertebrae. It is a cause of kyphosis, but is painless, and otherwise without symptoms.

DISORDERS OF THE STERNUM

Many of these are associated with concomitant changes in the ribs, as in the pigeon breast deformity. This condition is acquired and is found in children with hyperventilation since early in life. It is, therefore, common in frequent chest infections, as occur in congenital heart disease (the heart defect is not the primary cause of the defect) and in children with severe asthma, or as a result of mucoviscidosis.

Pectus Excavatum

This condition, which is familial, may be due to shortening of the diaphragmatic central tendon. In most instances it is asymptomatic, coming to attention for cosmetic reasons. If uncorrected, severe degrees of pectus excavatum may be associated with disordered lung function in later life.

Treatment. None is necessary for mild degrees. Appropriate surgical treatment is undertaken at the age of 10 or more years in the more severely affected.

DISORDERS OF THE FACIAL SKELETON

These are not very uncommon in the severer autosomal syndromes. Mandibular hypoplasia (Pierre-Robin syndrome) is described elsewhere as is craniofacial dysostosis (Crouzon's disease).

In mandibulofacial dysostosis (Treacher-Collins syndrome) the basic disorder is maldevelopment of the tissues derived from 1st and 2nd branchial arches. It is a familial condition, characterized by mandibular and zygomatic hypoplasia. The eyes are slanted downward and the jaw small. Ear abnormalities are common and notching of the lower eyelid is found. Deafness is common; the intelligence is, however, normal.

Allied to Treacher-Collins syndrome, is oculoauriculovertebral dysplasia (Goldenhaar's syndrome). This is characterized by malar hypoplasia, and dermoid or lipodermoid formation on the eye or cheek. Ear tags are frequent, as are pretragal pits. Various vertebral anomalies (hemivertebrae, occipitalization of atlas, spina bifida) are associations.

No specific treatment, other than plastic surgical procedures is indicated.

DISORDERS OF THE SKULL

These are frequently a complication of a generalized disease such as histiocytosis X, severe hemolytic anemias, and so on. Craniosynostosis has as its major manifestation, raised intracranial pressure and is covered in the section relating to that symptom. As already noted, congenital skull deformities are not uncommonly associated with similar disorders of the face, or vertebrae. Of the asymptomatic lesions (usually found on skull x-ray), *congenital foramina* are perhaps the more common. These have well-defined edges, and are usually in the parietal bone. They require differentiation from the lesions of histiocytosis X, of the eosinophilic granuloma variety.

More extensive defects are found in lacunar skull, which often accompanies meningomyelocele. In this the x-rays show multiple defects surrounded by bony ridges of varying density. Occipitalization of the atlas (*platybasia*) may be isolated, or form part of the Klippel-Feil complex. As the name indicated, the atlas is abnormally fused to, or may be assimilated into, the basal skull bones. In rare cases, the spinal cord is subjected to compression. Secondary platybasia occurs in conditions where the skull bones are soft, as in rickets, or where abnormal weight-bearing is demanded. The latter may occasionally be found in regurgitating infants who are nursed for a long time in the sitting position.

The commonest condition affecting the skull is *plagiocephaly*. This is probably acquired. In this the skull is asymmetrical, flattening of one side of the brow accompanying a corresponding asymmetry of the occiput. Some flattening of the chest may coexist. It is usually seen in infants who are less active, and who sleep persistently on one side. The condition is entirely harmless, although it may persist into later life, suitably disguised by hair growth. The sole treatment is reassurance.

PYOGENIC BONE INFECTIONS (OSTEOMYELITIS)

These may be due to the staphylococcus, streptococcus, *H. influenzae*, or salmonella species. The first is overwhelmingly the commoner cause.

Clinical features. Those in the newborn are described elsewhere. In the older child, the onset is sudden, with fever, anorexia, irritability, with pain and impaired function in the affected limb. As this is usually the leg, a limp, or refusal to walk is common. The cardinal finding is marked local tenderness. If the lesion is adjacent to a joint, as is frequently the case, limitation of movement is found. Swelling and fluctuation are relatively late signs, indicating rupture of the periosteal abscess.

Laboratory. Blood culture should always be done, and may indicate the offending organism. Polymorph leucocytosis is usual, and anemia may occur in patients in whom treatment is delayed.

Radiology. Definite changes are absent for 10-14 days. Thereafter an area of rarefaction is seen, followed by elevation of the periosteum with new bone formation.

Treatment. This is a matter of urgency. As the commonest organism is the staphylococcus, methicillin, and other broad-spectrum antibiotics (e.g., ampicillin) are given intravenously. The area of maximal tenderness is aspirated, as may be the adjacent joint if arthritis cannot be excluded clinically. If nothing can be aspirated, it is usual to explore the periosteum and bone directly, and to decompress by drill hole if necessary.

Prognosis. This depends upon the age of the patient, and the delay in establishing therapy. In the newborn and infant, epiphyseal involvement is usual, and joint destruction common. Accordingly, limb growth may be severely affected. At any age delay in treatment leads to necrosis of bone, sequestrum formation, persistent sinuses, deformity, and interference with limb growth.

OTHER INFECTIONS OF BONE

Tuberculosis

This is relatively uncommon nowadays, since hematogenous spread from the original site is less likely with modern chemotherapy. Clearly, any bone could be infected, but the commoner sites are the vertebrae, long bones and digits.

Vertebral tuberculosis. The infection is subacute and commonly painless; it gives rise to symptoms because of bone collapse, or through abscess formation with involvement of adjacent structures. In a few instances,the first problem is of spinal deformity—often scoliosis. This may be superimposed upon a known tuberculous state, or be associated with vague general ill health. In other children, the vertebral collapse and abscess formation may give rise to pressure upon the spinal cord. In rare instances, the abscess will rupture on the skin—within a wide area varying from close to the vertebral lesion, to a distant rupture, e.g., in the inguinal area. These have all the characteristics of a cold abscess—slow gathering, dilatory fluctuation, and an irregular indolent local reaction after rupture. The Mantoux reaction is positive, and the mycobacteria are readily seen in the exudates.

Tuberculosis of the long bones. This usually presents with local swelling with variable interference with function. The condition is of an osteomyelitis, so that, as in the acute pyogenic variety, an adjacent jcint may be involved. This is especially so in the common disease of the upper femur. The latter is more liable to cause relatively acute symptoms such as limp and some discomfort.

Tuberculous dactylitis. This may occur in the short bones of the hand or foot. Involvement of the latter is perhaps more characteristic. The finger swells symmetrically, loses function (particularly flexion), but is painless. It is unusual for more than 1 digit to be affected. The swelling feels solid, although caseation may ultimately give rise to a fluctuant mass. Eventually the underlying skin shows colour change (a mildly cyanotic tint). Ultimate perforation by an underlying abscess may occur, but is rare.

X-ray signs. The first sign is a localized area of sclerosis, followed by variable degrees of bone destruction.

Treatment. The sensitivity of the organism should, if possible, be ascertained. Full chemotherapy with streptomycin, isoniazid, and P.A.S. should then begin. In lesions of weight-bearing areas (spine, femur) traction should be used, using ordinary orthopedic principles.

Compression lesions of the spinal cord may require abscess drainage as well as traction.

Osseous syphilis

This too, is nowadays a rare disease, but can occur at any stage of the process. Thus, in early congenital syphilis of infancy, x-ray evidence of asymptomatic bone disease is not uncommon. The osteochondritis of the disease process may give rise to epiphyseal fracture with pain and limitation of movement (pseudoparalysis). In these children, the clinical features rather resemble those of scurvy, which is a principal differential diagnosis. In the older child who is walking, the bone softening may be associated with bending of the bone, giving a characteristic deformity (sabre shins, boomerang deformity).

X-ray changes. These are found in most bones, but are most readily appreciated in the epiphyseal areas of wrists and ankles. Here the osteochondritis causes widening and increased density of the epiphyseal plate, sometimes with separation. Periostitis is common, and osteomyelitic signs may also occur.

Treatment. A full course of penicillin is given, with orthopedic care when epephyseal separations have occurred.

TUMOURS OF BONE

In early life these are usually secondary, commonly from neuroblastoma. The latter probably gives rise to the so-called Ewing's tumour.

Osteosarcoma

This is the commonest osteogenic tumour. It affects older children and teenagers, and usually arises in the metaphyseal areas of the long bones (femur, tibia, humerus).

Clinical features. There is pain, which in the lower limbs causes a limp. Local swelling is invariable and this may be hot and tender. X-rays show an expanding osteolytic lesion with periosteal elevation. Bridging spicules of bone may be visible.

Treatment. The details will depend upon the presence of metastases to the lungs. If they are present, then radical amputation is contra-indicated. In most instances radiotherapy to the affected bone and a close watch for metastasis should continue for several months before amputations are carried out. The prognosis is generally unfavourable.

DISORDERS OF THE JOINTS

These may be affected in some of the osseous lesions already described. Additionally, joint manifestations are found in a variety of generalized disease processes such as rheumatic fever, rheumatoid arthritis, Henoch-Schönlein disease, and disseminated lupus erythematosus. Effusions into the joints occur in serum sickness and bleeding disorders such a haemophilia. Other entities which commonly occur in pediatric practice are described below.

Acute synovitis

This principally gives rise to problems when if affects the hip. There is often, but not invariably, a history of injury. The patient complains of pain, usually in the hip, sometimes in the knee, and develops a limp. Examination reveals limitation of hip movement, mainly internal rotation. The patient is afebrile, has no leucocytosis, and quickly recovers with rest. The x-rays are usually normal although an increased joint space may be seen.

Differential diagnosis. This is wide, ranging from septic arthritis, rheumatic fever, and serum sickness to Perthe's disease. In most instances, the absence of general signs, and the persistence of pain in only 1 joint in hip synovitis is sufficient guidance. The treatment is rest, occasionally with traction.

INFECTIONS OF THE JOINTS

Septic arthritis

The organisms responsible are those mentioned under osteomyelitis. Indeed, most of the features of septic arthritis are those of osteomyelitis. In the infant and younger child, osteomyelitis adjacent to a joint usually spreads into it because the epiphyseal plate is a less effective barrier at this age.

Clinical features. These closely resemble those of osteomyelitis, viz., fever, anorexia, and loss of function—commonly a limp. Movement of the joint is restricted in all directions. The one-finger tender spot of osteomyelitis may be absent.

A definitive diagnosis is made by aspiration of the joint. The treatment is that described for osteomyelitis.

Tuberculosis of the joints

In most instances this spreads from an adjacent focus of tuberculous osteomyelitis. The common variety which may occur (and it is rare), is tuberculosis of the hip joint. The usual clinical feature is of the onset of a limp, usually with relatively little discomfort, although nocturnal exacerbation may be noted as the splinting action of the muscle is relaxed. The diagnosis is not always easy. It should be suspected in the face of an appropriate history of exposure, and a positive Mantoux. In a few instances, biopsy of the synovium is necessary. The treatment is that described for tuberculous osteomyelitis.

Chronic destructive arthropathy

This is the response of a joint to multiple episodes of trauma sustained in the absence of a normal sensory supply. It occurs, therefore, in some children with meningomyelocele who can walk, in leprosy, and in some children with congenital syphilis. The first sign is a painless effusion and limitation of function. Gross deformity and disintegration of the joint follow, with genu recurvatum as a common sign. X-rays are confirmatory.

Treatment. If possible, this is of the primary disease. Local treatment consists in teaching the child the likely actions causing injury, and the provision of suitable orthopedic appliances.

23 Disorders of the muscles

Only the primary muscular diseases (myopathies) will be considered in this section. Secondary muscle disorders are mostly due to primary disease of the motor neurone and are covered in the section on nervous system disease.

MUSCULAR DYSTROPHY

This is an inherited disorder causing degeneration of skeletal muscle and thus weakness, wasting, and failure of function. Many varieties are described, some of these are noted in table 30.

Table 30. Muscular dystrophy types

Eponym	Inheritance
Duchenne (pseudohypertrophic) affecting pelvis	Usually sex-linked (affects males) Recessive Rarely can affect either sex (autosomal recessive)
Facioscapulohumeral (Landouzy-Déjérine)	Usually autosomal dominant Occasionally automsomal recessive
Limb–girdle dystrophy	Usually autosomal recessive

Pseudohypertrophic muscular dystrophy (Duchenne type)

Clinical features. The disease affects males, causing difficulty in walking (especially upstairs), stumbling, and frequent falls. Jumping, hopping, and running are impossible, although the ability to walk is preserved for some time, with the muscular weakness causing a wide-based, rolling walk, with lordosis (forward bending of the spine). The lower limb and gluteal muscles are symmetrically weak and wasting soon occurs, although it may be disguised at first by the accumulation of fat. This is particularly evident in the calves of the legs which may seem more prominent than usual (pseudohypertrophy). The true muscle mass is, however, much reduced. Sooner or later the chest muscles (pectorals) and the muscles of the shoulders and arms show weakness, wasting, and poverty of function.

These children are well aware of their disabilities, and develop trick movements for self help. This is the basis of the sign of climbing up the legs (Gower's sign), which is often found in muscular dystrophy when the patient gets up from the prone position. Weakness and loss of function gradually increase until the child is bedfast. Breathlessness and frequent chest infections occur when the respiratory muscles weaken. The myocardium (heart muscle) is involved also and congestive cardiac failure can occur in those who survive for a long time. The symptoms may wax and wane a good deal, but loss of function is accelerated by bedrest, as for the treatment of fractures or other illnesses.

Diagnosis. Some enzyme levels are increased in muscular dystrophy, e.g., serum creatine-phosphokinase (CPK). Electromyography (study of muscular electrical activity) and muscle biopsy are also helpful tests.

Management. There is no specific treatment, so every effort is made to keep the child active and walking. Simple physiotherapy is used to prevent muscle contractures, and undue bedrest strictly avoided. A normal education is given, with emphasis on reading, music and other cultural aspects which will help the child when he becomes bedfast. At this stage, postural deformities should be prevented, especially in the trunk (lordosis) and feet (equinovarus). Chest physiotherapy is done to prevent respiratory infections.

The family needs careful support, and genetic counselling since, if the carrier state is present in the family, there is a 50% chance of male children being affected. The carrier state may be suspected if the CPK levels are increased, or if electromyographic abnormalities are present.

Facioscapulohumeral dystrophy (Landouzy-Déjérine)

This is not very common in children. It is an autosomal dominant which usually begins to give trouble in the school-going years.

Clinical features. The face muscles become weak so that smiling fails and the eyes cannot be completely closed. The expression dulls, and the lips become pendulous, giving the tapir mouth appearance. Whistling is impossible and difficulties occur with eating. Weakness spreads to the shoulder and upper arms, so that normal movement becomes impossible. After a long delay, the pelvic and leg muscles are affected rather as in Duchenne dystrophy.

The CPK levels are variable, so that electromyography and biopsy are needed for a final diagnosis. The care of the patient is as already outlined.

Limb-girdle dystrophy

This is another autosomal recessive disorder which mostly begins at puberty, and involves the shoulder and pelvic muscles. The progress is slow, but ultimately the disorder closely resembles that described for Duchenne-type dystrophy. The enzyme changes are also similar, as is the treatment.

THE MYOTONIC DISORDERS

In these disorders, muscular weakness is found to be associated with abnormally prolonged muscular contraction. The main condition found in children is *dystrophia myotonica*.

In the newborn, facial weakness and difficulty in feeding are the main features. Flaccidity (hypotonia) is usual, and delay in milestones, difficulty in swallowing (due to palatal and tongue weakness) and drooping eyelids are common. Later examination may suggest retardation. The face is expressionless, the mouth open, and the eyelids droop. In many children the myotonia (prolonged contraction) can be elicited by tapping the affected muscles. In others, the myotonia can be confirmed only by electromyography. As in the adult form of the disease, a few older children may develop cataracts and premature baldness.

Myotonia congenita (Thomsen's disease)

This is an autosomal dominant which is rare in children. Inability to relax muscular movement may be noted by the parents or patient. This may lead to a certain degree of clumsiness, but specific complaints are not very common. The muscles may enlarge and myotonia is present as described above.

Arthrogryposis multiplex congenita

The cause of this disease is not known, but it causes muscle wasting and multiple contractures. Anterior horn cell disease (spinal muscular atrophy) can coexist.

Clinical features. These are present at birth and consist in multiple contractures causing an exaggerated fetal position. The hands are firmly flexed at the wrist, and the feet fixed in plantar flexion. The elbows and knees are often rigidly extended and hip movement is impaired. The arms are usually internally rotated, the thighs externally so. The skin is shiny and thickened. Other congenital defects (of bones, palate, or hips) may occur.

Treatment. This is entirely orthopedic.

Acute epidemic myositis (Bornholm disease)

This disease occasionally occurs in epidemics. The Coxsackie virus is the cause.

Clinical features. There is muscular pain in the chest, back, and belly. Breathing is painful and shallow. The muscles are tender to touch.

Differential diagnosis. This is principally from chest infections with pleurisy. Cough is seldom present in myositis, and crepitations and other chest signs are absent.

Treatment. General treatment such as analgesics and hot baths are useful in easing the pain. There is no specific treatment.

Congenital absence of muscle

In descending order of frequency, the following muscles may be lacking: *pectoralis major*, *trapezius*, *serratus anterior*, and the *biceps femorali*. These patients seldom have specific complaints other than the unusual appearance of the affected area. The more serious anterior abdominal wall deficits, the prune belly syndrome, is considered in the section on renal disease. More obvious problems are the following.

Congenital ptosis

In this condition, one or both upper eyelids droop. The appearance of the infant may suggest the diagnosis, or this may come to attention because of compensatory head tilting, giving a peculiar appearance. In a few instances, jaw movement will cause eyelid lift—jaw winking. Spontaneous recovery occurs. The treatment otherwise is surgical and depends on the degree of interference with vision.

Differential diagnosis. Ptosis may occur as part of defects of transmission of the neuromuscular junction as in myasthenia gravis, or poisoning by organophosphorus insecticides. Pseudoptosis occurs in male and female Turner's syndrome. In the newborn, the association of ptosis with myotonia dystrophica should be recalled.

Duane's syndrome

This condition is caused by fibrosis of the external rectus muscle of the eye. This causes a squint on lateral gaze, with retraction of the globe and apparent smallness of the eye. There is little risk of amblyopia in this condition, and treatment is made for purely cosmetic reasons.

Torticollis

This condition occurs in the infant. It is a hematoma in the sternomastoid which later calcifies, so that the first complaint is of a hard mass in the muscle. In some instances, the condition clears spontaneously; in others, shortening gives rise to the typical wry neck. In advanced cases, the face is deformed, and asymmetry of the skull occurs. Head tilt to the affected side is common. This may give rise to a compensatory head tilt or ocular ptosis.

Treatment. The infant's neck is treated by manipulation and stretching; if shortening has become permanent, surgical treatment is indicated.

MYOSITIS

Progressive myositis ossificans

This is a familial, happily rare, disease, often associated with other skeletal abnormalities.

Clinical features. Swellings appear, without apparent cause, on the head or trunk. These are painful, hot and tender, and ultimately may exude white material. The lesion then calcifies. The cycle is repeated, sometimes in association with minor injury. Ultimately the body is covered by a bony carapace which impairs eating (if on the face) or locomotion (if in the limbs and trunk). Ultimately the patient has dyspnea because of thoracic constriction, and dies of respiratory or cardiac failure.

Calcifying myositis (myositis ossificans conscripta)

This condition is always associated with trauma of, and hemorrhage into, the muscle. There is local pain and tenderness and x-ray shows calcium deposit. Physiotherapy is usually the treatment of choice, but the calcified mass may be removed surgically if local function is impaired.

24 Disorders of fluid and electrolytes

These are very important in paediatrics, since loss of water and salt (dehydration) occurs in many disorders.

PHYSIOLOGY

There are 2 body compartments or spaces which contain water and various salts. One is called the *intracellular* space, and the other the *extracellular* space. Water and salts can diffuse into and out of each, so that disorders of one will ultimately affect the other. *Total body water* is the sum of the water contained in each space. It's volume is greatest in the newborn (75% of body weight) and falls to 60% of body weight in the toddler. The extracellular water, which is contained in the blood volume, interstitial fluid and lymph, and fluids, e.g., intestinal, concerned in the transport of substances to and from cells, varies similarly, falling from 350 ml/kg body weight at birth to 250 ml/kg body weight in the 3-year old. The *total blood volume* is the most important component of the extracellular fluid, one half is made up of the *red cell mass* and the remainder as the *plasma volume*. Plasma is essentially an aqueous (watery) salt solution which also contains protein (total 6-8 g/l, albumin/globulin ratio about 2:1), and of course suspends the red cells, which are mainly composed of hemoglobin. The main cations (positively charged ions) in the extracellular fluid are sodium (Na^+ 140 mEq/1), potassium (K^+ 3.5 mEq/1), calcium (Ca^{++} 4.5 mEq/1), and magnesium (Mg^{++} 2.5 mEq/1). These cations must be chemically balanced by negatively charged ions (anions), of which the main one is chloride (Cl^{--} 105 mEq/1), together with small quantities of bicarbonate (HCO_3^-), phosphate (PO_4^{---}) and sulphate (SO_4^{---}).

The plasma acts not only as a solution in which essential nutrients and oxygen can be transported, but also acts as an important method by which marked variations in acid/base (alkali) body values can be avoided. This capability of maintaining normal acid/base balance is called buffering.

The extracellular volume has all of the properties of a simple solution. One of these is *osmolality* or *tonicity*. This is the force which tends to keep ions in solution against the barrier of a semipermeable membrane. In the case of the body, the membrane is the interface between the cells and the solution. If the concentration of ions (salts) in the solution were to increase greatly, then the water in the cells would be attracted out, and they would be damaged by shrinkage. On the other hand, if the solution was too weak, then the cells would absorb water, and could swell and rupture. Because of these dangers, the osmolality, or tonicity, of the extracellular fluid is maintained within very narrow limits. Aberrations in osmolality will occur through variations in the solvent (water) or in the solute (the contained salts), usually because of a disease which causes failure of intake of these, or which brings about their loss to an undue degree. The variations in osmolality are sensed by *osmoreceptors* in the brain, which in turn can control the kidney's release of water by the antidiuretic hormone mechanism. It is probable too that these receptors make us feel thirsty, giving an opportunity to renew the solvent.

Changes in solvent/solute (osmolality) relationships are often associated with changes in the extracellular volume. These are sensed in the kidneys which can then cause the adrenals to release a substance called aldosterone, which helps to control the reabsorption of water and sodium by the kidney.

Both of these mechanisms (osmolal sensing, volume sensing) work together in order to maintain the body's integrity. Thus, if we take in a lot of salt, this is absorbed, and temporarily increases the osmolality of the extracellular fluid. This increase is sensed by the osmoreceptors, which stimulate thirst and also the supply of antidiuretic hormone which slows the kidney's excretion of water. Both mechanisms restore the ratio of solvent to solute towards normal. However, the total volume of solution is now increased. This is determined by the receptors which activate the aldosterone mechanism, allowing the kidney to lose sodium. If the water is lost in the same ratio, then the situation is completely restored. The same mechanisms will operate in reverse when excess water intake tends to lower osmolality.

Clearly, diseases which interfere with the thirst mechanism (coma, delirium, severe illness), or kidney disease, will severely affect the body's ability to compensate for the primary variations noted above.

MAINTENANCE OF NORMAL ACID/BASE BALANCE

The acidity or alkalinity (pH value) of the body must be kept at about pH 7.4, otherwise death of the cells will occur. This buffering ability is closely bound up with fluid and electrolyte disorders, since the latter can impair the methods of compensation of acid/base variation.

The body faces 2 main problems: first, to get the acid products of metabolism out of the cells and into the extracellular fluid, and, second, to rid the extracellular fluid of these. Acids are substances which can supply hydrogen (H^+) ions, or protons, i.e., they are proton donors.

Alkalis are, in general substances which accept protons, or H^+ ions. Substances which can, in certain circumstances accept or donate protons are called *ampholytic*.

Proteins (including hemoglobin) fall into the last class and therefore are good buffering agents, well able to accept the products of cellular metabolism delivered by the process called the chloride shift.

Another method of buffering is the carbonic acid/bicarbonate system, which can deal both with acid and base excess. Hydrogen ion (acid) accumulation is dealt with through the equation ($H^+ + HCO_3^- \rightarrow H_2CO_3 \rightarrow H_2O + CO_2$). The end point of the reaction is dealt with by CO_2 excretion by the lungs, which in general act as the tactical reserve for acid/base regulation. However, the lungs cannot deal with unlimited hydrogen ion accumulation, so a strategic reserve is used. This is the kidney, which can excrete H^+ ion in a combined form. The 3 acceptors in the kidney are bicarbonate (HCO_3^-), phosphate (HPO_4^{--}) and ammonium (NH_3^-). Thus intracellular H^+ ion exchanges with kidney tubular Na^+ in the presence of tubular HCO_3^-, which can dissociate to H_2O and CO_2; at the pCO_2 values of the tubular fluid, CO_2, will be resorbed thus tending to conserve HCO_3^-. This mechanism can operate as long as tubular HCO_3^- is available. When this is not so, the intracellular H^+ ion exchanges with tubular Na^+ and is now available for addition to tubular HPO_4^{--} to form $H_2PO_4^-$ which is then excreted.

In the presence of tubular H^+ ions, the secretion of NH_3 will form NH_4^+, usually fixed as NH_4Cl. This mechanism is facilitated by the presence of tubular fluid which is already of low pH.

Acidosis and Alkalosis

These are rather archaic terms which imply retention of, or loss of H^+ ion respectively. The change in pH is small, and compensation rapidly occurs. The cause of the changes follow from the physiology, as described below.

Respiratory acidosis occurs when the blood pCO_2 increases. This can happen if breathing fails (as in paralysis of the respiratory muscles) or carbon dioxide cannot diffuse out of the body (as in hyaline membrane disease in newborns). The result of a high pCO_2 is an increase in H^+ ion (since H_2CO_3 shifts to $H^+ + HCO_3^-$). This acidosis can of course be compensated by the kidney so that pH shift is minimized.

Respiratory alkalosis. This occurs when there is an increase in respiratory rate (e.g., by fever, respiratory infection). The pCO_2 falls, and so does the availability of H^+ donor (H_2CO_3). This is compensated by the kidney which resorbs H^+ ion and increases the urinary excretion of HCO_3^-.

Metabolic acidosis will occur if we take in substances releasing H^+ ion, e.g. salicylates, or where there is excessive loss of hydrogen ion acceptor (HCO_3^-) as in diarrhea or high intestinal obstruction. Perhaps the most common cause, however, is interference with the renal mechanisms for excreting H^+ ion, as in most states of dehydration or chronic renal disease. The decrease in pH will cause respiratory compensation which will tend to decrease pCO_2. This will reduce the level of hydrogen ion donor (H_2CO_3), since one reactant in the equation ($H_2O + CO_2 = H_2CO_3$) is now deficient.

Metabolic alkalosis will occur with excessive ingestion of actual or potential hydrogen ion acceptor (e.g., sodium bicarbonate, sodium citrate). Excess loss of hydrogen ion by the kidney or gastrointestinal tract will lead to the same result. So too will the loss of chloride ion, by vomiting or other routes. In this circumstance, ionic balance is disturbed and is partially compensated by the retention of HCO_3^- ion.

If the respiratory mechanisms are intact, metabolic alkalosis will lead to a decrease in respiration (hypoventilation) although only to a limited degree, with a consequent increase in hydrogen ion donor (H_2CO_3). The kidney will tend to conserve H^+ ion and to lose HCO_3^- and to secrete an alkaline urine inimical to ammonia formation. Each of these would tend to compensate the alkalosis by conserving H^+ ion.

It is clear then that efficient lungs and kidneys are both essential for the maintenance of the normal buffering mechanisms. All treatments given to children must be based upon maintaining the integrity of the lungs and kidneys in relation to this activity of their cells.

CLINICAL PROBLEMS

Water and salt loss usually coincide, so dehydration implies salt loss and low salt syndrome implies water loss as well. Water and salt may be lost in unequal proportions and this will be reflected in the laboratory findings (see below). However, treatment will always include replacement of both items.

Causes of dehydration

These are many, and can roughly be divided into those associated with failure of intake, and those associated with excessive loss. Coma, due for example to head injury or drug overdosage, is an obvious cause of failure to take in salt and water, less obvious is the failure of appetite, or difficulty in drinking which occurs in childhood diseases such as tonsillitis or chest infections.

Excessive loss of water and salts are the more common problems. An obvious cause is gastroenteritis, in which large amounts of fluid and salts are lost in the diarrhea. In chest infections, such as bronchiolitis, there is a greatly increased respiration rate which causes water loss from the lungs. This in turn increases the salt content (osmolality) of the extracellular fluid. The body adjusts the osmolality towards normal by allowing the kidney to excrete salt. The whole process is aggravated by the breathlessness which discourages the patient from taking in food and water which could repair the deficits. In diabetic coma, the dehydration results from the excessive formation of urine associated with the excretion of sugar (glycosuria); vomiting also occurs, which not only aggravates the loss of body fluids, but prevents them being repleted. In adrenogenital syndrome, vomiting occurs and abnormalities of the aldosterone system cause excessive loss of sodium and water. Some of the more common causes of dehydration are shown in table 31.

Table 31. Common causes of dehydration

Situation	Example
Failure of ingestion	Coma: head injury; poisoning
Failure of retention	Vomiting: e.g., pyloric stenosis; intestinal obstruction; meningitis
Loss of fluid and electrolyte	Gut: gastroenteritis
	Kidney: diabetic coma; renal failure
	Lung: bronchiolitis; asthma
Failure of regulating mechanism	Adrenogenital syndrome (aldosterone)
	Diabetes insipidus (antidiuretic hormone)

The end result of dehydration is to reduce the extracellular volume which means that the heart cannot exert its full pumping capacity; in other words the cardiac output (circulatory effort) is impaired so that there is a reduction in the blood flow through the important organs of the body. The skin and muscles are usually affected first, then the kidneys, liver, and gut, and lastly the brain and the heart itself. If an organ does not receive enough blood then it cannot function properly. For example, the patient may become acidotic because his kidneys can no longer excrete H^+ ion by the methods already described. The younger the child the fewer are his reserves of salts and water, so the more rapidly does he deteriorate. On the other hand, young children respond more rapidly to proper treatment than do adults.

Ways of recognizing dehydration and salt loss

The child may have a disorder (gastroenteritis, bronchiolitis, meningitis, etc.) which could be complicated by dehydration. In addition to the features of the primary disease, the child fails to improve and then in general begins to look more ill; the speed of deterioration relates to his age, the younger he is the more rapidly he gets worse. An early sign is lessening of activity, a particularly helpful sign in an illness which is associated with irritability and restlessness such as meningitis. The skin becomes pale and cool, and sweating stops. There is a decrease in the amount of urine which is passed. The mouth and tongue dry out and the saliva becomes thick. As the extracellular volume decreases, the eyes look sunken, and, in some children, the abdomen becomes flat and empty looking (scaphoid appearance). The fontanelle, if open, becomes depressed. A very valuable sign is loss of tissue turgor—the skin feels doughy and inelastic, and if pinched up, retains its shape for some time. The failure of cardiac output is attested to by a rapid weak pulse, the onset of a greyish pallor, fall in the blood pressure, and an increase in the respiratory rate. The breathing may be aggravated by coincident acidosis which stimulates the respiratory centre. In older children this results in deep sighing respirations called Kussmaul breathing. Undue flaccidity of the limbs may suggest that potassium has been lost as well as sodium, chloride, and water.

If the patient has lost water, then he must lose weight. If he is under observation this weight loss may precede any of the signs noted above. Otherwise, it may be possible to get evidence of recent weight loss as part of the history of the illness.

Investigations

The most important of these is an accurate, frequent measurement of weight and blood pressure. The other things which are usually done are to measure the *concentrations* of sodium, chloride, and potassium in the blood. pH, pCO_2, and hence available alkali are also measured. Note that when sodium, etc. is measured as concentrations (mEq/l), this does not tell us the *total* quantity of the element in the body. So, a patient may be very ill, have lost equal quantities of water and sodium, and have *normal* serum and electrolyte (Na^+, K^+, Cl^-, etc.) values. This represents isosmolar dehydration. If more water than salt has been lost, then the *concentration* of salt will be high, although the *total body* salt is low—this is hyperosmolar (hypernatremic) dehydration. If more salt than water has been lost, then the salt concentration is low—this is hypoosmolar (hyponatremic) dehydration. Figure 54 shows diagrammatically what can happen. The important thing to recall is that in nearly every circumstance, the treatment is to give both salt *and* water.

Treatment

The principles of treatment are (1) to replace the lost water and salts so that the extracellular volume and circulation are restored, (2) to give the usual maintenance amount of fluid and electrolyte which the child needs, and (3) to treat the disorder which precipitated the dehydration.

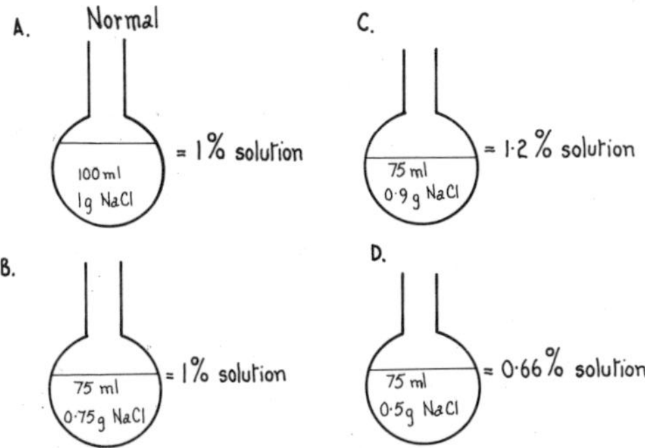

Fig. 54. Models of clinical situations: *a*, Normal body water and salt distribution (electrolyte concentration normal, e.g., Na 146mEq/1); *b*, symmetrical loss of water and electrolyte (electrolyte concentration normal, e.g., 146mEq/1 – isotonic dehydration); *c*, Dehydration and electrolyte loss, former predominates (electrolyte concentration high, e.g., Na 160mEq/1 – hypertonic dehydration); *d*, Loss of water and salt, latter predominates (electrolyte concentration low, e.g., Na 132mEq/1 – hypotonic dehydration).

Replacement

To do this we must try and calculate the loss of fluid, and decide what fluids are to be given and by what route. The actual loss of fluid is arrived at by estimating what the acute loss of body weight has been. If the patient has been in hospital before he became dehydrated, then the difference between the previous weight and the weight when he is dehydrated tells us what the fluid loss has been. However, the child may be dehydrated when he is admitted, so the best we can do is to make an intelligent guess. This is done in several ways. Firstly, find out from the parents if the child has been weighed recently. Otherwise, what can be done is to measure the child's length, assess his height percentile (see p. 6) and assume that his weight percentile would be about the same as that for his height. From the tables we can get a figure for weight. This is regarded as his normal (undehydrated) weight; his actual (dehydrated) weight is subtracted and the figure is an approximation of the weight, and hence the fluid loss. For example: A previously healthy body aged 9-12 develops diarrhea. His length is 71 cm (50th percentile), his dehydrated weight is 8.4 kg (25th percentile), his expected weight (at 50th percentile) is 9.1 kg. The approximate fluid deficit is

$$(9.1 - 8.4)\text{kg} = 0.7 \text{ kg} = 700 \text{ ml}$$

These approximate calculations are checked against the child's general appearance. Thus, if a child looks only mildly dehydrated but the calculation reveals a 10% weight loss, then something is wrong. On the other hand, if the child looks at death's door, and the calculation suggests only a 3% weight loss then this is wrong in the other direction.

Maintenance requirements of fluid

This is easily obtained from tables (see table 32) which give the requirement of fluid as ml/kg of *normal* body weight. Normal (undehydrated) body weight can be obtained from percentile tables as already described.

Table 32. Daily fluid requirements

Age	Weight (kg)	Water (ml) per kg Body Weight in 24 Hours
3 months	5.4	140–160 (750–850)
6 months	7.3	130–150 (950–1,100)
1 year	9.5	120–135 (1,150–1,300)
4 years	16.2	100–110 (1,600–1,800)
10 years	28.7	70–85 (2,000–2,500)

Daily ranges in parentheses – total intake.

Total fluid requirement

This is the total of the deficit and the 24-hour maintenance volume, each derived as described above. It should be emphasized that the prescription of fluid is not a fixed one. A child who has continuing diarrhea may require constant reevaluation and represcription of the fluid requirement.

What to give

The general requirement is for water, sodium, and chloride. Glucose is also usually given in order to supply some calories. Normal (0.9%) saline (NaCl) solution is the basis of treatment. It can be diluted to 0.5 N (normal) or 0.45% saline, 0.3 N (0.3% NaCl), or 0.2 N (0.18% NaCl). Solutions stronger than normal (0.9% NaCl) are NEVER given except in very special circumstances.

The volume of solution will have been approximated by the methods given. If there is evidence of severe sodium depletion—low blood pressure, suppression of urine (anuria), grayish cyanosis and low serum sodium—then 0.9% saline is given. In less severe circumstances, 0.5N (0.45%) saline may be adequate. Calories are supplied by adding dextrose to a final concentration of 5% *dextrose* in the *saline* solution.

The solution is given quickly, and always intravenously, until the patient has improved—looks better, has a normal blood pressure, warm extremities, a slower pulse, and has passed urine. He should also have gained weight at this stage. If the source of loss (e.g., diarrhea) has ceased, then it is usual to replace the 0.9% NaCl solution with one of 0.45% (0.5 normal) strength NaCl. If the first fluid given was 0.45% NaCl, then the follow on fluid will be 0.3% NaCl. When the patient is able to take normal amounts of fluid and electrolyte by mouth, then the intravenous fluid may be given as 0.18% (0.2 normal) NaCl.

Potassium

This is an important intracellular ion, which is often lost when a patient is dehydrated. The level of K^+ in the blood is controlled within fine limits by the kidney, because an excess (hyperkalemia) can cause death. Accordingly, potassium is not given until the intravenous saline solution has restored kidney function. The evidence that this has happened is the passing of urine by the patient. When this has happened then it is safe to add potassium (usually as potassium chloride—KCl) to the intravenous fluid. The normal daily requirment of potassium as KCl is 2.5 mEq/kg body weight/24 hours. This may be increased in certain circumstances. Potassium is always given in divided doses, commonly on a 4-6-hourly basis. Low blood potassium (hypokalemia) is a rare complication of dehydration. It is usually suspected by examining the electrocardiogram (E.C.G.). Hypokalemia causes flaccidity of the muscles, but is seldom a dangerous complication. Only in very exceptional circumstances is potassium given intravenously before urine has been passed.

Acidosis

This is the usual abnormality of acid/base balance found in dehydration. It is due to cessation of renal activity because of the poor cardiac output. Thus, in most instances, giving adequate fluid and electrolyte will restore renal circulation and correct the acidosis. If the blood pH is very low (<7.25) then an alkali (sodium bicarbonate) can be added to the saline solution. However, this is hardly ever necessary.

Alkalosis

This is a rather rare complication of dehydration. The respiratory variety may complicate salicylism, or occasionally, C.N.S. disease (e.g., encephalitis) where dehydration has supervened because of failure to ingest water and electrolytes. The commonest causes of metabloic alkalosis are those associated with vomiting, e.g., pyloric stenosis and high intestinal obstruction. Injudicious alkali therapy for acidosis is also a not uncommon cause. Chloride and potassium loss usually coexist and the condition may be difficult to compensate unless deficits of the latter are repaired. Otherwise, the relief of the primary disease and restoration of renal function is normally all that is necessary. The deliberate injection of actual or potential H^+ ion (e.g., NH_4Cl) should be avoided.

Route of infusion

The intravenous method is always used, normally by putting in a needle rather than by cut down and insertion of a cannula. Cut down destroys the vein—further use and conservation of veins is important especially in malnourished children who may require many drips. None the less, occasional cut downs will be necessary if a vein cannot be entered by needle, and the patient's condition is critical. Fluid may be given into the peritoneum in an emergency. Fluid should *not* be given subcutaneously in dehydrated patients, as the circulatory failure precludes its pick up from that area.

Speed of infusion

In extreme dehydration the fluid is given as rapidly as possible until the patient looks better, raises his blood pressure, passes urine, and gains weight. In less urgent circumstances, an *approximation* is to give the calculated deficit in 2-3 hours and to give the calculated 24-hour maintenance over 18 hours. The patient's condition and weight are, however, paramount over any rules: if fluid losses continue then prolonged rapid infusion may be needed.

PATIENTS WHO PRESENT SPECIAL DIFFICULTIES

Chronic malnutrition

Diarrhea is common in chronic malnutrition, and frequently coexists with acute or chronic respiratory infection. The patient may also have frank kwashiorkor with edema or hypoproteinemia, but more often this will occur after a week or more of intravenous glucose/electrolyte. Anemia and marked potassium loss are common. It should be realized that in these children recovery from diarrhea is a matter of weeks, unlike the few days of illness of the well nourished. It is fundamental then, that vein conservation is practised, and cut downs severely discouraged. The principles of treatment are those already noted. Assessment of height percentile will avoid overestimation of fluid need, and a close examination for edema will sensitize the clinician to a more serious situation than the scales indicate. In some instances, the gut infection results in a state akin to that found in ulcerative colitis, with continuous blood and protein loss. Accordingly, blood and plasma may be required early, although the principal infusions are of saline. Every effort should be made to treat any respiratory infection, as this is a continuing source of body water loss. Oral feeding should be well established before the intravenous is removed, and the food should be low in lactose as lactose intolerance is commonly found in such children, at least as an acute complication of diarrhea.

The major problem is not the acute repair of dehydration, but the rapid and disheartening return of diarrhea when the child is fed by mouth. This can often be treated only by a return to the gut resting drip. A careful watch should always be kept for the septicemias, which may occur in the course of treatment.

Chronic renal failure

These patients have, to a greater or lesser extent, lost the ability to conserve water. The urinary specific gravity is low and the ability to excrete H^+ is also impaired. A salt-losing state is rather unusual, but potassium retention occurs late in the disease. Such patients are liable to dehydration, often because intercurrent illness prevents the obligatory increased intake of fluid so necessary for them.

The general principles are those already noted. However, the patient's *maintenance* fluid requirement will be increased, usually by at least 25% above normal. Commonly, 0.45% (½N) saline is used as the initial rehydrating fluid. If the patient was previously known to be hypertensive, a normal blood pressure may indicate severe salt depletion. Saline infusion should be continued until a dilute urine has been passed and normal (i.e., sometimes hypertensive) blood pressure levels are reached.

The precautions concerning potassium administration should be redoubled in renal failure and it is best to divide this ion into fractional (x4-5 daily) doses, with previous E.C.G. check. This will avoid accidental hyperkalemia. The situation concerning acid/base balance is a ticklish one in renal failure. Attempts to change pH should be made with considerable deliberation and ordinarily guided by arterial samples. Thus, the giving of bicarbonate may precipitate a shift of H^+ ion level which will depress an already limited level of Ca^{++} ion. This in turn may cause a severe tetany (convulsions due to calcium imbalance). A similar situation (with the risk of K^+ intoxication) is also possible in rapid transfusion of blood containing the usual ACD anticoagulant.

Apart from the restoration of a dilute urine flow, a decrease in the blood urea values is a good guide to therapy. In general, dilute sodium containing fluids (e.g., 0.18% NaCl) are indicated as follow-on fluids, unless the plasma/urine studies indicate the rare salt losing states. Severe and symptomatic hyperkalemic syndromes cannot normally be relieved except by peritoneal dialysis.

The neonate

The newborn infant has certain disabilities in relation to the renal handling of water and solute. The mechanisms for water and electrolyte conservation also do not reach the efficiency levels of the older child, and his total exchangeable sodium is high. All of these disabilities are exaggerated in the premature infant. The normal newborn is relatively hydremic and the ranges of blood constituents are wider from those of the older child. Thus, micromethod ranges for sodium and chloride in the first 12 days are 125-45 mEq and 96-114 mEq respectively. Potassium ranges of 3.5-8.0 mEq/l are not uncommon in normal infants. In the first 24 hours of life pH values are lower than in later life.

Perhaps the commonest causes of neonatal water and salt loss are the intestinal obstructions and the respiratory distress syndromes. However, most of the other situations affecting the older child (e.g., gastroenteritis) can also affect the neonate; other less obvious causes include C.S.F. loss in ruptured meningomyelocele or through neurosurgical manoeuvre, or leaching of salt and water by repeated tapping of subdural effusions.

The clinical recognition of dehydration may not always be easy, especially in premature or dysmature infants. The most reliable sign is a *sudden* (over a few hours) loss of weight. This is in contrast to the relatively smooth weight loss which accompanies the adjustment of the neonatal hydremia. Loss of skin elasticity is usual, although less easy to be sure of in the dysmature infant. The fontanelle is depressed. Activity is limited and hypothermia, hypotension and greyish pallor are common in severe dehydration. In all instances, there is a definite route of loss, or block of the normal avenues of ingestion of fluid and electrolyte. *The principles of care are those already described.*

Thus the infant can normally be rehydrated to close to its birth weight. In general, 0.45% (½N) saline is useful initial rehydrating fluid, and follow-on solutions should be of the order of 0.18-0.3% NaCl. The infant should be *weighed at least every 4 hours*, and electrolyte estimations done at least thrice daily. The problems of control by such electrolyte values alone should be recalled. Blood pressure measurements are of great value in assessing therapy, as is the production of urine. Even with these precautions, it is, however, common enough to find that the infant develops some peripheral edema. If the general state (behaviour, blood pressure, urine output) is otherwise satisfactory, this complication may be looked upon with equanimity. Potassium therapy should be used with caution in the newborn, since plasma levels are normally quite high. Correction of acid/base balance should also be undertaken with care, and only if adequate samples (preferably arterial) show considerable derangement. Inessential sodium bicarbonate therapy may lead to potentially dangerous hypernatremia. Coincident hypoglycemia is common in dehydrated neonates and should be deliberately sought for and treated.

CONDITIONS CHARACTERIZED BY EXPANSION OF THE EXTRACELLULAR VOLUME

In most instances, this rare condition follows injudicious intravenous therapy, usually taking the form of excess of 5% glucose. This behaves as water and gives rise to a hypoosmolar (hypotonic) ECV expansion. Accordingly, plasma sodium and chloride values decrease. A similar condition will arise in hot, humid climates where excessive sweating is offset by drinking large amounts of water without added salt. Occasionally, the syndrome is associated with injudicious intravenous therapy in acute renal shut down. Central nervous system symptoms (irritability, convulsions, coma) occur, accounting for the synonym of water intoxication. Headache, nausea, and vomiting may be associated, and muscle cramps occur in older children. Muscle weakness is common but nonspecific. Terminally, degrees of raised intracranial pressure may occur, viz., hypertension, bradycardia and papilledema. *Weight loss does not occur in the syndrome* and this is the principal differentiating point in the diagnosis from other fluid electrolyte disturbances. At first much urine is passed then kidney function slows. The urine is dilute, and contains little sodium. All the blood constituents (Hb, Na^+, Cl^-, K^+) show low values because of dilution.

Treatment

This is based upon giving relatively strong saline solutions. In *severe* expansion, give 3% saline (contains 510 mEq/Na/litre) in volumes sufficient to raise the plasma sodium by 5 mEq/l to a maximum of 10 mEq/l. This will usually restore renal function to allow the excretion of excess water. A slow I.V. infusion of 0.9% (Normal) saline should be continued until the child again has normal water and electrolyte values.

Hypertonic expansion of the extracellular volume

Again this is usually the result of treatment and occurs when excessive amounts of 0.9% (or stronger) saline is given. It may complicate acute renal failure. It is much less common than the water intoxication syndrome already described, and is characterized by signs of high cardiac output, viz., normal blood pressure, loud venous hums, functional murmurs and third heart sounds. Urination is profuse and contains large quantities of sodium and chloride. There are no specific central nervous system signs. Dyspnea, hoarseness and edema occur if the condition is not recognized. The plasma sodium and chloride are increased but the hemoglobin and protein values suggest dilution. Weight gain is invariable.

The treatment consists in discontinuing, or markedly slowing down, intravenous therapy. No other treatment is indicated.

25 The allergic disorders

Allergic responses bear a resemblance to disturbances of immunological mechanism. Thus, an allergic reaction takes place when an antigenic substance (allergen) gains access to the body. It then promotes an immune response, characterized by stimulation of the lymphoreticular system and multiplication of specifically responding cells. This in turn produces immunoglobulins (IgG, IgA, IgM, or IgE) specific for the allergen. When this has occurred the person is *allergic*, i.e., capable of responding to further exposure to the allergen (antigen). Clearly in most instances the allergic state is physiological, and helpful to the individual. In certain circumstances, the response produces a disease state, i.e., the individual is hypersensitive. Symptoms will result from certain broad mechanisms, some of which may overlap. Thus in asthma and hay fever, the allergen may release pharmacological agents affecting the bronchi or nose, through reaction with cells such as basophils and mast cells. This reaction depends upon a reagin mechanism, of which immunoglobulin E (IgE) is a significant component. It seems likely that in man, histamine and bradykinin are among the pharmacological substances produced in the reaction. Cell damage can also result when antibody reacts with an antigen or a drug (hapten) in the presence of complement. This is the type of reaction seen in mismatched blood transfusion, and in drug induced hemolytic anemias.

Antigen/antibody complexes which localize in the blood vessels may also cause disease, e.g., serum sickness. This is also the basis of the Arthus phenomenon, in which a severe inflammatory cutaneous reaction follows an injection of a high concentration of antigen into an individual already sensitized to that antigen.

Delayed hypersensitivity does not depend upon antibody reaction, but initiates disease states of the type exemplified by contact dermatitis. The mechanism of this is not fully known, but would appear to involve lymphocytes which have specific receptors resembling antibodies.

GENERAL INVESTIGATION OF ALLERGIC DISORDERS

The most important investigation is a detailed history of the disease, related to such factors as time of occurrence, place of occurrence, and possible exposure to likely allergens. In this way one will establish whether the symptoms are seasonal or perennial. A simple environmental survey should also be made especially when the place of recurrence of symptoms can be reasonably located. The patient must of course be thoroughly examined for confirmatory signs of an allergic process, and to exclude other types of disease.

Skin testing

This is done to detect the presence of an allergic reagin and may be done by scratching in, or injection of, an antigen solution. The response is a flare or wheal in the tested area. Control scratch or injections of the vehicle must always be employed.

In general, the results of skin tests must always be interpreted with great caution, since a positive skin test may not indicate *clinical* sensitivity to the injected antigen. The converse also holds. Positive results may however stimulate further detailed history taking. Skin sensitivity to food products can often occur although the patient has no symptoms.

Passive transfer testing (Prausnitz-Küstner reaction)

This is used to demonstrate the presence of a reagin in the patient's serum. The test is done in a previously investigated volunteer, into whom intradermal infections of small volumes of the patient's serum are made. After 24-48 hours, the suspected agent is injected into the same area. This technique is of limited clinical value, although false-positive results are said to be less.

Provocative tests

This is a mode of determining clinical sensitivity to an allergen. It is of limited practical application and indicated perhaps only where the history is suggestive of a specific allergen, but where other tests are equivocal or contradictory. Such tests are principally indicated in hay fever and asthma. The object is more or less to reproduce the symptoms. Thus, in the case of asthma, an increase in airway resistance following inhalation of allergen, may be considered a positive result.

All provocative tests are potentially dangerous, and should only be employed in situations where full resuscitative measures are available. They should not be employed at all in serum sickness or other generalized allergic conditions.

Diet diary

This is sometimes of value when a response to an ingested allergen is suspected. A note is made of all foods eaten, together with any symptoms. In most instances it will readily be seen that there is no correlation between many foods and the appropriate symptoms. Again, this may help in evaluating the history, especially when symptoms are relatively infrequent. An extension of the diet diary is the *elimination diet*, in which suspect allergens are excluded from the food. Such diets should be continued only for a limited time, and without otherwise treating the patient or controlling his environment. Clearly, essential nutrients must always be included in the experimental diet. As in the investigation of all allergic disorders, the results should be regarded with reserve. Most of the commonly prescribed elimination diets are nutritionally inadequate for children, and should not be given over any lengthy period.

Other investigations

The white blood count may show an excess percentage of eosinophils. This is supportive evidence for an allergic state, it does not prove it. Many children have an eosinophilia which is not reflected in clinical allergic disease. An excess of eosinophils in the nasal mucosa is however characteristic of hay fever.

IgE

The level of this immunoglobulin is elevated in a substantial proportion of allergic subjects. As yet, IgE determination is hardly a routine test for allergic subjects.

SPECIFIC ENTITIES

Hay fever (allergic rhinitis and conjunctivitis)

This is a common disorder which may coexist with other allergic disease such as asthma. The sensitivity is usually to pollens and moulds and the disease is usually seasonal.

Clinical features. There is paroxysmal sneezing with itching, running eyes, and nose. The palate tickles and headache occurs in older children. Fever, in spite of the name, never occurs. The severity varies greatly. Thus in some children, sneezing, rhinorrhea, and lacrimation are continuous. In others there is only a minor degree of itching.

Signs. The eyes are blood shot, and conjunctival edema may be present. The eye lids are often swollen—usually after much rubbing by the patient. The nasal discharge is watery, and the nose is partly blocked. The mucosa itself is pale and swollen.

Treatment The allergen should be avoided if possible. A filtering air-conditioner may afford some relief indoors. Local treatment with vasoconstrictors (e.g. neosynephrine ¼% nose drops) may help the milder cases. A fair proportion of the severe cases are helped by oral antihistaminic drugs. In those who do not respond to these, sympathomimetic agents (e.g., ephedrine) are worthy of trial. In some, the sniffing of disodium cromoglycate may prevent attacks.

Where the allergen has been specifically determined, and when symptoms are severe, desensitization may be helpful.

Prognosis. This is good, except in those children with associated asthma.

Anaphylaxis and serum sickness

Etiology. The reaction can follow injections of animal products, usually sera, drugs such as penicillin, or follow insect bites.

Clinical features. In a few patients there is the rapid onset of hypotension, pallor, and tachycardia, followed by severe respiratory obstruction which may be fatal. In other children the main response is in the skin with urticaria, angioneurotic edema, and generalized itchiness. If the edema involves the larynx, there is dyspnea and stridor. Tightness in the chest and bronchospasm can occur. Fever, with pain and swelling of several joints, is also found.

Anaphylaxis due to insect bite

This is usually due to sensitivity to wasps, bees, hornets, and some species of ant. There is a history of an increasing local response to the bite, viz, an original simple papule is, on the next bite, a brawny swelling. On the next occasion, the whole limb is swollen and general anaphylaxis of the type described occurs at a subsequent bite.

Treatment:

1. Immediate. The allergen, if injected by mistake, or by insect bite, may be localized by tourniquet. Adrenaline should be injected and an antihistamine given. In respiratory obstruction, an endotracheal tube should be passed. In severe shock, an infusion of a drug to maintain blood pressure may be helpful.

2. Prevention. If due to a medication, the parents should be warned that the substance must not be given. In insect bite reactions, cautious desensitization is helpful.

Angioneurotic edema

This is the name given to allergic local swelling, with brawny edema. It may coexist with urticaria. The condition tends to affect the looser areas of skin such as that of the lips, eyes, and genitals, In a few instances the buccal mucosa and that of the larynx may be involved. The etiology is similar to that described for urticaria and the treatment is the same.

Cutaneous allergic disease

Atopic dermatitis (eczema) which begins early in life, tends to go away by itself by the second birthday. It may be followed by asthma. Contact dermatitis is more common in the older child and adolescent, except in countries where poison ivy (rhus toxicodendron) is found. Common allergens, apart from plants, are cosmetics, ointments, and substances (e.g., glues) used in the child's hobbies. Urticarial reactions with the characteristic wheal and papule are common in children and may be local or general. The latter are commonly due to ingestants, the former to insect bites.

The clinical features and treatment of these entities is discussed under skin disease.

Gastrointestinal allergy

The incidence of this entity is debateable. Many patients so labelled have subsequently been found to be sufferers from other conditions, particularly gut wall enzyme deficiency (e.g., alactasia). Accordingly, the diagnosis should be made only after careful consideration. Suggestive aspects are a recurrence of the symptom *soon* after the alleged allergen is introduced, and total disappearance of the problem if the allergen is avoided.

Bronchial asthma

The clinical features of this are described elsewhere. The disease may be superimposed upon other conditions with a definite allergic basis, such as hay fever and eczema. In many instances, however, the search for a precipitating allergen is not fruitful in perennial asthma, and treatments specifically against allergens (elimination diets, desensitization) are disappointing. Children with bronchial asthma show a large number of responses to skin tests. The avoidance of the test substance, or desensitization to it is, however, inconstantly associated with relief of the asthma. There is good clinical evidence that, in asthma sufferers, attacks can be precipitated by respiratory infections. It is as yet unclear as to whether this is an allergic reaction to the pathogen or one of its products, or a precipitant for some other factor.

26 Collagen diseases

This is the term applied to a group of disorders whose cause is imperfectly known. Superficially most appear to be inflammatory, but there is growing evidence that they may represent an abnormal antigen/antibody response, i.e., an autoimmune state.

SPECIFIC ENTITIES

Rheumatic fever

This is a disease associated with infection (or infestation) by the group A type of the beta-hemolytic streptococcus. It occurs at all seasons, perhaps more commonly in the winter months, bearing a close relationship to the community incidence of the streptococcus. There is some evidence of an inherited tendency to get rheumatic fever, but there is no predilection for either sex. It is very unusual before the fourth birthday.

Clinical features. Often there is a history of a streptococcal infection (throat, ears) in the preceding month. The most characteristic story is one of arthritis, which affects the larger joints making them painful, swollen, and sometimes red. Usually 1 joint is involved at a time, and disability varies from a mild ache to intolerable pain. Fever, lassitude, and anorexia are common. Epistaxis and abdominal pain occur often. The latter may be the presenting symptom, and be confused with an abdominal emergency. The polyarthritis may be accompanied by skin rashes, particularly erythema annulare, or nodosum. Neither rash is, of itself, specific for rheumatic fever.

Rheumatic carditis

This is the most important facet of rheumatic fever; fortunately, only a fraction of patients have cardiac involvement during the first attack. The evidence for carditis is variable. Thus one child may have obvious congestive cardiac failure, without any murmur. Another may develop the harsh constant apical systolic murmur of mitral insufficiency. This is probably the commonest objective sign. Some patients have variable, but always organic, murmurs—systolic or the diastolic of aortic insufficiency. These occasionally change from day to day, and while implying endocarditis, do not always result in fixed valvular deformity. A night and day tachycardia, usually with a prominent third heart sound (gallop rhythm) also ordinarily implies carditis, as does pericarditis. When the characteristic rub disappears, signs of valvular damage may be found, or a pericardial effusion may develop. In those with no murmur, congestive failure may occur even when the situation seems stable. Routine x-rays should always be made in rheumatic fever; unsuspected cardiomegaly may imply carditis.

Electrocardiography is only of moderate value in the diagnosis of rheumatic carditis. Usually more obvious signs are present, or the variability in normal children of the conduction time is underestimated.

In most patients whose heart is involved, there is some fever, and usually leucocytosis, rapid anemia, and loss of weight. Subcutaneous nodules may also occur, although they are found in those who have no carditis, or who have rheumatoid arthritis. They occur on the extensor tendons, the elbows, patella, spinous processes or scapulae.

Laboratory findings. There is no specific test for rheumatic fever. Leucocytosis, anemia and elevation of the sedimentation rate are common, but nonspecific. The C reactive protein reaction is often positive. The antistreptolysin titre (ASO) is evidence only of a precedent streptococcal invasion. Statistically speaking, while patients with a high ASO titre are likely to be sufferers from rheumatic fever, they are not bound to be.

Sydenham's chorea

This is a major manifestation of the rheumatic fever syndrome, either as a primary disorder, or following a typical attack of polyarthritis. Chorea is not constantly preceded by a streptococcal infection. The first symptom is usually clumsiness of movement or dropping things. In other cases, abnormal, uncontrollable movements are the first problem. These vary greatly in severity, from almost inobvious twitching to an uncontrollable incoordinate movement demanding heavy sedation. Grimacing and difficulty with writing are common symptoms, and weakness, sometimes of hemiplegic distribution (hemichorea) may occur. The speech may be indistinct, or disappear because of muscular weakness. Emotional instability is constant.

Characteristically the child loses the ability to perform fine movements such as buttoning, and unbuttoning. If asked to sit still the choreiform movements may be exaggerated. The hand grip is weak and variable, and the tongue cannot be kept out. If the arms and hands are held straight out, the child tends to overextend the fingers and wrists. Muscular hypotonia is common and the reflexes may be absent.

Treatment of rheumatic fever

The main end of treatment is to absolve the child from recurrences. This means the eradication of the streptococcus in the initial illness, and the maintenance of penicillin prophylaxis thereafter.

Rest in bed is needed while the disease is active, but normal movements in bed are useful in the prevention of foot drop and muscle wasting. Bedrest is continued until the temperature, the sleeping pulse, and the sedimentation rate are normal. In children with carditis, there should be no evidence of congestive failure, and the organic murmurs (if any) should have been constant for at least 3 months. Thereafter there is little point in continuing bedrest, and ambulation should be reasonably rapid, completed perhaps over 3-4 weeks. In those without evidence of carditis, the stage of ambulation should be reached within 3-4 weeks. In the patient with carditis, the period of bedrest should never exceed 4 months, unless there is congestive cardiac failure. All patients who are subjected to prolonged bedrest must have physiotherapy and education. In the absence of severe complications, most children need spend only a minimum of time in hospital. Thereafter they are best treated in their own home.

The child who has had rheumatic fever without carditis, and who has been clinically normal for 3 months, should be returned to normal activity (including sports) as soon as possible. The child who has a fixed valvular deformity, should be regarded as capable of exercise, and encouraged to find his own level of exercise tolerance.

The continued unreasoned application of restrictions, especially to the child with a valvular defect, is a fruitful source of cardiac necrosis. This may in turn defeat the future efforts of the cardiac surgeon.

Details of treatment

The acute attack. The child usually wishes to be in bed, and if the joints are very painful, he is given salicylates in an amount to relieve the arthritis. Symptoms and signs of salicylate intoxication should be watched for. Splinting of the limbs is seldom necessary. Steroids are equally effective in relieving the arthritis, but are not superior to salicylates. Infection with the streptococcus should be treated by penicillin injection.

There is no good evidence that steroids prevent the emergence of carditis. Therefore their routine use is to be deprecated. In the child who has evidence of carditis, there is perhaps more reason to use steroids, although controlled trials suggest that they have little superiority over salicylates. The prevention of further attacks resides in giving Bicillin for several years, or for life if endocarditis has occurred.

Rheumatoid arthritis

This is a disease of unknown etiology, which fortunately is relatively rare in children.

Clinical features. There are 2 basic types which may merge into each other. Perhaps the commoner is the following.

1. The early onset (2-4 years) systemic type. In this the features are continued fever, anorexia, loss of weight, and arthritis. Respiratory infections are common and abdominal pain not unusual. The arthritis may initially attack a large joint, but progression to smaller joints is usual. If the child is old enough, there may be a complaint of morning stiffness in the affected joints. In such children, lymphadenopathy and splenomegaly are common, and spindling of the finger joints ultimately develops. At some stage or another, the child develops a rheumatoid rash. This is not erythema multiforme, but consists in an evanescent but recurrent rash, often coincident with the peaks of pyrexia. The lesions are small, discrete macules with pallid centres, which often coalesce to give a morbilliform appearance. Subcutaneous nodules may be found at any stage. Muscle wasting is common, and in the neglected case, ankylosis occurs. Cardiac manifestations are rare, presenting usually as pericarditis.

Laboratory investigations. Anemia is usual, and leucocytosis common. The E.S.R. is increased. The gamma globulins are frequently above normal values. Agglutination tests (for latex particles, red cells, collodion), are nonspecific in this condition.

X-rays. Diminution of soft tissue shadows reflects muscular wasting. In the advanced and obvious case, the joint space is diminished, and osteoporosis evident.

2. Quasi-adult type rheumatoid arthritis. This is generally rarer than the infantile type described above. It occurs at 7-10 years of age and is characterized more by arthritis (often of a large joint), than by systemic disturbance. Wasting and fever are less apparent, although finger spindling and stiffness are usual. The laboratory and x-ray findings are somewhat more constant than in the younger patient.

Differential diagnosis. In the infantile type, the main differential is from a generalized infection, and in the older infant (4 years or so) from rheumatic fever. The latter is, of course, characterized by a precedent streptococcal infection, arthritis (usually of the larger joints), relatively little fever, and rapid response to salicylates. Useful differential points are the rheumatoid rash, and the finger spindling—each of which is not characteristic of rheumatic fever.

In the older child (7 +), rheumatic fever is again the likeliest cause of confusion. At this age too, disseminated lupus erythematosus (D.L.E.) becomes a consideration. Involvement of the kidney and myocardium are common in D.L.E., and the finding of L.E. cells in the blood diagnostic.

Treatment. A major point in therapy is support of the family. The nature of the condition is explained, and the need for long-term therapy emphasized, and the probability of cure made clear. Salicylates are the best drugs, and combined with heat treatment (hot baths, paraffin wax baths), are the mainstay of therapy. Physiotherapy is of minor value in the acute stage, but should be pushed when the child is free of pain. Steroids should be reserved for those with severe symptoms (gross weight loss, severe arthritis) and carefully supervised. Intercurrent respiratory infections should be vigorously treated.

Prognosis. Most children recover more or less completely over a period of years.

Henoch-Schönlein syndrome

This condition is also known as anaphylactoid or allergic non thrombocytopenic purpura. It affects many systems, principally the kidney, gut, and skin. The etiology is not fully known, but a coincidental streptococcal infection occurs in about half of the patients.

The clinical picture is variable and the features to be described may be initial or secondary ones. Gastrointestinal symptoms occur in most children and if they are the presenting phenomena, may simulate in intraabdominal catastrophe. The usual features are colicky abdominal pain, sometimes of considerable severity, and perhaps accompanied by vomiting. Abdominal tenderness and rigidity are found and may simulate the signs of appendicitis.

In other patients, the presenting feature is of an arthritis—with a hot, swollen joint which is painful on movement. The large joints of the legs are most frequently affected. Edema of the periarticular tissues is common, and the presence of fluid in the joint is usual.

A variable skin lesion may be the presenting symptom. In many children an itchy urticarial wheal appears, which then becomes petechial or frankly purpuric. A variety of skin lesions, urticarial, petechial, and purpuric is commonly present in the same patient. The hemorrhagic lesions go through the colour changes of a bruise, ending as a tobacco-coloured stain. These findings are commonest on the buttocks and the flexor aspects of the limbs. A minority of patients also show angioneurotic edema, with swelling of the eyelids, hands, feet, and the areas between the joints.

Renal involvement is rarely primary, although it occurs in more than half of the patients.

The syndrome is cyclic, and may extend over several weeks, with fresh episodes of abdominal pain, crops of skin lesions, or bouts of hematuria. Hypertension and signs of hypertensive encephalopathy may occasionally occur in those with renal involvement.

Laboratory findings. None is diagnostic. The E.S.R. is usually increased, polymorph leucocytosis is common, eosinophilia is rare. Platelet counts and the bleeding and clotting tests are normal. The hemoglobin decreases if there is massive bleeding into the skin, gastrointestinal or renal tracts. The ASO titre and latex tests are unhelpful.

Complications. A severe involvement of the gut may give rise to a situation of dehydration and salt loss because of vomiting. In this circumstance the jejunum is usually affected. Intussusception with obstruction rarely occurs.

Perhaps the most important complication is the kidney disorder, which rarely may cause persistent hematuria with ultimate chronic renal failure.

In a few cases the purpuric lesions of the skin may coalesce and become necrotic. There is never any permanent joint lesion.

Differential diagnosis. The principal problem arises when the patient presents with abdominal pain and vomiting. Appendicitis and gut obstruction are the main entities requiring exclusion. In all cases the rash, and evidence of hematuria should be sought. If there is abdominal pain and arthralgia, *rheumatic fever* deserves consideration.

Treatment. Most cases require no treatment. If there is evidence of streptococcal infection, penicillin should be given. The joint pain usually responds to rest and analgesics.

The abdominal colic may be so severe as to require morphine or pethidine. Vomiting and dehydration will demand intravenous fluids. Marked melena or hematuria may require blood transfusion. Hypertensive encephalopathy should be treated as in hemorrhagic glomerulonephritis. Steroids are indicated only in those cases where the course extends over more than 3-4 weeks without significant improvement. Return of symptoms after the cessation of steroid therapy is common.

Lupus erythematosus

This autoimmune disease usually occurs in school-age girls. It is occasionally familial. All mesenchymal tissues are affected, with marked changes in collagen and the development of fibrin-like deposits. A vasculitis is almost universal.

Clinical features. The onset may be preceded by fever, vague aches and pains, and purpuric rashes. In most children fever and symptoms in the larger joints are prominent. Pericarditis, cardiac murmurs and congestive cardiac failure are common. The involvement of the kidneys may be evident clinically as hematuria and albuminuria, or reveal itself by biochemical changes of renal failure in which hypertension is usual. Hepatomegaly and splenomegaly are common, especially in the younger patient. At any stage the classic butterfly rash ccurs on the nose, malar areas, and lower eyelids. It may spread to the neck and chest. Erythema punctata and petechial rashes are also common. Anemia is almost invariable.

Laboratory investigations. The most specific test is to demonstrate the LE cell phenomenon. A hemolytic anemia, thrombocytopenia, and leucocytosis may occur. Hypergammaglobulinemia is usual, and the E.S.R. increased, and flocculation reactions (e.g., a false positive Wasserman) common. The urine shows albumen, red cells, and casts. Kidney biopsy shows fibrinoid deposits and vasculitis.

Treatment. Steroids should be given in large dosage, with appropriate precautions to prevent severe side effects. If kidney involvement is marked, immunosuppressant drugs are given. Steroid treatment is long term, immunosuppression is usually intermittent.

As in leukemia, these patients are greatly at risk for unusual infections, e.g., herpes virus, cytomegalorivus, chicken pox infections, and fungal infections. These should be anticipated and diligently sought when unexplained symptoms arise during treatment.

Prognosis. This is still poor, since most children die within a year or two of the onset of the disease.

Dermatomyositis

This is a rare disease with inflammation of the unstriated muscle and skin.

Clinical features. The disease is seen in the school-age, and is of insidious onset with weakness, fatigue, and stiffness of the muscles, usually beginning in the legs. The weakness and stiffness spread ultimately involving the pharyngeal and respiratory muscles. The eyelids are characteristically bluish and may be swollen. An erythematous, scaling rash occurs in the butterfly facial distribution. As the disease progresses, muscle atrophy is severe and the skin binds to the deep tissues. The skin and muscle are tender and edema is common. Visceral involvement is reflected in enlarged glands, liver, and spleen. Subcutaneous calcification occurs in the late stage.

Course and prognosis. Many children ultimately recover, although remissions and exacerbations are usual. Death may occur from respiratory muscle involvement.

Laboratory signs. The muscle wasting is reflected in raised transaminase and aldolase levels; the electromyogram shows fibrillatory changes and the E.S.R. is high.

X-rays. X-rays may reveal the widespread subcutaneous calcification (calcinosis universalis).

Differential diagnosis. This is chiefly from rheumatoid arthritis or disseminated lupus erythematosus, where the skin lesions may cause confusion.

Treatment. This should be based on vigorous physiotherapy, and the prevention of contractures. Bedrest should be avoided and steroids are used principally to keep the patient comfortable and mobile.

27 Disorders of lymphatics, spleen, miscellaneous tumours

DISORDERS OF THE LYMPHATICS

Some of these are associated with other disorders, thus regional lymphadenitis is a common association of acute and chronic infections, or lymphatic problems may present primarily as a skin disease, or be a disorder of some other system.

Congenital disorders

Lymphangioma

In this condition there is dilatation and enlargement of the lymphatic vessels, to a degree suggesting a neoplasm.

Clinical features. They most frequently occur as a cystic *hygroma* which is usually found as a swelling in the posterior triangle of the neck. The edge of the swelling is poorly defined, but the overlying skin is normal, although often bluish in appearance. The mass is fluctuant and painless, but tends to infiltrate various tissue planes, giving rise to pressure symptoms, such as dyspnea and dysphagia. Similar lesions are found in the axillae and groins, and may cause severe local disfigurement.

Localized lymphangiomata may enlarge the lip, causing *macrocheilia*, and if in the tongue, one form of *macroglossia* (enlarged tongue). The latter may cause respiratory distress in the newborn.

Treatment. Surgical removal is usually necessary, and may be extremely difficult because of the risk to nerves and blood vessels. Lesions of the lip and tongue demand excision and plastic reconstruction.

Acute infections

Acute lymphangitis

This is a complication of some septic process such as cellulitis. The lymphatic vessels, usually invisible, become red, inflamed, and tender. The regional glands are also enlarged and painful.

Treatment. This is usually by antibiotics with surgical drainage of the primary focus of infection if necessary.

Lymphadenitis

This means enlargement, occasionally with suppuration of the lymphatic glands. By the nature of things, those of the groin and axillae seem most frequently to be affected. A primary site of infection is always present. Lymphangitis occurs, but in general is much less frequent than adenitis. The glands are painful to an extent which may inhibit movement of the limb. In *pyogenic* lymphadenitis, the enlarged glands are usually separate, in *tuberculous* lymphadenitis, pain is minimal or absent, and coalescence (matting) is common. The lymphatic glands may also be involved in secondary tumour (e.g., leukemia) or may be primarily affected as in lymphosarcoma.

Lymphatic malignancy

Primary tumours

These are regular occurrences in childhood, which bear a strong relationship to leukemia, itself a condition which is often a terminal stage of lymphatic tumours. It should be recalled too, that lymphatic malignancies are more common in disorders which have a primarily immunological basis, e.g., ataxia-telangiectasia (Louis-Bar syndrome), and Wiskott-Aldrich syndrome.

Although various histological types are described (Hodgkin's disease, lymphosarcoma, lymphoblastoma, reticular cell sarcoma), transformation from one type to another is not very uncommon.

Hodgkin's disease

Clinical features. The common presentation is with painless swelling of the lymph glands, most frequently in the posterior triangle of the neck. The inguinal and axillary nodes are next most commonly involved primarily, or secondarily. There is no redness or skin tenderness, and the individual glands can be felt. Their consistency varies from firmness (rubbery), to stony hardness.

Lymphatic gland involvement elsewhere will give rise to protean symptoms. Thus, invasion of the mediastinum will cause cough, and perhaps persistent signs of respiratory obstruction followed by lung collapse. Extensive intrathoracic infiltrates may involve the great veins to produce a superior vena cava syndrome. Invasion of the abdominal glands may cause enlargement of the belly, either through the accumulation of lymphatic tissue or of fluid.

Lymphosarcoma and lymphoblastoma

The clinical features of these are similar to those described for Hodgkin's disease, except that the speed of involvement and size of the glands is increased. In mesenteric glandular invasion, abdominal effusions, frequently hemorrhagic, are also found, and the features of leukemia may occur early in each.

Differential diagnosis. This is principally from lymphatic enlargement due to infection. In pyogenic infection which has been partially treated, tenderness may not be a marked feature; a precedent and appropriate history is, however, suggestive. In tuberculous lymphadenitis, the Mantoux reaction is positive, coalescence of the glands with adherence to the skin is common, and caseation may occur.

Diagnosis. This is entirely based upon biopsy. In Hodgkin's disease the multinucleated giant cell (Reed-Sternberg) coexists with a primitive reticular cell of large size.

In reticular cell sarcoma, large primitive cells occur, with little in the way of normal lymphatic architecture. In lymphoblastoma and lymphosarcoma, somewhat more differentiated cells are seen. At any stage leukemic cells may be seen in the glands, in the peripheral blood or bone marrow.

Treatment. The best mode is radiotherapy and useful adjuvants are the cytotoxic agents cyclophosphamide and vincristine. In leukemic transformation, appropriate therapy is indicated.

Prognosis. This is not good; few children survive more than a few years.

Malignant lymphoma (Burkitt's tumour)

This condition is commonly found in African children, but has been reported elsewhere. Its spread may be associated with an insect vector.

Clinical features. Most sufferers are in the age group 3-10 years, and invasion of the jaw is the usual presenting feature. The teeth are shed, and extensive soft tissue distortion occurs. Orbital invasion, or the presence of abdominal masses may appear in close association with the primary manifestations. Spread to the long bones, spinal column, parotids and other organs is common, and the secondary masses grow very rapidly.

Treatment. Cytotoxic drugs may cause a remission and x-ray therapy is of value in compressive lesions.

DISORDERS OF THE SPLEEN

Physiology. The spleen forms blood in the fetus, and may resume this function in later life if medullary hemopoiesis is compromised by disease. The spleen also culls abnormally shaped or damaged red cells from the circulation. This is done by phagocytes in the sinusoids. In conditions of persistent red cell anomaly, e.g., thalassemia, the spleen will greatly enlarge. The spleen also functions as a reservoir for red cells and platelets, and contributes to immunological competence.

Splenic abnormalities

The organ may be *congenitally absent*, especially in certain types of congenital heart disease, with situs inversus. Heinz bodies are seen in the red cells of these children, who are prone to severe infections.

Hypersplenism

This implies undue removal of red and white cells and platelets by the spleen, which is usually obviously enlarged. The most common background is hepatic cirrhosis, although the splenomegaly of storage disease may also be causal. The degree of destruction of the blood elements may be quantitated by appropriate cell labelling and counting over the spleen.

Splenic enlargement

This is found in a wide variety of pediatric diseases. The spleen may be physiologically palpable 2.5-3.8cm below the costal margin during the first 2 years of life. It is usually felt in the flank. Marked subcostal splenic enlargement is not physiological. Perhaps the commoner cause of minor splenomegaly is iron deficiency anemia of childhood. This is closely followed by viral diseases, especially infectious mononucleosis. Hematological disorders are also common causes of splenomegaly, as are the storage diseases, and neoplasms such as leukemia, lymphosarcoma, and Hodgkin's disease. In tropical areas, malaria and kala azar are likely causes.

Splenic enlargement is usually asymptomatic except for abdominal enlargement in the grosser forms. Older children may complain of vague abdominal discomfort. Acute pain of splenic origin may be due to infarction. This occurs most commonly in the infective splenomegalies such as that occurring in bacterial endocarditis.

Rupture of the spleen

In the newborn, this may occur merely as a complication of delivery, or it may rarely complicate the splenomegaly of erythroblastosis. In either case, there is sudden pallor, shock, and sometimes abdominal distension. Blood can be aspirated from the peritoneum.

In older children, splenic rupture is a common association with traffic accident. Pallor, shock, and signs of peritoneal irritation are usually present. Splenic injury should always be considered in the shocked unconscious victim of a road accident. Rupture of the spleen may occur with minor trauma in children with advanced malarial splenomegaly. The treatment of all forms of ruptured spleen is transfusion and laparotomy.

TUMOURS OF THE SOFT TISSUES

These arise from fat, connective tissue, or muscle. Elements of each may coexist. Such tumours make up 15-20% of pediatric neoplasms.

Simple tumours

The commonest of these is the lipoma which is composed of mature fat cells. It may occur anywhere, including the retroperitoneal space. The usual clinical feature is of a round local swelling. Fluctuation is usually absent, but the mass may be transilluminable. Midline lipomata of the back may connect with lesions in the nervous system or mediastinum. Rapid enlargement implies possible malignant change.

Fibromatoses

These are usually found in the fascia and muscle layers. They give rise to a slow growing mass. Palmar fibromatous transformation is the cause of Dupuytren's contracture; a similar lesion may occur in the plantar fascia.

Malignant tumours

These are usually sarcomata which may originate from fat, muscle, fibrous, or nervous tissue. The main form of presentation is as a rapidly growing, painless mass in the subcutaneous or mucosal areas, e.g., of the mouth and palate. Metastasis to bone and viscera is common and rapid.

Treatment. All soft tissue tumours should be biopsied. If malignant, widespread excision, followed by radiotherapy and cytotoxic drugs may be of value.

Sacrococcygeal tumour

This is a teratoma, which occurs most often in females.

Clinical features. Most present at birth as a mass at the coccygeal tip. It may extend to distort the buttocks. Anterior growth may press upon the anus and rectum, displacing them forward, but urinary or intestinal obstruction is uncommon. The tumour may be felt at rectal examination and x-rays often show calcification or premature bone formation within it.

Treatment. The teratoma is usually benign and should be removed surgically. Recurrence is not unusual, but yields to further surgery unless malignant transformation (carcinoma) has occurred in the teratoma.

Retroperitoneal tumours

These are principally derived from the common neuroblastoma of Wilm's tumour group. Occasionally the tumour is a retroperitoneal teratoma or sarcoma. The latter are especially to be suspected if the condition occurs in the first few months of life.

Clinical features. The principal, and often sole, complaint is of a mass in the belly, This may present an obvious abdominal enlargement, or may be felt by the parent, or less commonly by the physician. Growth is seldom greatly interfered with, and fever is uncommon. There are no specific laboratory findings.

X-rays. These will usually confirm the presence of a soft tissue mass; if it is a teratoma, calcification (usually inchoate, but sometimes clearly teeth or bones) may be seen. An intravenous pyelogram may suggest a primary renal or adrenal tumour; in the latter, urinary excretion of catecholamine end products may be increased.

Treatment. This is entirely surgical.

Chordoma

These are massive benign tumours of notochordal origin. They exist principally in the sacrococcygeal area and at the skull base. The principal symptom is of a local mass, or those of pressure upon adjacent structures such as the spinal cord. Primary excision is the treatment of choice; radiotherapy is used if recurrence takes place, or if surgery is technically impossible.

TUMOUR-LIKE LESIONS

Histiocytosis

This is the term applied collectively to Letterer-Siwe disease, eosinophilic granuloma and Hand-Schuller-Christian disease. As the name suggests, there is proliferation of the histiocytes in each. Accordingly, the lesions may be widespread and the symptoms protean. The condition is not a neoplasia. There is some evidence that it is inflammatory, but as yet the fundamental etiology is unknown.

Clinical features. Although protean, with entities shading into each other, there are several clinical pictures which warrant description. Common to each is a tendency to occur in the first 3 years of life, and to favour males. Perhaps the commonest situation is where there is a bone lesion (eosinophilic granuloma). This will present as a lump, if the bone is superficial, e.g., in mandible or skull. This swelling is painful and tender. In the inaccessible bones (e.g., pelvis) pain is commonly the first complaint, although pressure symptoms, varying with the anatomical site, may be the presenting feature. Where the mandible is affected, mouth ulcers and tooth shedding occur. In a number of the younger patients, the initial bone lesion is followed by invasion of the hypothalamic area, with resultant diabetes insipidus. This might approximate to the situation in some children with the Hand-Schuller-Christian syndrome.

The types so far described carry a relatively good prognosis. Much more serious is the extensive visceral involvement of young children. In these, the child usually signals the disease by showing pallor, infections, petechiae (all evidence of marrow depression) and a skin rash which resembles seborrhea. Abdominal enlargement (due to hepatosplenomegaly) may be the initial complaint. Lymphadenopathy is common, and miliary infiltrative lung lesions can be demonstrated by x-ray. The clinical picture described approximates that of Letterer-Siwe disease. Osseous lesions are occasionally clinically evident, more often they are found by x-ray survey.

Specific investigation. Anemia is common in all types. In the Letterer-Siwe type, thrombocytopenia and myeloid depression occur. The chest x-ray may reveal the classic honeycomb lung appearance, or smaller miliary type lung lesions.

Biopsy. This should be carried out in all cases and will demonstrate an infiltrative lesion with numerous large histiocytes.

Differential diagnosis. The principal problems arise with the disseminated visceral lesion (Letterer-Siwe disease). In the very young child, the clinical features may be simulated by generalized viral infections such as cytomegalovirus, and the rubella syndromes. In these the condition has usually existed since birth, and hemolysis with jaundice is usually prominent.

In the older child, leukemia and generalized dissemination of neuroblastoma are greater problems which can satisfactorily be resolved only by biopsy and skilled pathologic examination. The solitary osseous lesion may be mimicked by a true primary tumour of bone, by a secondary deposit (e.g., from neuroblastoma) or by infection of trauma. The battered baby syndrome may cause confusion, but is confidently diagnosed by x-ray demonstration of fractures, at various stages of healing, in other parts of the body.

Treatment. This is still unsatisfactory for the visceral forms, although steroids and cytotoxic agents appear to be of some value. In the solitary bone lesions, especially if pressure symptoms are present, radiotherapy is of help.

Prognosis. This is good in the older child with a solitary bone lesion. In the infant, with a widespread visceral problem, the prognosis is poor.

28 Miscellaneous disorders

BATTERED BABY SYNDROME

This is a growing problem in Western society and the end point of calculated neglect or hatred by one or both parents, or guardians. At the extreme, the infant dies of a blow to the head or abdomen—such tragedies are a legal, rather than a medical problem.

Clinical features. These vary greatly, but several general patterns are known. In most instances the infant is undersized and underweight; he may be dirty and neglected. The characteristic feature is injury without reasonable explanation. Common injuries are bruises of mysterious origin—but sometimes identifiable as the outline of adult finger marks. The face, chest, back, and buttocks are usual sites. Superficial burns, sometimes clearly due to a lighted cigarette, are frequent events. Another pattern is fever lassitude, and poverty of movement of 1 or more limbs. The bones are tender, and scurvy may be suspected. In these, as in the bruised infants, x-rays will reveal multiple fractures, often without displacement, and in unusual sites such as the ribs. Skull fractures are also found. These fractures are of different ages, reflecting several episodes of violence.

In the very young infant, injury to the head may cause a subdural hematoma (q.v.) and parental violence should always be suspected when this diagnosis is made in infancy.

Other suspicious circumstances are limb fractures without reasonable cause. These are usually transverse and without much displacement. An x-ray survey will sometimes reveal old fractures elsewhere.

There are many other variants on parental violence. It seems that parents usually seek some medical help for the child, and the diagnosis is suspected because the findings do not accord with the explanations given. Invariably the child is in the low growth percentiles.

If the diagnosis is suspected then the child must be carefully examined for bruising, cuts, burns, and the whole skeleton x-rayed. He should be admitted to hospital and kept there until his safety is assured, and the whole family situation reviewed. If bruising is the main finding, it is usual to exclude any bleeding disorder by appropriate tests. The evidence for the diagnosis is assembled and the parents interviewed separately and together. If, as is usually the case, one parent is responsible, the other may confirm the medical suspicions.

Treatment. The child must be protected until it is thought safe to re-expose him to the person responsible. Social and psychiatric help is given to the whole family. After discharge from hospital, close and frequent follow-up of the patient is necessary, since the pattern of violence may change, e.g., from bruising to deliberate starvation. Police action is not usually used in the first instance unless a charge has already been laid. If another episode of violence occurs, in spite of parental and family care, it is almost always necessary to take steps to remove the child from the hostile environment.

COT DEATH (SUDDEN UNEXPLAINED DEATH SYNDROME)

This is a problem of early infancy, most of the victims being aged 2-4 months. It occurs in the colder times of the year.

Clinical features. These are remarkably few. In some instances the baby has seemed irritable or even fevered but not acutely ill. He is put to bed and is found dead in the morning. Autopsy is essentially negative, although widespread petechiae in the lungs and elsewhere suggests an obstructive process in the respiratory tract. The bacteriological and virological examinations are negative. The principal value of the autopsy is to exclude other conditions as a cause of death.

There does not seem to be any way in which one can anticipate the onset of this tragic circumstance. Autopsy should always be insisted upon so that the parental guilt feelings can be dealt with.

Idiopathic hypercalcemia of infants

This curious condition is one which has been attributed to sensitivity to ingested Vitamin D. The disease begins in the first year of life, commonly about 6 months of age.

Clinical features. The usual complaints are of vomiting, refusal to feed, constipation, listlessness, and pallor. Weight loss is usual, and growth may be disturbed. The vomiting may be so severe as to cause dehydration.

Examination reveals an underweight, delicate-looking infant, with hypotonia. Fecal masses can be felt.

Laboratory studies. The serum calcium is increased, as may be the urinary excretion of calcium.

X-rays. There is increased density of the metaphyses, and of the periphery of the foot bones.

Treatment. A low calcium diet, together with steroids to promote the excretion of calcium, is the treatment. The intake of vitamin D should be kept at the usual levels (400 units daily).

Variant. Another less common type of hypercalcemia is that associated with mental defect and other congenital abnormalities. Nephrocalcinosis (calcification of the kidney) is often associated with symptoms (polyuria, polydipsia) and signs of renal failure. The prognosis is poor in this type. No specific treatment is available except for the renal failure.

Migraine

This disease is not very common in children, although it is familial. The condition is possibly due to some disturbance of the cerebral circulation.

Clinical features. In the full-fledged case there is a history of repeated attacks of headache, abdominal pain, and vomiting. The older child may describe preliminary complaints which consist usually in visual symptoms such as flashing lights and visual blind spots. Tingling and transient limb weakness also occur. These prodromata are followed by severe headache which is unilateral and frontal. Nausea, vomiting, and abdominal pain follow. Occasionally variable degrees of IIIrd nerve paralysis occur on the side of the headache (ophthalmoplegic migraine). In most instances, nothing is found on physical examination, and between attacks the child is perfectly normal. In the younger child, nausea, vomiting, and headache are the more common events.

Special investigations. Transient E.E.G. abnormalities in the temporal lobe leads may be seen at the beginning of the attack.

Treatment: The acute attack. The child is best put to bed in a darkened room and given a simple analgesic and plenty of fluids. The parents should be reassured as to the benign nature of the disease. In some children, the attacks may be rendered fewer by giving a mild tranquillizer. If the preliminary symptoms are readily recognized by the child or parents, early administration of an ergot preparation may abort the attack.

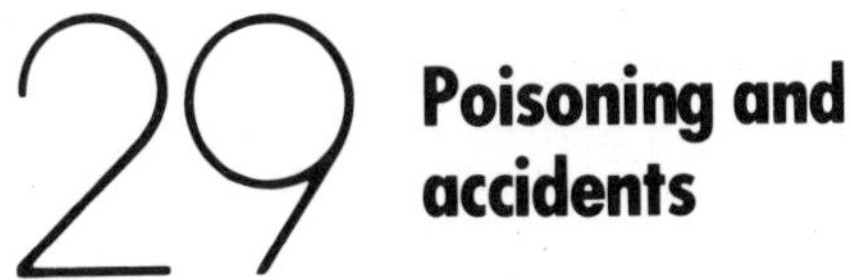

29 Poisoning and accidents

POISONING

This is one of the main causes of disease and death in children. The child is at risk as soon as he can crawl and although poisoning is commonest in the 2-year old, no age is immune. When the child is at the crawling stage he is more likely to swallow easily available liquids, such as house cleaning bleach and detergents. The inquisitive toddler will explore handbags and cupboards, and thus is more likely to be poisoned by drugs and pesticides, or indeed any substance which has been imperfectly concealed. Poisons stored in softdrink bottles are particularly dangerous, as the toddler has little sense of taste, and cannot read warning notices.

Common ingestants in the crawler and young toddler

These are bleach, detergents, furniture and floor polishes, deodorants, disinfectants, turpentine, kerosene, pesticides, weedicides, and products containing caustic soda. Kerosene (paraffin) tends to be the commonest liquid poison.

Common ingestants in the exploring toddler

Drugs, deodorants, cosmetics, poisonous berries, soldering flux, kerosene, as well as any of the products already mentioned.

Common drugs ingested

These will vary with the cultural pattern, and the prescribing habits of the medical community. Inevitably, however, aspirin and barbiturates are high on any list, followed by proprietary cough and cold suppressants, antihistamines, fluoride tablets, tranquillizers, and antidepressants, laxatives, oral contraceptives, anorectics (of the amphetamine series) and various externally applied agents, such as oil of wintergreen and other liniments.

Common cosmetic preparations which are swallowed

Setting lotions, hair colouring agents, shampoos, permanent wave solutions, nail care preparations, personal deodorants, and perfumes.

Common pesticides and weedicides

D.D.T., arsenicals, malathion and its congeners, dieldrin, chlordane, metaldehyde, rodenticides (anticoagulants, phosphorus).

Common industrial products

Soldering fluxes (HCL), plastic cement, fibreglass hardeners and thinners, wood stains and lacquers.

Common botanicals causing poisoning

Most of these are plants with poisonous berries, often of the belladonna group (e.g., deadly night shade), the castor oil bean (*Ricinus communis*), oleander and lantana. Mushroom poisoning is a constant risk. The exact sources of such ingestants will of course depend on local circumstances.

Symptoms of poisoning

These are legion, and the possibility of poisoning should always be considered in a previously well child who develops symptoms for which no obvious cause can be found. Accordingly, in the at risk age group, a searching enquiry into the possibility of obtaining drugs should always be made.

Coma

This is common in poisoning from barbiturates, opiates, alcohol, and antihistaminics, phenothiazine derivatives, and other antidepressants, aminophylline, piperazine, and quaternary ammonium detergents.

Convulsions

These are found in antihistaminic poisoning, are very common in severe poisoning from strychnine, phenothiazine derivatives, the tricyclic antidepressant drugs, and also the chlorobenzene insecticides, e.g., D.D.T., chlordane, and dieldrin.

Convulsions may occur in poisoning which causes severe anoxia, e.g., the late stage of barbiturate poisoning, or following the production of methemoglobin by aniline derivatives.

Drowsiness

As for coma, also salicylates, anticonvulsants, acetazolamide and iron containing compounds.

Ataxia

Alcohol, anticonvulsants, antihistaminics, phenothiazine, barbiturates, and indomethacin.

Vomiting

This is a common symptom and may occur with a very wide variety of poisons; it is a leading symptom in heavy metal poisoning and following phosphorus containing rodenticides, the petroleum distillates, alcohol, and iron derivatives.

Excitement and overactivity

Amphetamine derivates, organophosphorus insecticides, atropine, chlordiazepoxide, tricyclic antidepressants, and piperazine.

Extrapyramidal tract symptoms

Tricyclic antidepressants, chlordiazepoxide, phenothiazines, imipramine, and meprobamate.

Visual difficulties

Mushroom poisoning, tricyclic antidepressants, atropine, antihistamines, phenothiazines, diazepam, impramine, indomethacin, nalidixic acid, anticonvulsants, and piperazine.

Vomiting and diarrhea

Heavy metals, organophosphorus compounds, bacterial food poisoning, laxatives, fungi, petroleum distillates, digitalis, and nalidixic acid.

Corrosive poisons

Acids (soldering flux, battery acid), alkalis (cleaning compounds containing NaOH), bleaches, phenol, metallic salts ($CuSO_4$), deodorants, ammonia salts, formaldehyde, and strong detergents.

General principles of treatment

These include identification of the poison, its removal or dilution, prevention of further absorption from the alimentary tract, the use of specific antidotes, and general supportive measures.

Identification

Samples of any ingestant should be obtained, although not at the expense of delaying the transfer to hospital, or emergency treatment of the patient. Samples of blood, urine, vomit, and gastric washings should be kept until the patient has fully recovered.

Removal and dilution of poisons

Externally applied poisons (e.g., organophosporus insecticides) should be washed off with large amounts of water. Dilution of swallowed poisons with water is always in order unless the patient is severely dysphagic.

Emptying of the stomach is indicated in all situations of poisoning, *except* from strong acids, or alkalis, or following the ingestion of petroleum distillates or following any drug which has caused convulsions.

Methods of emptying the stomach

1. Vomiting. This is best induced by giving a draught of 20 ml of fluid containing 1.2 ml liquid extract of ipecacuanha B.P. This may be repeated in 20 minutes if vomiting has not occurred. Most other methods of inducing vomiting (mustard, hypertonic saline, stimulation of pharynx) are traditional rather than reliable.

Induced emesis is of little value in poisoning with powdered arsenic, or with drugs which have an antiemetic effect, e.g., the phenothiazines and antihistaminics. In these situations, the stomach must be washed out.

2. Gastric lavage. This is done by washing out the stomach with 300-400 ml of tap water. The washings should be retained for possible toxicological examination. If petroleum distillates have been swallowed, the patient should be anesthetized and intubated before gastric lavage is done.

If it is suspected that a large amount of tablets has been swallowed but the recovery is low, then x-ray of the stomach should be carried out. This may show a mass of material (e.g., iron tablets) which has resisted lavage. If so, continue the gastric lavage.

Preventing the absorption of poisons

Gastric lavage is best. Agents such as demulcents and kaolin are unreliable. Activated charcoal in solution will absorb the toxic alkaloids (atropine, digitalis, strychnine) as well as many of the metallic poisons, but is not a panacea.

Antidotes

Few of these are specific. Worthy of mention, however, are nalorphine for opiate poisoning, atropine and P.A.M. are useful in organophosphorus poisoning, and desferrioxamine in iron poisoning. Chelators (e.g., B.A.L.) are of value in mobilizing and aiding the excretion of heavy metals such as arsenic.

General measures

In most instances an intravenous drip should be set up. This will maintain hydration and increase urinary output. Blood and urine samples should be obtained and analyzed where the exact nature of the toxin is obscure. When convulsions require treatment, the safest drug to use is fresh paraldehyde (1.5 ml/kg body weight to a maximum of 5.0 ml and given *intramuscularly*). Diazepam should *not* be given as a routine anticonvulsant as it augments the action of such drugs as phenothiazines, tricyclic antidepressants, and antihistaminics. In appropriate circumstances, a general anesthetic with intubation and aided respiration may be the best mode of controlling severe convulsions.

Care of corrosive poisoning

This is considered in detail elsewhere (p. 194).

Some specific entities

Salicylate poisoning (sources—aspirin, headache powders, embrocations containing methyl salicylate, oil of wintergreen).

In most instances a few hours will pass before symptoms appear. The exception is the immediate corrosive action of methyl salicylate. The first symptom is an increase in the respiratory rate due to acidosis. Tinnitus occurs in the older child, and vomiting is usual, as is fever. Drowsiness progresses to coma, and dehydration is usual. The patient is found to have Kussmaul (acidotic) breathing from an early stage. Convulsions and circulatory failure are found in the terminal stage. A bleeding tendency, with hematemesis and melena may occur at any time.

Urinalysis may reveal blood and albumen, the ferric chloride test is positive but does not define the degree of poisoning. This is done by estimation of the serum salicylate level. An early acidosis is followed by a compensating alkalosis.

Differential diagnosis. This is principally from other dehydrating conditions with associated vomiting and dehydration such as diabetic coma. In the younger child *bronchiolitis* may have been the primary disorder which has been treated drastically with aspirin; the two may accordingly coexist.

Treatment. The stomach should be lavaged and an intravenous drip (e.g., 0.45 N saline with dextrose) administered. Blood transfusion may be necessary if much bleeding has occurred, and prophylactic vitamin K is in order. In severe acidosis (arterial pH < 7.2) bicarbonate may be given. These measures, together with anticipation of chest infections will deal with most cases. If coma is deep and urinary output low, consideration should be given to peritoneal or hemodialysis.

Barbiturate poisoning

The patient is usually drowsy, but may be excited or seem drunk since ataxia is common. In early coma, the patient can be roused and will reply to questioning. This situation will progress to failure to respond to pain, depression of the tendon reflexes. Last of all is depression of the respiration, circulation, and pharyngeal and laryngeal reflexes.

Treatment. In coma, the stomach should be lavaged only after an endotracheal tube has been passed. An intravenous saline drip is set up and a diuresis produced, provided the blood pressure is still reasonably normal. In severe respiratory depression, especially with low pO_2 and high pCO_2 values, monitored mechanical respiration should be carried out. A chest x-ray should be routine, as unsuspected lung collapse may be present, and require bronchoscopy.

Organophosphorus insecticides (malathion, parathion)

The onset of symptoms is very rapid with vomiting, diarrhea, abdominal pain, salivation, and respiratory obstruction. The pupils are small and the pulse is slow. Convulsions, coma, and respiratory paralysis are near-terminal events.

Treatment. The skin, if contaminated, should be washed with water. An intravenous dose of atropine (0.6 mg) is given or, if available, piralidoxime (PAM) 0.5-1 g I.V. The respiratory passages should be cleared and intubation and mechanical respiration set up.

Chlorinated hydrocarbon insecticides (D.D.T., dieldrin, aldrin, chlordane, lindane, methoxychlor)

These are very toxic substances (especially aldrin and dieldrin) which cause hyperexcitability, tremors, ataxia, convulsions, coma, and respiratory arrest. Absorption can readily occur from the skin.

Treatment. Wash out the stomach, control convulsions, protect the airway, intubate and respire mechanically as necessary.

Iron poisoning

This is generally due to swallowing medicinal iron tablets. These corrode the stomach and may cause a perforation. Vomiting, shock, and coma occur within a short time. Initial treatment may cause some improvement, but cerebral and hepatic problems follow. The former is evidenced by irritability, convulsions, and recrudescence of coma, the latter by jaundice and other signs of hepatic damage.

Treatment. The stomach should thoroughly be washed out, and intravenous saline or blood given. Desferrioxamine will aid the excretion of iron.

Lead poisoning

The metal is obtained from a variety of sources, principally from flaking paint. Symptoms resemble a slow onset meningitis with vomiting, irritability, anorexia, and sleepiness. Convulsions are common, and papilledema usual. Nerve palsies (cranial and peripheral) may occur in long-continued poisoning.

Special investigations. Lead lines are often visible on bone x-ray; the blood shows a hemolytic anemia, with stippling of the red cells (punctate basophilia). Chelating agents (calcium EDTA) are of value in mobilizing the lead into the urine.

Kerosene poisoning

This important disorder consists in cerebral excitation, gastroenteritis, and sometimes liver failure. The commonest problem is, however, an alveolitis. (see p. 254).

General prevention of poisoning

This depends largely on public and parental education, and legislative action. As most disasters occur with dispensed drugs, it is wise to give a word of warning to all persons receiving a prescription. The skill with which children can enter high cupboards and other supposed places of safety, is remarkable. This fact should be brought to the attention of all parents.

All tablets should be dispensed in safety packs which cannot be readily opened by the child. The storage of noxious fluids in softdrink bottles in particularly dangerous, and should be the subject of constant warning.

It is not very uncommon for children who have swallowed once to do so again. Accordingly, a sharp warning to the parents is very much in order in any instance of poisoning.

General sources of information concerning poisonous products

This is available at Poison Control Centres in many countries. Useful information is also found in the ubiquitous P.D.R. (Physician's Desk Reference).

ENVENOMATION BY ANIMALS

The usual sources are snakes, spiders, jellyfish, venomous octopi. Most dangerous bites inject neurotoxic venom which causes muscular weakness with respiratory paralysis (see p. 424). The toxin of viperine snakes causes hemorrhage and, in severe bites, circulatory failure.

General treatment of snake bite

A tourniquet is applied with the usual precautions. The bite should not be washed but inspected for signs of envenomation which consists in local pain, swelling, and enlargement of the regional lymph glands. Fang marks (never semicircular in pattern) are visible except in bites by certain small-toothed snakes which leave only linear scratches: such marks do not identify the responsible snake.

Vomiting, headache, abdominal pain, hematemesis, muscle weakness and visual difficulties are all positive signs of envenomation. As neurotoxic symptoms may be delayed for some hours, it is wise to observe such patterns for 12 hours before releasing them from medical attention.

Specific treatment

In neuroparalysis, all the apparatus for intubation and mechanical respiration should be available, as antiserum may not reverse the neurotoxins. Supportive intravenous therapy and blood transfusion are given as necessary.

Antivenene. If the snake has been reliably identified, and if definite signs of envenomation are present, a specific antivenene may be given. If any doubt exists, give a polyvalent preparation according to the general description of the snake. Reactions to antivenene are common, so that antihistamines and steroids are usually given at the same time.

ACCIDENTS

Burns and scalds

Scalds are more common in the younger child—he pulls pots from stoves or hot liquids from the table. Burns are more common in girls because of the inflammable nature of their nightwear, and the ease with which cotton and nylon garments catch fire at unprotected electric elements, or in the hot vapour of kerosene heaters. Explosive burns occur in children playing with fireworks and affect principally the hands and eyes.

Clinical features of burns. These are well known. In first degree burns, there is erythema and some blistering. In second degree burns, there is widespread blistering with sloughing of the superficial and middle layers of the skin. In third degree burns, there is destruction of the whole thickness of the skin. Each variety may coincide with the other.

The general features are of pain and shock, the severity of the latter depends upon the extent of the burns, and the consequent fluid loss. In older children, shock will occur when 10% of the skin is affected, but in infants it follows much smaller burns. Massive loss of protein, water, and electrolytes follows a burn and the exudate serves as an admirable culture medium for pathogens. Fluid loss is frequently underestimated so that intravenous infusions (of blood, plasma, and saline) should be liberal. Hypoglycemia and acid/base balance difficulties should be anticipated.

In general, the child with a widespread burn should be isolated, and burned areas exposed. In well-ventilated surroundings, an eschar forms from the exudates, and this limits bacterial invasion.

Simple occlusive dressings are indicated in burns of mobile areas such as the joints, the trunk, and so on. These dressings may be soaked with 0.25% aqueous chlorhexidine B.P. and allowed to dry. They should be renewed infrequently—once a week if infection is controlled. Antibiotics should not be given as a routine, but retained for use in a serious circumstance, such as septicemia.

Inhalation burns

Injury to the epiglottis and larynx causes closure of the airway. There is stridor and dyspnea, and intubation or tracheotomy may be necessary.

In burns of the smaller bronchioles, dyspnea and cyanosis are often severe, and pulmonary edema is present clinically and radiologically. The condition does not respond well to treatment, although humidified oxygen may tide the patient over.

Minor burns

A suitable first aid treatment is to immerse the area in cold, running water. A simple occlusive dressing may then be applied to prevent contamination.

Burns to the *fingers* are not minor, especially if they are *circumferential*. Such burns should be referred to a surgeon so that ischemic necrosis may be avoided.

Prevention of burns

As in poisoning, this largely depends upon public and parental education. Adequate standards for flame-resistant clothing, especially for girls' nightwear, is of considerable value, as is legislation for safety features in electric and kerosene heaters.

Constant vigilance is the only mode of prevention for young children. Obvious precautions, such as turning all pot handles inward on the stove and keeping tea and coffee pots off the table should be explained to all parents and constantly reiterated.

Vehicular accidents

This is an increasing source of severe injury to children, affecting all age groups except infants. Many injured children are pedestrians or bicycle riders. Death is usually due to head injury which is also a major source of chronic brain syndromes (aphasias, intellectual deterioration, various neurological disorders) in the survivors.

It is not possible to describe all of the clinical possibilities. Multiple injuries are usual, with a predominance of fractures, head injuries, and visceral rupture. The treatment demands a team approach with effective resuscitation a necessary preliminary. Flail chest injury, with rib and sternal fractures, dislocates the mechanism of breathing and requires early intubation and mechanical ventilation.

Prevention of vehicular accidents

In a sense, this is a social problem. So far success is elusive. Valuable measures include the provision of protected crossings for school children, the enforcement of speed limits, and, for older children, the provision of adequate driver training.

Suggestions for further reading

Chapter 1.

Normal Growth and Development

(a) Davis, J. A. and Dobbing, J., eds. *Scientific Foundations of Paediatrics.* London: William Heinemann Medical Books, 1974.

(b) Moore, K. L. *The Developing Human: Clinically Oriented Embryology.* London: W. B. Saunders, 1974.

(c) Sinclair, David. *Human Growth after Birth.* 2d ed. London: Oxford Medical Publications, 1973.

(d) Mitchell, Ross G., ed. *Child Life and Health.* 5th ed. London: J. and A. Churchill, 1970.

(e) Touwen, B. *Neurological Development in Infancy.* Clinics in Developmental Medicine, no. 58. London: SIMP and William Heinemann Medical Books, 1976.

(f) Egan, D. F.; Illingworth, R. S.; and MacKeith, R. C., eds. *Developmental Screening 0–5 Years.* Clinics in Developmental Medicine, no. 30. London: SIMP and William Heinemann Medical Books, 1969.

(g) Illingworth, R. S. *The Normal Child.* 6th ed. Edingburgh: Churchill Livingstone, 1975.

(h) Lowry, G. H. *Growth and Development of Children.* 6th ed. Chicago: Year Book Medical Publishers, 1973.

Chapter 2.

The Newborn

(a) Davies, P. A.; Robinson, R. J.; Slopes, J. W.; Tizard, J. P. M.; and Wigglesworth, J. S., eds. *Medical Care of Newborn Babies.* Clinics in Developmental Medicine, nos. 44–45. London: SIMP and William Heinemann Medical Books, 1973.

(b) Schaffer, A. J. and Avery, M. E. *Diseases of the Newborn.* 3d ed. London: W. B. Saunders, 1971.

(c) Brazelton, T. B., ed. *Neonatal Behavioural Assessment Scale.* Clinics in Developmental Medicine, no. 50. London: SIMP and William Heinemann Medical Books, 1973.

(d) Illingworth, Ronald and Cynthia. *Babies and Young Children.* Edinburgh: Churchill Livingstone, 1972.

Chapter 3.

Puberty and Adolescence

(a) Tanner, J. M. *Growth at Adolescence.* 2d ed. Oxford: Blackwell Scientific Publications, 1973.

(b) "Adolescent Medicine." *Pediatric Clinics of North America* 20, no. 4. London: W. B. Saunders, 1973.

Chapter 4.

Nutrition and its Disorders

(a) Davidson, S.; Passmore, R.; Brock, J. F.; and Truswell, A. S. *Human Nutrition and Dietetics.* 6th ed. London: Churchill Livingstone, 1975.

(b) *Handbook of Human Nutritional Requirements.* Geneva: World Health Organization, 1970.

Chapter 5.

Disease Due to Inborn Errors of Metabolism

Nyhan, W. L., ed. *Heritable Disorders of Amino Acid Metabolism.* London: J. Wiley and Sons, 1974.

Chapter 6.

The Chromosome and its Disorders

(a) Valentine, G. H. *The Chromosome Disorders.* London: William Heinemann Medical Books, 1968.

(b) Carter, C. O. *An ABC of Medical Genetics.* London: Lancet Publications, 1975.

Chapter 7.

Immunity and its Disorders

(a) Stiehm, E. R. and Fulginiti, V. A. *Immunologic Disorders in Infants and Children.* London: W. B. Saunders, 1973.

(b) Good, R. A. and Fisher, D. W., eds. *Immunobiology.* Stamford, Conn.: Sinauer Associates, 1972.

Chapter 8.

Disorders Due to Specific Infective Agents

Kurgman, S. and Ward, R. *Infectious Diseases of Children and Adults.* 5th ed. C. V. Mosby Co., 1973.

Chapter 9.

Infestation by Parasites

(a) Jelliffe, D. B., ed. *Diseases of Children in the Subtropics and Tropics.* London: Edward Arnold, 1970.

(b) Brown, H. W. *Basic Clinical Parasitology*. 3d ed. Appleton-Century-Croft, 1969.

Chapter 10.

Diseases of the Alimentary Tract

(a) Anderson, C. M. and Burke, V., eds. *Paediatric Gastroenterology.* Oxford: Blackwell Scientific, 1975.

(b) Dennison, W. M. *Surgery in Infancy and Childhood.* Edinburgh: Churchill Livingstone, 1974.

Chapter 11.

Disorders of the Respiratory System

(a) Williams, H. E. and Phelan, P. D. *Respiratory Illness in Children.* Oxford: Blackwell Scientific, 1975.

(b) Lough, M. D.; Doershuk, C. F.; and Stern, R. C., eds. *Pediatric Respiratory Therapy.* Chicago: Year Book Medical Publishers, Inc., 1974.

Chapter 12.

Disorders of the Heart and Circulation

Watson, H., ed. *Pediatric Cardiology*. London: Lloyd-Luke, 1968.

Chapter 13.

Disorders of the Urogenital System

(a) Smith, D. R. *General urology.* 8th ed. Los Altos, Cal.: Lange Medical Publications, 1975.

(b) "Pediatric nephrology." *Pediatric Clinics of North America* 23, no. 4. London: W. B. Saunders, 1976.

(c) Kolvin, I.; MacKeith, R. C.; and Meadow, S. R., eds. *Bladder control and enuresis.* Clinics in Developmental Medicine, nos. 48–49. London: SIMP and William Heinemann Medical Books, 1973.

Chapter 14.

Disorders of the Hemopoietic System

Nathan, D. G. and Oski, F. A., eds. *Hematology of infancy and childhood.* London: W. B. Saunders, 1974.

Chapter 15.

Disorders of the Endocrine System

(a) Gardner, L. I., ed. *Endocrine and Genetic Diseases of Children.* London: W. B. Saunders, 1969.

(b) Bacon, G. E.; Spencer, M. E.; and Keech, R. P. *Pediatric Endocrinology.* Chicago: Year Book Medical Publishers, 1975.

(c) Traisman, H. S. *Management of Juvenile Diabetes Mellitus.* St. Louis: C. V. Mosby Co., 1971.

(d) Parsons, J. A. and Potts, J. T. "Physiology and Chemistry of Parathyroid Hormone." *J. Clin. Endocrinol. and Metab.* 1, no. 33 (1973).

Chapter 16.

Disorders of the Eye

(a) Perkins, E. S. and Hansell, Peter. *An Atlas of Diseases of the Eye.* 2d ed. Edinburgh: Churchill Livingstone, 1971.

(b) Gardiner, P.; MacKeith, R.; and Smith, V., eds. *Aspects of Developmental and Paediatric Ophthalmology.* Clinics in Developmental Medicine, no. 32. London: SIMP and William Heinemann Medical Books, 1969.

Chapter 17.

Disorders of the Skin

Sneddon, I. B. and Church, R. E. *Practical Dermatology.* 3d ed. London: Edward Arnold, 1976.

Chapter 18.

Disorders of the Central Nervous System

(a) Nathan, Peter. *The Nervous System.* Ringwood, Vic.: Penguin Books, 1973.

(b) Vander, A. J.; Sherman, J. H.; and Luciano, D. S. *Human Physiology.* Sydney: McGraw-Hill, 1975.

(c) Ingram, T. T. S. *Paediatric Aspects of Cerebral Palsy*. Edinburgh: Livingstone, 1964.

(d) Ingram, T. T. S.; Jameson, S.; Errington, J.; and Mitchell, R. G. *Living with Cerebral Palsy.* Clinics in Developmental Medicine, no. 14. London: SSMEIU and William Heinemann Medical Books, 1964.

(e) Livingstone, Samuel. *Comprehensive Management of Epilepsy in Infancy, Childhood, and Adolescence.* Springfield: Chas. C. Thomas, 1972.

(f) Brown, J. K. and Habel, A. H. "Toxic Encephalopathy and Acute Brain Swelling in Children." *Developmental Medicine and Child Neurology* 17 (1975): 659–79.

(g) Brocklehurst, G., ed. *Spina Bifida for the Clinician.* Clinics in Developmental Medicine, no. 57. London: SIMP and William Heinemann Medical Books, 1976.

Chapter 19.

Disorders of Speech

(a) Morley, Muriel E. *The Development and Disorders of Speech in Childhood.* 3d ed. Edinburgh: Churchill Livingstone, 1972.

(b) Rutter, M. and Martin, J. A. M., eds. *The Child with Delayed Speech.* Clinics in Developmental Medicine, no. 43. London: SIMP and William Heinemann Medical Books, 1972.

(c) Critchley, Macdonald. *Developmental Dyslexia.* London: William Heinemann Medical Books, 1967.

Chapter 20.

Educational Difficulties

Wolff, P. and Mackeith, R., eds. *Planning for Better Learning.* Clinics in Developmental Medicine, no. 33. London: SIMP and William Heinemann Medical Books, 1969.

Chapter 21.

Mental and Emotional Problems

(a) Schulman, J. L. *Management of Emotional Disorders in Pediatric Practice.* Chicago, Year Book Medical Publishers, 1969.

(b) Carr, Janet. *Young Children with Down's Syndrome.* IRMMH Monograph 4. London: Butterworth, 1975.

(c) Apley, J. *The Child with Abdominal Pains.* Oxford: Blackwell Scientific, 1974.

Chapter 22.

Disorders of Bone

LLoyd-Roberts, G. C. *Orthopaedics in Infancy and Childhood.* London: Butterworth, 1971.

Chapter 23.

Disorders of the Muscles

Dubowitz, D. "Neuromuscular Disorders in Childhood: Old Dogmas, New Concepts." *Archives of Disease in Childhood* 50 (1975): 335–46.

Chapter 24.

Disorders of Fluid and Electrolytes

Winters, R. W., ed. *The Body Fluids in Pediatrics.* Boston: Little Brown, 1973.

Chapter 25.

The Allergic Disorders

"Pediatric allergy."
Pediatric Clinics of North America 22, no. 1, 1975. London: W. B. Saunders.

Chapter 26.

Collagen Diseases

Markowitz, M. and Gordis, L. *Rheumatic fever.* London: W. B. Saunders, 1972.

Chapter 27.

Disorders of Lymphatics, Spleen, Miscellaneous Tumours

Jones, P. G. and Campbell, P. E., ed. *Tumours of infancy and childhood.* Oxford: Blackwell Scientific, 1976.

Index